Second Edition

CARDIOVASCULAR AND PULMONARY PHYSICAL THERAPY

A Clinical Manual

JOANNE WATCHIE, PT, CCS

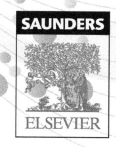

SAUNDERS

ELSEVIER

SAUNDERS
ELSEVIER

3251 Riverport Lane
St. Louis, Missouri 63043

Library of Congress Cataloging-in-Publication Data

Watchie, Joanne.
  Cardiovascular and pulmonary physical therapy: a clinical manual / Joanne Watchie. -- 2nd ed.
    p.; cm.
  Rev. ed. of: Cardiopulmonary physical therapy / Joanne Watchie. c1995.
  Includes bibliographical references and index.
  ISBN 978-0-7216-0646-0 (pbk.: alk. paper) 1. Cardiopulmonary system--Diseases--Physical therapy--Handbooks, manuals, etc. I. Watchie, Joanne. Cardiopulmonary physical therapy. II. Title.
  [DNLM: 1. Cardiovascular Diseases--rehabilitation--Handbooks. 2. Lung Diseases--rehabilitation--Handbooks. 3. Physical Therapy Modalities--Handbooks. WG 39 W324ca 2010]
  RC702.W38 2010
  616.1'2062--dc22

                                                                          2009008630

Vice President and Publisher: Linda Duncan
Executive Editor: Kathy Falk
Senior Developmental Editor: Melissa Kuster
Publishing Services Manager: Catherine Jackson
Project Manager: Jennifer Boudreau
Design Direction: Karen Pauls
Cover Designer: Karen Pauls

This book is dedicated to all physical therapists who appreciate the importance of the pulmonary and cardiovascular systems in designing treatment plans that not only achieve the treatment goals they establish for their patients, but also return them to optimal health.

CONTRIBUTORS

Jeffrey Rodrigues, PT, DPT, CCS
Instructor of Clinical Physical Therapy
Division of Biokinesiology and Physical Therapy
University of Southern California
Los Angeles, California
Chapter 7: Cardiovascular and Pulmonary Physical Therapy Treatment

Robin J. Winn, PT, MS, PCS
Head Physical Therapist
Morgan Stanley Children's Hospital of New York
Presbyterian Hospital/Columbia University Medical Center
Instructor in Clinical Rehabilitation Medicine (Physical Therapy)
Columbia University
College of Physicians and Surgeons
Program in Physical Therapy
New York, New York
Chapter 8: Pediatrics

Joel D. Hubbard, PhD, MT (ASCP)
Associate Professor
Clinical Laboratory Science
School of Allied Health Sciences
Texas Tech University
Lubbock, Texas
Chapter 9: Laboratory Medicine

PREFACE

The first edition of *Cardiopulmonary Physical Therapy: A Clinical Manual* came about as the result of discussions within the Executive Committee of the Cardiopulmonary Section of the American Physical Therapy Association in 1988. At that time, several members expressed frustration over the amount of time and effort required to find appropriate materials to use in the orientation and instruction of staff and students who would rotate onto services that served patients with cardiopulmonary diseases or dysfunction. In addition, some members received frequent requests for reference materials and bibliographies from practicing physical therapists interested in developing more expertise in cardiopulmonary physical therapy. *Cardiopulmonary Physical Therapy: A Clinical Manual* was created to address these needs.

The first edition of the book served as a ready reference for physical therapists and other care providers whose patients have primary or secondary cardiovascular or pulmonary conditions. It was designed to provide valuable information quickly and concisely for clinicians who require immediate understanding of a particular pathology, diagnostic test or procedure, therapeutic intervention, medication, or cardiopulmonary problem, as well as the important clinical implications of participation in exercise and rehabilitation activities.

The response to the book has been very positive, and the need for more current information has prompted the publication of a second edition. The title change to *Cardiovascular and Pulmonary Physical Therapy: A Clinical Manual* reflects the inclusion of pathologies and clinical manifestations involving the vascular system among the conditions affecting patients served by this area of clinical practice.

Like the first edition, this book is a quick and convenient resource, offering a clinical overview of a wide variety of diseases and disorders that affect the pulmonary and cardiovascular systems and the physical therapy management of patients with these conditions. It integrates information related to anatomy and physiology, diagnostic tests and relevant findings, significant pathophysiological features and clinical manifestations, and medical and surgical interventions, while offering important clinical implications for exercise and physical therapy interventions. Cross references to related information found in other chapters and bulleted lists make finding information quick and easy.

This edition includes an introduction to the oxygen transport pathway as it actually functions in the clinical setting and the implications of defects in the pathway. Updated material is provided on diagnostic tests and procedures, therapeutic interventions, pharmacology, and laboratory values and profiles used in the management of patients with cardiovascular and pulmonary dysfunction. There are many new and updated illustrations, including depictions of the pathophysiology and associated clinical manifestations of obstructive and restrictive lung disease and systolic and diastolic ventricular dysfunction. In addition, information on obesity and diabetes has been expanded, and material on metabolic syndrome and anthropometric measurements for determining obesity and associated level of health risk has been added.

Cardiovascular and Pulmonary Physical Therapy: A Clinical Manual is a unique and valuable resource for physical therapists practicing in all clinical settings, including acute and subacute care, home health care, pediatrics, and geriatrics, as well as in many rehabili-tation settings (e.g., orthopedics, oncology, and neurology) in which patients often have secondary diagnoses of hypertension, cardiovascular disease, obesity, diabetes, connective tissue disorders, and pulmonary disease. It will also appeal to physical therapy students who desire an integrated understanding of the many factors that influence the physical ther-apy management of patients with cardiopulmonary dysfunction.

ACKNOWLEDGMENTS

The revision of this book could not have been pulled off without the assistance of a whole lot of people. My friends and family have been the most important source of support through all stages of the revision of both the book and my life. I feel very blessed to have had so many "life lines" to call on when things were feeling particularly overwhelming! I especially want to thank Ellen Hillegass for all of her help, both professional and personal, throughout these years. I never could have succeeded without her encouragement and friendship! Others who have helped me hold it all together and maintain my forward momentum include my son, Tony; my sisters, Carolyn, Nancy, and Monica; my long-time friends, Marilyn, Phyl, Bonnie, Maribeth, Pat, Elena, Tana, Al, Pam, Mary Jean, and Lily; and my newer Pasadena friends, Kat, Sue, Liz, Rob, Rey, and Lynda. Thank you one and all for being there when I needed you!

The coauthors who contributed to several of the chapters also deserve my appreciation. This was the first adventure in chapter writing for Jeff Rodrigues and Robin Winn, younger physical therapists who offered fresh insights, clinical expertise, and a willingness to adapt to the modifications that must have seemed endless at times. I think all of us learned a great deal from this collaboration. In addition, Joel Hubbard provided valuable assistance and expertise with the chapter on Laboratory Medicine.

Lastly, I want to thank the professionals at Elsevier who were essential to the publication of this book—Kathy Falk, Melissa Kuster, and Jennifer Boudreau—as well as the artist who helped me create the new figures, Jeanne Robertson. I was very fortunate that Elsevier was challenged by staff changes and reorganization during the first few years of my book revision and so did not pressure me into progressing more quickly than the stresses in my life would allow. This work would never have been completed had this not been the case.

Alleluia! *Cardiovascular and Pulmonary Physical Therapy: A Clinical Manual*, Second Edition is done!

Joanne Watchie, PT, CCS

CONTENTS

The Oxygen Transport System: Why the Heart and Lungs Are Important to Physical Therapists

As physical therapists, we are concerned with the prevention, diagnosis, and treatment of movement impairments and the enhancement of physical health and functional abilities. Our clinical practices generally deal with movement impairments; that is, our patients usually have difficulty moving how and where they want. Most commonly, impairments are due to problems with the musculoskeletal, neuromuscular, and neurological systems. However, diseases affecting the pulmonary and cardiovascular systems also result in movement impairment because of their fundamental roles in the oxygen transport system, through which energy is provided for movement, as shown in Figure 1-1.[6]

When an individual wants to perform an activity, the central nervous system stimulates the appropriate muscles, and, if both systems are intact, the desired movements are produced. However, for activity to continue for more than a few minutes without local discomfort or shortness of breath, the muscles must receive adequate blood supply carrying enough oxygen to produce the energy required to sustain the activity. Under normal circumstances this oxygen is readily available in the air that we breathe; through the process of ventilation, it is inhaled through active contraction of the inspiratory muscles and flows through progressively smaller airways to the most distal units of the lungs, the alveoli. The oxygen then diffuses from the alveoli into the surrounding pulmonary capillaries, which are perfused by blood flow coming from the right ventricle via the pulmonary arteries. Most of the oxygen is bound to hemoglobin, and the oxygen-rich blood returns to the left atrium via the pulmonary veins and is pumped by the left ventricle to all the tissues of the body, including the contracting muscles. In the final steps of the oxygen transport system, the oxygen dissociates from arterial hemoglobin and diffuses across the capillary membrane into the muscle cells, where it enters the mitochondria to participate in the oxidative metabolic processes, which ultimately produce adenosine triphosphate, ATP, for energy.

Then the oxygen transport pathway proceeds in the reverse direction to eliminate metabolic by-products, particularly carbon dioxide, which diffuse from the muscle cells into the capillaries and are transported back to the heart via the systemic venous system. The right ventricle pumps the venous blood to the lungs, where carbon dioxide diffuses from the capillaries into the alveoli and, given adequate ventilation, is exhaled from the lungs.

Unfortunately, pathologies affecting any components of the respiratory and cardiovascular systems can interfere with normal function of the oxygen transport system.[1-6] Persons with neurological, neuromuscular, and musculoskeletal disorders affecting the thoracic cage may be incapable of moving (i.e., ventilating) enough air to meet the oxygen demands of many normal activities of daily living. Individuals with a number of lung pathologies, such as pneumonia, pulmonary edema, and pulmonary fibrosis, may have difficulty not only with delivering enough air to the alveoli but also with diffusion of oxygen from the alveoli into the bloodstream, particularly during activity. Conversely, persons with asthma and chronic obstructive pulmonary disease, such as emphysema and chronic bronchitis, are not limited in their ability to inspire adequate volumes of air, but exhibit airflow limitation during expiration and develop air trapping in the distal airways, which also interferes with effective gas exchange. In addition, abnormal gas exchange can result from impeded blood flow through the pulmonary capillaries, as in pulmonary embolism. Many individuals have normal pulmonary function, but abnormal heart function limits the amount of oxygen-carrying blood that can be pumped from the heart to the various tissues of the body, especially during exertion. Lastly, diseases such as atherosclerosis or the connective tissue diseases affect the patency of the arteries and can impede blood flow to active muscles and other tissues. Despite the wide variety of pathologies just mentioned, many of the clinical manifestations are often similar, including fatigue, weakness, and shortness of breath. Notably, these are also the limiting factors experienced by unfit sedentary individuals (i.e., your typical couch potatoes) during activity. Thus, disorders of the pulmonary system ultimately increase the work of breathing and interfere with gas exchange, while abnormalities of the cardiovascular system limit the amount of blood that can be pumped and delivered to the skeletal muscles. The result of both is manifested as exercise intolerance, which has direct implications for physical therapy interventions.

Because all of our clients depend on adequate cardiovascular and pulmonary function to participate effectively in rehabilitation activities, and diseases involving these systems are so prevalent in our society, assessment of the cardiovascular and pulmonary systems should be an essential component of every physical therapy evaluation. Clients with higher likelihood of cardiopulmonary impairment include those with two or more coronary risk factors (as presented in Chapter 4, Cardiopulmonary Pathology) and those over the age of 40 years. It is important to note that many individuals, especially those over 60 years of age, even though they have not been diagnosed with specific cardiovascular or pulmonary disease, may have some degree of dysfunction; thus, the absence of a specific cardiopulmonary diagnosis should not be taken as an indication that an individual has normal pulmonary and/or cardiovascular function. Through clinical monitoring at rest and during activity, physical therapists can detect any abnormal responses and make appropriate modifications in his or her treatment program in order to optimize both effectiveness and safety.

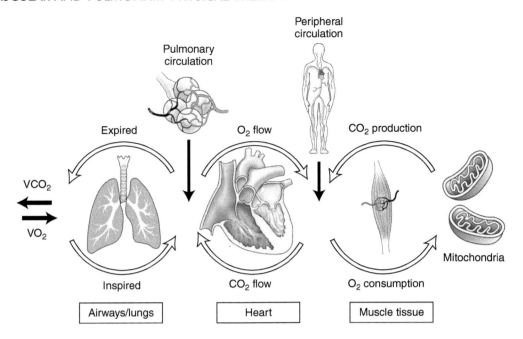

Figure 1-1: Scheme of the oxygen transport system showing the interactions of the respiratory, cardiovascular, and metabolic/tissue components.

The following chapters present information related to normal and abnormal respiratory and cardiovascular function, the diagnosis and treatment of dysfunction, and physical therapy assessment and treatment techniques. There are also chapters focusing on medications used to treat cardiovascular and pulmonary dysfunction and their effects on the physiologic responses to activity, pediatric evaluation and treatment procedures, and laboratory medicine and implications for physical therapy. The ultimate purpose of this book is to provide the clinician with an appreciation of how various pathologies affect the oxygen transport system, the resulting clinical manifestations, and the implications for activity and rehabilitation.

REFERENCES

1. DeTurk WE, Cahalin LP. *Cardiovascular and Pulmonary Physical Therapy: An Evidence-based Approach.* New York: McGraw-Hill; 2004.
2. Frownfelter DL, Dean E. *Cardiovascular and Pulmonary Physical Therapy: Evidence and Practice.* 4th ed. St. Louis: Mosby; 2006.
3. Hillegass EA, Sadowsky HS. *Essentials of Cardiopulmonary Physical Therapy.* 2nd ed. Philadelphia: Saunders Co; 2001.
4. Irwin S, Tecklin JS. *Cardiopulmonary Physical Therapy: A Guide to Practice.* 4th ed. St. Louis: Mosby; 2004.
5. McArdle WD, Katch FI, Katch VL. *Exercise Physiology—Energy, Nutrition, and Human Performance.* 5th ed. Philadelphia: Lea & Febiger; 2001.
6. Wasserman K, Hansen JE, Sue DY, et al. *Principles of Exercise Testing and Interpretation.* 4th ed. Philadelphia: Lippincott Williams & Wilkins; 2004.

CHAPTER 2

Pulmonology

To appreciate how abnormalities involving the respiratory system can produce movement impairment, one must first develop an understanding of normal respiratory function. Thus, this chapter begins with a review of basic anatomy and physiology, with emphasis on the factors that influence lung function. The remainder of the chapter presents the various diagnostic tests and procedures used to evaluate respiratory problems and the therapeutic interventions commonly used in the management of pulmonary dysfunction. Included are implications for physical therapy of important findings from the most common diagnostic tests, as well as for some therapeutic interventions. The most frequently encountered pulmonary diseases and disorders are described in Chapter 4 (Cardiopulmonary Pathology).

2.1 RESPIRATORY SYSTEM AND ITS FUNCTION

ANATOMY OF THE RESPIRATORY SYSTEM

The thoracic cage consists of 12 thoracic vertebrae, 12 ribs, the sternum, and costal cartilage. The respiratory passages, depicted in Figure 2-1, consist of the upper airways, including the nose, pharynx, and larynx; and the lower airways, referred to as the tracheobronchial tree, containing (a) the nonrespiratory conducting airways, or the anatomic dead space (i.e., the trachea, bronchi, and bronchioles), that channels inspired air to the gas exchange areas, and (b) the respiratory units, or acini, where gas exchange takes place. The two lungs with their various lobes and segments are illustrated in Figure 2-2.

- The major airways from the trachea through the 10 generations of bronchi have decreasing amounts of cartilaginous support surrounded by smooth muscle and elastic fibers; they have goblet cells for mucus production and are lined with ciliated columnar epithelium to facilitate secretion clearance.
- The five generations of bronchioles have no cartilage or goblet cells, but still have elastic tissue and smooth muscle fibers; they are lined with ciliated cuboidal epithelium.
- The functional unit of the lungs is the acinus, which participates in gas exchange. It includes the respiratory bronchioles, alveolar ducts and sacs, and the alveoli, whose walls consist of a thin epithelial layer over a connective tissue sublayer.

Muscles of Respiration

The respiratory muscles, their innervations, and their functions are listed in Table 2-1. The primary muscles of inspiration are the diaphragm, external intercostal muscles, and parasternal intercostals, as depicted in Figure 2-3. During deep or labored breathing, the accessory muscles of inspiration are recruited. At rest, expiration is a passive process, occurring as the inspiratory muscles relax and lung elastic recoil takes over. During forced expiration and coughing, the abdominal and internal intercostal muscles are activated. Respiratory muscle weakness and limited endurance can impair gas exchange and lead to respiratory insufficiency or failure, especially when the mechanics of breathing are altered by hyperinflation of the chest (e.g., emphysema, chronic bronchitis, and acute asthma attack).

Nervous Control

The lungs and airways are innervated by the pulmonary plexus (located at the root of each lung), which is formed from branches of the sympathetic trunk and vagus nerve. Sympathetic nervous system stimulation results in bronchodilation and slight vasoconstriction, whereas parasympathetic nervous system stimulation causes bronchoconstriction and indirect vasodilation.

The function of the lungs is controlled through complex interactions of specialized peripheral and central chemoreceptors, as well as the respiratory center with groups of neurons located in the medulla oblongata and pons, as illustrated in Figure 2-4.

- The respiratory center in the medulla contain chemosensitive areas that respond to changes in carbon dioxide levels (P_{CO_2}) and hydrogen ion (H^+) concentration, while other areas receive input from the peripheral chemoreceptors, baroreceptors, and several types of receptors in the lungs. They control inspiration and respiratory rhythm both at rest and during exercise.
- The pneumotaxic center in the pons limits the duration of inspiration and increases the respiratory rate.
- Peripheral receptors provide input to the respiratory center: stretch receptors in the lungs act to prevent overinflation; chemoreceptors located in the carotid and aortic bodies respond to hypoxemia and, to a lesser extent, to rising P_{CO_2} and H^+ concentration; and proprioceptors in the joints and muscles excite the respiratory centers in the medulla to increase ventilation.
- Higher centers in the motor cortex are responsible for voluntary control of breathing (e.g., voluntary breath holding or hyperventilation) and often stimulate respiration in anticipation of exercise.
- It is now recognized that the distribution of neural drive is a major determinant of which regions of the respiratory muscles are selectively activated and in what manner under various resting and exercise conditions, and thus of the actions they produce.[10]
- Disturbances in the control of breathing will result in abnormal blood gas values.

Blood Supply to the Lungs

The bronchial arteries arising from the descending aorta provide blood supply to the nonrespiratory airways, pleurae, and connective tissue, while the pulmonary arteries supply the respiratory

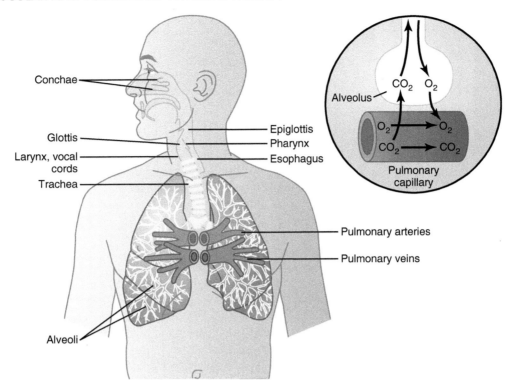

Figure 2-1: The respiratory passages, including gas exchange at the alveolus and pulmonary capillary. (From Guyton AC, Hall JE. *Textbook of Medical Physiology.* 11th ed. Philadelphia: Saunders; 2006.)

units (acini) and participate in gas exchange. Numerous pulmonary vasoactive substances can induce vasoconstriction or vasodilation of the pulmonary arterioles.

Defense of the Lungs

The lungs have a number of structures that serve to protect the lungs from inhaled organisms and particles, and they are assisted by several different types of cells that reside within the lungs.

- Nasal mucosa and hairs warm and humidify inhaled air and filter out particles.
- Goblet cells and bronchial seromucous glands produce mucus, which contains immunoglobulin A, to protect underlying tissue and trap organisms and particles. Mucus production is increased by inflammation (e.g., asthma and bronchitis) and its composition may be altered by various diseases (e.g., asthma and cystic fibrosis).
- Cilia are hairlike structures that wave mucus up to the carina and throat (mucociliary transport). Mucociliary transport is impaired by inhalation of toxic gases (e.g., cigarette smoke and air pollution), acute inflammation, infection, and other disease processes.
- Type II pneumocytes produce surfactant, which protects underlying tissue and repairs damaged alveolar epithelium.
- Alveolar macrophages roam the surface of the terminal airways and engulf foreign matter and bacteria. They also kill bacteria in situ by means of lysozymes. Their activity can be impeded by cigarette smoke, air pollution, alveolar hypoxia, radiation, corticosteroid therapy, and the ingestion of alcohol.

- B lymphocytes produce gamma globulin for the production of antibodies to combat lung infections, and T lymphocytes release a substance that attracts macrophages to the site of an infection.
- Polymorphonuclear leukocytes engulf and kill blood-borne gram-negative organisms.
- Mast cells, which are more numerous in distal airways, release mediators of the inflammatory response to alter epithelial and vascular permeability. Smokers and persons with asthma have greater numbers of mast cells.

RESPIRATORY PHYSIOLOGY

It is important for physical therapists to understand the factors that contribute to normal functioning of the respiratory system in order to appreciate normal versus abnormal physiological indicators, both at rest and during exercise, as well as the implications for physical therapy interventions.

Basic Functions of the Respiratory System

The basic functions of the respiratory system include oxygenation of the blood, removal of carbon dioxide, control of acid–base balance, and production of vocalization.

Mechanics of Breathing

Respiratory gas exchange requires the movement of sufficient volumes of air into the terminal airways to meet the oxygen needs of the body, whether at rest or during exercise. This occurs through active contraction of the inspiratory muscles with enough force to override the elastic recoil of the lungs and the resistance

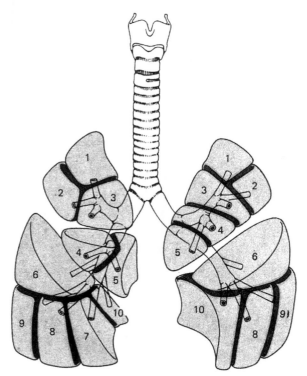

Figure 2-2: The bronchopulmonary segments. *Left and right upper lobes: 1,* apical; *2,* posterior; and *3,* anterior segments. *Left upper lobe: 4,* superior lingular and *5,* inferior linguinal segments. *Right middle lobe: 4,* lateral and *5,* medial segments. *Lower lobes: 6,* superior; *7,* medial basal (no medial basal segment in the left lung); *8,* anterior basal; *9,* lateral basal; and *10,* posterior basal segments. (From Weibel ER: Design and structure of the human lung. In Fishman AP, editor. *Pulmonary Diseases and Disorders.* Vol. 1. New York: McGraw-Hill; 1980.)

TABLE 2-1: Muscles of Respiration, Their Innervations, and Functions

Muscle (Innervation)	Functions
Primary Inspiratory Muscles	
Diaphragm (C_{3-5})	Expands thorax vertically and horizontally; essential for normal vital capacity and effective cough
Scalenes (C_{2-7})	When neck is fixed, elevate first two ribs to expand chest superiorly
Parasternal intercostals (T_{1-11})	Elevate ribs to expand upper half of rib cage
External intercostals (T_{1-11})	Anterior and lateral expansion of upper and lower chest
Accessory Inspiratory Muscles	
Sternocleidomastoid (cranial nerve XI and C_{2-3})	When head is fixed, elevates sternum to expand chest superiorly and anteriorly
Serratus anterior (C_{5-7})	When scapulae are fixed, elevates first eight or nine ribs to provide posterior expansion of thorax
Pectoralis major (C_5-T_1)	When arms are fixed, elevates true ribs to expand the chest anteriorly
Pectoralis minor (C_{6-8})	When scapulae are fixed, elevates third, fourth, and fifth ribs to expand the chest laterally
Trapezius (cranial nerve XI and C_{3-4})	Stabilizes scapulae to assist the serratus anterior and pectoralis minor in elevating the ribs
Erector spinae (C_1 down)	Extend the vertebral column to allow further rib elevation
Expiratory Muscles	
Abdominals (T_{7-12} + L_1 for some)	Help force diaphragm back to resting position and depress and compress lower thorax leading to ↑ intrathoracic pressure, which is essential for effective cough
Internal intercostals (T_{1-11})	Depress third, fourth, and fifth ribs to aid in forceful expiration

C_{1-8}, Cervical nerves 1 to 8; T_{1-12}, thoracic nerves 1 to 12; L_1, lumbar nerve 1. Data from de Troyer A: Actions of the respiratory muscles. In Hamid Q, Shannon J, Martin J, editors. *Physiologic Basis of Respiratory Disease.* Hamilton, ON, Canada: BC Decker; 2005.

to airflow offered by the airways. Thus, the respiratory cycle consists of:

- *Inspiration,* during which active muscle contraction results in expansion of the thorax and the lungs, a fall in alveolar pressure, and airflow into the lungs. At rest, inspiration is accomplished primarily by the diaphragm with some assistance from the parasternal and external intercostals and scalenes (the parasternal intercostals and scalenes act to lift the ribs and expand the upper half of the rib cage, which is important to counteract the inward motion of the upper chest that would result from an unopposed decrease in intrapleural pressure produced by diaphragmatic descent).[10] During deep breathing and exercise the accessory muscles of inspiration are recruited to increase tidal volume (see Table 2-1), which is assisted by passive relaxation of the expiratory muscles that are also activated.[10,29] The drop in intrathoracic pressure during inspiration also facilitates venous return to the heart.
- *Expiration,* during which passive relaxation of the inspiratory muscles to their resting positions and elastic recoil of the lungs cause alveolar pressure to rise, resulting in airflow out of the lungs. During exertion, forced expiration, and coughing, active

contraction of the expiratory muscles (plus closure of the glottis during coughing) causes a marked rise in intrathoracic pressure so that expiration occurs more rapidly and completely; in addition, passive relaxation of these muscles at end-expiration promotes descent of the diaphragm and induces an increase in lung volume toward its neutral resting position.

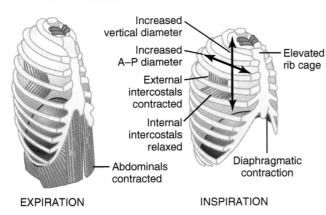

Figure 2-3: Contraction and expansion of the thoracic cage during expiration and inspiration, demonstrating contraction of the abdominals and depression of the rib cage that take place during active expiration and diaphragmatic and external intercostal muscle contraction (with relaxation of the internal intercostals), elevation of the rib cage, and increased vertical diameter that occur during inspiration. Not shown are the parasternal intercostals (which form the ventral part of the internal intercostal layer from the sternum and between the costal cartilages) and the scalenes, both of which also contract during normal quiet inspiration to produce elevation and expansion of the upper rib cage. (From Guyton AC, Hall JE. *Textbook of Medical Physiology.* 11th ed. Philadelphia: Saunders; 2006.)

A number of factors determine respiratory function and are described in Table 2-2.

- *Ventilation ($\dot{V}$):* The process by which air moves into and out of the lungs.
- *Airway resistance (R_{aw}):* The resistance to airflow through the airways; increased airway resistance can limit airflow, which is most noticeable during expiration when the airways are narrower.
- *Pulmonary compliance (C):* The ease with which the lungs expand during inspiration; normal lungs are very compliant and easily expand during inspiration, according to the specific compliances of both the lungs and the chest wall and their elastic properties, as well as the adequacy of thoracic pump function.
- *Diffusion:* The movement of gases into and out of the blood; because CO_2 is more readily diffusible than oxygen, diffusion abnormalities will result in hypoxemia long before hypercapnia develops.
- *Perfusion ($\dot{Q}$):* The blood flow through the pulmonary circulation that is available for gas exchange; hypoxic vasoconstriction is stimulated to reduce blood flow to alveoli that are not being ventilated (i.e., alveolar dead space).
- *Ventilation–perfusion ($\dot{V}/\dot{Q}$) matching:* The degree of physical correspondence between ventilated and perfused areas of the lungs; the optimal $\dot{V}/\dot{Q}$ ratio is 0.8 (4 parts ventilation to 5 parts perfusion) to maintain normal gas exchange.
- *Oxygen–hemoglobin (O_2–Hb) binding:* The level of oxygen saturation of the arterial blood, as shown in Figure 2-5; normal arterial oxygen saturation (Sao_2) is 95% or more.

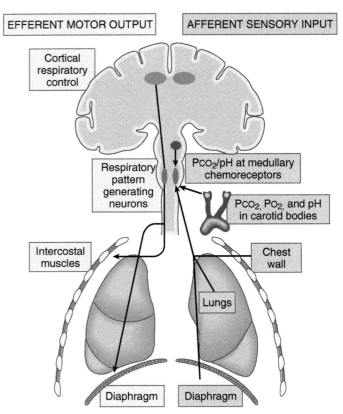

Figure 2-4: A simplified diagram of respiratory integration and control, showing the principal efferent *(left)* and afferent *(right)* pathways. The respiratory areas, as well as the central nervous system links to them, are shown using a section through the brain, brain stem, and spinal cord. (From Figure 86-1 in Goldman L, Ausiello D. *Cecil Textbook of Medicine.* 23rd ed. Philadelphia: Saunders; 2008.)

- Because the top portion of the O_2–Hb curve is fairly flat, it is not very sensitive to changes in Po_2 (e.g., at a Po_2 of 60, the Sao_2 is still 90%).
- Below a Po_2 of 60, the curve is much steeper and therefore much more sensitive to decrements in Po_2 (e.g., at a Po_2 of 40, the Sao_2 drops to 75% and at a Po_2 of 27, the Sao_2 decreases to 50%).
- Different conditions cause the O_2–Hb curve to shift to the right or left, which changes the ease with which oxygen binds to Hb in the blood and is released to the tissues, as described in Figure 2-5.

Lung Volumes and Capacities

As illustrated in Figure 2-6, it is possible to determine various lung volumes and capacities, which are described in Table 2-3.

- *Tidal volume (V_T)* represents the most efficient breathing pattern and volume and includes both dead space and alveolar volumes.
- *Functional residual capacity (FRC)* reflects the balance of the elastic forces exerted by the chest wall and the lungs and is the neutral resting volume of the respiratory system after a normal expiration.

TABLE 2-2: Factors Affecting Respiratory Function

Factor	Influenced by:
Ventilation ($\dot{V}$)	Gravity and differences in intrapleural pressure
	Ventilation is greatest in dependent/lower lung regions and least in upper lung regions
Airway resistance (R_{aw})	Upper airways
	Provides about 45% of total airway resistance
	Lower airways, which may be narrowed by:
	Normal expiration (airways are more expanded during inspiration)
	External pressure (e.g., tumor, pleural effusion)
	Bronchial smooth muscle contraction (i.e., bronchoconstriction)
	Mucosal congestion, inflammation, edema, mucus
	Loss of structural support (e.g., emphysema)
Compliance (C)	Lung compliance: How easily the lungs inflate during inspiration
	Opposed by the elastic properties of the lung, which tend to collapse the lungs if they are not acted on by external forces
	Decreased by fibrosis, edema, infiltrates, atelectasis, pleural effusion, tumor, etc., which increase the effort required to inflate the lungs
	Increased by age and emphysema, which result in loss of lung elasticity
	Chest wall compliance: How easily the chest wall expands during inspiration
	Assisted by the elastic forces of the chest wall, which cause it to expand if unopposed by the elastic recoil of the lungs
	Reduced by thoracic pump dysfunction due to chest deformity, splinting due to pain following injury or surgery, respiratory muscle weakness or paralysis or ↑ tone, obesity, pregnancy, ascites, and peritonitis
Diffusion	Interference at the alveoli, alveolar capillary interface, and capillaries
	Impaired by thickening, fibrosis, fluid, edema, etc.
	Surface area available for gas exchange
	Reduced by loss of surface area in emphysema, lung resection
Perfusion ($\dot{Q}$)	Body position/hydrostatic pressure
	Dependent/lower lung regions have greater perfusion than upper lung regions
	Interaction of alveolar, arterial, and venous pressures down the lungs
	Pulmonary arterial vasoconstriction (vasoconstriction triggered by hypoxia, acidemia, etc.)
Ventilation–perfusion ($\dot{V}/\dot{Q}$) matching	Uneven ventilation, which can result from:
	Uneven compliance due to fibrosis, emphysema, pleural effusion or thickening, pulmonary edema, etc.
	Uneven airway resistance due to bronchoconstriction, mucous plugs, edema, tumor, etc.
	Uneven perfusion, which can result from:
	Obstruction of part of the pulmonary circulation due to thrombosis, fat embolus, parasites, tumor, etc.
	Compression of blood vessels due to overexpanded alveoli, tumor, edema, etc.
Oxygen–hemoglobin (O_2–Hb) binding	Arterial oxygen concentration (P_{O_2}, or more precisely Pa_{O_2})
	A decrease in Pa_{O_2} results in ↓ association + ↑ dissociation of O_2–Hb (so less O_2 is bound to Hb, but the bound O_2 is more easily given off to the tissues)
	A number of other factors that cause a shift of the oxyhemoglobin curve:
	↓ pH, ↑ P_{CO_2}, ↑ temperature (all of which occur in the muscle capillaries during vigorous exercise), and ↑ 2,3-DPG cause a shift to the right so there is greater release of O_2 to the muscle at lower P_{O_2} levels
	↑ pH, ↓ P_{CO_2}, ↓ temperature (all of which occur in the lungs during vigorous exercise), and ↓ 2,3-DPG cause a shift to the left so the amount of O_2 that binds with Hb at any given P_{O_2} is increased in the lungs
	Amount and adequacy of hemoglobin; red blood cell count

↓, Decreased (lower than normal); ↑, increased (higher than normal); 2,3-DPG, 2,3-diphosphoglycerate.

ARTERIAL OXYGENATION

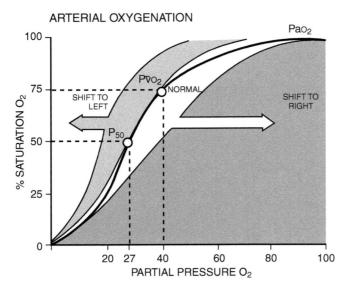

Figure 2-5: The oxyhemoglobin (O_2–Hb) dissociation curve. Various factors cause the curve to shift to the left (e.g., acute alkalosis, hypocapnia, hypothermia) or right (e.g., acute acidosis, hypercapnia, increased body temperature), as described in Table 2-2. Pao_2 = partial pressure of oxygen in arterial blood, Pvo_2 = partial pressure of oxygen in venous blood (normally 40 mm Hg), P_{50} = partial pressure of oxygen when hemoglobin is 50% saturated with oxygen (normally 27 mm Hg). (From Frownfelter DL, Dean E. *Cardiovascular and Pulmonary Physical Therapy: Evidence and Practice.* 4th ed. St. Louis: Mosby; 2006.)

TABLE 2-3: **Lung Volumes and Capacities**

Volume or Capacity	Description
Tidal volume (V_T)	Amount of air inspired or expired during normal breathing
Inspiratory reserve volume (IRV)	Extra volume inspired over and above the tidal volume
Expiratory reserve volume (ERV)	Extra amount of air forcefully expired after the end of a normal tidal expiration
Residual volume (RV)	Volume of air still remaining in the lungs (i.e., in the anatomic dead space and the acini) after a maximal forced expiration
Inspiratory capacity (IC)	Maximal volume of air that can be inspired after a normal tidal expiration = TV + IRV
Functional residual capacity (FRC)	Amount of air remaining in the lungs after a normal tidal expiration = RV + ERV
Vital capacity (VC)	Maximal volume of air that a person can forcefully expire after taking in a maximal inspiration = IRV + TV + ERV
Total lung capacity (TLC)	Maximal volume of air that the lungs can contain following a maximal inspiration = RV + ERV + TV + IRV

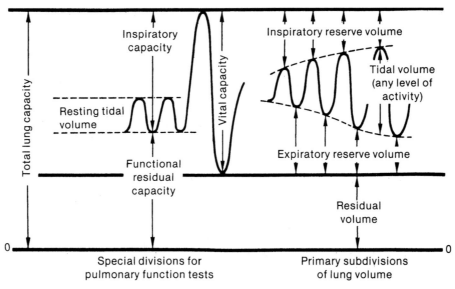

Figure 2-6: A spirogram showing the lung volumes and capacities during normal breathing and during maximal inspiration and expiration. To the right are the changes in primary lung volumes that occur during progressively more intense activity. (Modified from Pappenheimer JR, Comroe JH, Cournand A, et al. *Fed Proc.* 1950;9:602. Used with permission.)

- At *total lung capacity (TLC)*, the elastic forces of the lungs are balanced by the maximal inspiratory muscle forces during a very deep breath.
- At *residual volume (RV)*, the elastic forces of the chest wall are balanced by the maximal expiratory muscle forces at the end of a forced expiration; it is normally about 20% to 30% of V_T.

For additional information on the various lung volumes and capacities, as determined by pulmonary function testing, and how they are affected by various types of lung disease, refer to pages 11 to 12.

Exercise Physiology

During exercise the respiratory system must increase the volume of air (oxygen) that is ventilated by the lungs (i.e., minute ventilation, $\dot{V}$, which is usually measured during expiration and thus referred to as $\dot{V}_E$) and diffused into the blood for delivery to the exercising muscles. There are a number of factors that affect respiratory function and the ability of the respiratory system to meet the oxygen demands of the exercising muscles during vigorous exertion (see Table 2-2).

- At rest, $\dot{V}_E$ is usually 5 to 10 L/min and it often increases 15- to 20-fold during maximal exercise.
- At the onset of mild to moderate exercise, $\dot{V}_E$ typically increases via increasing tidal volume.
- During more strenuous exercise, rising respiratory rates further augment $\dot{V}_E$.
- $\dot{V}_E$ increases in direct proportion to oxygen consumption ($\dot{V}_{O_2}$) and carbon dioxide production ($\dot{V}_{CO_2}$) until exercise intensity exceeds the ventilatory threshold (generally about 50% to 70% of $\dot{V}_{O_{2max}}$, when there are abrupt nonlinear increases in lactate and $\dot{V}_{CO_2}$). At this point $\dot{V}_E$ also increases disproportionately with $\dot{V}_{O_2}$.
- At rest, the energy cost of breathing is 1% to 4% of total body $\dot{V}_{O_2}$, and at maximal exercise it increases to 8% to 11% of total $\dot{V}_{O_2}$ in healthy individuals and as high as 40% in those with severe pulmonary disease.
- Ventilation is not normally a limiting factor to aerobic capacity.

Effects of Aging

Many of the changes that were once attributed to the normal aging process are now known to be effects of deconditioning and can be retarded or reversed with exercise conditioning. However, there are a number of physical and functional changes that do occur with normal aging that affect pulmonary function and increase the work of breathing.

- The thoracic cage becomes less compliant due to increased stiffness of the costovertebral joints and chest wall, so thoracic expansion is reduced.
- A decrease in the number and thickness of elastic fibers impairs elastic recoil during expiration, which increases RV and FRC.
- The diaphragm assumes a lower and less mechanically efficient position in the chest, causing a reduction in its force-generating ability.
- Airway resistance increases, so expiratory time is prolonged.
- Diffusing capacity decreases as a result of reductions in alveolar surface area (the alveoli and alveolar ducts become enlarged)

and the number of pulmonary capillaries, which reduces the efficiency of gas exchange.
- Recruitment of the accessory muscles of respiration occurs more often and at lower levels of exertion, leading to an increase in the work of breathing.
- The peripheral and central chemoreceptors become less sensitive to increasing levels of carbon dioxide and hypoxemia, so they are less likely to stimulate ventilation to compensate for abnormalities.

2.2 EVALUATION OF THE PULMONARY SYSTEM

Although physical therapists seldom generate or read the raw data of most diagnostic tests and procedures, we are frequently challenged to interpret the results of these investigations and their implications for the patients we treat. Through better appreciation of the information in a patient's chart, we can grasp more completely the patient's status and the possible pathophysiological effects of our treatment interventions and can provide appropriate modifications as needed.

SIGNS AND SYMPTOMS OF PULMONARY DISEASE

An important component of a patient evaluation is the patient's subjective complaints related to respiratory function and exercise tolerance and any abnormal physical signs that are detected on physical examination. Table 2-4 describes the most common signs and symptoms and their pulmonary causes. There may be other explanations for some of these symptoms; the cardiovascular causes are listed in Chapter 3 (Cardiovascular Medicine; see Table 3-3 on page 46), and other causes are presented in Chapter 6 (Cardiopulmonary Assessment; see Table 6-5 on page 228). The physical examination findings relevant to physical therapy evaluation and their implications for treatment are also discussed in Chapter 6.

CYTOLOGIC AND HEMATOLOGIC TESTS

Cytologic and hematologic tests are used to identify disease-causing organisms and their sensitivity to antibiotics, to assess the impact of pulmonary disease on gas exchange, and to monitor responses to treatment.

Sputum Analysis

Collection and examination of expectorated sputum obtained from a deep cough, especially first thing in the morning, is the most common method of obtaining a sample for cytologic evaluation. Samples can also be obtained invasively, via suctioning, bronchoscopy, or transtracheal or needle aspiration, which are described on page 25. The sample is sent to the laboratory for sputum culture and sensitivity testing to provide definitive identification of the pathologic agent and to determine the most effective antimicrobial agent(s). In patients with chronic obstructive pulmonary disease

TABLE 2-4: Signs and Symptoms of Pulmonary Disease

Sign or Symptom	Common Pulmonary Causes
Anorexia, weakness, fatigue, weight loss	Chronic respiratory disease (probably caused by ↑ work of breathing), pulmonary infection
Bradycardia	Profound hypoxemia
↓ Breath sounds	Atelectasis, emphysema, fibrosis, pleural effusion, pneumothorax, local bronchial occlusion, hypoventilation of any cause, diaphragmatic paralysis, obesity
Bronchial breath sounds	Consolidation, tumor, fibrosis in close approximation to a patent bronchus
↓ Chest expansion (focal or generalized)	Pulmonary consolidation, fibrosis, atelectasis, pleural effusion, pneumothorax, obesity, kyphoscoliosis, obstructive lung disease, respiratory muscle weakness
Chest pain	Pleurisy, pneumonia, cancer, tuberculosis, pulmonary emboli or infarction, pneumothorax, violent coughing, rib fracture or other trauma, tracheobronchial infection, inhalation of noxious fumes, intercostal neuritis, pulmonary hypertension
Coma, convulsions	Rapid ↑ $Paco_2$
Confusion, ↓ concentration, restlessness, irritability	Hypoxemia, hypercapnia
Cough	Stimulation of airway mucosal irritant receptors by inflammation, secretions, foreign bodies, chemical substances, and intrabronchial masses
Crackles, or rales	Interstitial fibrosis, atelectasis, pulmonary edema, COPD
Cyanosis	Hypoxemia
Diaphoresis	Infection (fever), ↑ sympathetic nervous system activity (e.g., anxiety concerning SOB), night sweats (unknown mechanism)
Digital clubbing	Unknown; seen in bronchogenic carcinoma, chronic infections (empyema, lung abscess, bronchiectasis, cystic fibrosis), interstitial pulmonary fibrosis, hepatopulmonary syndrome, and right-to-left shunting (pulmonary arteriovenous malformations)
Dullness to percussion	Pleural effusion, lobar consolidation, lobar or whole lung atelectasis
Dyspnea, shortness of breath (SOB) (air hunger)	*Acute onset:* Pulmonary embolism, pneumothorax, acute asthma, pulmonary congestion caused by CHF, pneumonia, upper airway obstruction
	Subacute or chronic: Airflow limitation/COPD, ↓ lung volume, impaired gas exchange, ↓ lung compliance (e.g., pneumonia, congestion, atelectasis, pleural effusion, pulmonary fibrosis), ↓ chest wall compliance (e.g., kyphoscoliosis, obesity, neuromuscular impairment), ↑ oxygen consumption (as with exertion)
Fever	Pulmonary infection, tissue degeneration, trauma
Hemoptysis (expectoration of bloody or blood-streaked secretions)	Acute exacerbation of chronic bronchitis, bronchial carcinoma, tuberculosis, bronchiectasis, pulmonary hypertension, pulmonary infarction, pneumonia (especially pneumococcal)
Hypercapnia (↑ $Paco_2$)	↑ Ventilation–perfusion mismatching, alveolar hypoventilation, pulmonary arteriovenous malformations
Hypoxemia (↓ Pao_2)	↑ Ventilation–perfusion mismatching, diffusion defect, alveolar hypoventilation, pulmonary arteriovenous malformations, ↓ Fio_2 (e.g., altitude)
Mediastinal shift	Severe kyphoscoliosis (toward side of compressed lung)
Toward affected side	Pulmonary fibrosis, atelectasis, lobectomy or pneumonectomy
Away from affected side	Pneumothorax, pleural effusion, hyperinflation of one lung caused by check-valve obstruction of a bronchus
↑ Nasal secretions	Infection, irritants, allergens
Orthopnea (SOB when recumbent)	Paralysis of both hemidiaphragms, pulmonary edema
Paroxysmal nocturnal dyspnea (PND), or awakening with SOB in the middle of the night	Pooling of secretions, gravity-induced ↓ lung volumes, sleep-induced ↑ airflow resistance

Continued

TABLE 2-4: Signs and Symptoms of Pulmonary Disease—Cont'd

Sign or Symptom	Common Pulmonary Causes
Pleural friction rub	Irritation of the pleurae (e.g., pneumonia, pleurisy)
↑ Resonance to percussion	Pneumothorax, emphysema, chronic bronchitis, possibly acute asthma
↓ Resonance to percussion	Atelectasis, consolidation, fibrosis, pleural effusion
Rhonchi, wheezes	↑ Secretions in airway(s)
Sputum production	Pulmonary suppuration, lung abscess, acute or chronic bronchitis, bronchiectasis, neoplasm, pulmonary edema, pneumonia
Stridor	Narrowing of the glottis, trachea, or major bronchi, as by foreign body aspiration, external compression by tumor, or tumor within the airways
Tachycardia	Hypoxemia
Tachypnea	Pneumonia, pulmonary edema, pulmonary infarction, diffuse pulmonary fibrosis
↑ Vocal fremitus	Consolidation, just above level of pleural effusion
↓ Vocal fremitus	Asthma, atelectasis, COPD, fibrosis, pleural effusion, pneumothorax, obesity, ↑ chest musculature
Wheezes	Narrowing of a bronchus (e.g., bronchoconstriction, stenosis, ↑ secretions, edema, inflammation, tumor, foreign body aspiration)

↓, Decreased (lower than normal); ↑, increased (higher than normal); CHF, chronic heart failure; COPD, chronic obstructive pulmonary disease; Fio_2, fraction of inspired oxygen; LV, left ventricular; $Paco_2$, partial pressure of arterial carbon dioxide; Pao_2, partial pressure of arterial oxygen; SOB, shortness of breath.

(COPD), the appearance of purulent green sputum has been found to be 94% sensitive and 77% specific for a high bacterial load that usually benefits from antibiotic therapy, whereas the presence of white mucoid sputum during acute exacerbation is likely to improve without antibiotics.[39]

Hematologic Tests

Blood tests that may aid in the assessment of pulmonary disease include arterial blood gases (see page 17), as well as complete blood counts and coagulation studies, which are described in Chapter 9 (Laboratory Medicine; see pages 401 and 405). In addition, blood cultures may be obtained in cases of suspected acute bacterial pneumonia.

CHEST RADIOGRAPHY

Despite the development of a variety of newer imaging modalities, the standard chest radiograph (CXR) remains a critical element in the detection, diagnosis, and follow-up of thoracic disease.
- The various projections that may be used are described in Table 2-5. The most common are the posteroanterior (PA) and lateral views.
- The structures that can be identified in a normal PA CXR are shown in Figure 2-7.
- The differences between an inspiratory CXR and an expiratory CXR are illustrated in Figure 3-9 on page 47.
- Physical therapists working in cardiopulmonary care often become familiar with the basic principles of CXR interpretation and use the results to anatomically locate the patient's pathologic condition and direct treatment interventions.

Digital (or Computed) Radiography

Digital chest x-rays are acquired most commonly with reusable plates and are electronically displayed.
- The main advantages are the ability to manipulate and process the images, allowing improved diagnostic value, and to store images and view them in remote locations.
- Digital imaging is particularly useful for viewing the denser portions of the thorax and the lung in front of or behind these dense areas. They may not be as effective at visualizing fine lung detail, line shadows, pneumothoraces, and interstitial lung disease.

PULMONARY FUNCTION TESTS

Pulmonary function tests (PFTs) consist of a series of inspiratory and expiratory maneuvers designed to assess the integrity and function of the respiratory system. The information provided by PFTs is helpful to the therapist in establishing realistic treatment goals and an appropriate treatment plan according to the patient's current pulmonary problems and degree of impairment.

Data Available From PFTs

PFTs include measurements of lung volume and capacity, ventilation, pulmonary mechanics, and diffusion, many of which are described subsequently.

Lung Volumes and Capacities
- The various lung volumes and capacities are described in Table 2-3.
- Normal values vary depending on age, gender, height, and ethnicity.

TABLE 2-5: **Various Projections Used for Chest Radiography**

Projection	Description
Posteroanterior (PA)	The x-ray beam passes back to front with the subject standing or sitting with the chest against the film plate, usually with the breath held following a deep inspiration
Anteroposterior (AP)	The x-ray beam passes front to back with the patient's back against the film; most often obtained with a portable x-ray machine when patients are too ill or unable to travel to the radiology department
Lateral (Lat.)	The beam passes side to side, usually right to left, with the side of the chest against the film plate in an upright position; commonly obtained along with a PA film
Oblique	The beam passes PA or AP with one of the patient's sides in contact with the film plate and the chest rotated 10 to 45 degrees
Decubitus	The beam travels PA or AP with the patient lying on one side. Used to confirm the presence of pleural fluid or suspected foreign body in small children
Lordotic	The x-ray is taken in the PA position with the patient tilted backward. Because structures change their relative positions, this view allows better visualization of subapical, posterior, middle lobe, and lingular lesions
Expiratory	The x-ray is obtained following expiration or forced expiration to document focal air trapping or delayed emptying

- Total lung capacity is not measured directly during PFTs but is extrapolated from other measurements. It may be decreased in disease processes with space-occupying lesions (such as edema, atelectasis, tumors, and fibrosis) and in pleural effusion, pneumothorax, and thoracic deformity. It may be normal or increased in obstructive lung diseases, being elevated in hyperinflation.
- Vital capacity (VC) is reduced if there is a loss of distensible lung tissue (such as in atelectasis, pneumonia, pulmonary fibrosis, pulmonary congestion or edema, bronchial obstruction, carcinoma, and surgical excision) or impairment of thoracic pump function. It is also affected by patient effort and motivation.
- Residual volume (RV) and functional residual capacity (FRC) are reduced in restrictive lung dysfunction, when there is interference with either lung or thoracic expansion. They are

increased (>120% of predicted normal) in chronic obstructive lung disease, indicating air trapping.
- Examples of proportional changes typically seen in obstructive and restrictive lung disorders compared with normal function are illustrated in Figure 2-8.

Ventilation

The parameters that describe ventilatory function include the following:
- Tidal volume (V_T)
  - ▸ Values should always be assessed within the context of respiratory rate and minute ventilation.
  - ▸ Values of 400 to 700 mL are typical, although there is considerable variation.
  - ▸ Values may be decreased in severe restrictive lung dysfunction and respiratory center depression, in which case a greater proportion of the volume serves as dead space and less volume reaches the acini for participation in gas exchange; values are increased during exertion and at rest in some patients with pulmonary disease.
- Respiratory rate (RR, f)
  - ▸ Normally, RR = 12 to 20 breaths/min in adults. Values are increased with exertion, hypoxia, hypercapnia, acidosis, increased dead space volume, and decreased lung compliance; they are often decreased in central nervous system depression and carbon dioxide narcosis.
  - ▸ RR is often considered to be a good indicator of the stimulus to breathe and of normal versus abnormal ventilatory status.
- Minute ventilation, expired ($\dot{V}_E$)
  - ▸ $\dot{V}_E = V_T \times RR$ and is usually between 5 and 10 L/min. $\dot{V}_E$ will be increased (>20 L/min) in hypoxia, hypercapnia, acidosis, increased dead space volume, anxiety, and exercise and will be decreased in hypocapnia, alkalemia, respiratory center depression, and neuromuscular disorders with ventilatory muscle involvement.
  - ▸ $\dot{V}_E$ is the primary index of ventilation when used in conjunction with arterial blood gases.
    - ⊙ *Hypoventilation* is defined as inadequate ventilation to eliminate normal levels of carbon dioxide (CO_2), resulting in hypercapnia and respiratory acidosis.
    - ⊙ *Hyperventilation* is ventilation in excess of that needed to maintain adequate CO_2 removal, and produces hypocapnia and respiratory alkalosis.
- Dead space (V_D)
  - ▸ V_D is the volume of lungs that is ventilated but not perfused by pulmonary capillary blood flow, and is usually 125 to 175 mL.
  - ▸ V_D can be divided into the volume in the nonrespiratory conducting airways, or the anatomic dead space, and that in the nonperfused alveoli, or the alveolar dead space. Anatomic dead space is increased in larger individuals and in bronchiectasis and emphysema and is decreased in asthma, bronchial obstruction, and mucous plugging. V_D is increased during normal exercise and in pulmonary embolism and pulmonary hypertension.

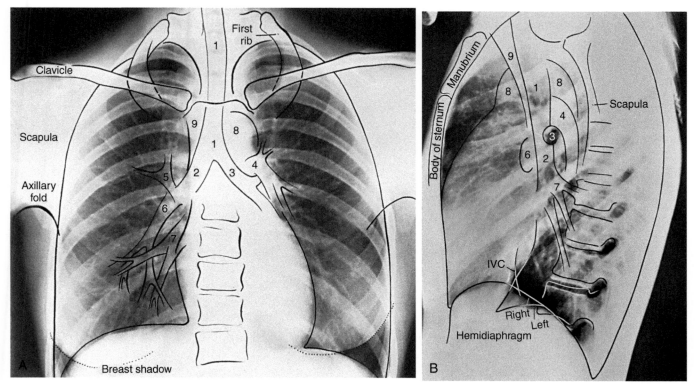

Figure 2-7: Normal chest radiographs. **A,** Posteroanterior view. *1,* Trachea; *2,* right main bronchus; *3,* left main bronchus; *4,* left pulmonary artery; *5,* right upper lobe pulmonary artery; *6,* right interlobar artery; *7,* right lower and middle lobe vein; *8,* aortic knob; *9,* superior vena cava. **B,** Lateral view. *1,* Trachea; *2,* right main bronchus; *3,* left main bronchus; *4,* left interlobar artery; *6,* right main pulmonary artery; *7,* confluence of pulmonary veins; *8,* aortic arch; *9,* brachiocephalic vessels. (From Fraser RG, Paré PD. Principles of chest x-ray interpretation. In Fraser RG, Paré JAD, Paré PD, Fraser RS, Genereux GP, editors. *Diagnosis of Diseases of the Chest.* 3rd ed. Vol. 1. Philadelphia: Saunders; 1988.)

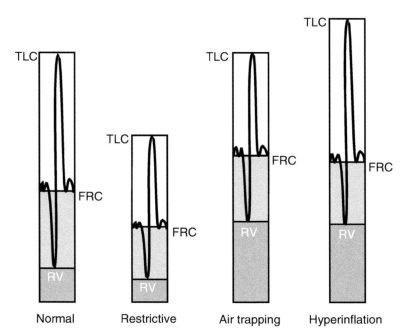

Figure 2-8: Examples of absolute lung volumes in a normal person, a patient with restrictive lung disease (all volumes are decreased), and patients with air trapping and hyperinflation (↑ RV and FRC without reduction in VC) due to obstructive airway disease. FRC, Functional residual capacity; RV, residual volume; TLC, total lung capacity; VC, vital capacity. (From Ruppel GL. *Manual of Pulmonary Function Testing.* 9th ed. St. Louis: Mosby; 2008.)

- Ratio of dead space to tidal volume (V_D/V_T)
  - ▸ Normally, the derived value is 0.2 to 0.4.
  - ▸ V_D/V_T decreases in normal individuals during exercise because of increased cardiac output and enhanced perfusion of the alveoli at the lung apices (despite an absolute increase in V_D) and increases in pulmonary embolism and pulmonary hypertension. The failure of V_D/V_T to decrease during exercise may be an early sign of pulmonary vascular disease.
- Alveolar ventilation ($\dot{V}_A$)
  - ▸ $\dot{V}_A$ is the volume of air that participates in gas exchange. $\dot{V}_A = f(V_T - V_D)$ and is usually about 4 to 5 L at rest, with large variations in healthy individuals. Decreased $\dot{V}_A$ can result from absolute increases in dead space, as well as decreases in $\dot{V}_E$.
  - ▸ $\dot{V}_A$ is one of the major factors determining gas exchange, the adequacy of which can be measured only through determination of arterial blood gases.

Pulmonary Mechanics

Because studies of pulmonary mechanics (e.g., flow rates, compliance, and airway resistance) are dynamic in nature, the validity of their measurement is dependent on patient effort and cooperation. Tests of pulmonary mechanics are often performed before and after the administration of bronchodilators to detect reversibility of airflow limitation and to determine the efficacy of their use.

- Spirometric and pulmonary mechanics measurements are described in Table 2-6. Normal values vary depending on age, gender, height, and ethnicity, as well as on level of cooperation and effort.

- Flow–volume curves depict the flow generated during a forced vital capacity (FVC) maneuver; typical curves illustrating obstructive and restrictive lung disease compared with normal function are shown in Figure 2-9.
  - ▸ In obstructive lung disease, the TLC and RV points are displaced to the left (indicating increased volumes), peak expiratory flow rate is significantly reduced (e.g., the volume expired in the first second [FEV_1] is decreased), the FEV_1/FVC is reduced to less than 65%, and the curve is flattened or concave.
  - ▸ In restrictive lung disease, the TLC and RV points are shifted to the right (indicating decreased volumes), the FVC and peak expiratory flow are reduced, but the FEV_1/FVC is usually normal and the shape of the curve is preserved.
  - ▸ Some patients have both obstructive and restrictive defects and therefore will exhibit a combination of low volumes and reduced expiratory flow rates.

Typical patterns for flow–volume loops, showing both forced inspiration and expiration curves, for obstructive and restrictive dysfunction compared with normal function are shown in Figure 2-10. See preceding comments regarding typical abnormalities.

Gas Distribution Tests

Tests that measure the distribution of ventilation are useful in detecting the presence of early stages of abnormalities, when other tests are normal, or to confirm the presence of airflow obstruction when other tests are only mildly abnormal.

- The single-breath nitrogen washout test assesses the evenness of the distribution of ventilation by measuring the change in nitrogen concentration during an FVC following a single inhalation of 100% oxygen.

TABLE 2-6: **Spirometric and Pulmonary Mechanics Measurements**

Parameter	Comments
Forced vital capacity (FVC) (the maximal volume that can be expired as forcefully and rapidly as possible after a maximal inspiration)	Normally FVC and vital capacity (VC) should be within 200 mL of each other.
	FVC may be <VC in chronic OLD if forced expiration causes bronchiolar collapse or is reduced by mucous plugging and bronchiolar narrowing
	Both FVC and VC are similarly ↓ in RLD
Forced expiratory volume in 1 sec (FEV_1) (the volume of gas expired over the first second of an FVC)	As a measure of flow, FEV_1 is valuable in assessing the severity of airway obstruction (see FEV_1/FVC)
	FEV_1 is ↓ in both RLD and OLD; in RLD the ↓ is proportional to that of the FVC, whereas it is more marked in OLD
FEV_1/FVC (the forced expiratory volume in 1 sec expressed as a percentage of forced vital capacity)	Younger subjects can normally expire 50%-60% of FVC in 0.5 sec, 75%-85% in 1 sec, 94% in 2 sec, and 97% in 3 sec. The FEV_1/FVC is typically 70%-75% in healthy older adults
	FEV_1/FVC <65% is diagnostic of OLD, the severity of which can be gauged by the extent of the ↓, as are the degrees of functional limitation and morbidity
	In RLD, FVC is often ↓ and FEV_1 may be similarly ↓, normal, or ↑, so FEV_1/FVC is normal or ↑

Continued

TABLE 2-6: Spirometric and Pulmonary Mechanics Measurements—Cont'd

Parameter	Comments
Forced expiratory flow from 25% to 75% of vital capacity ($FEF_{25\%-75\%}$) (the average flow rate in L/sec during the middle half of an FVC)	$FEF_{25\%-75\%}$ was formerly referred to as the maximal midexpiratory flow rate (MMFR)
	It indicates the status of the medium and small airways. ↓ Values are seen even in the early stages of OLD and provide confirmation when FEV_1/FVC is borderline or low. Sometimes it is ↓ in moderate to severe RLD when the cross-sectional area of the small airways is ↓
Flow–volume curve/loop (a graph of flow generated during an FVC maneuver plotted against volume; when it is followed by a forced inspiratory maneuver, a flow–volume loop is produced)	Although the initial 25%-30% of the expiratory phase is effort dependent, the remainder of the curve is not and is very reproducible, being determined by lung elastic recoil and flow resistance
	Abnormal loops with significantly ↓ flow are seen in obstruction due to small airway disease (e.g., emphysema and asthma) or large airway disease (e.g., tumors of trachea and bronchi)
	Abnormal loops with significantly ↓ volume are seen in moderately severe RLD
	The highest point on the expiratory curve is the PEFR (see the next entries)
Peak expiratory flow rate (PEFR) (the maximal flow rate attainable during an FVC maneuver)	PEFR is effort dependent and measures primarily large airway function
	Together with the FVC and FEV_1, it provides a good indication of subject effort
	In healthy young adults, PEFR may exceed 10 L/sec (600 L/min)
	Assessment from an expiratory flow–volume curve helps to define both the severity and site of large airway obstruction
	Home monitoring of PEF can provide early detection of asthmatic episodes
Maximal voluntary ventilation (MVV) (the largest volume that a subject can breathe per minute using forced rapid deep breaths)	MVV measures the overall function of the respiratory system, including airway resistance, respiratory muscle function, pulmonary compliance, and ventilatory control mechanisms
	It is often extrapolated from values obtained in 12–15 sec
	MVV is highly dependent on subject cooperation and effort
	Normal values in healthy young males average 150-200 L/min and slightly lower in females, then ↓ with age
	↓ MVV is seen in moderate or severe OLD and neuromuscular disease or paralysis but is often normal in RLD
Compliance (C) (the change in volume produced by a unit change in pressure for the lungs [C_L], the thorax [C_T], or the lungs–thorax system [C_{LT}])	Measurements of C describe the elasticity of the lungs, thorax, and the two combined
	C_L varies with the end-expiratory volume, or functional reserve capacity (FRC)
	It is usually ↓ in pulmonary edema or congestion, atelectasis, pneumonia, loss of surfactant, and pulmonary fibrosis; it is also ↓ with age
	C_L is often ↑ in emphysema due to loss of elastic tissue
	C_T may be ↓ due to thoracic disease, such as kyphoscoliosis, and obesity
Airway resistance (R_{aw}) (the pressure difference required for a unit of flow change)	Measurement of R_{aw} is helpful in distinguishing between RLD and OLD; it is usually ↑ in acute asthma and other OLDs as well as large airway obstruction but not in RLD

↓, Decreased (lower than normal); ↑, increased (higher than normal); OLD, obstructive lung disease; RLD, restrictive lung disease.

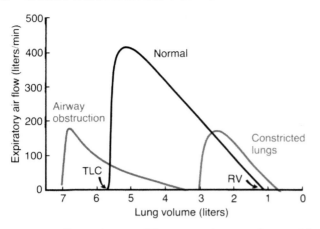

Figure 2-9: Effect of two different respiratory abnormalities, obstructive disease and restricted lung dysfunction, on the maximal expiratory flow–volume curve, compared with normal. (From Guyton AC, Hall JE. *Textbook of Medical Physiology.* 11th ed. Philadelphia: Saunders; 2006.)

- Closing volume is that portion of the VC that can be expired from the lungs after the onset of airway closure (usually expressed as a percentage of VC) and is used to document pathologic changes in small airways (<2 mm in diameter) and to measure the uniformity of gas distribution within the lungs.
  - ▸ In healthy young adults, airway closure begins after 80% to 90% of the VC has been expired, which is a volume below the FRC, indicating that the airways are open throughout the lungs during tidal breathing.
  - ▸ When airway closure occurs above the FRC, early onset of airway closure leads to underventilation of the affected alveoli and air trapping. This may occur in the elderly, in chronic smokers, and in patients with asthma, chronic bronchitis, and emphysema, some restrictive diseases, or congestive heart failure when edema compresses the small airways.

Diffusion Studies

Physiological tests for the measurement of diffusion permit the diagnosis of impaired surface area for gas exchange, sometimes even during the early stages of disease.

The parameters that describe diffusing capacity include the following:

- Carbon monoxide diffusing capacity ($D_{L_{CO}}$), which measures all the factors that affect diffusion of gases across the alveolar–capillary membrane. Values decrease with anemia, interference at the alveolar–capillary membrane (e.g., alveolitis, pulmonary fibrosis, and pulmonary edema), and decreased surface area for gas exchange (e.g., emphysema and lung resection) (see Table 2-2).
- Transfer factor for carbon monoxide ($T_{L_{CO}}$), which is proposed to be more accurate terminology, because the diffusion process includes the rate of reaction of carbon monoxide with hemoglobin as well as its diffusion across the alveolar–capillary membrane.
- Diffusion coefficient (K_{CO}), which is the transfer factor per unit lung volume.

Individuals with a $D_{L_{CO}}$ less than 60% of the predicted normal value are likely to exhibit oxygen desaturation during exertion and should be monitored via pulse oximetry (see page 18).

Maximal Respiratory Pressures

Measurements of the static pressures developed by inspiratory and expiratory muscle contraction are particularly valuable for assessing possible respiratory muscle weakness.

- Maximal inspiratory pressure (MIP) is the maximal negative pressure developed during a forceful inspiration against an occluded airway and is normally measured at RV. It provides a good indication of inspiratory muscle strength.
  - ▸ Normal adults can achieve MIP values of at least −60 cm H_2O.
  - ▸ MIP is decreased in neurologic disorders and neuromuscular diseases and other abnormalities affecting the diaphragm, intercostals, or accessory muscles (e.g., hyperinflation in emphysema or thoracic trauma or deformities).

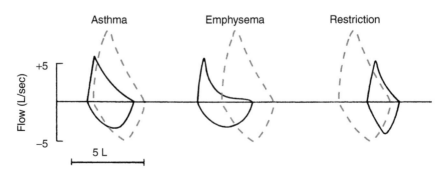

Figure 2-10: Examples of flow–volume loops in patients with asthma, emphysema, and restrictive disease as compared with a normal individual *(dashed lines).* Volumes on the axis are absolute values to better demonstrate the relation of flows to volume. The forced expiratory curve is shown above the *x* axis, and the forced inspiratory curve is shown below the *x* axis. In asthma and emphysema, the curves are displaced to the left because of air trapping and/or hyperinflation, and the portion of the expiratory curve from the peak flow to residual volume is characteristically concave due to airflow limitation. In restrictive disease, the shape of the inspiratory and expiratory curves is preserved but the reduced lung volumes shift the curve to the right. (From Ruppel GL. *Manual of Pulmonary Function Testing.* 9th ed. St. Louis: Mosby; 2008.)

- Maximal expiratory pressure (MEP) measures the maximal pressure generated during forced expiration and is usually measured at TLC. It depends on the strength of the expiratory muscles as well as the elastic recoil of the lungs and thorax.
  - ▸ Normal values usually exceed 80 to 100 cm H_2O and sometimes 200 cm H_2O.
  - ▸ MEP is reduced in neuromuscular diseases, spinal cord injury, other cases of generalized muscle weakness, and diseases causing hyperinflation.
  - ▸ Decreased values are associated with ineffective cough and may complicate chronic bronchitis, cystic fibrosis, and other conditions with increased mucus production.

Chemical Control of Ventilation

The change in $\dot{V}_E$ caused by breathing various concentrations of CO_2 under normoxic conditions (i.e., the CO_2 response) or various concentrations of oxygen (O_2) under isocapneic conditions (i.e., the oxygen response) is used to assess a patient's responses to hypoxemia and/or hypercapnia. Abnormal responses identify:

- Patients with COPD who increase their ventilation to maintain normal levels of carbon dioxide (Pco_2) versus those who do not
- Patients with chronic CO_2 retention who receive their primary stimulus for breathing from hypoxia (e.g., some patients with COPD, especially if severe, and those with respiratory muscle weakness and neurologic diseases)
- Patients with little intrinsic lung disease who show markedly decreased response to hypoxemia or hypercapnia (e.g., myxedema, obesity–hypoventilation syndrome, obstructive sleep apnea, and primary alveolar hypoventilation)

Interpretation of PFT Results

- For appropriate clinical interpretation of PFTs, pulmonary history and radiographic information are essential.
- PFT data are usually presented in absolute terms along with the predicted normal values (based on patient age, gender, height, weight, and race); in addition, the data are often presented as percentages of the predicted normal reference values. Levels at which the results of individual tests should be considered abnormal are not universally accepted.
  - ▸ Sometimes a standard of 80% to 120% of normal reference values is considered normal and all other values are considered abnormal. However, this standard of ±20% of normal reference values may cause older, shorter individuals without lung disease to be classified as abnormal, whereas taller, younger individuals with lung disease may be erroneously classified as normal.
  - ▸ A more accurate approach is to base the lower limit of normal (LLN) on some number of standard deviations from the normal reference values (e.g., 1.65 SD when only the LLN is significant versus ±1.96 SD when abnormalities can cause either high or low values). Thus, the LLN for $FEF_{25\%-75\%}$ (forced expiratory flow from 25% to 75% of vital capacity) and $\dot{V}_{max}$ may be as low as 50% of the predicted value, depending on the reference set used, because of the wide variability among healthy individuals.

- The diagnosis of obstructive pulmonary disease or restrictive pulmonary defects is based on the pattern of abnormal values exhibited, as seen in Figures 2-8, 2-9, and 2-10; a simplified sequence for examining PFT data is summarized in Chapter 6 (see Table 6-7 on page 230).
- The results of PFTs offer physical therapists valuable information, which may have direct implications for rehabilitation:
  - ▸ The greater the degree of impairment, the greater the likelihood that the patient will exhibit abnormal physiological responses to activity and will require treatment modifications.
  - ▸ The specific treatment modifications that are indicated vary according to the patient's pathology and type of PFT abnormality (see Chapter 4 and Chapter 7 [Cardiovascular and Pulmonary Physical Therapy Treatment]).

ARTERIAL BLOOD GASES

Arterial blood is often analyzed to obtain information related to a patient's oxygenation, ventilatory, and acid–base status. Values can be obtained by analysis of an arterial blood sample or by direct-reading electrodes after arterial cannulation.

- The data obtained from arterial blood gases (ABGs) and normal values are listed in Table 2-7.
- The interpretation of ABGs is achieved by following four simple steps, as presented in Chapter 6 (see Table 6-5, page 228 and Figure 6-1, page 229).
- Sudden acute changes in the levels of $Paco_2$ and pH are more dangerous than gradual chronic changes and tend to be associated with more serious clinical manifestations.
- It is important for physical therapists to appreciate normal versus abnormal values for ABGs and how abnormalities affect an individual's ability to perform exercise and rehabilitation activities.
- Patients with chronic pulmonary disease and low oxygen saturations often benefit from the use of supplemental oxygen, especially during exertion (see page 26).[11]
- Although ABGs provide the most accurate method of assessing a patient's oxygenation, current technology does not allow continuous monitoring of a patient's status.

TABLE 2-7: **Parameters Measured in Arterial Blood Gas Analysis**

Parameter	Normal Value (Range)
Partial pressure of oxygen (Po_2, Pao_2)	97 mm Hg (>80)
Partial pressure of carbon dioxide (Pco_2, $Paco_2$)	40 mm Hg (35-45)
Hydrogen ion concentration (pH)	7.40 (7.35-7.45)
Arterial oxygen saturation (Sao_2)	>95%
Bicarbonate level (HCO_3^-)	24 mmol/L (22–26)
Base excess/deficit (BE)	0 (−2 to +2)

PULSE OXIMETRY

Arterial oxygen saturation of hemoglobin (SaO_2) can be estimated via pulse oximetry (SpO_2), which employs spectrophotometry in a sensor typically placed on an ear lobe or finger to measure the differential absorption of light by oxyhemoglobin and reduced hemoglobin.

- Assessment of SpO_2 is strongly advised for all patients with an FEV_1 less than 50% of predicted normal or a $D_{L_{CO}}$ less than 60% of predicted, because of the increased likelihood of desaturation.
- Pulse oximeters tend to have an accuracy of $\pm 2\%$ when resting SaO_2 is 80% to 100%, but accuracy may be reduced during exercise and when oxygen saturation is less than 70% to 80%.[13,22,45] Inaccuracies are especially likely to occur during rapid or severe desaturation, in patients requiring intensive care, and those with poor peripheral perfusion due to peripheral arterial disease, vasoconstriction, or low cardiac output, as well as a number of other conditions, as listed in Table 2-8 (also refer to Chapter 6, page 280).[43]
- When discrepancies are found between the SpO_2 results and the patient's clinical presentation, blood gas analysis is indicated.
- In infants, transcutaneous oxygen ($tcPO_2$) electrodes are often used to monitor oxygenation in neonatal respiratory distress syndrome and for apnea and sleep studies.

AMBULATORY OXIMETRY

Ambulatory oximetry monitoring uses a pulse oximeter with computer software to continuously record the SpO_2 and often the pulse rate waveform for up to 24 hours. These small, lightweight units typically collect and store data every 15 seconds via a finger probe.

TABLE 2-8: Factors That Limit the Accuracy of Pulse Oximetry Results

Factor	Examples
Interfering substances	Carboxyhemoglobin (COHb) (e.g., smokers, carbon monoxide inhalation)
	Methemoglobin (MetHb) (e.g., with nitrate, nitroprusside, or lidocaine therapy)
	Fetal hemoglobin
	Intravascular dyes (e.g., methylene blue, indocyanine green)
	Nail polish or synthetic nails (if finger sensor)
Interfering factors	Motion artifact, shivering
	Bright ambient light
	Hypotension, low perfusion (at sensor site)
	Increased bilirubin
	Severe anemia
	Hypothermia
	Vasoconstrictor drugs
	Increased venous pulsations
	Dark skin pigmentation

The goal is to document SpO_2 values, particularly desaturation events, during activities of daily living and sleep and to correlate them with symptoms and use of supplemental oxygen.

- Computer software generates a report on the mean, maximal, and minimal SpO_2 and the percentage of time that the SpO_2 falls below various values between 90% and 86%, and some show the percentage of time during which the SpO_2 is greater than 95%.
- Research suggests that the use of ambulatory oxygen monitoring might provide a more realistic, physiological assessment of oxygen requirements in the outpatient setting than the current practice of using a measurement of SpO_2 at one point in time when assessing the need for long-term oxygen therapy.[12,28]

ELECTROCARDIOGRAPHY

A 12-lead electrocardiogram is commonly obtained to ascertain the presence of right ventricular hypertrophy (RVH) and/or strain in patients with chronic lung disease, acute asthma, and pulmonary embolism.

- Specific indicators of RVH and/or strain include right axis deviation, P pulmonale (a tall, peaked P wave >2.5 mm in leads II, III, and aVF), and a dominant R wave in leads aVR and V_1, as seen in Figure 2-11 (see also Figure 6-2 on page 232).
- In addition, hypoxemia and acidosis are often associated with atrial and ventricular arrhythmias.

EXERCISE TESTING

Exercise testing can be performed using standardized protocols on a treadmill or cycle ergometer in order to document the cardiovascular, and sometimes respiratory, responses to physiological stress (see page 49 for a description of standard exercise testing). Alternatively, walk tests are often used to evaluate functional status.

Pulmonary Exercise Testing

Pulmonary exercise testing, more often called cardiopulmonary exercise testing (CPX or CPET), incorporates the analysis of respiratory gases, including the measurement of oxygen uptake ($\dot{V}O_2$) and carbon dioxide production ($\dot{V}CO_2$), and other ventilatory parameters, in addition to the usual parameters monitored during standard exercise testing (see Chapter 3, pages 49 to 50), in order to assess the integrative exercise responses involving the pulmonary, cardiovascular, and other systems.[3]

- During testing the patient breathes through a one-way nonrebreathing valve with nose plugged so that expired air can be analyzed and airflow can be measured while the patient performs graded exercise on a treadmill or stationary cycle ergometer. CPX may also include insertion of an arterial line for periodic blood gas analysis or the use of pulse oximetry for documentation of oxygen saturation.
- Among the data that can be provided, in addition to that from a standard exercise test, are the following:
  - Respiratory rate *(f)*
  - Tidal volume (V_T)
  - Expired, or minute, ventilation ($\dot{V}_E$)
  - Maximal oxygen uptake ($\dot{V}O_{2\ max}$)

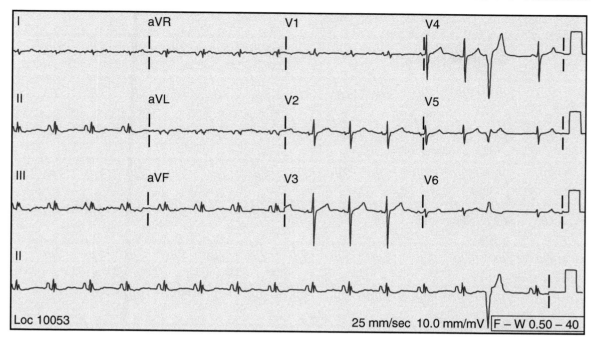

Figure 2-11: An electrocardiogram of a patient with chronic cor pulmonale reveals prominent P pulmonale in leads II, III, and aVF, as well as right ventricular hypertrophy and right axis deviation. (From Mason RJ, Murray JF, Broaddus VC, Nadel JA, editors. *Murray & Nadel's Textbook of Respiratory Medicine.* 4th ed. Philadelphia: Saunders; 2005.)

- ▸ CO_2 production ($\dot{V}CO_2$)
- ▸ Ventilatory or anaerobic threshold (AT)
- ▸ Respiratory exchange ratio (RER = $\dot{V}CO_2/\dot{V}O_2$)
- ▸ Breathing reserve (BR); calculated as maximal voluntary ventilation (MVV) – $\dot{V}E$ at maximal exercise
- ▸ Oxygen uptake–work rate (WR) relationship ($\Delta\dot{V}O_2/\Delta WR$) and oxygen difference
- ▸ Respiratory dead space (VD) and ratio to tidal volume (VD/VT)
- ▸ Alveolar ventilation ($\dot{V}A$)
- ▸ Alveolar–arterial oxygen difference [P(A–a)O$_2$]
- ▸ Arterial–end tidal carbon dioxide difference [P(a–ET)CO$_2$]
- ▸ Ventilatory equivalents for oxygen ($\dot{V}E/\dot{V}O_2$) and carbon dioxide ($\dot{V}E/\dot{V}CO_2$)
- ▸ Expiratory flow patterns
- ▸ Oxygen pulse ($\dot{V}O_2$/heart beat)
- ▸ Maximal MET (metabolic equivalent of energy expenditure) capacity
- ▸ Cardiac output ($\dot{Q}$)
- • In addition, blood sampling can be performed to determine plasma bicarbonate and acid–base responses as well as lactate levels.
- • These data allow for the differentiation of cardiovascular versus pulmonary limitations as the cause of exercise-induced dyspnea or impaired exercise tolerance. Suggested normal guidelines for the interpretation of CPX results are provided in Table 2-9.[2] Conditions that are often associated with exercise intolerance and the measurements that usually deviate from normal are listed in Table 2-10.
- • In some facilities physical therapists are involved in conducting and supervising cardiopulmonary exercise tests.

Walk Tests

Because formal laboratory testing is complicated, time-consuming, expensive, and not always available, a number of "field tests" have been developed to indirectly assess exercise capacity. Walk tests are objective exercise tests that are used to measure functional status, monitor treatment effectiveness, and establish prognosis in patients with limited exercise tolerance, including those with lung disease.
- • A variety of walk tests are available[35]:
  - ▸ Time-based tests (e.g., 6-min walk test and 12-min walk test)
  - ▸ Fixed-distance tests (e.g., 100-m, half-mile, and 2-km walk tests)
  - ▸ Velocity-determined walk tests (e.g., self-paced walk test)
  - ▸ Controlled-pacing incremental tests (e.g., incremental shuttle walk test)
- • The walk tests used most commonly in the assessment of patients with lung disease, as well as other chronic diseases, are the 6-min and 12-min walk tests (6MWT and 12MWT, respectively), during which clients are asked to walk as far as they can during the time of the test, with rests allowed as needed. Although these tests are often considered submaximal, they may be near maximal in patients with severe obstructive lung disease. A description of the procedures involved in administering the 6MWT is presented in Chapter 6 (see page 257).

PULMONARY IMAGING STUDIES

A wide variety of methods exist to image the pulmonary system besides standard chest radiography. These include fluoroscopy, computed tomography, magnetic resonance imaging, and ultrasonography, as well as scintigraphic imaging studies, all of which are described in the following sections.

TABLE 2-9: Suggested Normal Guidelines for Interpretation of Cardiopulmonary Exercise Testing Results*

Variable	Criteria of Normality
Peak oxygen consumption ($\dot{V}o_{2peak}$)	>84% of predicted $\dot{V}o_{2max}$
Anaerobic threshold (AT)	>40% of predicted $\dot{V}o_{2max}$; wide range of normal (40%-80%)
Heart rate (HR)	HR_{max} >90% age-predicted value
Heart rate reserve (HRR)	Predicted HR_{max} − HR_{peak}: <15 bpm
Blood pressure (BP)	<220/90 mm Hg
O_2 pulse ($\dot{V}o_2$/HR)	>80%
Ventilatory reserve (VR)	
• MVV − $\dot{V}_{Emax}$	>11 L
• $\dot{V}_{Emax}$/MVV	<85%; wide range of normal: 72 ± 15%
Respiratory rate or frequency (RR, f)	<60 breaths/min
$\dot{V}_E$/$\dot{V}co_2$ (at AT)	<34
V_D/V_T	<0.28; <0.30 for age >40 yr
Pao_2	>80 mm Hg
P(A–a)o_2	<35 mm Hg

From American Thoracic Society/American College of Chest Physicians. ATS/ACCP statement on cardiopulmonary exercise testing. *Am J Respir Crit Care Med.*2003;167:211-277.
bpm, Beats per minute; MVV, maximal voluntary ventilation; Pao_2, partial pressure of arterial oxygen; P(A–a)o_2, alveolar–arterial oxygen difference; V_D, dead space volume; V_T, tidal volume; $\dot{V}co_2$, carbon dioxide production; $\dot{V}_E$, minute ventilation; $\dot{V}_{Emax}$, $\dot{V}_E$ at maximal exercise; $\dot{V}o_{2max}$, maximal oxygen consumption.
*Maximal or peak cardiopulmonary responses except for anaerobic threshold and $\dot{V}_E$/$\dot{V}co_2$ at AT.

Fluoroscopy

Fluoroscopy produces radiographic images with real-time display of a patient's breathing that may be highlighted with a radio-opaque contrast agent.

- Fluoroscopy offers a quick and inexpensive method of detecting lesions that are obscured by ribs or that can be seen clearly only in an unusual oblique projection (e.g., some pleural plaques, retrocardiac nodules), as well as pulsatile nodules and masses.
- It is used most commonly to guide interventional procedures, such as needle or transbronchial biopsies or catheter angiography, to detect minor variations in symmetry of diaphragmatic motion seen in phrenic nerve damage, as shown in Figure 2-12, and to diagnose air trapping in small children with suspected foreign body aspiration.

Computed Tomography

With computed tomography (CT), x-ray beams pass through a body part in multiple projections in order to produce clear cross-sectional images of various body tissues with good contrast resolution (Figure 2-13). Chest CT is valuable in evaluating mediastinal masses, hilar abnormalities, thoracic aortic dissection, diffuse lung disease, pleural abnormalities, presence of metastatic lesions, and resectability of bronchial carcinoma, and in quantifying the severity of emphysema and its appropriateness for lung reduction surgery.

- During conventional CT scanning, patient movement on the table alternates with data acquisition via the rotating x-ray source (i.e., data are acquired from one tissue plane, and then the patient is moved into position for the next image plane).
- During helical or spiral CT, both the patient and the x-ray source move continuously (i.e., the data are acquired continuously as the x-ray source traces a spiral path relative to the patient), which allows a study to be completed during a single breath-hold.
- Multidetector-row CT (MDCT) uses helical or spiral CT with thinner collimation to increase the sensitivity of images. Its accuracy has made it a first-line study in the diagnosis of pulmonary embolism and venous thrombosis.[37] It is also able to evaluate all other thoracic structures, including the lungs and heart, allowing multiplanar and three-dimensional image reconstruction, as shown in Figure 2-14.
- Interventional CT is widely used to guide percutaneous biopsy or drainage of thoracic lesions and to localize fluid collections or pneumothoraces that are not responding to blindly placed thoracostomy tubes.
- High-resolution CT (HRCT) uses thinner slices at more frequent intervals to provide improved visualization of small structures and detailed anatomic features, producing images that correlate closely with the macroscopic appearance of pathologic specimens (see Figure 2-13). It is most valuable in diagnosing diffuse lung disease in patients with a normal CXR, detecting parenchymal abnormalities involving a small volume of lung obscured by superimposed structures, monitoring disease processes, and indicating which type of biopsy procedure is likely to be successful in obtaining diagnostic material.

Magnetic Resonance Imaging

Magnetic resonance imaging (MRI) uses radiofrequency pulse sequences with the patient positioned in a strong magnetic field to generate and then amplify electromagnetic signals. These signals are spatially mapped to create images of body tissues. The usefulness of MRI for imaging the lung parenchyma is limited by extremely low proton density.

- However, thoracic MRI is useful for imaging mediastinal masses, thromboses of the superior vena cava and great vessels, central pulmonary emboli, vascular stenoses, aneurysms, and dissections, and soft tissues of the chest wall.
- Magnetic resonance angiography (MRA) and magnetic resonance perfusion studies, including direct thrombus imaging (MR-DTI), are valuable tools for assessing suspected pulmonary embolism, particularly in those patients with iodinated contrast allergy or pregnancy. Magnetic resonance methods are also expected to play a significant role in the assessment of patients with chronic thromboembolic hypertension, vasculitis, and arteriovenous malformations.[27]

TABLE 2-10: Typical Cardiopulmonary Exercise Testing Response Patterns Seen in Common Disorders Associated With Impaired Exercise Tolerance

Disorder	$\dot{V}O_2$ max or $\dot{V}O_2$ peak	AT	Peak HR	O_2 Pulse	VR	$\dot{V}_E/\dot{V}CO_2$ at AT	V_D/V_T	PaO_2	$P(A{-}a)O_2$	Other
Pulmonary										
COPD	→	nl, ↓, indeter	↓, nl if mild	nl or →	↓	↑	↑	var	var, us. ↑	↑ HRR
RLD										
↓C_L	→	nl, ↓, indeter	→	nl or →	nl or →	↑	↑	→	↑	RR >50, ↑ V_T/IC
↓C_T	→	nl, ↓, indeter	→	→	nl or →	↑	↑	→	↑	RR >50, ↑ V_T/IC, ↑ HRR
Pulmonary vascular disease	→	→	nl, sl ↓	↓	nl	↑	↑	→	↑	
Cardiac										
CAD	→	nl	→	↓, rising post ex	nl or ↑	nl	→	nl	nl	abnl ECG, poss angina, ↓ HRR, ↓ ΔVo$_2$/ΔWR at onset of ischemia
LV failure	→	→	var, us. nl if mild	→	nl or ↑	↑	↑	nl	us. nl	
Anemia	→	→	nl	→	↑	↑	nl	nl	nl	↑ symptoms when acute onset vs. chronic
Peripheral arterial disease	→	→	→	→	↑	↑	nl	nl	nl	leg pain, ↑ BP, ↑ HRR, ↓ ΔVo$_2$/ΔWR
Obesity	↓ for actual wt, nl for ideal wt	nl	nl, sl ↓	nl	nl or ↓	nl	nl	nl, may ↑	may ↓	↑ ΔVo$_2$/ΔWR
Anxiety	nl or near nl	nl	↓ or nl	nl or ↓	nl or ↓	↑	nl	nl	nl	↑ $\dot{V}_E$, ↓ PaCO$_2$, ↑ pH
Malingering	→	nl or indeter	→	→	↑	→	nl	nl	nl	↑ or ↓$\dot{V}_E$, irreg RR, ↑ HRR
Deconditioning	→	nl or ↓	nl, sl ↓	↓	nl	nl	nl	nl	nl	

Data from American Thoracic Society/American College of Chest Physicians. ATS/ACCP statement on cardiopulmonary exercise testing. *Am J Respir Crit Care Med.* 2003;167:211-277; Antonelli M, Pennisi MA, Montini L. Clinical review: Noninvasive ventilation in the clinical setting—experience from the past 10 years. *Crit Care.* 2005;9:98-103.

↓, Decreased (lower than normal); ↑, increased (higher than normal); abnl, abnormal; AT, anaerobic threshold; BP, blood pressure; CAD, coronary artery disease; C_L, lung compliance; C_T, thoracic compliance; HR, heart rate; HRR, heart rate reserve; IC, inspiratory capacity; irreg, irregular; LV, left ventricular; indeter, indeterminate; nl, normal; poss, possible; post ex, postexercise; RR, respiratory rate; sl, slightly; us, usually; var, variable; wt, weight; VR, ventilatory reserve (equals peak $V_E/MVV \times 100$); WR, work rate. For explanation of other abbreviations, see text.

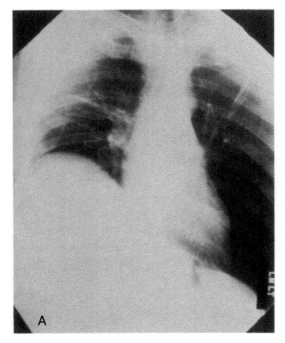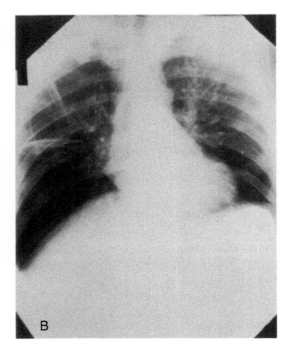

Figure 2-12: Fluoroscopic image showing diaphragmatic function in a patient with right hemidiaphragm paralysis: **A,** Paradoxical upward motion of the paralyzed right hemidiaphragm during sudden inspiration; **B,** paradoxical downward motion during expiration. (From Baum GL, Wolinsky E, editors. *Textbook of Pulmonary Diseases.* 4th ed. London: Little, Brown & Company; 1989.)

- The most significant advantage of MRI over other cross-sectional imaging is its excellent contrast resolution of soft tissues. In addition, its multiplanar imaging capability allows a truly three-dimensional view of complex regions, such as the hila and mediastinum. An example is seen in Figure 3-22 on page 56.

Ultrasonography

The use of sound waves (ultrasound) has limited value in thoracic imaging, because of the reflection of the ultrasound beam at the air–soft tissue interface around the lungs. However, it is useful for detecting, localizing, and characterizing pleural effusions and guiding thoracentesis, for differentiating pleural fluid from pleural thickening, and for assessing areas of consolidated lung or masses contacting or invading the chest wall. In addition, flexible bronchoscopy with an ultrasound probe is being investigated as a means of mapping the airways and surrounding tissues.

NUCLEAR MEDICINE/SCINTIGRAPHIC IMAGING STUDIES

Scintigraphic studies employ radioactive imaging agents to "light up" various tissues during imaging, using a gamma counter.

Ventilation–Perfusion Scanning

Ventilation–perfusion ($\dot{V}/\dot{Q}$) scans use radionuclides to evaluate and compare the distribution of ventilation and perfusion within the lungs.
- Perfusion and ventilation studies are obtained separately and then the images are compared, as shown in Figure 2-15.

- $\dot{V}/\dot{Q}$ scans are used most commonly to diagnose pulmonary embolism, predict postoperative lung function after pneumonectomy, diagnose early airflow obstruction, and assess the potential benefit of surgical excision of emphysematous bullae.
- $\dot{V}/\dot{Q}$ scans do not confirm or exclude pulmonary embolism; rather, they give an estimate of its likelihood, as described in Table 2-11. However, a normal perfusion scan virtually excludes clinically relevant pulmonary embolism.
- Parenchymal lung diseases, whether obstructive or restrictive, usually produce matched defects in both ventilation and perfusion or a reverse mismatch in which ventilation is reduced compared with perfusion.
- Abnormal findings indicate that significant mismatch between ventilation and perfusion exists and the patient is likely to have limited tolerance for activity.

Single-photon Emission Computed Tomography

Single-photon emission computed tomography (SPECT) imaging involves the injection of a radiolabeled tracer, the photon emissions of which can be detected much like x-rays in CT to produce three-dimensional images of the distribution of the tracer in a particular organ; these images are often shown with a color scale.
- SPECT images reflect functional information, including blood flow, oxygen or glucose metabolism, or dopamine transporter concentration.
- In pulmonary medicine, SPECT is commonly used for $\dot{V}/\dot{Q}$ studies and produces better characterization of the lobes and segments than two-dimensional imaging.

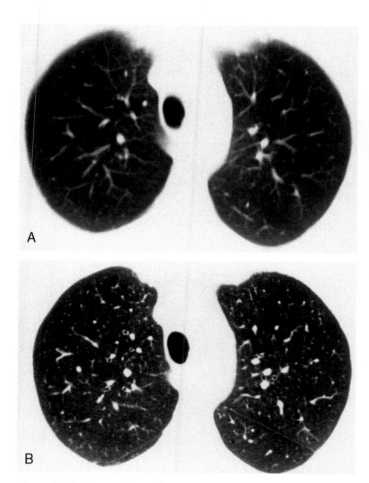

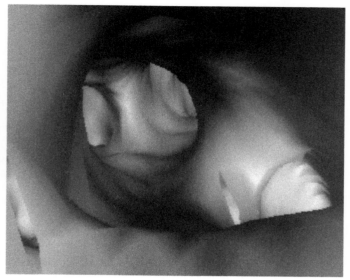

Figure 2-14: Three-dimensional reconstruction of computed tomography data simulating a bronchoscopic view of the segmental bronchi. (From Gibson GJ, Geddes DM, Costabel U, Sterk PJ, Corrin B, editors. *Respiratory Medicine.* 3rd ed. Vol. 1. Philadelphia: Saunders; 2003.)

Figure 2-13: Comparison of images obtained at the same level from conventional computed tomography (CT) **(A)** and high-resolution CT (HRCT) **(B)**. HRCT demonstrates better visibility of bronchial walls and fissures as well as small vessels. (From Gold WM, Murray JF, Nadel JA. *Atlas of Procedures in Respiratory Medicine: A Companion to Murray and Nadel's Textbook of Respiratory Medicine.* Philadelphia: Saunders; 2002.)

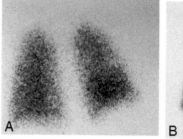
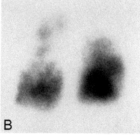

Figure 2-15: High-probability lung scan. This patient with metastatic cancer developed sudden dyspnea and unexplained hypoxemia after prolonged bed rest. **A,** The ventilation scan is normal. **B,** The perfusion scan demonstrates multiple bilateral perfusion defects consistent with pulmonary emboli. (From Hess DR, MacIntyre NR, Mishoe SC, et al. *Respiratory Care: Principles and Practice.* Philadelphia: Saunders; 2002.)

Positron Emission Tomography

Positron emission tomography (PET) scanning uses biologically active positron emission radiopharmaceuticals (i.e., ^{18}F-deoxyglucose, FDG) to display and quantify metabolic processes, receptor occupancy, and blood flow. In pulmonary medicine, PET is used mostly for evaluating newly discovered pulmonary nodules, staging of confirmed non–small cell lung cancer, and sometimes for monitoring response to therapy.

Other Scintigraphic Imaging Studies

• Gallium scans use radioactive gallium (^{67}Ga), which has a high affinity for tumor cells and white blood cells, to detect areas of hidden inflammation. In pulmonary medicine, it is used to detect pulmonary infections, lung involvement in AIDS, and interstitial lung disease; it is also valuable in staging pulmonary sarcoidosis.

• Other radionuclides can also be used to detect opportunistic infections seen in immunocompromised patients and to measure mucociliary clearance (e.g., indium-111–labeled white blood cells, ^{111}In WBCs; technetium 99m–labeled diethylenetriaminepentaacetic acid, ^{99m}Tc-DTPA; or thallium-201, ^{201}Tl).

INVASIVE DIAGNOSTIC TECHNIQUES

Some pulmonary disorders are best evaluated through invasive diagnostic techniques, which may involve the injection of contrast medium into the airways or blood vessels; endoscopic viewing of the bronchi, pleural space, or mediastinum; transbronchial or percutaneous needle aspiration or biopsy of the lungs or pleurae; or open lung biopsy or exploratory thoracotomy.

TABLE 2-11: Interpretation of Ventilation–Perfusion ($\dot{V}/\dot{Q}$) Scans

Category	$\dot{V}/\dot{Q}$ Scan Pattern*	Approximate Incidence of Pulmonary Embolism[†]
Normal	No perfusion defects	0
Low probability	Small $\dot{V}/\dot{Q}$ mismatches $\dot{V}/\dot{Q}$ mismatches without corresponding roentgenographic changes Perfusion defect substantially smaller than roentgenographic density	10
Intermediate probability	Severe, diffuse COPD with perfusion defects Perfusion defect of same size as roentgenographic changes Single medium or large $\dot{V}/\dot{Q}$ mismatch[‡]	30
High probability	Two or more medium or large $\dot{V}/\dot{Q}$ mismatches Perfusion defect substantially larger than roentgenographic density.	90

Reprinted with permission from Biello DR. Radiological (scintigraphic) evaluation of patients with suspected pulmonary thromboembolism. *JAMA*. 1987;257:3257-3259. Copyright © 1987, American Medical Association.

COPD, Chronic obstructive pulmonary disease.

*A small perfusion defect involves less than 25% of the expected volume of a pulmonary segment; medium, 25% to 90%; and large, 90% or more.

[†]Detected by pulmonary angiography.

[‡]Controversy exists regarding whether single large $\dot{V}/\dot{Q}$ mismatches are categorized as high or intermediate probability. The more conservative interpretation has been used in this table.

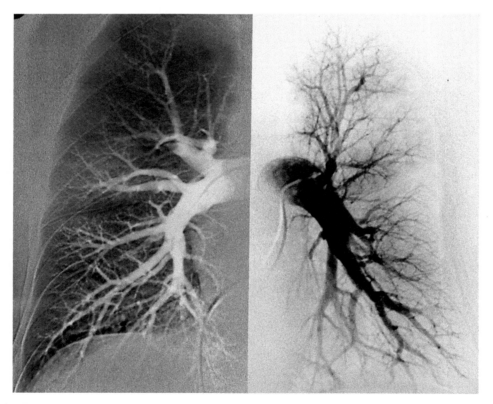

Figure 2-16: Normal pulmonary angiograms from selective injections into the main pulmonary arteries. The right lung is imaged by the conventional technique; the left lung by digital subtraction angiography. (From Gibson GJ, Geddes DM, Costabel U, Sterk PJ, Corrin B, editors. *Respiratory Medicine*. 3rd ed. Vol. 1. Philadelphia: Saunders; 2003.)

Pulmonary Angiography

The injection of contrast material into the thoracic blood vessels allows them to be depicted on x-ray film. Digital subtraction angiography uses fluoroscopy and image intensification, along with computer processing, to subtract interfering background body parts, leaving only the intravascular contrast materials, as depicted in Figure 2-16.

- Pulmonary angiography is used to diagnose pulmonary emboli, arteriovenous malformations, pulmonary varices, and occasionally to delineate the anatomy of the pulmonary vessels before lung surgery.
- It can also be used therapeutically to inject thrombolytic agents to dissolve pulmonary emboli and to embolize arteries supplying the bleeding sites in severe hemoptysis.

Bronchography

Images of the bronchopulmonary tree can be obtained by instilling contrast medium directly into the airways and then obtaining radiographs or tomographs. Although bronchography has been largely replaced by fiberoptic bronchoscopy, HRCT, and spiral CT, it is occasionally used in combination with bronchoscopy for defining bronchopleural fistulae.

Bronchoscopy

Using a flexible or rigid fiberoptic endoscope, the larger airways down to the third or fourth divisions of the segmental bronchi can be visualized directly.

- Because flexible fiberoptic bronchoscopy requires only topical anesthesia and the range of visible airways is greater, it is the more commonly used method, as pictured in Figure 2-17.
- However, rigid bronchoscopy allows for greater airway patency; maintenance of ventilatory support; better removal of blood, secretions, and tissue samples with less impairment of ventilation; greater ease and safety in removal of foreign bodies; and local tumor therapy (e.g., placement of radioactive seeds, laser therapy, and cryotherapy).
- If abnormalities are noted during bronchoscopy, additional diagnostic maneuvers may be performed:
  - ▸ *Bronchial brushings* are done to obtain cells for the diagnosis of neoplasms and infectious pulmonary infiltrates.
  - ▸ *Bronchoalveolar lavage* is used to sample cells, inhaled particles, and infectious agents from the terminal bronchioles and alveoli in order to diagnose infectious agents and sometimes malignant infiltrates. In addition, examination of cellular composition and extracellular proteins is useful in defining sarcoidosis, extrinsic allergic alveolitis, idiopathic pulmonary fibrosis, tuberculosis, and many other lung diseases.
  - ▸ *Transbronchial needle aspiration/lung biopsy* can be performed with a small-gauge needle or biopsy forceps passed through a bronchoscope in order to acquire tissue samples from within the walls of the trachea and major bronchi or through these structures to peribronchial lymph nodes. The

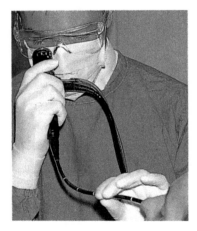

Figure 2-17: Fiberoptic and video-bronchoscopy are typically performed on the conscious patient. The bronchoscope is usually passed through the nose. (From Forbes CD, Jackson WF. *Color Atlas and Text of Clinical Medicine.* 3rd ed. St. Louis: Mosby; 2003.)

diagnostic yield is highest in diffuse lung diseases with specific recognizable histologic patterns (e.g., sarcoidosis, metastatic cancer, lymphoma, and lymphangitic carcinoma).

- Bronchoscopy can also be used as a therapeutic intervention, such as in removing retained secretions or aspirated foreign bodies, assisting in difficult intubation and bronchodilation, and managing malignant obstruction (e.g., bronchodilation, placement of stents, laser therapy, and brachytherapy). In addition, bronchial thermoplasty involving bronchoscopic radiofrequency ablation of airway smooth muscle is under investigation for the treatment of asthma (see page 35).

Percutaneous Transthoracic Needle Aspiration/Lung Biopsy

In some cases, a needle is inserted through the skin to obtain tissue samples from peripheral lung and sometimes mediastinal masses, usually with guidance via fluoroscopy, CT, or ultrasound imaging. It is used most commonly to diagnose solitary pulmonary nodules or masses suspected of being malignant, particularly in patients who are clearly inoperable because of disease extent, significant cardiorespiratory disease, or poor performance status.

Thoracentesis and Pleural Biopsy

The insertion of a needle into the pleural space allows for the removal of pleural fluid or acquisition of a pleural biopsy.

- Pleural fluid is analyzed to determine whether it is a transudate or an exudate. In addition, it may be sent for a variety of cytologic, biochemical, hematologic, immunologic, molecular, and microbiologic studies.
- Pleurocentesis is also performed therapeutically to relieve respiratory impairment caused by pleural effusions.
- Blind, or closed, needle biopsy is performed, usually with image guiding, when tuberculosis, malignant effusion, or other pleural pathology is suspected.

Rehabilitation activities should be postponed until a postprocedure chest radiograph has ruled out a pneumothorax.

Thoracoscopy/Pleuroscopy

Thoracoscopy, often with video, can be used to visualize most intrathoracic structures, including the pleurae. It is used most commonly as an alternative to open pleural biopsy when malignant disease is suspected and a diagnosis has not been made despite repeated thoracenteses and pleural biopsies. Furthermore, therapeutic interventions are often performed thorascopically, using video-assisted thoracic surgery (VATS), including debridement in tuberculosis and empyema; diathermy, laser coagulation, or endostapling in recurrent pneumothorax; pleurodesis (see page 36) in malignant effusion and pneumothorax; as well as visual placement of drains.[19]

Mediastinoscopy and Mediastinotomy

Exploration of the mediastinum can be achieved with an endoscope inserted through an anterior cervical or parasternal incision (i.e., mediastinoscopy), using VATS, or by direct visualization via an anterior incision (i.e., mediastinotomy). These procedures are used most commonly to detect mediastinal lymph node involvement by lung cancer and to biopsy abnormal lymph nodes noted on chest radiography.

Open Lung Biopsy/Explorative Thoracotomy

Open lung biopsy via an exploratory thoracotomy is performed in patients with hilar abnormalities in which overlying vascular structures impede other approaches and when transbronchial biopsy has been unsuccessful in providing a diagnosis in chronic interstitial lung disease. It may also useful in determining the nature of the underlying disease in pulmonary heart disease.

- After surgery, two chest tubes are usually inserted: a lower one to drain fluids and an upper one, which requires a water seal and is often set to gentle suction, to evacuate air from the pleural space and to create the negative pressure required for reexpansion of the lung.
- For more information on chest tubes, management, and implications for physical therapy, see page 32.

2.3 THERAPEUTIC INTERVENTIONS IN PULMONARY MEDICINE

Advances in pulmonary research continue to affect the therapeutic options available to patients with pulmonary diseases.[3] Some of these are purely palliative, whereas others may be curative. The more common interventions, as well as some of the newer ones, are described briefly in the following sections.

MEDICAL MANAGEMENT

The medical management of pulmonary disease includes pharmaceuticals, oxygen therapy, airway adjuncts, mechanical ventilation, bronchial hygiene and other physical therapy techniques, smoking cessation, pulmonary rehabilitation, and social services.

Pharmacologic Therapy

The various medications used to treat pulmonary disease are described in Chapter 5 (Pharmacology); however, oxygen therapy is presented here.

Oxygen Therapy

Oxygen therapy is indicated for the treatment of acute or chronic hypoxemia and can be administered via a variety of devices, which achieve different concentrations (or fractions) of inspired oxygen (FIO_2), as indicated in Table 2-12. Alternatively, some patients with COPD on long-term oxygen therapy (LTOT) choose transtracheal oxygen (TTO) delivery via a microcatheter inserted into the anterior tracheal wall, which they feel is more comfortable and less conspicuous than supplemental oxygen via a nasal cannula.

- As with other medications, oxygen is prescribed to provide the proper dose that maximizes benefits while minimizing toxicity; an increased dose may be indicated during exertion.
- Oxygen sources include compressed gas stored in a cylinder, liquid oxygen stored in a vessel similar to a thermos, and oxygen concentrators that extract oxygen from the air and concentrate and store it. The first two can be used for ambulation; however, compressed gas cylinders are bulky and heavy and liquid oxygen canisters, although small and lightweight, may not contain enough oxygen for longer periods of use.
- Oxygen-conserving devices in the form of demand delivery devices, or pulsed-dose systems, sense the onset of inspiration

TABLE 2-12: Approximate FIO_2 Achieved With Various Oxygen Delivery Devices

Device	Oxygen Flow Rate	FIO_2
Nasal cannula*	1 L/min	0.24
	2 L/min	0.28
	3 L/min	0.32
	4 L/min	0.36
	5 L/min	0.40
	≥6 L/min	0.44
Simple face mask	5-6 L/min	0.35
	6-7 L/min	0.45
	7-10 L/min	0.55
Partial rebreathing mask	6-10 L/min	0.40-0.60[†‡]
Nonrebreathing mask	≥10 L/min	About 0.60-0.80
Aerosol face mask	10-12 L/min	0.35-1.0[†]
Venturi mask[§]	4-10 L/min	0.24-0.50[‖]

Data from Baum GL, Crapo JD, Celli BR, et al. *Textbook of Pulmonary Diseases.* 6th ed. Philadelphia: Lippincott-Raven; 1998; and Burton GG, Hodgkin JE, Ward JJ. *Respiratory Care: A Guide to Clinical Practice.* 4th ed. Philadelphia: Lippincott Williams & Wilkins; 1997.
FIO_2, Fraction of inspired oxygen.
*Estimated FIO_2, assuming normal minute ventilation (typically measured during expiration, $\dot{V}E$); values may be 10% lower, or more, with increased $\dot{V}E$.
†FIO_2 depends on setting.
‡Reservoir bag should always be at least one-third to one-half full on inspiration.
§Oxygen flow rates are minimums to be used with specific-sized orifice for desired FIO_2.
‖FIO_2 depends on the size of the orifice or the entrainment ports, which vary among manufacturers.

before delivering a bolus of oxygen, which ceases during expiration, thus reducing oxygen wastage.

- Because therapeutic oxygen is stored with all water vapor removed, humidity is often added in order to prevent irritation of the pulmonary mucosa, particularly when flow is 5 L/min or more. In addition, when the upper airway is bypassed (e.g., endotracheal intubation or tracheostomy) or when flow rates exceed 10 L/min, the oxygen may be heated to increase its water vapor–carrying capacity.
- Large-scale clinical trials are needed to define which patients should receive LTOT (e.g., patients with mild, moderate, or severe hypoxemia) and under what conditions (e.g., exercise, airline flights, and sleep).[15]
- Heliox, a mixture of 80% helium and 20% oxygen, is sometimes used in emergency rooms and intensive care units for the treatment of acute respiratory distress associated with croup, asthma, COPD, bronchiolitis, and respiratory acidosis. Because helium is less dense than nitrogen, it reduces airway turbulence and thus airway resistance, increasing the delivery of oxygen to distal airways and decreasing the work of breathing.

The goals of oxygen therapy are to slow the progression of COPD, improve survival, reduce dyspnea, and increase exercise tolerance by reducing or eliminating exercise-induced hypoxemia and desaturation. Medicare and other insurers generally cover the cost of oxygen therapy in patients with a Pao_2 of 55 mm Hg or less, or an oxygen saturation (Sao_2) no greater than 88% while seated at rest or a Pao_2 of 56 to 59 mm Hg or Sao_2 of 89% in the presence of cor pulmonale or polycythemia. In these patients, survival benefits may be gained only if the oxygen is used continuously, 24 hours/day, and not just when dyspnea develops, so that Pao_2 remains above 60 mm Hg (Sao_2, $\geq$90%).[26] In patients who desaturate only during activity (Sao_2, $\leq$88%), the use of supplemental oxygen during activity tends to reduce dyspnea and improve exercise.[11]

The use of supplemental oxygen carries important implications for physical therapy in all clinical settings:

- If a patient requires oxygen at rest, he/she will definitely need it during exertion and all rehabilitation activities.
- Because the additional demands of rehabilitation activities may cause oxygen desaturation, physical therapists must be able to recognize the signs and symptoms of hypoxemia (see Table 6-13 on page 241).
- Patients with a history of lung disease, especially those with an FEV_1 less than 50% or a DL_{CO} less than 60% of the predicted normal value, are likely to exhibit oxygen desaturation during exertion and should have their oxygenation status monitored initially (see pages 17 to 18).
- A drop in oxygen saturation to less than 86% to 90% (chronic versus acute disease, respectively) during activity indicates that the patient needs additional oxygen; an order to institute oxygen therapy or to increase the oxygen dose during exertion should be requested from the physician (be certain to return the flow back to resting level at the end of each treatment session).
- Home physical therapists should be aware of the oxygen therapy prescription for their patients and ensure that they are using their oxygen as prescribed.

Airway Adjuncts

There are a variety of different types of accessory airways, which may be used to maintain or protect a patient's airway, to provide mechanical ventilation, or to facilitate airway clearance (Figure 2-18):

- An *oral pharyngeal airway* is a semirigid oral plastic tube, or open-sided channel shaped to fit the natural curvature of the soft palate and tongue, that holds the tongue away from the back of the throat and thus maintains the patency of the airway.

- A *nasal pharyngeal airway*, a soft latex or rubber tube inserted through the nose, is commonly used to maintain airway patency and allow nasotracheal suctioning with less mucosal trauma to the nares and pharynx.
- A *laryngeal mask airway* consists of a semirigid plastic tube with an inflatable rubber cuff with slits that is inserted in the posterior hypopharynx, displacing the tongue anteriorly while keeping the glottis open. Once inflated, it allows limited positive-pressure ventilation, if needed, and permits insertion of an endotracheal tube via fiberoptic bronchoscopy.
- The *endotracheal (ET) tube* is a semirigid plastic tube inserted into the trachea via the mouth or nose (i.e., an orotracheal tube or a nasotracheal tube) to provide an airway, protect the lungs from aspiration, and allow mechanical ventilation. Adult ET tubes usually have a low-pressure, large-volume inflatable cuff near their distal end to prevent aspiration of secretions; neonatal and pediatric tubes usually do not have cuffs because of the small size of the airways.
- A *transtracheal catheter* can be used to provide supplemental oxygen or jet ventilation in emergent situations when other approaches have failed and improvement in oxygenation is critical. A microcatheter is inserted through the anterior tracheal wall with the tip lying just above the carina. It can also serve as an alternative way to provide long-term oxygen therapy.
- The *tracheostomy tube,* an artificial airway inserted into the trachea via an anterior cervical incision below the level of the vocal cords, is used in patients requiring prolonged mechanical ventilation and those with upper airway obstruction, absence of protective reflexes, or a number of other problems; most have inflatable cuffs to prevent aspiration, which may be deflated to assess a patient's ability to handle secretions. There are several types, as illustrated in Figure 2-19:
  - ▸ A *standard tracheostomy tube,* shown in Figure 2-18, has a neck flange, body, and usually a cuff; some have a removable inner cannula. Cuffed tracheostomy tubes are used primarily with positive-pressure ventilators to reduce the risk of aspiration. They are available in a variety of styles, sizes, and materials. Cuffless tracheostomy tubes permit speech in continuously ventilated patients who are not at risk for aspiration.

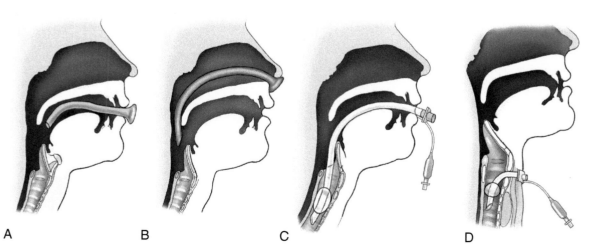

A   B   C   D

Figure 2-18: Common airway adjuncts. **A,** Oropharyngeal tube. **B,** Nasopharyngeal tube. **C,** Oral endotracheal tube. **D,** Tracheostomy tube.

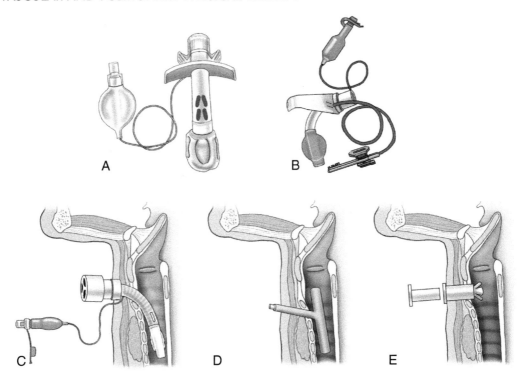

Figure 2-19: Some types of tracheostomy tubes. **A,** Fenestrated. **B,** Portex speaking or talking. **C,** Passy-Muir valve connected to a tracheostomy tube. **D,** Montgomery T-tube. **E,** Tracheostomy button.

▸ A *fenestrated tracheostomy tube* consists of a double cannula with an opening in the superior aspect of the outer cannula so that air can pass through the vocal cords and upper airway when the inner cannula is removed, the tracheal opening is plugged, and the cuff is deflated.

▸ *Speaking, or phonation, valves,* such as the *Passy-Muir valve,* are one-way valves that can be attached to a standard tracheostomy tube during periods of free breathing; they open during inspiration only, while forcing exhalation through the vocal cords and upper airway, thus permitting speech.

▸ The *Montgomery T-tube* is a bifurcated silicone rubber stent that is used to maintain patency of the airways in patients with tumors or injuries causing major airway obstruction.

▸ A *tracheostomy button* is a short, straight, externally plugged tube extending from the anterior neck to the inner tracheal wall, which maintains the tracheal stoma for suctioning and emergency ventilation during weaning from prolonged mechanical ventilation.

Mechanical Ventilation

Patients with severe pulmonary dysfunction resulting from primary lung disease or secondary to other disorders often require ventilatory support. The main indications for mechanical ventilation are acute respiratory failure (66% of patients, including those with acute respiratory distress syndrome, heart failure, pneumonia, sepsis, complications of surgery, and trauma), coma (15%), acute exacerbation of chronic obstructive pulmonary disease (13%), and neuromuscular disorders (5%).[39]

Invasive Mechanical Ventilation

Invasive mechanical ventilation involves intubation of the patient or tracheotomy along with the use of an automatic cycling ventilator to generate air pressure and thus assist or take over the breathing function of the patient. The goals are to improve oxygenation and reduce the work of breathing.

• The main variables that determine the amount of mechanical ventilation provided are the ventilator's pressure, volume, flow, and time.

• There are many types of positive pressure mechanical ventilators that can provide a variety of modes of ventilation, as described in Table 2-13.

▸ The vast majority of patients receiving ventilatory assistance undergo assist-control, intermittent mandatory ventilation, or pressure-support ventilation, with the latter two often being used in combination.

▸ In addition, dual control modes are now available, which use a feedback loop to allow the ventilator to control pressure or volume. In the *dual control within-a-breath mode,* the ventilator switches from pressure control to volume control during each breath, whereas the *dual control breath-to-breath mode* operates in either the pressure-support or pressure-control mode, with the pressure limit increasing or decreasing as needed to achieve a preset V$_T$.

• The goal of mechanical ventilation is to strike a balance between excessive respiratory muscle rest, which causes deconditioning and muscle atrophy, and excessive stress, which promotes respiratory muscle fatigue.

▸ Invasive mechanical ventilation is commonly associated with poor nutrition, psychological depression, poor patient motivation, lack of restful sleep, and lack of mobility, which contribute to the vicious cycle that often occurs in respiratory failure.

TABLE 2-13: Types and Modes of Positive-Pressure Mechanical Ventilation

Type and Mode of Ventilation	Description
Conventional Positive-Pressure Ventilation: Volume or Time Cycled, Preset Tidal Volume (V_T)	
Augmented minute or assisted mechanical ventilation (AMV) or Assist/control (A/C) ventilation (ACV)	Delivers a preset V_T when the patient triggers the ventilator by spontaneous inspiratory effort; if less than required or no inspiratory effort is provided, the machine delivers a preset minute ventilation
Controlled mechanical ventilation (CMV), Volume-controlled ventilation (VCV)	Delivers a preset V_T at a predetermined rate without regard to patient's spontaneous breathing pattern
Intermittent mandatory ventilation (IMV)	Allows the patient to breathe spontaneously between the "mandatory" ventilator breaths, which are delivered at the preset rate regardless of the phase of the patient's spontaneous breathing. Mandatory minute ventilation (MMV) can be used with IMV to ensure a minimal minute ventilation with low IMV rates in case the spontaneous ventilation becomes inadequate
Synchronous intermittent mandatory ventilation (SIMV)	As for IMV, except that SIMV allows the mandatory breaths to be triggered by the patient's spontaneous inspiratory efforts
Conventional Positive-Pressure Ventilation: Flow or Time Cycled, Preset Peak Pressure	
Pressure-support ventilation (PS, PSV)	Augments the inspiratory phase of a patient's spontaneous ventilatory efforts with a preset amount of positive pressure in order to reduce the work of breathing imposed by the endotracheal tube. PSV can be added during volume-controlled ventilation, as in PIMV or PSIMV
Pressure control ventilation (PCV)	Delivers a preset number of breaths per minute with fixed inflation pressure and time but allows patient's pulmonary compliance to determine V_T
Pressure control with inverse ratio ventilation (PCIRV)	As for PCV, except with inspiratory time exceeding expiratory time to prevent collapse of the alveolar units; raises the mean airway pressure without increasing the peak inspiratory pressure
Positive end-expiratory pressure (PEEP)	Applies a threshold-like resistance at the end of expiration to prevent early closure of the distal airways and alveoli
Continuous positive airway pressure (CPAP)	Maintains pressure, usually above ambient levels during both inspiration and expiration in a spontaneously breathing patient. It is often used to wean patients off mechanical ventilation
Airway pressure-release ventilation (APRV)	In spontaneously breathing patients receiving a high level of CPAP, allows brief passive exhalation to occur by periodically releasing the CPAP to a lower level so that functional reserve capacity (FRC) is reduced and CO_2 is excreted
Proportional assist ventilation (PAV)	Delivers positive pressure into the airways of spontaneously breathing patients in direct proportion to instantaneous effort; no preset frequency, Vt, pressures, or flows
High frequency ventilation	Uses small tidal volumes at frequencies of >100 breaths/min to increase the kinetic energy of the gas molecules and thus their diffusion movement

▸ Other complications associated with invasive positive pressure ventilation include barotrauma, possible pneumothorax, diminished cardiac output, and hypotension.

• Physical therapy treatments for a patient receiving mechanical ventilation invariably trigger the ventilator alarms. Therapists should become familiar with the various ventilator settings (Table 2-14) and alarms so they can differentiate between real clinical problems and activity-induced false alarms.

  ▸ Low-pressure alarms warn of disconnection of the patient from the ventilator or of circuit leaks.

  ▸ High-pressure alarms indicate rising pressures (e.g., excessive secretions in the airways, kinked tubing, tubing filled with water, patient–ventilator asynchrony, or splinting of chest because of pain during movement).

  ▸ Condensation of water in the corrugated tubing leading to the patient increases the resistance in the circuit and generates positive end-expiratory pressure (PEEP); if it accumulates near the endotracheal tube, the patient can aspirate the water, which may be contaminated by bacterial growth. Therefore, this moisture should be drained into a receptacle, not back into the sterile humidifier, at the beginning of each treatment session.

• Mechanical ventilation is not a contraindication for aggressive physical therapy, including ambulation, as long as the patient is hemodynamically stable, receiving PEEP of 5 cm H_2O or less, tolerating a weaning mode of ventilation, and does not exhibit abnormal signs and symptoms in response to pre-gait activities (see Chapter 6, pages 261, 278, and 282).[6] Exercise training of both the respiratory and peripheral muscles is recommended to prevent deconditioning and the adverse effects of medications and has been shown to increase muscle strength and ventilator-free time and thus improve functional outcomes. During ambulation mechanical ventilation can be maintained by bagging, sometimes provided by a nurse or respiratory therapist, or with a portable ventilator.

TABLE 2-14: Ventilator Settings

Ventilator Settings	Comments
Tidal volume (V_T)	Typically set at 10-15 mL/kg of body weight
Frequency (cycles/min)	Usually set at 8-16, depending on desired P_{CO_2} or pH
Mode	Several are available as listed in Table 2-13
Oxygen concentration (F_{IO_2})	Usually 100% initially unless it is apparent that a lower F_{IO_2} would provide adequate oxygenation ($P_{aO_2} \geq 60$ mm Hg); hopefully <40%-50% within 20 min to ↓ toxicity
Inspiratory flow rate ($\dot{V}_I$)	Typically set at 40-60 L/min unless patient has COPD, in which case it is set at 80-100 L/min to allow more expiratory time
Positive end-expiratory pressure (PEEP)	PEEP is generally initiated at 5 cm of H_2O and increased by increments of 2-5 cm to maintain the P_{aO_2} at ≥ 60 mm Hg
Inspiratory time (T_I)	The time interval between the start of inspiratory flow and the start of expiration
Inspiratory triggering pressure (P_{tr})	The airway pressure that must be generated by the patient to initiate the ventilator inspiratory phase in assisted or intermittent ventilator modes
Inspiratory triggering response time (T_{tr})	The time delay between triggering of the ventilator and the start of inspiratory flow
Inspiratory triggering volume (V_{tr})	The volume change required to initiate the ventilator inspiratory phase
Maximal safety pressure	The highest gauge pressure that is allowed during the inspiratory phase when the ventilator is malfunctioning so that the safety relief valve opens

IMV, Intermittent mandatory ventilation; MMV, mandatory minute ventilation; SIMV, synchronous intermittent mandatory ventilation. For explanation of other abbreviations, see text.

Noninvasive Mechanical Ventilation

Noninvasive ventilation is a form of ventilatory assistance that does not require intubation, yet provides partial ventilatory support in order to maintain appropriate levels of arterial P_{O_2} and P_{CO_2} while also unloading the respiratory muscles. It is used most commonly in patients with chronic or acute respiratory failure, where it has been shown to reduce the need for invasive mechanical ventilation as well as complications and mortality[4,17,18,44]; it is also used in the treatment of obstructive sleep apnea, where positive pressure pneumatically splints open the upper airway to prevent collapse.

- Noninvasive positive pressure ventilation employs a positive-pressure ventilator connected to a mask that applies positive air pressure to the nose, mouth, or both. Because the nasal mask permits talking and eating, it is often preferred by patients with chronic disease.
  - *Continuous positive airway pressure (CPAP)* provides positive pressure throughout the respiratory cycle.
  - *Bilevel positive airway pressure (bi-PAP)* is similar to CPAP except that the inspiratory and expiratory pressures are set separately and the difference between the two is the driving pressure for ventilation.
  - *Airway pressure-release ventilation (APRV)* may be added for patients receiving high-level CPAP in order to allow greater passive exhalation to occur by intermittently releasing the CPAP to a lower level; thus, functional reserve capacity (FRC) is reduced and additional CO_2 is eliminated.
- Negative-pressure ventilation involves the intermittent application of subatmospheric pressure, using an airtight enclosure around the thorax, to assist in expanding the chest wall.

- The *tank ventilator, or iron lung,* is a rigid tank into which the patient's entire body, except for the head, is placed.
- A *cuirass* is a rigid shell that fits over the patient's chest and abdomen.
- The *body wrap ventilator* consists of a sealed garment that encompasses the chest and abdomen.
- Noninvasive mechanical ventilatory assistance can also be achieved through mechanical displacement of the abdominal contents, in order to augment movement of the diaphragm, or by electrical stimulation of the diaphragm.
  - A *rocking bed* rocks the patient back and forth, head to toe, through an arc of 45° so that the force of gravity produces movement of the diaphragm.
  - A *pneumobelt* consists of a rubber bladder, contained in an abdominal corset, that periodically inflates to force the diaphragm upward.
  - *Diaphragm pacing* or *electrophrenic respiration* involves electrical stimulation of the phrenic nerve to elicit contraction of the diaphragm, which can be used with patients in whom the neuromuscular apparatus is intact (e.g., those with central alveolar hypoventilation or high cervical spinal cord injuries).

Extracorporeal Ventilation

Ventilatory support can also be provided by extracorporeal membrane oxygenation (ECMO), also called extracorporeal life support (ECLS), which involves the circulation of venous blood outside of the body through a carbon dioxide scrubber and membrane oxygenator (thus, it is sometimes referred to as veno-venous ECMO or ECLS), so that it is returned to the body as arterial blood with the desired P_{aCO_2} and P_{aO_2}. Alternatively, low-frequency positive-pressure ventilation can be used to achieve oxygenation while CO_2 removal is accomplished outside of the body, using a CO_2 scrubber. Both ECLS and extracorporeal CO_2 removal are used for patients with severe respiratory and/or cardiac failure (e.g., neonatal or acute respiratory distress syndrome, pneumonia, trauma, primary graft failure in lung transplantation). Patients can be supported with ECLS for days to weeks while waiting for organ recovery, and its use allows for reduction of other forms of support, thereby minimizing iatrogenic injury from high mechanical ventilation pressures, high fraction of inspired oxygen, and vasopressor medications for severe heart failure (see page 66). However, full systemic heparinization is required because of platelet activation in the circuit and commonly leads to bleeding complications.

Airway Suctioning

Suctioning involves the application of subatmospheric pressure through a flexible catheter or rigid tube inserted into the airway for the removal of secretions. Indications for suctioning include loss of airway control, increased secretion production, inadequate cough, and thickened secretions, usually in patients with artificial airways.

- Suctioning can be applied in a few different ways:
  - ▸ Using a rigid oral suction catheter (e.g., Yankauer device, tonsillar) to remove secretions from the oropharynx
  - ▸ Using a flexible catheter inserted through the nares and nasopharynx and into the trachea (nasotracheal suctioning)
  - ▸ By inserting a flexible catheter through artificial airways (e.g., nasopharyngeal airway, ET tube, or tracheostomy tube; see page 27) and into the trachea
- Therapists who work with neurologic and ventilator-dependent patients should be familiar with, if not skilled in, suctioning techniques and other treatment procedures for secretion mobilization and clearance (see Chapter 7, page 336).

Airway Clearance Techniques

Various airway clearance techniques aimed at mobilizing and removing secretions are performed by physical therapists and other health care professionals involved in the care of patients with acute and acute on chronic pulmonary dysfunction. These include bronchial drainage, chest percussion, vibration, shaking, assisted coughing techniques, breathing exercises, active cycle of breathing, autogenic drainage, positive expiratory pressure therapy, and high-frequency oscillation techniques. These techniques are described in Chapter 7 (see page 323).

Incentive Spirometry

Incentive spirometry involves the use of a device that provides visual and/or auditory feedback regarding inspiratory effort (e.g., rising cylinder or balls) as a means of encouraging patients to take slow, deep breaths several times an hour. It is commonly used postoperatively to prevent or reverse atelectasis. Instruction is required for patients to use the device correctly; emphasis should be place on taking slow deep breaths, using the diaphragm and lower chest, rather than quick inspirations using the upper chest. The motivated patient can then continue with little supervision. Physical therapists are often in an excellent position to encourage patients to use their incentive spirometers and also to cough after rehabilitation activities, which often stimulate the mobilization of secretions.

Smoking Cessation

Smoking is a major health problem in the United States, which is associated with increased risk of morbidity and mortality due to atherosclerotic heart disease; stroke; COPD; lung cancer; peptic ulcers; cancer of the mouth, larynx, esophagus, stomach, breast, and bladder; respiratory tract infections, and adverse effects during pregnancy. Smoking also increases the prevalence of asthma, respiratory infections, and sudden infant death syndrome.

- Many techniques with wide variability in success rates are used to assist patients in smoking cessation, including patient education programs, group or individual counseling, hypnosis, acupuncture, aversive conditioning, behavior modification, nicotine replacement therapy (NRT), and some medications. Some programs also provide reinforcement via the Internet and cellular phone text messaging.
- The vast majority of individuals who attempt to quit smoking do so on their own, which has a success rate of only 3% to 5% at 1 year. However, because of sheer volume alone, it has the greatest impact in terms of numbers of quitters (684,000 quitters out of 22.8 million attempts).[32]
- NRT is the mainstay of smoking cessation treatment and comes in the form of chewing gum, skin patches, tablets, nasal spray, and inhalers. It is designed to decrease withdrawal symptoms by replacing nicotine in the blood and nearly doubles the long-term success rates. The highest success rates (40% to 44% at 1 yr) for the general public have been reported with a combination of NRT and behavior modification.[33,41] Greatest success is achieved by those who have suffered an acute myocardial infarction and those who have previously failed attempts at smoking cessation.
- Other medications used to treat nicotine dependence include bupropion hydrochloride and nortriptyline, which are tricyclic antidepressants with adrenergic and dopaminergic actions that essentially replace nicotine's neurochemical effects, and varenicline, a selective nicotinic receptor partial antagonist, which may alleviate cravings and the reinforcing effects of smoking. All of these drugs increase the success rates for smoking cessation, but their use is often limited by adverse side effects.[14]
- The advantages of smoking cessation include the following[42]:
  - ▸ Decreased risk of stroke and heart attack, beginning immediately and returning to that of a nonsmoker in approximately 5 years[40]
  - ▸ Reduced risk of developing lung cancer and emphysema, approaching that of a nonsmoker in about 15 years
  - ▸ Declining rate of deterioration of lung function
  - ▸ Increased survival among patients with COPD
  - ▸ Decreased respiratory infections
  - ▸ Financial savings
- Physical therapists can play a key role in offering encouragement and support to patients who are trying to quit smoking. Helpful information to share includes the following:
  - ▸ Individuals who have attempted to quit previously and failed have a greater chance of success with each attempt; most people succeed on their third or fourth attempt, but it may take up to seven or more attempts.
  - ▸ Individual responses to the various forms of NRT (e.g., nicotine patch, gum, inhaler, and nasal spray) vary a great deal,

so patients might have better success with one dosing form than another. The use of NRT doubles a smoker's chances of successfully quitting smoking.[33]

- ▸ Cravings usually last only a couple of minutes; strategies to cope with them include chewing gum, taking a walk, playing a harmonica or singing, and so on.
- ▸ Smoking a single cigarette is just a mistake, not a failure; patients should be encouraged to simply renew the commitment to quit and carry on their efforts.

Pulmonary Rehabilitation

Pulmonary rehabilitation is an individually tailored, multidisciplinary treatment program that employs diagnosis, therapy, emotional support, and education to stabilize or reverse both the physiological and psychological problems associated with chronic pulmonary disease and attempts to return the patient to the highest possible functional capacity.

- The essential components of a comprehensive program consist of:
  - ▸ Assessment by appropriate pulmonary rehabilitation team members
  - ▸ Patient education (see Chapter 7, page 310)
  - ▸ Exercise training (see Chapter 7, pages 298-309)
  - ▸ Psychosocial intervention
  - ▸ Follow-up
- The demonstrated benefits of pulmonary rehabilitation include the following[30]:
  - ▸ Reduced hospitalizations and use of medical resources
  - ▸ Increased quality of life
  - ▸ Decreased respiratory symptoms (e.g., dyspnea)
  - ▸ Amelioration of psychosocial symptoms (e.g., anxiety and depression)
  - ▸ Enhanced exercise tolerance and performance
  - ▸ Improved ability to perform activities of daily living
  - ▸ Ability to return to work for some patients
  - ▸ Increased knowledge about pulmonary disease and its management
  - ▸ Improved survival in some patients
- Because of our expertise in exercise prescription and modification, as well as our knowledge of pulmonary diseases and treatments, physical therapists are valued members of many multidisciplinary pulmonary rehabilitation teams.

Social Services

Social services are often an important element in the care of pulmonary patients who have become debilitated. Some services that may be required include arrangements for home health services, home oxygen equipment, vocational rehabilitation, and patient and family support services.

SURGICAL INTERVENTIONS

As noted previously, surgery sometimes plays a role in the diagnosis of pulmonary disease. In addition, surgical interventions are sometimes valuable for the treatment of some pulmonary diseases or their complications. For certain types of pulmonary disease, particularly localized primary lung cancer, surgery may be the best means of effecting a cure. The surgical procedures frequently used to treat pulmonary disease are listed in the following sections.

Tracheotomy

As illustrated in Figure 2-18, tracheotomy involves the insertion of a tube through the third tracheal ring or cricothyroid membrane (i.e., below the level of the vocal cords) and into the trachea, usually for the purpose of allowing prolonged mechanical ventilation or providing airway protection or maintenance. Tracheotomy is sometimes required to relieve upper airway obstruction due to tumor, edema, trauma, or foreign body. Tracheostomy tubes reduce the risk of vocal cord injury and tracheal damage that may occur while the patient is intubated with a nasotracheal or orotracheal tube.

Cricothyroidotomy

A cricothyroidotomy, or minitracheotomy, is a procedure by which a small incision is made through the cricothyroid membrane followed by the insertion of a small endotracheal tube. It is sometimes performed in patients who have difficulty clearing secretions from the trachea. It allows for saline irrigation of the bronchial tree and suctioning of secretions and, even more importantly, it can be used to stimulate a strong cough reflex.

Excision of Pulmonary Emboli

Pulmonary embolism (PE) obstructs pulmonary arterial flow. Surgical excision is performed via a median sternotomy in patients with hemodynamically significant massive PE who have an absolute contraindication to anticoagulant or thombolytic therapy and in those who develop severe PE despite aggressive medical therapy. The goal is to relieve the obstruction and thus reduce pulmonary hypertension and RV afterload.

- *Pulmonary thromboembolectomy or thrombectomy* is performed as an emergency procedure in patients with severe acute PE. It requires cardiopulmonary bypass (CPB) in order to divert blood from the pulmonary vasculature and provide gas exchange without respiratory movements so the blood clot can be safely removed.
- *Pulmonary thromboendarterectomy (PTE)* is a much more complex surgery that is used for the treatment of chronic thromboembolic pulmonary hypertension resulting from recurrent/chronic PE. In addition to CPB, this surgery requires deep hypothermia and periods of full cardiac arrest, because chronic PE are organized and adhere to the arterial wall, eventually causing severe intimal thickening and webbing within the lumen, so they require complete visualization in a totally bloodless surgical field to remove completely. PTE is performed at a limited number of centers around the world because of its technical complexity. Recovery is often complicated by reperfusion injury necessitating ventilatory support and the mortality rate is generally 4% to 7%.[5,14]

Catheter or Chest Tube/Drain Placement

Disruption of the integrity of the lungs and chest cavity (e.g., trauma, surgery, or as the result of preexisting lung disease) can be treated by simple manual needle aspiration, insertion of an intrapleural small-caliber catheter, or placement of a large chest tube (i.e., a *tube thoracostomy*).[20] All of these methods serve to remove air, fluid, or blood from the pleural space, restore negative intrapleural pressure, and reexpand a collapsed or partially collapsed lung; in addition, the latter two techniques allow continued drainage, prevent reflux of drainage back into the chest, and can accommodate a water seal device and negative-pressure suction.

- An intrapleural catheter is usually inserted in the second or third intercostal space at the midclavicular line and attached to a Heimlich one-way valve or water seal device as treatment for a primary and sometimes secondary spontaneous pneumothorax; suction is added if full reexpansion of the lung is not achieved within 24 to 48 hours. It is associated with less pain and anxiety and allows greater early mobilization than standard chest tube placement.
- Intrapleural chest tubes require an underwater seal to prevent outside air from entering the chest. Gentle suction is often added to remove air leaking from damaged lung tissue and to create the desired negative intrapleural pressure.
  - ▸ A two-chamber system has a water seal and a collection chamber. The water level is usually set at 2 cm and should fluctuate during respiration (rising during inspiration and falling during expiration). Bubbling should be seen in the underwater seal chamber only during expiration, unless the patient is receiving positive-pressure ventilation; constant bubbling indicates either an air leak in the system or a bronchopleural fistula.
  - ▸ Most systems contain three chambers because of the addition of a suction control chamber, as shown in Figure 2-20. In this system, the height of the water column in the third chamber, not the amount of wall suction, determines the amount of suction applied to the chest tube (most commonly −20 cm H_2O, so that a gentle rolling bubbling is produced).
  - ▸ Suction applied to the underwater seal device results in bubbling within the water chamber, as described previously, which may diminish as the air leak seals off. If bubbling ceases completely, the tube has become kinked or blocked; if a change in position and release of the chest tube does not result in bubbling, the nurse or physician should be notified immediately to prevent the development of a tension pneumothorax. Likewise, a sudden increase in the amount of bubbling also should be reported.
  - ▸ Chest tube suction is usually avoided after pneumonectomy or in patients with emphysema and a prominent air leak, such as those undergoing lung volume reduction surgery.
  - ▸ Fluid often pools in the dependent portion of the tubing connecting to the underwater seal device, which increases the resistance to proper drainage of air and fluid and could delay healing. Physical therapists should carefully drain any pooled fluid into the drainage chamber before the initiation of each treatment. Care should be exercised not to elevate the drainage system or tube above the level of the chest, as this may cause the fluid to drain back into the chest.
  - ▸ There is no contraindication to rolling the patient onto the side of a chest tube; in fact, patients should be encouraged to intermittently assume this position (with assistance) to preserve normal drainage and expansion of the uninvolved lung.
  - ▸ If a chest tube falls out or is accidentally pulled out, the insertion site should be sealed off quickly by pressing a gloved hand over it and help should be summoned immediately.
- When a patient develops a prolonged air leak, which is not amenable to surgical repair but is expected to eventually heal spontaneously, a Heimlich flutter valve may be used to allow a patient to be discharged home with close follow-up. It provides a passive drainage system with a one-way flutter

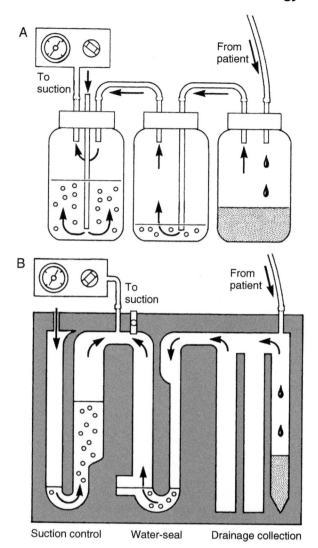

Figure 2-20: Schematic drawing of chest drainage systems. **A,** A three-bottle system. **B,** A commercially available system that combines all components in one device. The collection chamber collects fluid drainage from the pleural space. The underwater seal serves as a one-way valve between the pleural space and the atmosphere. The suction control chamber controls the amount of pressure applied to the pleural space.

valve that allows air and fluid to be expelled from the chest cavity while preventing air from entering the pleural space.
- An open tube inserted to drain an empyema is an intracavitary drain and does not require a water seal.
- When an individual develops a spontaneous pneumothorax associated with shortness of breath, the first choice of treatment may be the insertion of a needle into the intrapleural space in order to extract the air (i.e., a needle aspiration).

Pulmonary Resection/Thoracotomy

Surgical resection of part or all of a lung may be indicated for the treatment of bronchogenic carcinoma, bronchiectasis, fungal infections, tuberculosis, and benign tumors. In addition, surgery is sometimes performed to excise emphysematous bullae (see the next section).

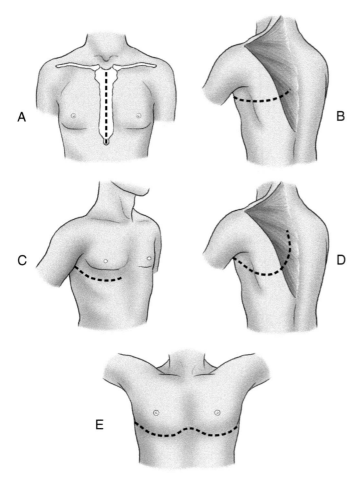

Figure 2-21: Surgical incisions of the thorax. The median sternotomy **(A)** is commonly used for cardiac surgery, including heart and heart–lung transplantation, although some mitral valve surgery is performed via a posterolateral thoracotomy **(B)**. Lung surgeries are usually performed via the anterolateral **(C)** or posterolateral thoracotomy incision **(D)**, except for bilateral lung and live donor lobar transplantations, which use the clamshell incision **(E)**.

- Resections are performed by means of an anterolateral or posterolateral thoracotomy incision, as illustrated in Figure 2-21, and involve the following:
  ‣ An incision made through the intercostal space corresponding to the lesion, and
  ‣ Division of the muscle fibers of the serratus anterior and intercostal muscles, and sometimes the latissimus dorsi and rhomboid muscles
- The surgical procedures are named for the portion of the lung removed:
  ‣ *Wedge resection:* Removal of a small localized lesion
  ‣ *Segmentectomy:* Excision of a bronchopulmonary segment
  ‣ *Lobectomy:* Resection of an entire lung lobe
  ‣ *Bilobectomy:* Removal of the middle lobe along with an upper or lower lobe
  ‣ *Bronchoplastic/sleeve resection:* Excision of a lobe and part of the main stem bronchus followed by anastomosis of the lower lobe(s) to the proximal bronchus

  ‣ *Pneumonectomy:* Resection of an entire lung
- For the treatment of cancer, the amount of lung resected is not always related to the size of the tumor but is determined by any extension of the tumor into adjacent pulmonary lobes, lymph nodes, hilar structures, or blood vessels.
- After pulmonary resection, two chest tubes are usually placed: one at the apex of the lung to remove air and one at the base and/or mediastinum to drain blood and serous fluid (see page 32).
- There are specific implications for physical therapy after thoracotomy:
  ‣ Because of significant postoperative pleural and musculoskeletal pain resulting from the operative position as well as the large number of muscles incised, adequate pain control is essential for patients to perform effective deep breathing and coughing and other physical therapy interventions. Therefore, if patients are not receiving epidural anesthesia, physical therapy treatments should be coordinated with the patient's pain medication schedule.
  ‣ Patients who have undergone thoracotomy are prone to developing postural abnormalities and ipsilateral shoulder range of motion restrictions caused by splinting of the incision. Thus, it is important to encourage full range of motion and postural exercises as healing occurs.

Bullectomy

Bullae, or intrapulmonary air spaces greater than 1 cm in diameter, may occur as isolated lesions in otherwise normal lungs or in lungs with generalized emphysema. Excision or plication of giant bullae may be performed via thoracotomy, median sternotomy, or thoracoscopy in hopes of releasing relatively normal lung tissue being compressed by the bullae, which act as space-occupying lesions, and thus improving lung function. Patients with a large bulla occupying at least 33% to 50% of the hemithorax, an FEV_1 not exceeding 50% predicted, reasonably well-preserved diffusing capacity, and normocapnia tend to gain the most benefit from this procedure.[1,5]

Lung Volume Reduction Surgery

Lung volume reduction surgery (LVRS) is a palliative procedure involving the resection of 20% to 35% of the lung tissue most damaged by emphysema. It is usually performed via thoracotomy or median sternotomy, although video-assisted thoracoscopy is being used at some centers. The aim of LVRS is to improve the expansion and recruitment of more functional lung tissue and to reduce intrathoracic volumes. The goals are to restore the dome shape of the diaphragm and to improve the mechanical advantage of the inspiratory muscles, so that patients can breathe more comfortably at a lower functional residual capacity and perform routine activities of daily living without significant limitation.

- Patients who benefit most from LVRS are those with significant dyspnea and severe fixed expiratory obstruction (i.e., FEV_1 less than 40% to 45% of predicted) despite maximal medical therapy, as well as predominantly upper lobe disease and low maximal exercise tolerance. However, those with FEV_1 not exceeding 20% predicted combined with either very low diffusing capacity ($\leq$20%) or diffuse emphysema on CT do not appear to be good candidates because of higher mortality rates.[23,25]

- The natural history following LVRS is currently unclear: Although improvements are seen in FEV_1, FVC, RV, diffusing capacity, exercise tolerance, and quality of life after surgery, with peak values obtained at 6 months to 1 year, they may be short-lived except for a select group of patients.[7,23,46]

Lung and Heart–Lung Transplantation

Lung transplantation (LTx) may be used to treat patients who have end-stage COPD, interstitial pulmonary fibrosis, cystic fibrosis, primary pulmonary hypertension, bronchiectasis, bronchiolitis obliterans, and other rare diseases affecting the lungs, but no serious comorbidities (e.g., morbid obesity, severe hypertension, heart failure, cancer, or cachexia).[9] Some patients with primary pulmonary hypertension or other primary lung disease with severe biventricular failure may be treated with combined heart–lung transplant rather than with lung transplantation alone. In general, transplant candidates must be less than 65 years of age, nonsmokers, ambulatory, and able to participate in pulmonary rehabilitation.

- The usual procedures are single-lung transplantation (SLTx) or bilateral sequential (single) lung transplantation (BLTx), although some centers are performing living donor lobe transplants in selected patients, where two individuals each donate one lower lobe to a recipient.[9] SLTx is performed via a thoracotomy or sternotomy incision whereas BLTx and living donor lobe transplants usually involve a clamshell incision (see Figure 2-21). Postoperative pain is managed with epidural anesthesia.
- In heart–lung transplantation (HLTx), the heart and either one or two lungs are transplanted as a unit. Fortunately, research has revealed that the right ventricle is remarkably resilient and capable of recovery within 3 to 6 months when LTx alone is performed for many types of end-stage primary lung disease, so the heart can be made available for a patient on the heart transplant waiting list.
- Immunosuppression is required to avoid organ rejection. The highest levels of immunosuppression are required immediately after surgery; the doses are then decreased over time until the lowest maintenance levels of suppression necessary to prevent rejection are identified for each patient.
  - ▸ Less than half of LTx patients currently receive induction therapy aimed at reducing the incidence of early acute rejection and bronchiolitis obliterans syndrome seen in chronic rejection. The agents most commonly used are the new anti–interleukin-2 receptor antibodies, daclizumab and basiliximab, and less frequently OKT3 and rabbit anti-thymocyte globulin (rATG).[24,31]
  - ▸ Maintenance immunosuppression typically involves a three-drug regimen based on a calcineurin inhibitor (either cyclosporine A or tacrolimus [FK 506]), an antimetabolite (either mycophenolate mofetil or azathioprine) or sirolimus, and corticosteroids (see Chapter 5, page 205).
  - ▸ Episodes of rejection requiring increased immunosuppression, usually corticosteroids or occasionally rATG or daclizumab, occur in about 40% of patients.[30]
  - ▸ Newer immunosuppressive agents and modalities are currently under investigation.
- The most common causes of early mortality after LTx are acute graft failure and reperfusion injury, whereas infection and bronchiolitis obliterans syndrome due to chronic rejection are the major causes of morbidity and mortality in the first 5 years after transplantation.

Patients who undergo LTx are usually in poor physical condition with low muscle mass and reduced skeletal muscle oxidative capacity.[3] In addition, major surgery, sepsis, and medications (especially cyclosporine A, tacrolimus, and corticosteroids) often confound these problems. Therefore, patients benefit from beginning physical therapy as soon as possible in their recovery, often while still in the intensive care unit, and typically continue rehabilitation for several weeks.

- Early treatment consists of breathing exercises; coughing; progressive mobility; light range of motion, callisthenic, and postural exercises; and advances to walking and/or stationary cycling. Exercise limitations are usually due to chronic deconditioning and peripheral muscle dysfunction rather than ventilatory capacity.
- Patients should be encouraged to regain full range of motion of their shoulders, trunk, and neck, which may be limited by splinting of the incision, and to practice good posture.
- Careful monitoring of the physiological responses to exercise, especially oxygen saturation and blood pressure, is important in these patients even as outpatients, as a drop in either of these parameters, especially during exercise, may be an indication of acute rejection. In addition, a 10% reduction in vital capacity and forced expiratory volume in 1 second (FEV_1) may indicate rejection or infection.
- After LTx, the majority of patients have marked improvements in resting pulmonary function, functional capacity, and quality of life.[34,36] However, maximal oxygen uptake is significantly reduced compared with age-matched control subjects, attaining only 40% to 60% of predicted values at 3 to 6 months after transplant and then remaining level. The major factor associated with this exercise impairment is diminished peripheral skeletal work capacity with a reduced lactate threshold, particularly involving the lower extremities, which is due predominantly to deconditioning and immunosuppressive therapy.[16,21,24,31] There is some evidence that aerobic endurance training may increase exercise capacity in long-term survivors of LTx.[38]
- Specific resistance training is also recommended, as it has been shown to prevent vertebral osteoporosis in LTx recipients and may also improve skeletal muscle function.

Bronchial Thermoplasty

Because patients with asthma often develop bronchoconstriction despite conventional drug therapy, radiofrequency ablation of airway smooth muscle is currently under investigation. Bronchial thermoplasty involves the bronchoscopic application of radiofrequency energy to circumferentially heat the airway walls in order to disrupt the arterial smooth muscle, which is later replaced by loose connective tissue. Thus, chronic symptoms may be ameliorated and acute exacerbations inhibited.[8]

Decortication

Decortication is a major thoracic surgery involving the excision of the parietal pleurae and residual clot and/or organizing scar tissue that forms after a hemothorax or empyema, or occasionally for symptomatic patients with pleural thickening due to rheumatoid arthritis. This procedure allows expansion of the underlying lung tissue and obliterates the pleural space to prevent further infection.

Pleurodesis, Pleurectomy, and Pleuroperitoneal Shunt

Obliteration of the pleural space, or *pleurodesis*, can be achieved by instilling a sclerosing agent (e.g., tetracycline derivatives, talc slurry, or bleomycin) into the pleural space thorascopically or by severely abrading the pleurae at thoracotomy. *Pleurectomy* consists of the stripping away and removal of the parietal pleurae from the chest wall to obliterate the pleural space and thus prevent the reaccumulation of air or fluid. Another alternative for the management of rapidly accumulating pleural effusion, where lung reexpansion is impossible due to tumor, is the insertion of a *pleuroperitoneal shunt*, where the pleural fluid drains into the abdominal cavity.

Pulmonary Metastasectomy

Excision of pulmonary metastases may be performed in selected patients with curable cancer and no evidence of metastatic disease in other sites, especially if there is a long interval between diagnosis and the appearance of the pulmonary metastases. More than 50 metastases may be removed during a single surgical procedure.

Tracheal Resection

The excision of a portion of the trachea with end-to-end anastomosis of the remaining trachea is most commonly performed for localized tumors and benign strictures. Resection is usually performed via a cervical incision. If resection of the carina or main stem bronchus is indicated, a right lateral thoracotomy is required.

REFERENCES

1. American Thoracic Society. Standards for the diagnosis and treatment of patients with chronic obstructive pulmonary disease. *Am J Respir Crit Care Med.* 1995;152:S77-S120.
2. American Thoracic Society/American College of Chest Physicians. ATS/ACCP statement on cardiopulmonary exercise testing. *Am J Respir Crit Care Med.* 2003;167:211-277.
3. American Thoracic Society/European Respiratory Society. Skeletal muscle dysfunction in chronic obstructive pulmonary disease. *Am J Respir Crit Care Med.* 1999;159:S1-S40.
4. Antonelli M, Pennisi MA, Montini L. Clinical review: Nonivasive ventilation in the clinical setting – experience from the past 10 years. *Crit Care.* 2005;9:98-1203.
5. Benditt JO. Surgical options for patients with COPD: sorting out the choices. *Respir Care.* 2006;51:173-186.
6. Chiang L-L, Wang L-Y, Wu C-P, et al. Effects of physical training on functional status in patients with prolonged mechanical ventilation. *Phys Ther.* 2006;86:1271-1281.
7. Ciccone AM, Meyers BF, Guthrie TJ, et al. Long-term outcome of bilateral lung volume reduction in 250 consecutive patients with emphysema. *J Thorac Cardiovasc Surg.* 2003;125:513-525.
8. Cox PG, Miller J, Mitzner W, et al. Radiofrequency ablation of airway smooth muscle for sustained treatment of asthma: preliminary investigations. *Eur Repir J.* 2004;24:659-663.
9. DeMeo DL, Ginns LC. Clinical status of lung transplantation. *Transplantation.* 2001;72:1713-1724.
10. de Troyer A. Actions of the respiratory muscles. In: Hamid Q, Shannon J, Martin J, eds. *Physiologic Basis of Respiratory Disease.* Hamilton, Ontario: BC Decker Inc; 2005.
11. Emtner M, Porszasz J, Burns M, et al. Benefits of supplemental oxygen in exercise training in nonhypoxemic chronic obstructive pulmonary disease patients. *Am J Respir Crit Care Med.* 2003;168: 1034-1042.
12. Fussell KM, Ayo DS, Branca P, et al. Assessing need for long-term oxygen therapy: a comparison of conventional evaluation and measures of ambulatory oxygen monitoring. *Respir Care.* 2003; 48:115-119.
13. Jensen LA, Onyskiw JE, Prasad NGN. Meta-analysis of arterial oxygen saturation monitoring by pulse oximetry in adults. *Heart Lung.* 1998; 27:387-408.
14. Johnson BA. New weapon to curb smoking: No more excuses to delay treatment. *Arch Int Med.* 2006;166:1547-1550.
15. Kim V, Benditt JO, Wise RA, et al. Oxygen therapy in chronic obstructive pulmonary disease. *Proc Am Thorac Soc.* 2008;5:513-518.
16. Lands LC, Smountas AA, Mesiano G, et al. Maximal exercise capacity and peripheral skeletal muscle function following lung transplantation. *J Heart Lung Transplant.* 1999;18:113-120.
17. Lanuza DM, Lefaiver CA, Fracas GA. Research on the quality of life of lung transplant candidates and recipients: an integrative review. *Heart Lung.* 2000;29:180-195.
18. Lightowler JV, Wedzicha JA, Elliott MW, et al. Non-invasive positive pressure ventilation to treat respiratory failure resulting from exacerbation of chronic obstructive pulmonary disease: Cochrane systematic review and meta-analysis. *BMJ.* 2003;326:185-187.
19. Luh S, Liu H. Video-assisted thoracic surgery—the past, present status and the future. *J Zhejiang Univ SCIENCE B.* 2006;7:118-128.
20. Marquette C-H, Marx A, Leroy S, et al. Simplified stepwise management of primary spontaneous pneumothorax: a pilot study. *Eur Respir J.* 2006;27:470-476.
21. Mathur S, Reid WD, Levy RD. Exercise limitation in recipients of lung transplants. *Phys Ther.* 2004;84:1178-1187.
22. Mengelkoch LJ, Martin D, Lawler J. A review of the principles of pulse oximetry and accuracy of pulse oximeter estimates during exercise. *Phys Ther.* 1994;74:40-49.
23. Meyers BF, Yusen RD, Guthrie TJ, et al. Results of lung volume reduction surgery in patients meeting a National Emphysema Treatment Trial high-risk criterion. *J Thorac Cardiovasc Surg.* 2004;127:829-835.
24. Moffatt SD, Demers P, Robbins RC, et al. Lung transplantation: a decade of experience. *J Heart Lung Transplant.* 2004;24:145-151.
25. National Emphysema Treatment Trial Group. A randomized trial comparing lung-volume-reduction surgery with medical therapy for severe emphysema. *New Engl J Med.* 2003;348:2059-2073,
26. Nocturnal Oxygen Therapy Trial Group. Continuous or nocturnal oxygen therapy in hypoxemic chronic obstructive lung disease. *Ann Intern Med.* 1980;93:391-398.
27. Pedersen MR, Fisher MT, van Beek EJR. MR imaging of the pulmonary vasculature – an update. *Eur Raidol.* 2006;16:1374-1386.
28. Pilling J, Cutaia M. Ambulatory oximetry monitoring in patients with severe COPD – a preliminary study. *Chest.* 1999;116:314-321.
29. Reid WD, Dechman G. Considerations when testing and training the respiratory muscles. *Phys Ther.* 1995;75:971-982.
30. Ries AL. Position paper of the American Association of Cardiovascular and Pulmonary Rehabilitation: Scientific basis of pulmonary rehabilitation. *J Cardiopulm Rehabil.* 1990;10:418-441.
31. Shapiro R, Young JB, Milford EL, et al. Immunosuppression: evolution in practice and trends, 1993–2003. *Am J Transplant.* 2005;5(Part 2):874-886.
32. Shiffman S, Mason KM, Henningfield JE. Tobacco dependence treatments: Review and Prospectus. *Annu Rev Public Health.* 1998;190:335-358.
33. Silagy C, Mant D, Fowler G, Lodge M. Meta-analysis of efficacy of nicotine replacement therapies in smoking cessation. *Lancet.* 1994;343:139-142.
34. Smeritschnig B, Jaksch P, Kocher A, et al. Quality of life after lung transplantation: a cross-sectional study. *J Heart Lung Transplant.* 2005;24: 474-480.
35. Solway S, Brooks D, Lacasse Y, Thomas S. A qualitative systematic overview of the measurement properties of functional tests used in the cardiorespiratory domain. *Chest.* 2001;119:256-270.
36. Stavem K, Bjortuft O, Lund MB, et al. Health-related quality of life of lung transplant candidates and recipients. *Respiration.* 2000;67: 159-165.
37. Stein PD, Fowler SE, Goodman LR, et al. Multidetector computed tomography for acute pulmonary embolism. *N Engl J Med.* 2006;354:2317-2327.

38. Stiebellehner L, Quittan M, End A, et al. Aerobic endurance training program improves exercise performance in lung transplant recipients. *Chest.* 1998;113:906-912.
39. Stockley RA, O'Brien C, Pye A, et al. Relationship of sputum color to nature and outpatient management of acute exarbations of COPD. *Chest.* 2000;117:1638-1645.
40. Taylor CB, Miller NH. Smoking cessation in patients with cardiovascular disease. *Qual Life Cardiovasac Care.* 1989; Spring: 229-236.
41. Tonneson P, Fryd V, Hansen M, et al. Effect of nicotine chewing gum in combination with group counseling on the cessation of smoking. *N Engl J Med.* 1988;318:15-18.
42. U.S. Department of Health and Human Services. *Health consequences of smoking cessation report of the surgeon general.* Washington D.C.: U.S. Government Printing Office; 1990.
43. Van de Louw A, Cracco C, Cerf C, et al. Accuracy of pulse oximetry in the intensive care unit. *Intensive Care Med.* 2001;27:1606-1613.
44. Winck JC, Azevedo LF, Costa-Pereira A, et al. Efficacy and safety of non-invasive ventilation in the treatment of acute cardiogenic pulmonary edema – a systemic review and meta-analysis. *Crit Care.* 2006;10:R69.
45. Yamaya Y, Bogaard HJ, Wagner PD, et al. Validity of pulse oximetry during maximal exercise in normoxia, hypoxia, and hyperoxia. *J Appl Physiol.* 2002;92:162-168.
46. Yusen RD, Lefrak SS, Gierada DS, et al. A prospective evaluation of lung volume reduction surgery in 200 consecutive patients. *Chest.* 2003;123: 1026-1037.

ADDITIONAL READINGS

Albert RK, Spiro SG, Jett JR. *Clinical Respiratory Medicine.* 2nd ed. Philadelphia: Mosby; 2004.

American Association of Cardiovascular and Pulmonary Rehabilitation, Connors G, Hilling L, eds. *Guidelines for Pulmonary Rehabilitation Program.* 3rd ed. Champaign, IL: Human Kinetics; 2004.

Barnes TA. *Respiratory Care Principles—A Programmed Guide to Entry-Level Practice.* 3rd ed. Philadelphia: F.A. Davis Co; 1992.

Barnes PJ, Drazen JM, Rennard S, Thomson NC. *Asthma and COPD—Basic Mechanisms and Clinical Management.* Boston: Academic Press; 2002.

Baum GL, Crapo JD, Celli BR, Karlinsky JB, eds. *Textbook of Pulmonary Diseases.* 6th ed. Philadelphia: Lippincott-Raven; 1998.

Burton GG, Hodgkin JE, Ward JJ, eds. *Respiratory Care: A Guide to Clinical Practice.* 4th ed. Philadelphia: Lippincott Williams & Wilkins; 1997.

Cherniack NS, Altose MD, Homma I, eds. *Rehabilitation of the Patient with Respiratory Disease.* New York: McGraw-Hill; 1999.

Crapo JD, Glassroth JL, Karlinsky JB, Talmadge EK. eds. *Baum's Textbook of Pulmonary Diseases.* 7th ed. Philadelphia: Lippincott Williams & Wilkins; 2003.

Fink JB, Hunt GE. *Clinical Practice in Respiratory Care.* Philadelphia: Lippincott Williams & Wilkins; 1999.

Fraser RS, Muller NL, Colman N, Pare PF. *Fraser and Pare's Diagnosis of Diseases of the Chest.* 4th ed. Philadelphia: Saunders Co; 1999.

Frownfelter D, Dean E. *Cardiovascular and Pulmonary Physical Therapy: Evidence and Practice.* 4th ed. St. Louis: Mosby; 2006.

Gershwin ME, Albertson TE. *Bronchial Asthma—Principles of Diagnosis and Treatment.* 4th ed. Totowa, NJ: Human Press; 2001.

Gibson GJ, Geddes DM, Costabel U, et al., eds. *Respiratory Medicine.* 3rd ed. Philadelphia: Saunders; 2003.

Gold WM, Murray JF, Nadel JA. *Atlas of Procedures in Respiratory Medicine: A Companion to Murray and Nadel's Textbook of Respiratory Medicine.* Philadelphia: Saunders Company; 2002.

Goldman L, Ausiello D. *Cecil Textbook of Medicine.* 22nd ed. Philadelphia: Saunders; 2004.

Guyton AC, Hall JE. *Textbook of Medical Physiology.* 10th ed. Philadelphia, Saunders; 2000.

Hansen JE, Sue DY, Casaburi R, Whipp BJ, Wasserman K, eds. *Principles of Exercise Testing and Interpretation.* 3rd ed. Philadelphia: Lippincott Williams & Wilkins; 1999.

Hess DR, MacIntyre NR, Mishoe SC, et al. *Respiratory Care: Principles and Practice.* Philadelphia: Saunders; 2002.

Hillegass EA, Sadowsky HS, eds. *Essentials of Cardiopulmonary Physical Therapy.* 2nd ed. Philadelphia: Saunders; 2001.

Humes HD, ed-in-chief. *Kelley's Textbook of Internal Medicine.* 4th ed. Philadelphia: Lippincott Williams & Wilkins; 2000.

Irwin S, Tecklin JS. *Cardiopulmonary Physical Therapy.* 4th ed. St. Louis: Mosby; 2004.

Mason RJ, Broaddus VC, Murray JF, Nadel JA. *Murray and Nadel's Textbook of Respiratory Medicine.* 4th ed. St Louis: Mosby; 2005.

McArdle WD, Katch FI, Katch VL. *Exercise Physiology—Energy, Nutrition, and Human Performance.* 5th ed. Philadelphia: Lea & Febiger; 2001.

Ruppel GL. *Manual of Pulmonary Function Testing.* 8th ed. St. Louis: Mosby; 2003.

Wasserman K, Hansen JE, Sue DY, et al. *Principles of Exercise Testing and Interpretation.* 4th ed. Philadelphia: Lippincott Williams & Wilkins; 2004.

Weinberger SE. *Principles of Pulmonary Medicine.* 2nd ed. Philadelphia: Saunders; 1992.

CHAPTER 3

Cardiovascular Medicine

This chapter begins with a review of basic cardiovascular anatomy and physiology, with emphasis on the factors that influence cardiac function, both at rest and during activity. The remainder of the chapter presents the various diagnostic tests and procedures and therapeutic interventions most commonly used in the management of cardiovascular disease. In many instances the implications for physical therapy treatments for important diagnostic findings and therapeutic interventions are included. The cardiovascular diseases and disorders frequently encountered in rehabilitation patients are described in Chapter 4 (Cardiopulmonary Pathology), and the clinical applications of many of the physiological principles are expanded in Chapter 6 (Cardiopulmonary Assessment).

 3.1 THE HEART AND CIRCULATION

A brief review of cardiac anatomy and the physiological principles essential for understanding cardiac function are offered in this section. It is only through a sound grasp of normal cardiovascular anatomy and physiology that therapists can appreciate the effects of disease and dysfunction and how to appropriately modify treatment.

ANATOMY

This section describes the normal anatomy of the heart, its blood and nervous supply, as well as its conduction system, and the vasculature of the body.

The Heart

The heart is essentially a muscle pump, or more accurately two separate muscle pumps in one organ. The right side receives blood from the venous system and pumps blood to the lungs for gas exchange, while the left side receives oxygenated blood from the lungs and pumps it out to the tissues of the body.

- The heart chambers and valves are shown in Figure 3-1.
  - Right atrium (RA): Receives venous blood from the superior and inferior vena cavae
  - Tricuspid valve (TV): Prevents backflow of blood from the right ventricle into the RA during systole
  - Right ventricle (RV): Pumps blood via the pulmonary arteries to the lungs for gas exchange
  - Pulmonary valve (PV): Prevents backflow of blood from the pulmonary artery into the RV during diastole
  - Left atrium (LA): Receives oxygen-rich blood from the lungs via the pulmonary veins
  - Mitral valve (MV): Prevents backflow of blood from the LV into the LA during systole
  - Left ventricle (LV): Pumps blood to the body via the aorta
  - Aortic valve (AoV): Prevents backflow of blood from the aorta into the LV during diastole
- The terminology used to describe the regions of the heart includes:

- Basal: Posterior, superior aspect of the heart (mostly LA and some RA)
- Apical: Anterior, inferior tip of the heart (tip of the LV)
- Anterior: Sternocostal surface of the heart (primarily RA and RV)
- Diaphragmatic: Inferior, posterior surface of the heart (mainly RV and LV)
- Lateral: Left lateral surface of the heart (lateral LV)
- The four layers of cardiac tissue are known as the:
  - Endocardium: Innermost mesothelial lining of the heart
  - Myocardium: Middle layer consisting of muscle tissue
  - Epicardium: Outer layer of the heart and inner visceral layer of the serous pericardium
  - Pericardium: Thick outer layer of the fibrous sac around the heart

The Conduction System of the Heart

The heart contains several areas of specialized cells that have the inherent ability to spontaneously generate electrical impulses: the sinoatrial (SA) node, the atrioventricular (AV) node and AV bundle (bundle of His), and ventricular pacemaker cells.

- Conduction of the electrical activity of the heart normally occurs along the pathway illustrated in Figure 3-2.
- Cells in the SA node depolarize fastest, at a rate of 60 to 100 beats per minute (bpm), and a wave of depolarization is sent through the atria along the internodal pathways, causing atrial contraction.
- After a brief delay in the AV node to allow for active ventricular filling, the impulse is conducted through the AV bundle (bundle of His), the left and right bundle branches, and the Purkinje fibers to the ventricular muscle cells, which then contract to initiate systole.
- During diastole, the ventricles repolarize and refill with blood.
- Damage to any part of the conduction system of the heart results in impaired initiation or conduction of the impulse.
  - If the SA node becomes damaged and does not function, the role of pacemaker is taken over by the AV node at 40 to 60 bpm or ventricular pacemaker cells at 25 to 40 bpm.
  - Damage to the AV node results in AV, or heart, block (i.e., first degree [1°], 2°, or 3°/complete), which results in delayed or failed conduction of some or all of the impulses from the atria to the ventricles (see Chapter 6, page 270).
  - Damage to one of the bundle branches or a subdivision creates right or left bundle branch block or interventricular conduction delay, which leads to late activation of one of the ventricles, as shown on page 232.

Innervation of the Heart and Blood Vessels

- The cardiovascular system is innervated by the autonomic nervous system, consisting of two antagonistic parts, the sympathetic and parasympathetic nervous systems (SNS and PNS,

HEAD AND UPPER EXTREMITY

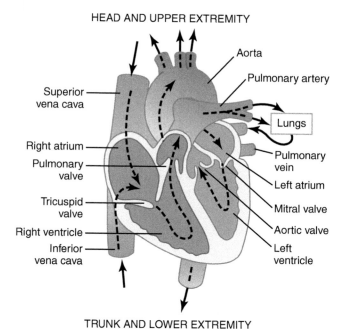

TRUNK AND LOWER EXTREMITY

Figure 3-1: The heart chambers and valves. Blood flows into the right atrium from the superior and inferior vena cavae, and then through the tricuspid valve to the right ventricle and out through the pulmonary valve and pulmonary arteries to the lungs; blood returns to the left atrium via the pulmonary veins, and then passes through the mitral valve to the left ventricle. It is finally ejected through the aortic valve into the aorta and the coronary arteries to supply all tissues of the body. (From Guyton AC, Hall JE. *Textbook of Medical Physiology.* 11th ed. Philadelphia: Saunders; 2006.)

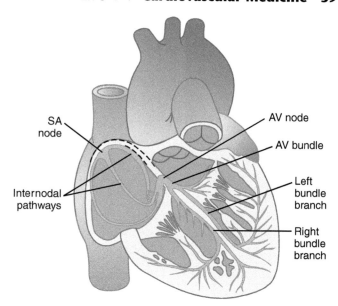

Figure 3-2: The conduction system of the heart. Impulses travel from the sinoatrial (SA) node through the atria via the internodal pathways to the atrioventricular (AV) node, and then through the bundle of His, right and left bundle branches, and Purkinje fibers to the ventricular muscle. (From Guyton AC, Hall JE. *Textbook of Medical Physiology.* 11th ed. Philadelphia: Saunders; 2006.)

respectively), which are controlled by the vasomotor center in the medulla and lower pons, as illustrated in Figure 3-3. The vasomotor center receives input from higher brain centers, including the reticular substance, hypothalamus, and cerebral cortex.

- The PNS, via the vagus nerves, is dominant during basal conditions, when the SNS is inhibited. It acts to decrease the heart rate (negative chronotropic effect), decrease the strength of atrial contraction (negative inotropic effect), and slow conduction through the AV node.
- The SNS becomes dominant during any form of stress and affects many complex changes involving most systems of the body.
  ▶ Effects of the SNS on the heart include increased heart rate (positive chronotropic effect), enhanced force of contraction in both the atria and the ventricles (positive inotropic effect), and accelerated conduction velocity throughout the atria, AV node, and ventricles.
  ▶ SNS stimulation of the small arteries and arterioles results in vasoconstriction to reduce blood flow to the tissues they supply, while constriction of the veins increases venous return to the heart. SNS nerves to the skeletal muscles contain a small number of vasodilator fibers, in addition to the vasoconstrictor fibers, which may play a role in increasing blood flow in anticipation of activity.

Blood Supply of the Heart

- The heart muscle receives its blood supply via the coronary arteries, which arise just above the right and left cusps of the aortic valve.
- The most common angiographic views of the coronary arteries (CAs) are shown in Figure 3-4, which depicts the major CAs and their branches:
  ▶ Right coronary artery (RCA)
  ▶ Left main coronary artery (LMCA)
  ▶ Left anterior descending (LAD) artery
  ▶ Circumflex (Cx, Circ)
  ▶ Posterior descending artery (PDA)
- The most common distribution of blood supply is described in Table 3-1; however, there is a fair degree of individual variability.
- In addition, coronary collateral channels provide communication between the major coronary arteries and their branches. With slowly developing occlusions, further development of these channels may occur to bypass the lesions.
- It is now recognized that vascular endothelium is actively involved in many physiological and pathological processes that mediate vascular inflammation, plaque stability, thrombus formation, and vascular tone. This is particularly important in the coronary arteries.
- Venous drainage of the heart occurs via the cardiac veins to the coronary sinus, which drains into the RA, and through the small thesbian veins, which empty directly into the chambers of the heart.

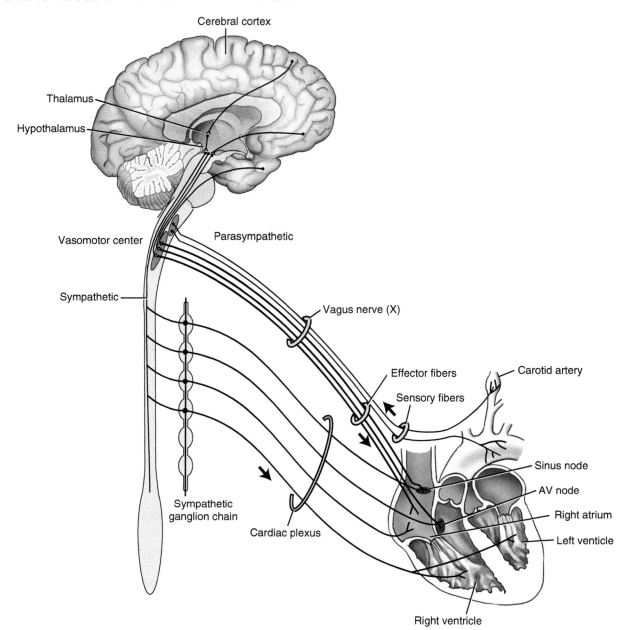

Figure 3-3: Autonomic nervous system innervation of the heart. Sympathetic nervous system (SNS) stimulation reaches the heart via the sympathetic chain, whereas the parasympathetic nervous system (PNS) acts through the vagus nerves (cranial nerve X). Both are controlled by the vasomotor center, which receives input from higher brain centers and the periphery.

The Systemic Circulation

The vascular system consists of a series of blood vessels that transport blood from the heart to the tissues and back:

- Arteries: The largest, most muscular and elastic vessels, which carry oxygen-rich blood away from the heart to the arterioles
- Arterioles: Small, thinner walled arteries with circular layers of smooth muscle, which constrict and relax to regulate blood flow to the tissues (e.g., during exercise, blood flow is reduced to some organs and increased to active muscle)
- Capillaries: Microscopic blood vessels with a single layer of epithelial cells for easy diffusion of gases and other nutrients to and from the tissues

- Venules: Small veins receiving deoxygenated blood and metabolic waste products from the capillaries
- Veins: Thinner, less muscular blood vessels than arteries; they return blood to the heart with the aid of flaplike valves and act as capacitance vessels, or blood reservoirs, when cardiac output needs are low

PHYSIOLOGY

It is important for physical therapists to understand the factors that contribute to normal functioning of the cardiovascular system in order to appreciate normal versus abnormal physiological

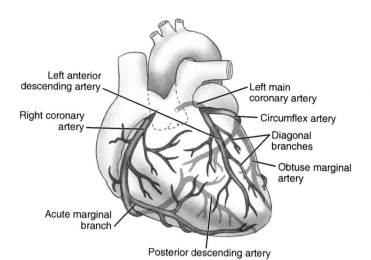

Left anterior descending artery

Left main coronary artery

Right coronary artery

Circumflex artery

Diagonal branches

Obtuse marginal artery

Acute marginal branch

Posterior descending artery

Figure 3-4: The coronary arteries.

TABLE 3-1: Common Distribution of the Coronary Arteries

Coronary Artery	Distribution
Right coronary artery (RCA)	Right atrium, SA node, posterior right ventricle, AV node, bundle of His, and usually serves as origin of the posterior descending artery (≈80%–90% of people)
Left main coronary artery (LMCA)	Bifurcates within 2–10 mm into the left anterior descending and circumflex arteries
Left anterior descending (LAD) artery	Anterior left ventricle, anterior intraventricular septum and adjacent right ventricle, portions of both bundle branches, and often the proximal inferior portion of both ventricles and apex
Circumflex (Cx) artery	Left atrium, lateral and inferior walls of the left ventricle, and sometimes serves as origin of the posterior descending artery (≈10%–20% of people)
Posterior descending artery (PDA)	Posterior intraventricular septum, plus at least half of the inferior left ventricle

AV, Atrioventricular; SA, sinoatrial.

responses, both at rest and during exercise, as well as their implications for physical therapy interventions.

Basic Functions of the Cardiovascular System

- Circulation of blood
- Delivery of oxygen, nutrients, and water
- Circulation of hormones
- Regulation of body temperature
- Removal of metabolites
- Maintenance of acid-base balance (pH)

Important Relationships

Cardiovascular function is determined by a number of factors and relationships.

- *Cardiac output* (CO, or $\dot{Q}$) is the volume of blood pumped by the heart per minute and is the product of heart rate (HR) and stroke volume (SV) (i.e., CO = HR × SV).
  - ▸ Normal resting HR is 60 to 100 bpm and stroke volume is usually 50 to 80 mL, being higher in the supine position than upright; thus, resting CO is typically 4 to 5 L/min.
  - ▸ Factors that influence HR and SV, and therefore CO, are listed in Table 3-2.
  - ▸ During exertion, HR increases proportional to intensity, and there is a modest increase in SV during low and moderate intensity upright exercise, which then plateaus. In the supine position, SV is nearly maximal at rest and changes very little with activity. A maximal CO of 15 to 22 L/min is seen in healthy sedentary individuals, whereas elite athletes can achieve values of 35 to 40 L/min.
- *Preload* is the resting tension or stretch on the myocardial cells, which correlates with the volume of blood in the ventricle at the end of filling (i.e., the end-diastolic volume, EDV).
  - ▸ An increase in preload, up to a certain point, results in an increase in stroke volume due to more powerful ventricular contraction, as shown in the various ventricular function curves depicted in Figure 3-5.
  - ▸ Preload increases with exercise training and also as a compensatory mechanism involving the kidneys in poorly functioning hearts.
- *Afterload* refers to the load or pressure against which the ventricle must work in order to eject blood, which corresponds to the pressure resisting the ejection of blood during systole (i.e., for the LV, it is initially the diastolic aortic blood pressure and then increases during systole with the rising blood pressure as ejection into the aorta continues).
  - ▸ An increase in afterload (e.g., systemic hypertension or aortic valve stenosis) effects a decrease in SV.
  - ▸ A decrease in afterload (e.g., during aerobic exercise or with vasodilator medications) leads to greater SV.
- *Contractility, or inotropic state* is the innate rate and intensity of force development during contraction.
  - ▸ An increase in the inotropic state, as occurs during exercise or with anxiety or fear, causes faster myocardial shortening at any given preload and afterload, as well as a greater degree of shortening and force development, so that a greater stroke volume of blood is ejected at any given preload or afterload.
  - ▸ Inotropism is affected by numerous factors, as listed in Box 3-1.
- *Ventricular compliance* refers to the ease with which the ventricle distends when it is filled with blood.
  - ▸ If compliance is reduced (i.e., the ventricle is stiffer, as in left ventricular hypertrophy), a given volume of filling will result in a higher end-diastolic pressure.
  - ▸ If compliance is increased (i.e., the ventricle is less stiff, like an overstretched deflated balloon, as occurs in left ventricular dilation and systolic failure), a given filling volume will effect a lower end-diastolic pressure.

TABLE 3-2: Factors That Influence Heart Rate and Stroke Volume and Therefore Cardiac Output

Factor	Influenced by:
Heart rate	The intrinsic rate of spontaneous pacemaker function
	The balance of SNS and PNS stimulation
	Levels of circulating catecholamines and other substances
Stroke volume	*Preload* ($\uparrow$ preload $\rightarrow$ $\uparrow$ SV), which is affected by:
	Active atrial contraction ($\rightarrow$ $\uparrow$ EDV by 10%–25%)
	Heart rate ($\uparrow$ HR $\rightarrow$ $\downarrow$ diastolic filling time $\rightarrow$ $\downarrow$ EDV and vice versa)
	Venous blood return ($\uparrow$ venous return $\rightarrow$ $\uparrow$ EDV and vice versa)
	Total blood volume, state of hydration ($\uparrow$ total blood volume $\rightarrow$ $\uparrow$ preload and vice versa)
	Ventricular compliance ($\uparrow$ compliance $\rightarrow$ $\uparrow$ preload and vice versa)
	Afterload ($\uparrow$ afterload $\rightarrow$ $\downarrow$ SV), which is affected by:
	Total peripheral resistance ($\uparrow$ TPR $\rightarrow$ $\uparrow$ afterload and vice versa)
	Aortic compliance ($\downarrow$ Ao compliance $\rightarrow$ $\uparrow$ afterload and vice versa)
	EDV and SV ($\uparrow$ EDV and SV $\rightarrow$ $\uparrow$ CO + afterload and vice versa)
	Blood viscosity ($\uparrow$ blood viscosity $\rightarrow$ $\uparrow$ afterload and vice versa)
	Presence of outflow obstruction (e.g., AS, HOCM) ($\uparrow$ outflow obstruction $\rightarrow$ $\uparrow$ afterload)
	Contractility ($\uparrow$ contractility $\rightarrow$ $\uparrow$ SV and vice versa), which is affected positively and negatively by multiple factors*

$\rightarrow$, Leads to; $\uparrow$, increased (more than normal); $\downarrow$, decreased (less than normal); Ao, aortic; AS, aortic stenosis; CO, cardiac output; EDV, end-diastolic volume; HOCM, hypertrophic obstructive cardiomyopathy; HR, heart rate; PNS, parasympathetic nervous system; SNS, sympathetic nervous system; SV, stroke volume; TPR, total peripheral resistance.
*See Box 3-1.

- *Ejection fraction (EF)* is the percentage of ventricular filling that is ejected with each heart beat (EF = SV/EDV).
- *Myocardial oxygen consumption* is the amount of oxygen the heart is using for energy, which is related to the HR and the *intramyocardial wall tension* or *stress* each ventricle must develop in order to eject blood against its afterload.
  - As ventricular pressure rises during systole, intramyocardial wall tension increases in direct proportion to pressure within the ventricle and its radius and in inverse proportion to its wall thickness (i.e., $T = P \times r/h$, as depicted in Figure 3-6). Thus, a heart challenged by excessive pressure or volume loads will increase its ventricular wall thickness (i.e., hypertrophy) as a compensatory mechanism to reduce wall stress and oxygen demand.
  - A commonly used indirect index of myocardial oxygen demand is the rate-pressure product (RPP), or double product, which is equal to the product of HR and systolic blood pressure (SBP) (i.e., RPP = HR $\times$ SBP). A healthy, physically fit individual will be able to achieve a higher RPP before the onset of discomfort or fatigue compared with a healthy, sedentary individual and particularly an individual with heart disease, who will likely develop signs and symptoms of exercise intolerance at a much lower RPP (see Chapter 6, page 282).
- *Arterial blood flow* through a tissue is determined by the difference between the arterial and venous pressures in the vessels supplying it and its vascular resistance. Some important points to keep in mind when considering blood flow through the coronary arteries are the following:

- *Coronary blood flow (CBF)* is determined by the difference between the aortic diastolic pressure, where the flow originates, and the pressure resisting flow through the small subendocardial vessels (i.e., the resistance within the vessels, as well as the diastolic pressure within the LV chamber).
  - ⊙ The presence of coronary disease increases coronary arterial resistance so that CBF is diminished distal to the lesion. Coronary spasm also has the same result.
  - ⊙ As the penetrating coronary arteries become smaller, their arterial pressure drops, so that the pressure gradient and blood flow are diminished, creating the risk of subendocardial ischemia.
  - ⊙ Higher ventricular filling pressures further reduce the pressure gradient determining CBF and increase the likelihood of subendocardial ischemia.
  - During systole CBF is interrupted by increased intraventricular pressures as well as compression of the penetrating coronary arteries by contracting myocardium. Thus, CBF occurs almost exclusively during the diastolic phase of the cardiac cycle.
- *Systemic arterial blood pressure* is a factor of cardiac output and total peripheral resistance (TPR). The determinants of cardiac output are described in Table 3-2. TPR is influenced by:
  - The caliber of the arterial bed (i.e., the degree of arteriolar contraction/relaxation and the presence of any atherosclerotic lesions)
  - The viscosity of the blood
  - The elasticity versus stiffness (i.e., compliance) of the arterial walls

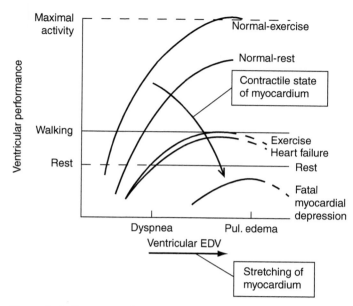

Figure 3-5: Illustration showing a number of ventricular function curves, which depict the relationship between ventricular end-diastolic volume (EDV) through stretching of the myocardium (i.e., the Frank-Starling law of the heart), and the effects of various states of contractility. Sympathetic stimulation, as normally occurs during exercise, increases stroke volume at a given level of ventricular filling, whereas heart failure results in lower stroke volume at a given level of ventricular filling, which may or may not increase during exercise. The dashed lines are the descending limbs of the ventricular performance curves, which are seen only rarely in patients. Levels of ventricular EDV associated with filling pressures that induce dyspnea and pulmonary edema are indicated, along with levels of ventricular performance required during rest, walking, and maximal activity. (Modified from Braunwald E, Ross J Jr, Sonnenblick EH. *Mechanisms of Contraction of the Normal and Failing Heart.* Boston: Little, Brown;1979:9.)

Cardiac Cycle

The cardiac cycle includes all of the events that occur within the heart during the relaxation and filling phase (i.e., diastole) and the pressure-development and ejection phase (i.e., systole). These events are illustrated in Figure 3-7 and occur as follows:

- During *diastole,* blood flows continuously into the RA and LA via the vena cavae and pulmonary veins, respectively, and continues its flow across the atrioventricular (AV) valves (i.e., the TV on the right and MV on the left) into the RV and LV, respectively.
- Spontaneously, the SA node initiates a wave of *depolarization* that travels through the atria and is depicted as the P wave on the electrocardiogram (ECG).
- Depolarization is followed by *atrial contraction,* the final event of diastole (note the *a* wave in Figure 3-7), which forces a last increment of blood into the ventricles and results in the RV and LV end-diastolic volumes and pressures.
- The wave of depolarization then traverses the AV node, bundle of His, bundle branches, and Purkinje fibers to excite the RV

BOX 3-1: Factors That Influence Contractility/Inotropism

Positive Inotropic Influence	Negative Inotropic Influence
• ↑ Sympathetic tone	• β-Blockers
• ↑ Endogenous catecholamines	• Calcium antagonists
• Digitalis	• Barbiturates
• Sympathetic amines	• Acidosis
• ↑ Heart rate	• Hypoxia
• Glucagon	• General anesthesia
• Angiotensin	• Antiarrhythmic agents
• Aldactone	• Heart failure
• Corticosteroids	• ↓ Functional ventricular muscle mass
• Hyperthyroidism	• ↓ Myocardial oxygen supply: demand
• Serotonin	• Circulating myocardial depressant factors

↑, Increased (higher than normal); ↓, decreased (lower than normal).

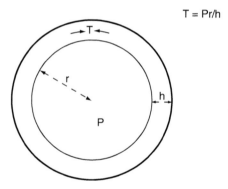

Figure 3-6: The determinants of circumferential wall tension: Wall tension (T) is a factor of pressure (P) and radius (r) divided by ventricular wall thickness (h). (From Irwin S, Tecklin JS. *Cardiopulmonary Physical Therapy.* 3rd ed. St. Louis: Mosby; 1995.)

and LV muscle fibers, causing *left, then right, ventricular contraction* (normally 20 to 30 msec apart).
- With the onset of contraction, the respective *ventricular pressures* begin to *rise* so that they exceed the pressures in the atria and force *MV and TV closure.*
- Now all of the heart valves are closed and there is a fixed volume of blood in each ventricle. Ventricular contraction continues against this fixed volume (*isovolumic contraction*) until the pressures within the ventricles exceed that in the aorta on the left and in the pulmonary artery (PA) on the right.
- At this point, the *ejection valves* (i.e., the AoV on the left and PV on the right) *open* and *ejection of blood* begins. Additional ventricular contraction results in ejection of the final stroke volume for that heart beat.

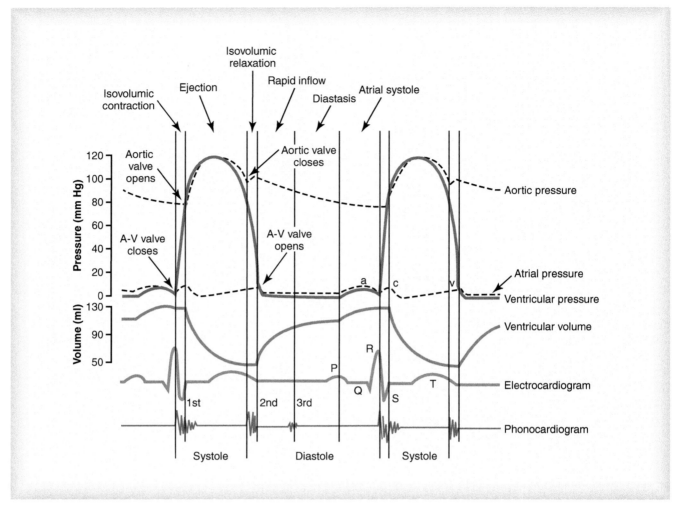

Figure 3-7: The events of the cardiac cycle, showing changes in left atrial pressure, left ventricular pressure, aortic pressure, and ventricular volume in relation to the electrocardiogram; and heart sounds via a phonocardiogram. (From Guyton AC, Hall JE. *Textbook of Medical Physiology.* 11th ed. Philadelphia: Saunders; 2006.)

- Ventricular contraction is followed by *relaxation* with *repolarization* of the myocardial cells and diminution of ventricular pressures. When the ventricular pressures fall below that in the aorta and PA, the *ejection valves close.*
- Further decline in ventricular pressures *(isovolumic relaxation)* to the level of the atrial pressures results in *MV and TV opening* so that the *diastolic filling phase* begins again.
- The atria, which have been filling with blood throughout the ejection phase, initially empty rapidly into the ventricles *(early rapid passive filling).* Continued slower ventricular filling (diastasis) occurs until the next atrial contraction occurs *(active filling).*

Heart Sounds

Usually, only two heart sounds can be auscultated, but on occasion a third and/or fourth heart sound may be present. In addition, extra sounds are sometimes heard (see Chapter 6, page 248).

▸ S_1: The first heart sound is associated with MV and TV closure and corresponds with the onset of ventricular systole; separate MV (M_1) and TV (T_1) sounds can sometimes be appreciated, particularly during expiration.

▸ S_2: The second heart sound is associated with AoV and PV closure and corresponds with the start of ventricular diastole; splitting of S_2 is common, especially during inspiration with the AoV component (A_2) preceding the PV component (P_2).

▸ S_3: The third heart sound is associated with early rapid passive filling of the ventricles immediately after the MV and TV open and is called a "ventricular gallop"; it is most frequently associated with heart failure although it may occur normally in children and young adults up to age 40 years.

▸ S_4: The fourth heart sound is associated with active ventricular filling due to atrial contraction and is called an "atrial gallop"; it is often heard in hypertension with LV hypertrophy, ischemic heart disease, and acute myocardial infarction.

▸ *Adventitious heart sounds:* Additional sounds may be heard during the cardiac cycle, including murmurs, clicks, snaps, and friction rubs, which are associated with increased turbulence of blood flow or abnormal movement or inflammation of the valves or pericardium.

Exercise Physiology

During exercise the cardiovascular system is challenged to deliver increasing amounts of blood (i.e., cardiac output) to meet the metabolic demands of exercising muscles. It accomplishes this by tapping into the body's cardiovascular reserves through increases in HR and SV (see Table 3-2).

- As soon as exercise begins, or even in anticipation of the exercise, HR increases, mostly because of withdrawal of PNS stimulation. As exercise becomes more intense, further increases in HR are produced by SNS stimulation, reflex stimulation of pulmonary stretch receptors, and increasing levels of circulating catecholamines. During very strenuous exercise, HR can reach its maximal level, in beats per minute (bpm), of approximately 220 minus the individual's age.
- Augmented stroke volume also contributes to increased cardiac output and is achieved mainly by enhanced venous return (i.e., increased preload) and more forceful ventricular contractions (i.e., increased contractility or inotropy).
- The ability of the body to increase blood flow to exercising muscles is also facilitated by the redistribution of cardiac output away from the majority of organs that are not necessary to exercise performance (e.g., kidneys, gut, and nonexercising muscle) to those that are (heart, brain, skin [for body cooling], and exercising muscle).
- Different types of exercise produce different physiological responses, as discussed on page 263. Briefly, dynamic, or isotonic, exercise creates a volume load on the heart, which results in significant increases in cardiac output and oxygen consumption and a fall in systemic vascular resistance, whereas isometric and intense resistance exercise create a pressure load on the heart, which causes significant increases in systemic vascular resistance and blood pressure but minimal increases in cardiac output and oxygen consumption. Less intense resistance exercise can produce both volume and pressure loads on the heart, depending on intensity. Most activities contain elements of all three types of exercise.
- With regular exercise training, cardiovascular (and respiratory) function improves in efficiency, leading to increased maximal cardiac output and oxygen consumption ($\dot{V}O_{2 \, max}$), as well as enhancements in a number of other parameters (see page 309). However, these improvements are quickly lost if training is halted.

Effects of Aging

As with the respiratory system, many of the changes that were once attributed to the normal aging process are now known to be effects of deconditioning and can be retarded or reversed with exercise conditioning. Nevertheless, there are physical and functional changes that do occur with normal aging.

- The blood vessels lose elasticity, becoming thicker and stiffer, and therefore blood pressure rises.
- The left ventricle becomes more hypertrophied and less compliant, which leads to slower ventricular filling.
- The heart valves become thickened and calcified, which may cause abnormal function (i.e., stenosis or incompetence).
- The conduction system exhibits degenerative changes, which reduces HR and increases the incidence of arrhythmias.

- The baroreceptors become less sensitive, leading to orthostatic hypotension.
- Adrenergic responsiveness declines, resulting in lower exercise and maximal HRs.
- Changes within the myocardial cells affecting energetics lead to slower force development and diastolic dysfunction.
- The combination of cardiovascular and respiratory changes that occur with aging results in a decline in $\dot{V}O_{2max}$ and higher relative stress for submaximal activities.

◻ 3.2 EVALUATION OF CARDIAC FUNCTION

Although physical therapists rarely participate in or read the data produced by most of the diagnostic tests and procedures described in this section, we are frequently challenged to interpret the results of these investigations and determine the implications for our patients. By appreciating the information presented in a patient's chart, we can develop a fairly accurate perception of the patient's status and anticipate probable or possible physiological responses to our interventions even before we begin our assessment. At the least, we should be able to determine when caution is particularly warranted.

SIGNS AND SYMPTOMS OF CARDIOVASCULAR DISEASE

In general, the first information that is presented in a patient's medical history is a description of his/her clinical complaints. Table 3-3 tabulates the most common patient complaints and their cardiovascular causes. There may be other explanations for some of these complaints, including pulmonary disease (see Chapter 2 [Pulmonology], page 10) or other problems, as presented in Chapter 6 (see Figure 6-5, page 233).

PHYSICIAN'S PHYSICAL EXAMINATION

The history and physical examination section of a patient's chart is a valuable source of important information relating to the patient's status and level of function. The relevant data and their implications are discussed in Chapter 6 (see Table 6-3, page 224).

BLOOD PRESSURE MEASUREMENT

Arterial blood pressure is a factor of cardiac output and peripheral vascular resistance and therefore provides important information about cardiovascular function (see Chapter 6, page 275). Unfortunately, BP measurements are highly prone to error, both at rest and during exercise, due to faulty equipment and improper technique, as well as a high degree of intrinsic variability (see page 275).

- Arterial blood pressure is usually measured indirectly with a sphygmomanometer. In critical care units it may be obtained directly by means of an indwelling arterial catheter.
- Ambulatory BP monitoring involves automatic recordings of BP, usually every 15 to 30 minutes, over a 24-hour period or longer, during which the individual performs her/his usual daily activities, including sleep. It is particularly useful in

TABLE 3-3: Signs and Symptoms of Cardiovascular Diseases

Sign or Symptom	Cardiovascular Causes
Chest pain or discomfort	Mismatch between myocardial oxygen supply and demand (due to coronary disease, LV hypertrophy, LV outflow obstruction, coronary spasm, microvascular angina), autonomic dysfunction, MV prolapse
Claudication	Peripheral arterial disease with mismatch between peripheral O_2 supply and demand
Clubbing of digits	Right-to-left shunting in congenital heart disease
Cough	Acute pulmonary edema, MS
Cyanosis	Right-to-left shunting in congenital heart disease, significant ↓ cardiac output
Dizziness	Inadequate cardiac output resulting in ↓ perfusion of the brain (due to LV dysfunction, LV outlet obstruction, arrhythmias, blood pooling in lower extremities)
Dyspnea, SOB	↑ Pulmonary venous pressure caused by LV diastolic or systolic dysfunction (due to coronary ischemia, hypertension, valvular disease, cardiomyopathy), peripheral arterial disease with lactic acidosis
Edema	↑ Systemic venous pressure due to ↑ RA pressure (e.g., LV failure, MS, cor pulmonale, TS, TR, constrictive pericarditis)
Fatigue	Low cardiac output (due to LV dysfunction, LV outlet obstruction, arrhythmias), drugs
Abnormal funduscopic examination	Hypertension, diabetes mellitus, sometimes infective endocarditis
Hemoptysis	Acute pulmonary edema, MS
Hypotension	↓ Cardiac output, vasodilation
Jugular venous distension	↑ Systemic venous pressure caused by ↑ RA pressure (see preceding entry for Edema)
Nocturia	CHF with peripheral edema
Orthopnea	In CHF, SOB when lying flat due to ↑ pulmonary venous pressure caused by ↑ venous return to heart, which is not able to handle ↑ workload
Palpitations	Arrhythmias
Paroxysmal nocturnal dyspnea	In CHF, sudden onset of SOB that awakens patient at night because of ↑ pulmonary pressures caused by the gradual reabsorption of edema fluid from the LEs (which are no longer dependent), resulting in ↑ venous return to heart, which is not able to handle ↑ workload
Pulmonary rales	CHF, exercise-induced ↑ pulmonary pressures
Abnormal pulse rate or rhythm	Arrhythmias
S_3, S_4	*
SOB	See preceding entry for Dyspnea
Syncope	Profoundly ↓ cardiac output (see preceding entry for Dizziness)
Weakness	See preceding entry for Fatigue

↑, Increased (more than normal); ↓, decreased (less than normal); CHF, congestive heart failure; LE, lower extremity; LV, left ventricle; MS, mitral stenosis; MV, mitral valve; O_2, oxygen; RA, right atrium; S_3, third heart sound; S_4, fourth heart sound; SOB, shortness of breath; TS, tricuspid stenosis; TR, tricuspid regurgitation.
*See earlier section on Heart Sounds.

identifying "white coat" hypertension; is a strong predictor of left ventricular hypertrophy, cardiac function, and secondary complications; and is a very strong predictor of future cardiovascular events.[30,31]

CHEST X-RAY

As in pulmonology, the chest x-ray is the most common radiographic study performed for patients with cardiac disease. Because of the low density of the air-filled lungs, it is possible to determine the size of the heart, its various chambers, and the major blood vessels on the basis of a standard posteroanterior chest x-ray (Figure 3-8).

- The size of the heart is usually determined by measuring the transverse diameter of the heart relative to the transverse thoracic diameter from a posteroanterior (PA) chest film taken at full inspiration, as shown in Figure 3-9. Normally, the ratio is usually between 0.45 and 0.50.
- Portable chest x-rays, which are typically anteroposterior (AP) views, produce greater magnification of the cardiac structures and result in an apparent 10% to 20% increase in the transverse cardiac diameter and thus should be interpreted with caution.

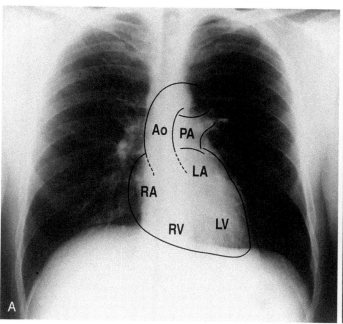
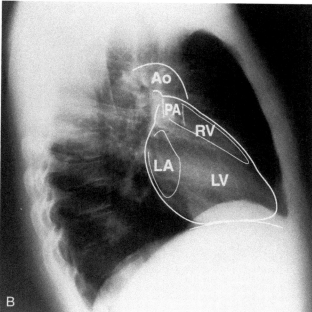

Figure 3-8: Schematic illustration of the parts of the heart, the outlines of which can be identified on a routine chest radiograph. **A,** Posteroanterior view. **B,** Lateral view. Ao, aorta; LA, left atrium; LV, left ventricle; PA, pulmonary artery; RA, right atrium; RV, right ventricle. (From Andreoli TE, Carpenter CCJ, Griggs RC, Benjamin IJ, editors. *Andreoli and Carpenter's Cecil Essentials of Medicine.* 7th ed. Philadelphia: Saunders; 2007.)

- Chest radiographs also depict the pulmonary vasculature, especially on the right, and can reveal increased pulmonary blood flow, pulmonary hypertension, and pulmonary (vascular) congestion due to impaired pump function of the left ventricle.
- Prominence of particular parts of the cardiac silhouette suggests structural enlargement.

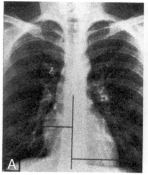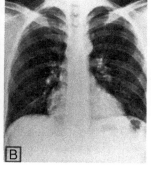

Figure 3-9: Measurement of the transverse cardiac diameter on a posteroanterior inspiration chest radiograph **(A),** using the spinous processes to draw the vertical reference point and the longest distances to the right and left heart borders. The normal value of 50% is not valid in an expiration film **(B),** in which the heart is raised by the diaphragm to a more horizontal position. (From Harrington DP. Chest radiograph in the evaluation of acquired cardiac disease. In Kloner RA, editor: *The Guide to Cardiology.* 2nd ed. New York: Le Jacq Communications; 1990.)

ELECTROCARDIOGRAPHY

An electrocardiogram (ECG) records the electrical activity of the heart on a graph of voltage versus time. It can be obtained with a single lead, as in a rhythm strip, or with multiple leads, as in the standard 12-lead ECG, which provides 12 different "views" of the heart's electrical activity.

Rhythm Strips

An ECG recording obtained from one to three leads can be acquired via hard wiring (where wires connect the patient to the monitor) or telemetry (where a radiotelemeter worn by the patient transmits the ECG signal to a monitor).

- Rhythm strips are used mainly to monitor HR and rhythm and are commonly acquired in intensive care units and step-down or transitional care units, as well as in cardiac and pulmonary rehabilitation programs.
- A rhythm strip showing normal sinus rhythm is depicted in Figure 3-10.
- Information related to ECG lead setups and basic interpretation of rhythm strips is presented in Chapter 6 (see page 264).

Twelve-lead ECG

The electrical activity of the heart is usually recorded from 12 specific leads, as shown in Figure 3-11, to provide a "map" of the electrical voltages created by the different areas of the heart.

- Lead placement for a 12-lead ECG is depicted in Figure 3-12.
- Information that can be obtained from a 12-lead ECG, in addition to rate and rhythm, includes the following:
  - ▶ The electrical axis of the heart

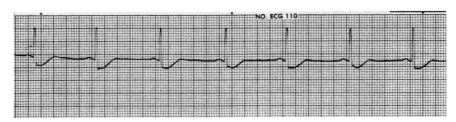

Figure 3-10: Rhythm strip showing normal sinus rhythm. Abnormal ST-T changes are also present.

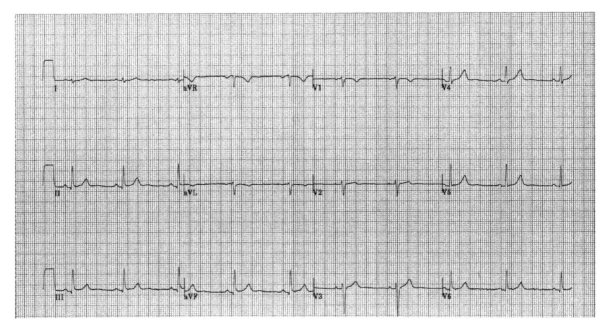

Figure 3-11: A normal 12-lead electrocardiogram. Note the progression of the QRS waves across the precordium (leads V_{1-6}) as the deflections transition from predominantly negative to totally positive. (Courtesy of Ellen Hillegass.)

▶ The presence of specific abnormalities (see Chapter 6, page 232):
  ⊙ Left ventricular hypertrophy (LVH)
  ⊙ Right ventricular hypertrophy (RVH)
  ⊙ Left atrial abnormality
  ⊙ Right atrial abnormality
  ⊙ Left bundle branch block (LBBB)
  ⊙ Right bundle branch block (RBBB)
  ⊙ Myocardial ischemia (ST segment depression, shown in Figure 3-13)
  ⊙ Myocardial infarction (MI) (see Figure 6-5 on page 233)

Ambulatory/Holter Monitoring

Ambulatory or dynamic ECG monitoring permits the recording of a patient's ECG while he carries on his usual daily activities. It can be performed either as a continuous 24- to 48-hour recording of one or more ECG leads or as an intermittent event monitor, worn for several days to weeks at a time, that the patient activates when he/she experiences a significant arrhythmia, allowing occasional events to be captured. It is useful for the diagnosis of cardiac arrhythmias and myocardial ischemia as correlated with patient symptoms (see Figure 3-13), the evaluation of efficacy of antiar-rhythmic drug therapy, and the assessment of artificial pacemaker function.

By knowing the type(s) of arrhythmias a patient demonstrates on ambulatory monitoring and their frequency and whether any therapeutic interventions have been instituted, the therapist may be able to anticipate the rhythm changes that may occur during activity and can inform the physician about any changes in the patient's status and the effectiveness of treatment.

Signal-averaged ECG

The signal-averaged ECG (also called a high-resolution ECG or late potential study) averages 100 to 200 QRS complexes obtained from orthogonal XYZ ECG leads (a three-dimensional system depicting the horizontal [x] axis, frontal [y] axis, and sagittal or anteroposterior [z] axis) in order to improve signal-to-noise ratio and identify reproducible, low-amplitude, high-frequency potentials at the end of the QRS complex (ventricular late potentials).

• These potentials are predictive of ventricular tachycardia in patients with previous myocardial infarction, independent of left ventricular function and other risk predictors.

• Other uses include identification of patients whose unexplained syncope may be caused by tachycardia and detection of P wave abnormalities that are predictive of atrial fibrillation and other atrial arrhythmias and their response to drugs.

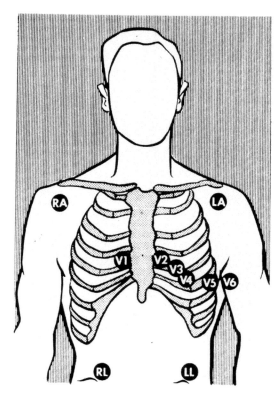

Figure 3-12: Placement of electrodes for the standard 12-lead electrocardiogram (ECG), in this case for exercise testing. For a standard 12-lead ECG, the RA electrode would be attached to the right arm, the LA electrode on the left arm, the RL electrode on the right leg, and the LL electrode on the left leg. (Modified from Wilson PK, Fardy PS, Froelicher VF. *Cardiac Rehabilitation, Adult Fitness, and Exercise Testing.* Philadelphia: Lea & Febiger;1981:261.)

Spatial Vectorcardiography

A modified ECG that records the electrical activity of the heart, using the three-dimensional orthogonal lead system, creates a vectorcardiogram, depicting the sum of spatial orientation and magnitude of force at any instant of time.

- Using a special camera and instant film, a vectorcardiogram produces four different vector loops instead of a simple graph of voltage versus time: a small atrial *P loop,* a large ventricular depolarization *QRS loop,* a smaller ventricular repolarization *ST-T loop,* and a very small *U loop.*
- A vectorcardiogram is particularly informative for patients with right ventricular hypertrophy and myocardial infarction involving the inferior or posterior wall of the left ventricle.

EXERCISE AND STRESS TESTING

Stress testing involves the application of physiological stresses to increase the workload of the heart as a means of documenting the cardiovascular, and sometimes respiratory, responses. The most common modalities are exercise and pharmacologic stress. In addition, a variety of field tests, usually based on walking, can be used to screen groups of people and to assess functional status in patients with cardiovascular disease.

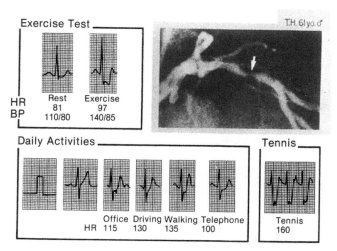

Figure 3-13: Myocardial ischemia induced by an exercise stress test: 4-mm ST segment depression at stage 2 of a Bruce protocol treadmill test. Ambulatory ECGs from lead V_5 also show ischemic changes during a number of activities, especially while playing tennis, during which he was asymptomatic. Coronary angiography revealed severe left anterior descending stenosis *(see arrow).* (From Nabel EG, Rocco MB, Selwyn AB. Characteristics and significance of ischemia detected by ambulatory electrocardiographic monitoring. *Circulation.* 1987;75:V74-V83, Used with permission of the American Heart Association, Inc.)

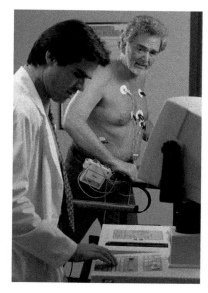

Figure 3-14: A patient peforming a treadmill exercise stress test with 12-lead ECG monitoring. (From Getty Images.)

Exercise Testing

Graded exercise testing, typically using a treadmill or bicycle ergometer, is commonly performed in order to evaluate the physiological responses to increasing demands on the body (Figure 3-14).

- The parameters most commonly monitored during exercise testing include the following:
  - ▶ Heart rate
  - ▶ Blood pressure

- 12-lead ECG
- Signs and symptoms
- Rating of perceived exertion
- The purpose of exercise testing may be to assess any of the following:
  - Functional work capacity
  - Possible presence and extent of coronary disease
  - Prognosis
  - Effects of therapeutic interventions
- In addition, ancillary techniques such as radionuclide imaging and echocardiography can provide supplementary information and augment the diagnostic value of exercise testing in selected patients, particularly women, for whom standard exercise testing is of limited value.
- The energy expenditure associated with the various stages of some common exercise test protocols is depicted in Figure 3-15. Note that stage 1 of the standard Bruce protocol begins at 1.7 mph at a 10% grade; the two stages that appear in the figure (1.7 mph at 0% grade and 1.7 mph at 5% grade) are part of the modified Bruce protocol, which is often used in patients with limited exercise tolerance due to cardiopulmonary dysfunction or other chronic medical problems.

- The information obtained from exercise testing is extremely valuable to physical therapists (PTs), as it documents the patient's exercise tolerance and physiological responses to increasing exercise and gives a good indication of how well the patient will tolerate vigorous rehabilitation activities (for norms, see page 284). Testing data may also reveal the factor(s) that limit(s) exercise tolerance.
- Exercise testing parameters that are associated with an adverse prognosis and multivessel coronary artery disease (CAD) include the following:
  - Exercise capacity less than 6 metabolic equivalents (METs)
  - Maximal SBP less than 140 mm Hg
  - Sustained drop in SBP of at least 10 mm Hg or to below resting level
  - ST segment depression of at least 2 mm, downsloping ST segment, and ST depression starting at less than 6 METs, involving five or more leads, or persisting for at least 5 minutes into recovery
  - Exercise-induced ST elevation (excluding lead aVR)
  - Angina pectoris at low workloads
  - Reproducible sustained (>30 sec) or symptomatic ventricular tachycardia

Functional class	Clinical status	O₂ cost mL/kg/min	METS	Bicycle ergometer	Bruce (3-min stages) mph	Bruce %GR	Balke-Ware %GR at 3.3 mph 1-min stages	Ellestad (3/2/3 min stages) mph	Ellestad %GR	McHenry mph	McHenry %GR	Naughton (2-min stages 3.0 mph) %GR	METS
				1 watt = 6 kpds	5.5	2.0							
Normal and I	Healthy, dependent on age, activity	56.0	16	For 70 kg body weight, kpds	5.0	18		6	15			32.5	16
		52.5	15									30.0	15
		49.0	14	1500			26 25	5	15	3.3	21	27.5	14
		45.5	13		4.2	16	24 23			3.3	18	25.0	13
		42.0	12	1350			22 21					22.5	12
		38.5	11	1200			20 19 18	5	10	3.3	15	20.0	11
	Sedentary healthy	35.0	10	1050			17 16					17.5	10
		31.5	9	900	3.4	14	15 14 13	4	10			15.0	9
		28.0	8	750			12 11			3.3	12	12.5	8
	Limited	24.5	7		2.5	12	10 9	3	10	3.3	9	10.0	7
II		21.0	6	600			8 7 6					7.5	6
	Symptomatic	17.5	5	450	1.7	10	5 4	1.7	10	3.3	6	5.0	5
		14.0	4	300			3 2					2.5	4
III		10.5	3	150	1.7	5	1			2.0	3	0.0	3
		7.0	2		1.7	0							2
IV		3.5	1										1

Figure 3-15: Common exercise testing protocols, their stages, and the predicted oxygen cost of each stage. Stage 1 of the conventional Bruce treadmill protocol starts at 1.7 mph and a 10% grade; the modified Bruce protocol may start at 1.7 mph and a 0% or 5% grade, as shown, to allow low-level testing of symptomatic and limited patients. (From Fuster V, Alexander RW, O'Rourke RA. *Hurst's The Heart.* 11th ed. New York: McGraw-Hill; 2004.)

Cardiopulmonary Exercise Testing

Cardiopulmonary exercise testing incorporates the analysis of respiratory gases, including the measurement of oxygen uptake ($\dot{V}_{O_2}$), carbon dioxide production ($\dot{V}_{CO_2}$), and other ventilatory parameters during exercise testing and is described in Chapter 2 (see page 18).

Walk Tests

As presented in Chapter 2 (see page 19), walk tests can be used to measure functional status, monitor treatment effectiveness, and establish prognosis in patients with limited activity levels and exercise tolerance.

- Standardization of testing procedures is critical for optimal reliability, sensitivity, and interpretation of walk test results. The procedures for performing the 6-minute walk test are described in Chapter 6 (refer to page 257).
- The 6-minute walk test has been studied in patients with heart failure, pacemakers, and peripheral arterial disease, among others.[27]
  - ▸ In patients with heart failure, strong correlations have been reported between distance walked and $\dot{V}_{O_{2max}}$ and exercise ergometry performance, and moderate to strong associations have been made with the New York Heart Association (NYHA) functional classifications (see Chapter 6, Table 6-2 on page 223), oxygen cost, and various activity scales and questionnaires. In addition, distance walked (≤ 300 m) may be used to identify patients at high risk for increased morbidity and mortality within 3 months to 1 year.
  - ▸ In patients with peripheral arterial disease, distance walked has been correlated with oxygen cost and exercise ergometry performance.
  - ▸ In patients with pacemakers, the distance walked has been demonstrated to discriminate between pacing modes and rates, and improvements in distance walked have been related to diminished shortness of breath.

Pharmacologic Stress Testing

When patients are unable to tolerate an adequate level of exercise stress (e.g., because of peripheral vascular, neurologic, chronic respiratory, orthopedic, or other disease), pharmacologic agents can be used as an alternative means of challenging the cardiovascular system to aid in noninvasive diagnosis and functional evaluation of patients with known or suspected CAD. As with exercise testing, the physiological responses of the patient are monitored to determine the presence and degree of dysfunction.

- The agents currently used include dipyridamole and adenosine, which produce vasodilator stress that results in maximal or near-maximal coronary blood flow increases, and dobutamine, which induces inotropic stress and is usually reserved for patients with asthma or chronic obstructive pulmonary disease or those who have ingested caffeine before testing. Sometimes a combination of dobutamine and atropine is used.[11]
- Pharmacologic stress testing is usually combined with echocardiography or radionuclide studies (e.g., myocardial perfusion SPECT [single-photon emission computed tomography]),[13a] or it may be applied during cardiac catheterization.

ECHOCARDIOGRAPHY

Echocardiography uses inaudible, variable-frequency sound waves to depict cardiac structures and function, similar to ultrasound used for fetal imaging. In its simplest form, the ultrasonic beam produces a one-dimensional view of the heart, where the amplitude of the signals varies with the density of elements encountered. These signals are displayed as dots, the brightness of which is proportional to the intensity of the reflected energy (B-mode echo).

M-mode Echocardiography

If repetitive B-mode scan lines are produced and swept across the screen over time, the movement of the heart can be obtained as a time-motion (or M-mode) recording, providing dynamic cardiac images, showing time on the x axis, distance on the y axis, and intensity of echocardiography on the z axis, as depicted in Figure 3-16. The ECG is recorded for timing of events.

- M-mode echo serves mostly a secondary role in echocardiography, having been supplanted by two-dimensional and Doppler technology. However, its more precise measurements may be used to calculate the LV dimensions and wall thicknesses, comparing end-diastole with end-systole, especially for the evaluation of pericardial effusions, mitral valve disease, and hypertrophic obstructive cardiomyopathy.
- The normal adult ranges for echocardiographic measurements are listed in Table 3-4. Higher chamber values indicate dilation due to a higher volume load, whereas greater wall thicknesses indicate hypertrophy and thus decreased compliance.

Two-dimensional Echocardiography/Sector Scanning

When a B-mode echocardiographic tracing is rapidly and sequentially scanned across a sector field at a rate sufficiently fast to provide a continuous picture, two-dimensional images are produced, as shown in Figure 3-17. These images, when viewed on a monitor, provide dynamic images of cardiac motion and are recorded on videotape or converted to digital format.

- Different views of the heart structures and chambers can be produced by varying the transducer position and orientation to scan the different planes of the heart. The four standard views are the parasternal long-axis, parasternal short-axis, apical four-chamber, and apical two-chamber.
- Common clinical uses of two-dimensional echocardiography include evaluation of LV function, including end-systolic volume (ESV), end-diastolic volume (EDV), and ejection fraction (EF); calculation of LV mass; assessment of wall motion; detection of complications after acute MI; evaluation of valve structure and motion; identification of vegetations in infective endocarditis; detection of intracavitary masses; and assessment of congenital heart defects.
- Many abnormalities noted on echocardiography have direct implications for physical therapy because of possible exercise intolerance. For example, patients with an EF less than 40%, large areas of abnormal wall motion, significant valvular abnormalities, and increased LV mass are likely to exhibit abnormal physiological responses to activity and require treatment modifications.

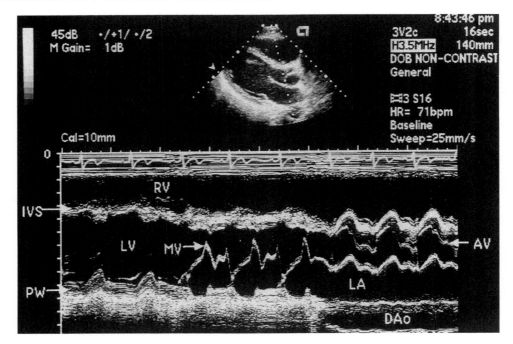

Figure 3-16: A normal M-mode echocardiogram in which the M-mode beam is swept from the aortic valve through the mitral valve and to the level of the papillary muscles. AV, Aortic valve; Dao, descending aorta; LA, left atrium; LV, left ventricle; MV, mitral valve; RV, right ventricle. (From Zipes DP, Libby P, Bonow RO, Braunwald E, editors. *Braunwald's Heart Disease: A Textbook of Cardiovascular Medicine.* 7th ed. Philadelphia: Saunders; 2005.)

TABLE 3-4: Normal Adult Values for M-mode Echocardiographic Measurements

Structure	Range
RV dimension: flat	7–23 mm
RV dimension: left lateral	9–26 mm
LV dimension: flat	37–56 mm
LV internal dimension: left lateral	35–57 mm
Posterior LV wall thickness	6–11 mm
Posterior wall amplitude	9–14 mm
IVS thickness	6–11 mm
Mid-IVS amplitude	3–8 mm
Apical IVS amplitude	5–12 mm
Left atrial dimension	19–40 mm
Aortic root dimension	20–37 mm
Aortic cusp separation	15–26 mm
Fractional shortening	34%–44%

From Armstrong WF: Echocardiography. *In* Zipes DP, Libby P, Bonow RO, Braunwald E (eds.): *Heart Disease: A Textbook of Cardiovascular Medicine,* 7th ed. Philadelphia, Saunders, 2005.
IVS, Intraventricular septum; LV, left ventricular; RV, right ventricular.

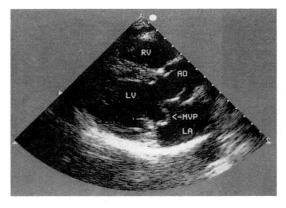

Figure 3-17: A two-dimensional echocardiogram (parasternal long-axis view) showing mitral regurgitation due to mitral valve prolapse in systole. Note the open cusps of the aortic valve and the backward prolapsing of the posterior leaflet of the mitral valve (MVP) into the left atrium. Ao, aorta; LA, left atrium; LV, left ventricle; RV, right ventricle. (From Forbes CD, Jackson WF. *Color Atlas and Text of Clinical Medicine.* 3rd ed. Philadelphia: Mosby; 2003.)

been of particular value in providing quantitative precision in unusually shaped ventricles and accurate anatomic description of complex anatomy such as complex congenital heart disease.

Three-dimensional Echocardiography

Three-dimensional images can be obtained in several different ways, all of which can be displayed as two-dimensional tomographic cuts with three-dimensional spatial orientation, as wire runs, or with surface rendering. Three-dimensional images have

Doppler Echocardiography

Doppler echocardiography uses ultrasound to determine the velocity and direction of blood flow by measuring the change in frequency produced when sound waves are reflected from red

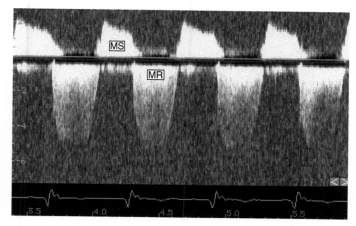

Figure 3-18: Continuous wave Doppler study through the mitral valve in combined mitral stenosis (MS) and mitral regurgitation (MR). (From Smiseth OA, Bjørnerheim R, Nitter-Hauge S. Noninvasive assessment of valvular function. In Crawford MH, DiMarco JP, Paulus WJ, editors. *Cardiology.* 2nd ed. Edinburgh; Mosby; 2002.)

blood cells. Doppler data can be displayed as a velocity profile, often called spectral Doppler, or a color flow image.

- Doppler echocardiography can be used to measure cardiac output from the aorta and pulmonary artery, blood flow through heart valves, including the regurgitant volume through an incompetent valve (as shown in Figure 3-18), valve orifice cross-sectional area, and peak velocity of blood flow across the valves, including the pressure gradient across a stenotic valve.
- Color flow mapping depicts the direction of blood flow and therefore provides documentation of valvular incompetence with regurgitant flow, and is often used intraoperatively to assess the adequacy of surgical reconstruction.
- Tissue Doppler imaging uses Doppler principles to measure the velocity of myocardial motion.
- Patients with significant valve disease often exhibit abnormal responses to activity and have reduced exercise tolerance. Those with moderately severe aortic stenosis and obstructive hypertrophic cardiomyopathy affecting the aortic valve (>75-mm Hg gradient) are usually restricted to only mild exertion because of increased risk of syncope and sudden death.

Transesophageal Echocardiography

High-quality two-dimensional and Doppler images of the heart and nearby structures can be obtained by placing a miniaturized transducer with an array of ultrasound crystals at the end of a flexible endoscope and inserting it in the esophagus. Image resolution is improved over standard transthoracic echocardiography because of the proximity of the heart and aorta to the esophagus and the absence of air-filled lung tissue in the imaging window; however, sedation or anesthesia is required. Transesophageal echocardiography is particularly useful in assessing prosthetic valve function, infective endocarditis and its complications (e.g., valvular vegetations or chordal rupture), and aortic dissections. It is also used to monitor cardiac function during heart surgery.

Contrast Echocardiography

The use of microbubbles as an ultrasonic contrast agent is based the fact that the gas-fluid interface is a potent reflector of ultrasonic waves. Initially, room air microbubbles served as the contrast agent, but newer contrast agents using a dense, high molecular weight gas surrounded by a shell or surface-modifying agent have been developed.

- Room air microbubbles injected into the venous system are too large to pass through the pulmonary capillary bed, and thus their appearance in the left side of the heart can be used to diagnose pathological intracardiac shunts.
- Intravenous injection of stabilized solutions of microbubbles that are small enough to traverse the pulmonary capillary bed in high concentration allows for imaging of both sides of the heart.
- Contrast echo can be used to enhance the application of stress echo as well as Doppler recording of flow abnormalities.

Intravascular Ultrasound

An ultraminiaturized ultrasound transducer can be incorporated into the tip of an intracardiac catheter and inserted into the cardiac chambers, epicardial coronary arteries, or other blood vessels. Most commonly, it is used to provide high-resolution views of intracardiac anatomy and the morphology and composition of coronary lesions, which can assist in determining the most appropriate interventional technique (e.g., angioplasty for intimal/medial hypertrophy vs. atherectomy for calcified lesions). This technique is particularly useful in identifying diffuse disease without focal lesions, diagnosing aortic dissection, and determining the success of interventions such as stent deployment.

Stress Echocardiography

Echocardiography during or immediately following stress testing is effective in diagnosing coronary disease, due its ability to detect stress-induced regional ischemia and abnormalities of contraction resulting in impaired wall motion. Stress echo is especially useful for detecting ischemia in women and other situations in which exercise ECG may be inaccurate or falsely positive (e.g., left ventricular hypertrophy and chronic digitalis therapy). It is also of value in assessing global changes in LV function during stress and the hemodynamic status and functional severity of valvular heart disease.

- The stress employed can be in the form of either exercise or a pharmacologic agent (see pages 47 to 51).
- Results revealing increased ventricular end-diastolic volume, wall motion abnormalities, or valvular dysfunction during or immediately after exercise may indicate significant exercise intolerance and the need for careful monitoring during activities of limited intensity.

Duplex Ultrasound

Duplex ultrasound combines Doppler and conventional ultrasound to provide noninvasive information about blood vessel structure and flow characteristics. The addition of color Doppler further enhances the imaging. Duplex studies are commonly used to detect deep venous thrombosis in the lower extremities and to assess atherosclerotic occlusive disease of the upper and lower extremities, as well as in the aorta and carotid arteries.

CARDIAC IMAGING TECHNIQUES

Various diagnostic tests using other sophisticated methods of imaging the cardiac structures are becoming increasingly popular. Some of them involve the injection of specially prepared radiopharmaceuticals that can be detected in the bloodstream or tissues and imaged by nuclear scanning devices.

Computed Tomography

Computed tomography (CT), as described in Chapter 2 (see page 20), can also be used to image the heart. High-resolution images of the heart usually require the use of injected contrast agents. Two types of scanners are used to image the heart: an electron beam CT (EBCT), which uses a magnetically focused electron beam rotating through a 210 degree arc to acquire images in one tenth of a second; and a multidetector or multislice spiral CT (MDCT or MSCT, respectively), which acquires multiple parallel slices during each 360 degree rotation taking about one half of a second.

- CT images are most often used to document thoracic aorta disease and paracardiac and intracardiac masses, to image cardiac valves in patients who are difficult to echo (e.g., those with emphysema or obesity), and to differentiate constrictive from restrictive pericarditis.
- EBCT is particularly useful in evaluating bypass graft patency and congenital lesions, and in quantifying ventricular mass, chamber volume, and systolic and diastolic function. It can also measure calcium deposits in the coronary arteries and is being marketed directly to the public as a way of screening for CAD. Although the detection of coronary artery calcification provides an accurate assessment of overall atherosclerotic plaque burden, it does not directly identify or localize coronary artery stenoses. In addition, early lesions associated with soft plaques and vessel remodeling are not detected by EBCT, and therefore a negative test does not necessarily rule out coronary disease.[9a,9b,15]
- Three-dimensional reconstruction from contrast-enhanced EBCT or MDCT data can produce angiographic images of the coronary arteries and bypass grafts,[14] as shown in Figure 3-19. With MDCT, the administration of β-receptor blocking agents before scanning is often done to prolong diastole and minimize motion artifacts. MSCT using 64-slice CT allows for the detection of clearly discernible noncalcified coronary plaques.

Myocardial Perfusion Imaging

Radioisotopes that accumulate in the myocardium according to regional blood flow can be used to determine relative myocardial perfusion. Imaging can be performed at rest or immediately after peak exercise or pharmacologic stress.

- During maximal exercise, coronary vascular reserve is recruited in order to meet the demand for increased blood flow. Coronary flow will be maximal in myocardium supplied by normal coronary arteries as indicated by excellent deposition of radioisotope in these regions; however, zones supplied by stenotic coronaries will show substantially less radionuclide deposition because of the limited ability to augment blood flow.

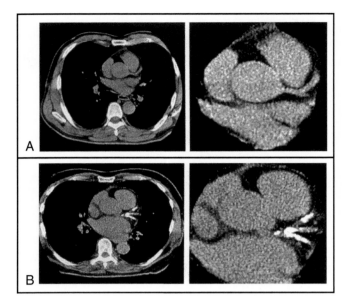

Figure 3-19: Single-level noncontrast electron beam computed tomography (EBCT) scan of a normal subject *(top)* and an individual with severe coronary artery calcification *(bottom)*. Calcium is shown as intensely white areas within the coronary arteries. (From Heller GV, Papaiouannou GI, Pennell DJ, et al. Chronic coronary heart disease. In St. John Sutton MG, Rutherford JD, editors. *Clinical Cardiovascular Imaging: A Companion to Braunwald's Heart Disease.* Philadelphia: Saunders; 2004.)

Thus, the relative distribution of radioisotope indicates the relative perfusion in various portions of the myocardium.
- A repeat scan can be performed 3 to 24 hours after a stress scan to distinguish between reversible defects resulting from ischemia and permanent defects resulting from previous myocardial infarction.
  ‣ Patients with reversible defects require careful monitoring during activity in order to avoid ischemia, whereas those with permanent defects are more likely to exhibit abnormal physiological responses to exercise.
- The most common radioisotope employed for cardiac imaging is technetium-99m, which can be used to label sestamibi (99mTc-sestamibi) and other agents, such as tetrofosmin (99mTc-tetrofosmin). Thallium-201 (201Tl) is still used in some centers.

Single-photon Emission Computed Tomography

Single-photon emission computed tomography (SPECT) uses a rotating gamma camera to detect radiolabeled isotope emissions to localize and quantify regional myocardial perfusion defects (Figure 3-20). Myocardial perfusion SPECT currently accounts for more than 95% of all nuclear cardiology studies.
- SPECT can be used to acquire multiple planar images around an object in order to reconstruct the three-dimensional object by "back projection," and thus permits the identification of disease in specific coronary artery distributions.

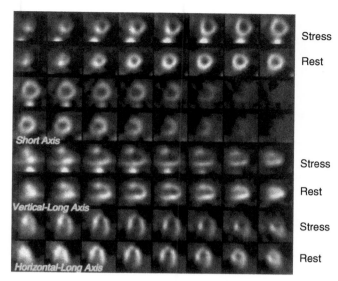

Stress

Rest

Short Axis

Stress

Rest

Vertical-Long Axis

Stress

Rest

Horizontal-Long Axis

Figure 3-20: Myocardial perfusion single-photon emission computed tomography (SPECT) imaging with ^{99m}Tc-sestamibi in multiple views. Stress images demonstrate transient cavity dilation and extensive ischemia involving the anterior, anteroseptal, anterolateral, and anteroapical distribution. Rest images reveal normalization of the cavity size and resolution of the perfusion abnormalities. (From Heller GV, Papaiouannou GI, Pennell DJ, et al. Chronic coronary heart disease. In St. John Sutton MG, Rutherford JD, editors. *Clinical Cardiovascular Imaging: A Companion to Braunwald's Heart Disease.* Philadelphia: Saunders; 2004.)

- Other uses for myocardial perfusion imaging include documenting acute myocardial infarction, determining the size of an infarction to provide prognostic information, and demonstrating reversible defects and thus viable myocardium in unstable angina and postinfarction chest pain that would benefit from revascularization (Figure 3-20).

Infarct-avid Imaging

Using radiotracers, such as technetium-labeled pyrophosphate or radiolabeled anti-myosin antibody, which bind selectively to necrotic myocardial cells, it is possible to establish a diagnosis of acute MI when the clinical presentation is not clear.

- These scans are most valuable in patients who present several days after the onset of symptoms, when other studies are equivocal, or when a perioperative MI is suspected.
- The intensity of the image is greatest at approximately 72 hours after infarct and lasts up to 7 to 10 days.

Radionuclide Angiography and Ventriculography

Assessment of cardiac performance can also be provided by radionuclide angiography (RNA) or ventriculography (RNV). Because of its accuracy and reproducibility, RNA is considered one of the "gold standards" for assessing left ventricular ejection fraction (EF). RNA can be performed by two different techniques.

First-pass Technique

- A bolus of ^{99m}Tc-sestamibi or ^{99m}Tc-tetrofosmin is injected intravenously and followed through the heart chambers; the ratio of the number of counts at end-systole and end-diastole is then used to determine these two volumes, as well as the ejection fraction.
- With a data acquisition time of less than 30 seconds, it is possible to define rapidly changing physiological states. The first-pass technique is particularly useful for evaluating RV function and intracardiac shunts, cardiac function in acutely ill patients who cannot remain in a stable position for long periods of time, and cardiac performance during upright exercise.

Gated Equilibrium Technique

- After injection of ^{99m}Tc, which is allowed to equilibrate with the blood volume for 5 to 10 minutes, images "gated" to the ECG can be obtained that define specific events within the cardiac cycle, as demonstrated in Figure 3-21. Data from several hundred beats are stored in a computer to obtain signals of adequate intensity; thus, it is sometimes called a MUGA (multiunit gated acquisition) scan.
- The equilibrium technique allows for multiple studies after a single radionuclide injection so that regional assessment can be performed in as many views as are relevant for analysis, and sequential and serial data can be obtained in a variety of control, physiologic, and/or pharmacologic states. However, to obtain meaningful data, cardiac performance must be relatively stable, and the patient must remain fairly still beneath the detector for up to 10 minutes of data acquisition per position.
- To enhance the assessment of regional function, SPECT acquisition can be combined with equilibrium RNA or RNV.
- The most common uses for gated equilibrium RNA and RNV include the measurement of resting cardiac function in patients with CAD, the detection of cardiotoxicity in patients receiving doxorubicin (Adriamycin) or other anthracycline chemotherapy, and the determination of timing for valve replacement in aortic regurgitation.
  - ▸ The normal response to activity is an increase in EF. If a patient exhibits a rise in EF during activity, he or she will usually exhibit more normal responses to exertion and better exercise tolerance, even if the initial EF is low.
  - ▸ A significant drop in EF with activity is abnormal regardless of the initial EF; the lower the EF and the more pronounced the drop, the greater will be the impairment of an individual's exercise tolerance and thus the need for careful monitoring during physical therapy activities.
  - ▸ Patients with a resting EF less than 40% are more likely to exhibit abnormal physiological responses to exertion.

Cardiac Magnetic Resonance Imaging

In magnetic resonance imaging or spectroscopy (MRI and MRS, respectively) of the heart, two techniques, ECG-gated spin echocardiography and fast gradient echocardiographic imaging (cine MRI), produce high-contrast images that are extremely valuable for noninvasively defining cardiac anatomy (Figure 3-22). Cardiac magnetic resonance (CMR) is particularly helpful in documenting wall thickness, chamber volumes, valve areas, and vessel cross-sections

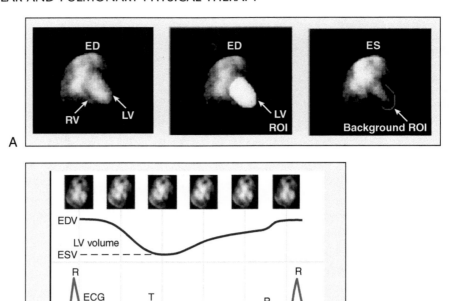

A

B

Figure 3-21: Quantitative analysis of equilibrium ECG-gated radionuclide ventriculography. **A,** The left anterior oblique view of the left ventricle (LV) and right ventricle (RV) is shown at end-diastole (ED) *(left),* with the region of interest (ROI) identifying the LV contour at ED *(middle),* and a "background" ROI drawn at end-systole (ES) *(right),* which is used to correct for count activity in front of and behind the LV. **B,** A time–activity curve illustrates the change in counts within the ROIs shown in **A** across a cardiac cycle. EDV, end-diastolic volume; ESV, end-systolic volume. (From Green MV, Bacharach SL, Douglas MA, et al. Measurement of left ventricular function and the detection of wall motion abnormalities with high temporal resolution ECG-gated scintigraphic angiocardiography. *IEEE Trans Nucl Sci.* 1976;23:1257–1263.)

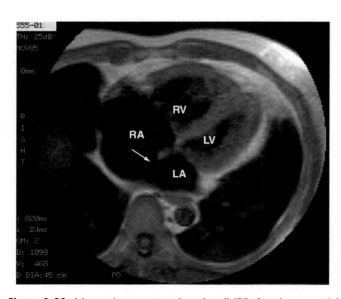

Figure 3-22: Magnetic resonance imaging (MRI) showing an atrial septal defect. The right ventricle (RV) and right atrium (RA) are dilated. LA, Left atrium; LV, left ventricle. (From Forbes CD, Jackson WF. *Color Atlas and Text of Clinical Medicine.* 3rd ed. Philadelphia: Mosby; 2003.)

and lesion sizes; identifying pericardiac and intracardiac masses; evaluating regional and global function of the ventricles; and determining the severity of valvular insufficiency.

- Angiographic forms of MRI are useful for evaluating the carotid and intracerebral vasculature, the great vessels of the chest and abdomen, and the arteries and veins of the extremities. Evaluation of coronary artery anatomy and patency of coronary artery bypass grafts is also possible.
- Multiphasic MRI techniques comparing end-systole with end-diastole allow for the estimation of ejection fraction.
- CMR can detect regions of decreased LV systolic wall thickening caused by ischemic heart disease, distinguish acute from subacute and chronic myocardial infarctions and define their size, and discern viable from nonviable myocardium after MI.
- In addition, CMR is particularly useful in the evaluation of patients with severe pulmonary hypertension and all forms of cardiomyopathy.
- Phosphorus-31 nuclear MRS cardiac stress testing has been shown to be valuable in the assessment of women with chest pain, in whom at least half do not show any flow-limiting coronary lesions at angiography.[24] Detection of a reduced phosphocreatine-to-adenosine triphosphate ratio suggests a shift toward anaerobic metabolism consistent with myocardial ischemia.

Positron Emission Tomography

Positron emission tomography is an imaging technique that uses biologically active positron emission radiopharmaceuticals (e.g., rubidium-82, ^{18}F-labeled 2-fluoro-2-deoxyglucose [FDG], ^{13}N-ammonia, and ^{11}C-acetate) to display and quantify metabolic processes, receptor occupancy, and blood flow. In cardiology, it is being used to assess coronary perfusion, quantify coronary reserve, determine regional myocardial substrate utilization and oxygen consumption, diagnose and localize CAD (Figure 3-23), demonstrate ischemic but viable myocardium (hibernating myocardium) that would benefit from revascularization surgery, and assess autonomic innervation of the heart.

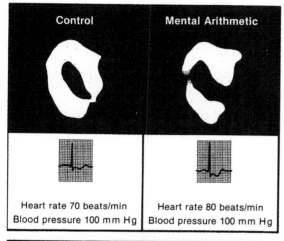

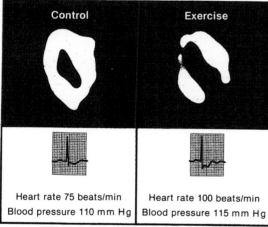

Figure 3-23: Positron emission tomography scan of the heart, showing regional myocardial uptake of rubidium-82 in a patient with chronic stable angina, a positive exercise test, and proven coronary disease. The two control images show uniform perfusion to the posterior wall, free wall, anterior wall, and septum of the left ventricle. However, regional perfusion abnormalities and ST segment depression on ECG are evident during both mental arithmetic and exercise. Notably, the patient evidenced no symptoms during the mental arithmetic. (From Deanfield JE, Shea M, Kensett M, et al. Silent myocardial ischemia due to mental stress. *Lancet.* 1984;2:1001–1005.)

INVASIVE MONITORING

Monitoring of cardiovascular status can be performed with specially designed intravascular catheters capable of measuring temperature, pressure, and volume.

Intraarterial Catheterization

Catheters, placed usually within the brachial or femoral artery, are often used in intensive care units for acquiring arterial blood gas samples and for directly monitoring arterial blood pressure, which is displayed on the bedside monitor. Physical therapists can use the direct BP values to monitor a patient's responses to activity as long as the arterial line insertion site is positioned at the level of the heart while measurements are taken.

Pulmonary Artery Catheter

A balloon-tip catheter (often referred to as a Swan-Ganz catheter, after the original brand) can be placed into the pulmonary artery (PA) via a large central vein, usually the subclavian or internal jugular, in order to obtain the PA wedge pressure (PAWP; formerly referred to as the pulmonary capillary wedge [PCW] pressure). It can also provide an indirect indication of the left atrial pressure (LAP) when significant pulmonary vascular disease is not present.
- Patients with mean pulmonary pressures exceeding 20 mm Hg are likely to become symptomatic during exertion.
- A pulmonary artery pressure of 35 mm Hg or more is often considered to be a contraindication to exercise; however, this may not be the case (see page 97 on exercise for patients with pulmonary hypertension).

Thermodilution Catheter

A special thermodilution catheter, inserted like a pulmonary artery catheter, can be used to measure cardiac output. Cold saline is injected through the proximal lumen lying in the right atrium and then the resulting temperature change is measured by means of a thermistor bead embedded in the catheter wall near the tip of the catheter in the PA. Calculation of the volume of blood required to produce this temperature change yields the cardiac output.

Combination Catheters

Combination catheters, which contain two or more lumens and ports serving different purposes (as described previously), are commonly found in intensive care units. An example of a triple-lumen catheter is depicted in Figure 3-24.

Central Venous Pressure Line

An intravenous line in the subclavian, basilic, jugular, or femoral vein and passed to the right atrium (RA) can be used to measure the pressure in the vena cavae or RA. This central venous pressure (CVP) line provides information about the adequacy of right heart function, effective circulating blood volume, vascular tone, and venous return.
- A CVP line is especially useful in assessing fluid volume and replacement needs.
- However, if the patient has chronic obstructive pulmonary disease or myocardial ischemia or infarction, CVP measurements may reflect pathological changes rather than fluid volume.

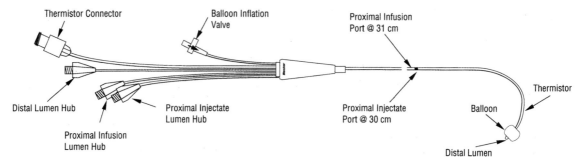

Figure 3-24: A typical triple-lumen pulmonary artery catheter. (VIP-831 catheter courtesy of Baxter Healthcare Corporation, Edwards Critical-Care Division, Santa Ana, CA.)

CARDIAC CATHETERIZATION

Using one or more fluid-filled catheters inserted into the heart through the venous and/or arterial systems, cardiac anatomy and function can be evaluated. Through these catheters, intracardiac pressures can be measured to assess the hemodynamic function of the heart (Table 3-5) and dye can be injected to study ventricular performance and intracardiac and coronary arterial anatomy (see Figure 3-11).

- Because of the improved sensitivity and specificity of newer noninvasive cardiac tests, standard diagnostic cardiac catheterization is used less frequently than in the past; it is often reserved for patients who need further quantification of the severity of their disease or for the determination of the appropriateness of surgical intervention.
- Yet, the use of cardiac catheterization has been expanded to include intracardiac electrophysiological testing, endomyocardial biopsy, percutaneous transluminal angioplasty and atherectomy, and percutaneous balloon valvotomy (see later in this chapter).

Right Heart Catheterization

Right heart catheterization involves the insertion of a catheter into the venous system, usually through the femoral or basilic vein, which is passed into the RA, RV, and PA. It is used primarily to:

- Determine RA, RV, and PA pressures
- Document the pulmonary artery wedge pressure (PAWP) if the catheter is advanced so that it "wedges" in the distal PA; in addition, in the absence of pulmonary vascular disease, the PAWP reflects the LA pressure, and if there is no significant mitral valve disease, it also reflects the LV diastolic pressure
- Sample blood from the RV to evaluate shunts
- Measure cardiac output
- Assess LV function in patients with an atrial septal defect (ASD) or ventricular septal defect (VSD) is present

Left Heart Catheterization

Left heart catheterization involves the insertion of a fluid-filled catheter into the arterial system, usually through the femoral or brachial artery; the catheter is passed up through the aorta to the coronary arteries or LV. It can be used to:

- Evaluate mitral and aortic valve disease
- Assess regional and global LV function
- Measure LV and aortic pressures
- Document pressure gradients across the aortic and mitral valves
- Perform coronary angiography (imaging of the coronary arteries, using injected dye and high-speed x-ray cinematography)

TABLE 3-5: Normal Resting Hemodynamic Values

Parameter	Range	Mean Value
Cardiac index (L/min/m^2)	2.6–4.2	3.4
Stroke index (mL/beat)	35–55	47
Systemic arteries: systolic/end diastolic (mm Hg)	100–140/60–90	70–105
Left ventricle: systolic/end diastolic (mm Hg)	100–140/3–12	—
Left atrium (mm Hg)	3–15	1–10
Pulmonary artery: systolic/end diastolic (mm Hg)	16–30/4–12	10–16
Right ventricle: systolic/end diastolic (mm Hg)	16–30/0–8	—
Right atrium (mm Hg)	2–10	0–8
Systemic vascular resistance (mm Hg/L/min)	700–1600	1150
Systemic vascular resistance (Wood units)	10–20	16
Pulmonary vascular resistance (mm Hg/L/min)	20–120	70
Pulmonary vascular resistance (Wood units)	0.25–1.5	0.90
Oxygen consumption (mL/min/m^2)	110–150	—
Arteriovenous oxygen difference (mL/L)	30–45	—

Patients with coronary occlusions greater than 70% to 75% usually exhibit symptoms during activity and often benefit from carefully prescribed exercise training, which has been shown to increase exercise tolerance and reduce symptoms.

Endomyocardial Biopsy

Small samples of ventricular endocardium can be acquired during cardiac catheterization with specially designed forceps call a *biotome*. Typically, the biotome is introduced into the venous system through the right internal jugular vein and guided into the right ventricle by fluoroscopy. The endomyocardial samples are then sent for histologic evaluation. Endomyocardial biopsy is most commonly used to assess and detect rejection after cardiac transplantation and to document cardiotoxicity due to anthracycline chemotherapy; it can also be used to diagnose myocarditis, sarcoidosis, amyloidosis, and secondary causes of cardiomyopathy, and to distinguish between restrictive and constrictive cardiomyopathy.

ELECTROPHYSIOLOGICAL STUDIES

Electrophysiological studies (EPSs) can be employed to assess the electrical activity and responses of the heart. An EPS involves the insertion of multipolar catheter electrodes into the right and/or left sides of the heart, after which they are positioned at various intracardiac sites to stimulate and record electrical activity from portions of the atria or ventricles, His bundle region, bundle branches, or accessory pathways, depending on the purpose of the study.

- EPSs are commonly performed in patients with symptomatic, recurrent, or drug-resistant supraventricular or ventricular tachyarrhythmias, particularly when they produce serious hemodynamic consequences, and in patients with unexplained syncope.
- Electrophysiological studies are used therapeutically to terminate a tachycardia by electrical stimulation or electroshock, to evaluate the therapeutic efficacy of a particular intervention, and to ablate myocardium involved in initiating or perpetuating tachyarrhythmias and thus to prevent further episodes (see page 62).

 ## 3.3 THERAPEUTIC INTERVENTIONS

As in most areas of medicine, the types of therapeutic interventions in cardiology continue to expand. The more common ones encountered by physical therapists are described briefly in the following pages.

MEDICAL MANAGEMENT

Generally speaking, most types of cardiac dysfunction are treated medically for as long as possible, using pharmacologic agents, diet modification, risk factor reduction, rehabilitation, and other interventions. When symptoms become disabling, surgery may be warranted.

Pharmacologic Therapy

The various medications used to treat cardiovascular dysfunction are described in Chapter 5 (Pharmacology).

Diet Modification

Specific diet modifications may be advised for patients with cardiovascular disease.

- A low-cholesterol, low saturated fat diet is usually recommended for patients with known atherosclerotic cardiovascular disease and those at high risk for its development. In addition, the American Heart Association has issued preventative dietary guidelines for healthy adults that emphasize the importance of a healthy diet that is low in saturated fat and trans-fat, and rich in fruits, vegetables, whole grains, fat-free and low-fat dairy products, and lean meat, fish, and poultry. These guidelines also address appropriate body weight and desirable blood pressure.
- High-fiber intake (25 to 35 g/d) is recommended for the prevention of atherosclerosis as well as colon cancer.
- Sodium restriction is often used to reduce preload in heart failure (along with fluid restriction to avoid hyponatremia) and to lower blood pressure in hypertension.
- Caloric restriction is usually recommended to achieve weight loss in overweight and obese individuals, reduce the workload of the heart for those with heart failure, and decrease blood pressure in hypertensive individuals.
- Because of the extended contact we have with patients, physical therapists are in an ideal position to reinforce the importance of diet modification and share the findings of current literature and good low-fat, low-cholesterol foods and recipes with our patients.

Risk Factor Reduction

Because the atherosclerotic process has been linked to specific risk factors, their reduction is often recommended for patients with atherosclerotic coronary, cerebrovascular, and peripheral vascular disease.

- Risk factor reduction includes cessation of smoking, treatment of hypertension, exercise training, diet modification, weight control, stress reduction training, and control of blood glucose levels.
- There is a great deal of scientific data to support risk factor reduction both for primary prevention of atherosclerotic disease as well as for secondary prevention of recurrent events.[4,11,19,28]
- As physical therapists practice more independently, we have an increasing responsibility to assess the overall health status of the patients we treat and make appropriate recommendations for their general health and well-being. Risk factor reduction for cardiovascular disease, the leading cause of death in the United States, is a critical element.

Cardiac Rehabilitation

Cardiac rehabilitation (CR) is a multidisciplinary program aimed at restoring the cardiac patient to optimal physiologic, social, vocational, and emotional status. It usually includes patient assessment, case management, and the development of an individualized treatment plan, patient and family education, risk factor modification, exercise training, psychological counseling, and patient reassessments to document progress.[5] A great deal of research has documented that optimal reduction of coronary risk factors results in stabilization and possibly regression of the atherosclerotic process.[11,19] In patients with CAD, CR, particularly exercise training, has demonstrated favorable effects on plasma lipids, fasting glucose levels, body composition, peak aerobic capacity, depression, and quality of life.[4,27] In patients receiving CR after heart transplantation and heart valve surgery and for chronic heart failure, demonstrated benefits include increased functional capacity, favorable modification of disease-related risk factors, amelioration of symptoms, identification of signs and symptoms of disease before they become serious complications, and improved quality of life.[18,25,28,29]

Because physical therapists have unequaled expertise in prescribing exercise, especially for patients with chronic medical problems, and in the prevention and treatment of exercise-related injuries, we are assets to the cardiac rehabilitation team.

Enhanced Extracorporeal Counterpulsation

Enhanced extracorporeal counterpulsation (EECP) is a noninvasive technique involving the sequential inflation of pressure cuffs applied to the lower extremities, which gently compresses the veins to assist blood return to the heart during diastole. EECP results is increased preload, decreased afterload, and improved coronary perfusion pressure during diastole. It is performed over a series of several weeks in patients with myocardial ischemia to improve the balance between myocardial oxygen supply and demand and thus relieve chest pain and in patients with heart failure to improve LV function and exercise tolerance.

Cardiopulmonary Resuscitation

Physical therapists are required to be trained in cardiopulmonary resuscitation (CPR) in the event that a patient experiences cardiac arrest. The goal is to support a small amount of blood flow to the heart and brain to "buy time" until normal heart function is restored. Frequently, cardiac arrest is due to ventricular fibrillation (see page 272), which requires the delivery of an electrical shock (i.e., defibrillation) to restore normal rhythm. The availability of small portable defibrillators, called automated external defibrillators (AEDs), has improved the ability to provide rapid defibrillation in many medical buildings and public places.

Cough CPR

A coughing procedure widely publicized on the Internet, cough CPR involves the use of repeated forceful coughing when a conscious, responsive person experiences a sudden arrhythmia. The theory is that it may maintain enough blood flow to the brain to allow the person to remain conscious for a few seconds until the arrhythmia disappears or is treated. In the hospital setting, it is used mainly during cardiac catheterization.

Cardioversion and Defibrillation

Direct current (DC) electrical energy is used to correct serious tachyarrhythmias and ventricular fibrillation.

- Cardioversion is used to treat hemodynamically significant tachyarrhythmias (see page 113) that are refractory to medications or to convert atrial fibrillation to normal sinus rhythm. The patient must be connected to an electrocardiogram (ECG) so the electrical shock can be synchronized with the R wave to avoid delivery during the T wave, which can induce ventricular fibrillation (VF). It is often performed as an elective procedure with patients under general anesthesia or sedation.

- Defibrillation is used emergently to treat patients with VF or pulseless ventricular tachycardia. The electrical discharge is used to overwhelm and suppress chaotic ectopic impulses so the intrinsic conduction system can take over. Automatic external defibrillators (AEDs) can be found in most physical therapy departments and many public facilities to allow immediate resuscitation of individuals who collapse with cardiac arrest.

SURGICAL INTERVENTIONS

A variety of surgical interventions are used in the treatment of patients with heart disease, many of which are described briefly in the following pages.

Myocardial Revascularization

Several procedures exist to increase myocardial blood flow through stenotic coronary arteries. These include a number of catheter-based percutaneous techniques as well as surgical revascularization via coronary artery bypass grafting (CABG) or transmyocardial revascularization.

Percutaneous Transluminal Coronary Angioplasty

During percutaneous transluminal coronary angioplasty (PTCA), a balloon-tip catheter is passed through the femoral artery, up the aorta, and then into a diseased coronary artery, using fluoroscopic guidance. The balloon is positioned across a stenotic lesion and inflated. The goal is to increase the intraluminal diameter by fracturing the plaque and disrupting the vessel intima, as illustrated in Figure 3-25.

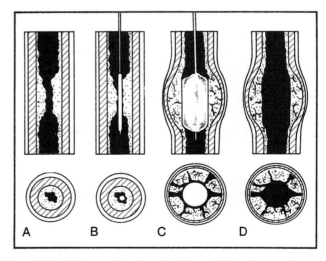

Figure 3-25: Likely mechanism of balloon dilation in percutaneous transluminal coronary angioplasty (PTCA). Serial panels show the baseline stenosis **(A)**, passage of the deflated balloon catheter **(B)**, balloon inflation **(C)**, and the postdilation appearance **(D)**, as drawn in longitudinal and transverse cross-sectional views. Note fracture and outward displacement of atherosclerotic plaque and stretching of the media and adventitia (**C** and **D**). (From Castaneda-Zuniga WR, Formanek A, Tadavarthy M, et al. The mechanism of balloon angioplasty. *Radiology.* 1980;135:565–571.)

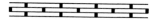
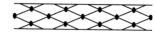

Unexpanded stent   Expanded stent

Figure 3-26: An intracoronary stent before inflation and in its expanded configuration, used to maintain the patency of a vessel after PTCA.

Restenosis occurs in 10% to 50% of patients undergoing PTCA, usually within the first 6 months; therefore, about 70% to 90% of PTCAs also involve placement of a stent (see the next section).

Percutaneous transluminal angioplasty can also be applied to the renal, mesenteric, and peripheral arteries and to diseased saphenous vein coronary artery bypass grafts.

Intracoronary Stents

Coronary stents are intraluminal metallic mesh tubes (Figure 3-26), which are usually inserted after PTCA via a balloon-tipped catheter in order to maintain vessel patency. Simple stents decrease the rate of restenosis to approximately 20%, and newer *drug-eluting stents* that provide for the local delivery of immunosuppressive or antiproliferative agents slash the restenosis rate to approximately 5%; however, there have been some reports of a small increase in risk of late stent thrombosis associated with the use of these stents. Another treatment option that reduces restenosis within stents by approximately 50% is intravascular radiation therapy *(brachytherapy)*, using radioactive γ- or β-emitters.

Atherectomy

Atherectomy involves the insertion of intracoronary catheters with special tips that shave, grind, or slice the atherosclerotic plaque within a coronary artery, somewhat like a little "Roto-Rooter" or "Pac Man" with suction. It is usually combined with PTCA in order to increase lumen size.

Laser Angioplasty

In laser angioplasty, a catheter with a laser at its tip is inserted into a coronary artery and advanced to a blockage, where it emits pulsating beams of light in order to vaporize the plaque. This procedure may be used alone or with balloon angioplasty.

Coronary Artery Bypass Graft Surgery

Coronary artery bypass graft (CABG) surgery, also referred to as aorto-coronary bypass (ACB) surgery, uses autogenous saphenous vein or arterial grafts (usually the internal thoracic/mammary artery or occasionally the radial or gastroepiploic artery) to bypass stenotic lesions of the coronary arteries. Figure 3-27 shows the common types of bypass grafts. Multiple lesions in the same coronary artery can be bypassed by sequential grafting, particularly when an internal thoracic artery graft is used.

- CABG is performed primarily via a median sternotomy, and at closing, the sternum is wired back together again.
  - ▸ Immediately after surgery, the patient commonly has two chest tubes in place: one to drain the mediastinum and an intrapleural tube to reinflate the left lung, which was collapsed during surgery (see Chapter 2, page 32, for information related to chest tubes and their implications for physical therapy).

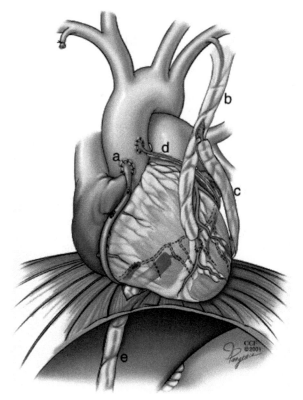

Figure 3-27: Coronary artery (CA) bypass graft surgery showing a reverse saphenous vein graft from the ascending aorta to the right CA *(a)*, an in situ left internal mammary artery graft to the left anterior descending CA *(b)*, a Y-graft of the right internal mammary artery from the left internal mammary artery to the circumflex CA *(c)*, a radial artery graft from the aorta to the circumflex CA *(d)*, and an in situ gastroepiploic graft to the posterior descending branch of the right CA *(e)*. (From Goldman L, Ausiello D. *Cecil Textbook of Medicine.* 23rd ed. Philadelphia: Saunders; 2008.)

- ▸ Reasonable healing of the sternum usually takes approximately 6 to 8 weeks. Although there are no controlled studies documenting their efficacy, sternal precautions related to the amount of weight patients are allowed to lift are commonly prescribed during this interim period to avoid excessive sternal stress; the amount of restriction and the time period vary widely from surgeon to surgeon but normally fall in the range of not more than 10 to 20 pounds for 6 to 12 weeks. Patients are also restricted for 3 to 4 months, or more, from doing pushups and other strenuous resistive exercises that involve the pectoralis muscles. Furthermore, most physicians require modifications of assisted transfers and ambulation with a walker or crutches to minimize sternal stress.
- Although CABG is usually performed while the patient is supported by extracorporeal cardiopulmonary bypass (CPB), some centers use *beating heart* or *off-pump coronary artery bypass (OPCAB)* when only one or two grafts are needed, particularly in elderly patients and patients with calcified ascending aortas, carotid disease, or previous stroke or coronary artery bypass grafting.

- An alternative to standard CABG via sternotomy is *minimally invasive direct coronary artery bypass surgery (MIDCAB)*, which is performed endoscopically and off-pump through a combination of small holes in the chest and a small incision made directly over the coronary artery to be bypassed. In this method the internal thoracic artery is often employed to bypass the left anterior descending (LAD) coronary artery. During *port-access coronary artery bypass (PACAB or PortCAB)*, the patient is placed on CPB and the heart is stopped while bypasses are performed endoscopically through small ports or incisions. Computer, or robotic, enhancement of minimally invasive techniques is also possible using totally endoscopic, robot-assisted coronary artery bypass grafting (TECAB).

Besides the sternotomy precautions mentioned previously, there are other implications pertaining to physical therapy treatment of patients who have undergone CABG surgery:

- During the immediate postoperative period, arrhythmias are not uncommon and usually do not cause hemodynamic compromise; however, clinical monitoring of the patient's HR, BP, and any signs of exercise intolerance should be performed to detect any serious problems (see Chapter 6, pages 261, 278, and 282).
- Patients should be encouraged to maintain full range of motion of their shoulders, trunk, and neck and to practice good posture, and they should be discouraged from crossing their legs when they sit, especially if saphenous vein grafts were harvested.
- In addition, cardiac rehabilitation with exercise training is important for these patients, both to increase exercise tolerance and to reduce the rate of atherogenesis and restenosis in their bypass grafts.

Hybrid Revascularization

For patients with complex lesions not fully amenable to any of the aforementioned approaches, both percutaneous coronary intervention and minimally invasive CABG surgery can be performed during the same procedure. Typically, it consists of anastomosis of the left internal mammary artery (LIMA) to the LAD artery with stenting of the right coronary and/or circumflex arteries.

Transmyocardial Revascularization

For patients with severe angina who are not candidates for other treatment options, transmyocardial revascularization (TMR) can be used to increase blood flow to the myocardium. TMR is usually performed through a small incision in the left chest, through which the surgeon uses a laser to drill a series of holes from the outside of the heart into the LV. Pressure from the surgeon's fingers is sufficient to stop the epicardial bleeding from the laser channels within a few minutes. The mechanism by which TMR reduces angina is not fully understood, but may be due to stimulation of new blood vessel growth (angiogenesis) by the laser and destruction of sympathetic nerve fibers so the patient simply no longer feels his chest pain. A worldwide registry of more than 3000 patients treated with TMR found that 80% show improvement in angina class and 30% had no angina a 1-year follow-up.[16] Other studies report reductions in cardiac events and rehospitalization as well as improved exercise tolerance and quality of life.[2]

Treatment of Arrhythmias

Cardiac Ablation

Cardiac, or catheter, ablation involves the use of energy to destroy (ablate) areas of endocardium that are related to the onset or maintenance of tachyarrhythmias. It is used in patients with supraventricular tachycardia, atrial flutter or fibrillation, and ventricular tachycardia with focal sources of the arrhythmia or an accessory pathway that perpetuates it, as identified through an EPS. It is typically performed in patients with tachyarrhythmias that cannot be controlled with medication or who cannot tolerate or prefer not to take antiarrhythmic medications and has very high success rates.

- Radiofrequency ablation causes resistive heating in cells near the catheter tip, resulting in irreversible damage and tissue death.
- Cryoablation uses nitrous oxide delivered to the catheter tip to cause tissue damage by freezing the nearby cells.
- Chemical ablation with alcohol or phenol may be performed in patients who fail other ablation procedures or when other approaches cannot be done.

Pacemaker Insertion

Pacemakers are electronic devices that use an external energy source to stimulate the heart when disorders of impulse formation and/or transmission create significant hemodynamic problems. They are surgically implanted, usually in the left infraclavicular area, as depicted in Figure 3-28; in a subxiphoid pocket; or in the left anterior chest wall.

- Modern pacemakers have a variety of functions, which can be programmed according to patient need. Pacemaker modes and functions are described according to an established five-letter code, described in Table 3-6.
  - The first letter designates the chamber being paced (A for atrium, V for ventricle, and D for dual-chamber).

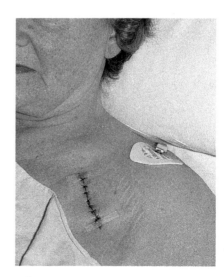

Figure 3-28: The most common site of implantation of a permanent pacemaker is the left pectoral region, but it may be placed elsewhere if necessary. (From Forbes CD, Jackson WF. *Color Atlas and Text of Clinical Medicine.* 3rd ed. Philadelphia: Mosby; 2003.)

TABLE 3-6: The NASPE/BPEG Generic Code for Antibradycardia Pacing

I. Chamber Paced	II. Chamber Sensed	III. Response to Sensing	IV. Rate Modulation	V. Multisite Pacing
V = ventricle	V = ventricle	I = inhibited	O = none	O = none
A = atrium	A = atrium	T = triggered	R = rate modulation	A = atrium
D = dual (A + V)	D = dual (A + V)	D = dual (atrium triggered and ventricle inhibited)		V = ventricle
	O = none			D = dual (A + V)
		O = none		

BPEG, British Pacing and Electrophysiology Group; NASPE, North American Society of Pacing and Electrophysiology.
Note: The top three features are most commonly used to identify pacemaker modes (e.g., a VVI pacemaker), often with an indication of rate modulation; the last feature is included on occasion.

▸ The second letter indicates the chamber being sensed (A, V, D, or O for no sensing).

▸ The third letter specifies the response to sensing: I if the sensed signal inhibits pacemaker discharge, or T if the sensed signal triggers pacemaker discharge, D if both functions are available, or O for none.

▸ The fourth letter refers to the programmability of the pacemaker for rate modulation independent of atrial activity (R) or not (O) (see later section on rate-responsive pacemakers).

▸ The fifth letter indicates multisite pacing in none of the chambers (O), one or both of the atria (A), one or both of the ventricles (V), or any combination of A and V (D).

• There are several types of pacemakers, the most common of which are briefly described here. In addition, the pacemaker modes recommended by the British Pacing and Electrophysiology Group (now Heart Rhythm UK, London, UK) for various conduction disturbances are listed in Table 3-7.

▸ *Dual-chamber pacemakers* have the ability to sense both the atrium and the ventricle, or just the ventricle, and to pace both the atrium and the ventricle, or just the ventricle, according to specific need. They can be programmed to either inhibit or trigger a discharge.

⊙ DDD pacemakers provide optimal sequential pacing because they sense and pace both the atrium and the ventricle and adapt to the underlying rhythm automatically, according to a specific scheme, to either inhibit or trigger a discharge as needed; they are best for patients with both sinus and AV nodal dysfunction, providing AV synchrony.

⊙ VDD devices are designed for patients with AV block and normal sinus node function, sensing both the atrium and ventricle and providing a ventricular stimulus when an excessive delay occurs after a spontaneous atrial discharge.

⊙ DDI pacemakers sense and pace both the atrium and the ventricle, inhibiting pacemaker discharge when spontaneous activity is sensed.

⊙ DVI devices pace both the atrium and the ventricle while sensing only the ventricle. This mode is rarely used because the asynchronous atrial pacing it produces can precipitate atrial fibrillation.

⊙ Mode switching allows dual-chamber pacemakers to change the pacing mode automatically and reversibly to eliminate atrial sensing during atrial fibrillation and flutter or other supraventricular tachyarrhythmias (i.e., they change to VVI, VDI, or DDI mode).

▸ *Single-chamber pacemakers* are demand pacemakers, which sense and pace either the atrium or ventricle.

⊙ VVI pacemakers deliver automatic pacing of the ventricles unless spontaneous ventricular activity is sensed. Because this type of pacing disturbs normal atrioventricular synchrony, it is used only for patients with chronic atrial fibrillation or flutter.

⊙ AAI pacemakers provide automatic pacing of the atrium unless inhibited by spontaneous atrial activity. It is used for

TABLE 3-7: Recommended Pacemaker Modes

Diagnosis	Optimal	Alternative	Inappropriate
Sinus node dysfunction	AAIR	AAI, DDDR	VVI, VDD, VDI, DDI
AV block	DDD	VDD	AAI, DDI
Sinus node dysfunction and AV block	DDDR	DDD	AAI, VVI
Chronic AF with AV block	VVIR	VVI	AAI, DDD, VDD
Hypersensitive carotid sinus and neurally mediated syndromes	DDI	DDD, VVI*	AAI, VVI,* VDD

From Andersen HR, Nielsen JC. Cardiac pacing. In Crawford MH, DiMarco JP, Paulus WJ, editors. *Cardiology.* 2nd ed. Edinburgh: Mosby; 2004.
A, Atrium; AF, atrial fibrillation; AV, atrioventricular; D, dual; I, inhibited; O, none; R, rate responsive; T, triggered; V, ventricle.
*VVI pacing should be used only in cases of chronic atrial fibrillation or other chronic atrial tachyarrhythmias.

patients with sick sinus syndrome and no signs of AV conduction disturbances.

▸ *Rate-responsive pacemakers* allow for more normal physiological function by producing increases in the paced HR in response to various stimuli detected by special sensors.

⊙ The most common type of sensors use piezoelectric crystals or accelerometers to detect activity. Other types use sensors of minute ventilation, Q-T interval, and temperature. Sensor activity is programmable.

⊙ New pacemaker models use sensor combinations (e.g., activity and minute ventilation in the same pacemaker) and self-adjusting sensors that automatically adjust upper and lower rates and sensor activity. In addition, automatic rate reduction during sleep is available in some models.

▸ Rate-responsive pacing is available on most current pacemakers and is recommended for all but the most inactive patients.

- Pacemakers are occasionally used to control certain tachyarrhythmias, although the success of catheter ablation techniques and implantable cardioverter/defibrillators has nearly eliminated this application.

- Implantation of a pacemaker carries implications for physical therapy, both acutely and long term.

▸ Immediately after pacemaker insertion, patients usually have a chest x-ray taken to rule out pneumothorax. Once this has been cleared, they can usually resume physical therapy activities, although many physicians limit ipsilateral shoulder range of motion for days to weeks in order to avoid dislodging the pacemaker leads. However, the need for restricted shoulder range of motion has not been scientifically validated, and some physicians have their patients ambulate with their upper extremity fully stretched overhead by holding onto an intravenous pole the day after surgery.

▸ Once the incision has healed, there are no surgical precautions. However, it is advantageous for physical therapists to know the type of pacemaker a patient has so that his or her physiological responses to activity can be anticipated and appropriate modifications included in the treatment plan.

▸ In addition, therapists should be aware that the onset of weakness, lightheadedness, exercise intolerance, or palpitations might indicate dysfunction or failure of the pacemaker.

Automatic Implantable Cardioverter-Defibrillator

An automatic implantable cardioverter-defibrillator (AICD or ICD) is a self-contained system that both detects and treats serious arrhythmias. The device is surgically implanted similar to a pacemaker, usually in the left pectoral area.

- AICDs provide arrhythmia prevention or termination, including antitachycardia pacing or low-energy synchronized cardioversion for the termination of ventricular tachycardia, unsynchronized cardioversion for the termination of atrial fibrillation, and/or defibrillation for resuscitation of ventricular fibrillation.

- Refer to comments regarding pacemaker insertion for important implications for physical therapy management. In addition, therapists should recognize that urgent evaluation is necessary if patients begin to experience flurries of discharges.

- If a patient with an AICD experiences a cardiac arrest, the patient should be treated with standard resuscitation procedures (e.g., CPR and defibrillation).

Surgical Treatment of Tachyarrhythmias

Surgical treatment of resistant atrial fibrillation and flutter (see the next section) and of tachyarrhythmias that have failed catheter ablation includes excision, isolation, or interruption of cardiac tissue critical for the initiation, maintenance, or propagation of tachycardias.

- Surgery usually involves endocardial resection or ablation of trigger sites or reentry pathways.

- Patients undergo preoperative electrophysiological studies, as well as intraoperative intracardiac recordings and programmed stimulation, in order to achieve successful results.

- Other indirect surgical approaches, including aneurysectomy, coronary artery bypass grafting, and valve surgeries, may provide relief from tachyarrhythmias by improving cardiac hemodynamics and myocardial blood flow.

Maze Surgery

The maze, or Cox maze, procedure is a surgical intervention that involves the strategic placement of incisions or ablative lesions in both atria as a means of curing medically refractory atrial flutter and atrial fibrillation (AF).[6,17] When the lesions heal through scar formation, a maze is created that blocks the formation and conduction of abnormal electrical impulses and allows conduction of normal electrical impulses down only one path from the SA node to the AV node.

- The standard maze procedure, which has evolved over the years to the Cox maze III procedure, is performed through a median sternotomy on a cooled, nonbeating heart with cardiopulmonary bypass. Precisely located incisions or ablations (using radiofrequency, ultrasound, laser, cryothermy, or microwave energy) are made in the endocardial walls of the atria. This surgery is usually performed in conjunction with other open-heart surgeries, such as coronary artery bypass grafting, mitral valve repair, and valve replacement.

- Some centers use minimally invasive keyhole incisions or a completely endoscopic approach with video and sometimes robotic assistance to create the lesions that block abnormal electrical conduction in the atria.

- An alternative approach employs catheter ablation techniques on the ectopic foci that trigger AF (usually in the left atrium, pulmonary vein, superior vena cava, and coronary sinus) and on specific sites in the left atrial wall. It is most useful for the treatment of paroxysmal AF rather than for permanent or persistent AF.

Maze surgery is highly effective in curing atrial fibrillation, with success rates for sinus rhythm conversion of 75% to 90% for the Cox maze III procedure when performed by experienced surgical groups and slightly less when alternative energy sources are used.[6,17] The mortality rate of these surgeries is approximately 2% to 4% and about 5% to 6% of patients require postoperative pacemaker insertion.

Valve Repairs and Replacement

Abnormalities of the cardiac valves are usually well tolerated by patients for several years to decades before myocardial dysfunction becomes significant enough to warrant surgical intervention, which is sometimes performed through a central sternotomy or keyhole incision, as a totally endoscopic procedure, or using catheter technology. A number of procedures can be used to repair or replace defective cardiac valves, several of which are presented in the following sections.

Percutaneous Balloon Valvuloplasty

Percutaneous balloon valvuloplasty uses a balloon-tip catheter, which is inserted into the orifice of a stenotic valve and inflated, to increase the area of the valve orifice. Percutaneous balloon valvuloplasty is most successful in mobile, minimally calcified, minimally thickened valves without severe subvalvular fibrosis.

Open Valvotomy and Commissurotomy

Valvotomy and commissurotomy involve an incision into the chest (either median sternotomy or left thoracotomy) followed by surgical cutting or digital manipulation of a valve or its adherent diseased commissures in order to relieve stenosis. Direct visualization of the stenotic valve during cardiopulmonary bypass allows for removal of atrial thrombi, incision of commissures, separation of fused chordae, splitting of underlying papillary muscle, and debridement of valvular calcium.

Physical therapy recommendations for patients with sternotomy incisions can be found on pages 61 to 62, and recommendations for patients with thoracotomy are located on page 34.

Valvectomy

Complete excision of right-sided heart valves without insertion of a replacement may be performed for some congenital defects or for infective endocarditis in drug abusers in whom reinfection is likely.

Annuloplasty

Annuloplasty consists of the surgical repair or reconstruction of a defective valve ring and its leaflets.

- Annuloplasty may be possible in patients with mitral or tricuspid valvular incompetence caused by myxomatous degeneration, rupture of chordae tendineae or papillary muscle, or dilation of the valve annulus. During ring annuloplasty, a prosthetic ring is sutured into place to restore the normal proportions of the annulus and correct dilation, and to improve durability of valve repair.
- Valve reconstruction offers the advantages of avoiding the problems associated with chronic anticoagulation and thromboembolism, as well as eventual valve failure (see the next section). It is generally the treatment of choice for mitral or tricuspid regurgitation, where the valve apparatus is important for coordinated ventricular contraction and helps to maintain normal ventricular ellipsoid shape.

Valve Replacement

When other interventions have failed or are not possible, excision of a heart valve and replacement with a prosthetic valve is performed. Surgery is usually performed through a median sternotomy or left thoracotomy incision, although some cardiac surgery centers use minimally invasive partial upper sternotomy, or keyhole or endoscopic incisions; and new percutaneous catheter-based techniques are being developed.

- Valve replacement is commonly performed for severe mitral and aortic diseases and occasionally for pulmonary valve or tricuspid valve disease.

- ▸ Access to the aortic valve is through a transverse aortotomy at the base of the ascending aorta.
- ▸ The mitral valve is accessed via an incision through the left atrium.
- Prosthetic valves can be either mechanical or tissue-based (Figure 3-29), with each offering its own advantages and disadvantages.
  - ▸ Mechanical prosthetic valves are either ball-in-cage (e.g., Starr-Edwards), tilting disc (e.g., OmniCarbon, Medtronic-Hall, Lillehei-Kaster, and Björk-Shively), or bileaflet (e.g., Mira, On-X, ATS Open Pivot, CarboMedics, and St. Jude) in design. The major advantage of mechanical prostheses is their durability (up to 40 yr for the Starr-Edwards valve). However, they require long-term anticoagulation and aspirin therapy because of the increased risk of thromboembolic complications. On rare occasions, thrombosis develops in a mechanical valve.
  - ▸ Tissue valves (bioprostheses) consist of autografts (removal and translocation of one of a patient's valves to another valve site; see the next section, Ross Procedure), homografts (or allografts, acquired from a cadaver), or heterografts (or xenografts, transplanted from another species, as in porcine valves). In addition, biological valves can be constructed from pericardium (either autograft or bovine) that is inserted into a valve frame. Tissue prostheses have a low risk of thromboembolic complications and therefore chronic anticoagulation is often not required. However, structural deterioration occurs more rapidly, especially in children and young adults, necessitating reoperation for progressive prosthetic regurgitation and/or stenosis.
  - ▸ On occasion, endocarditis develops in prosthetic valves, which is serious and often fatal. Refer to page 127 for information regarding its prevention.
- Sometimes, mitral valve replacement can be performed with preservation of the continuity between the native valve leaflets and the papillary muscles *(mitral valve replacement with apparatus preservation),* which serves to maintain the LV functional aspects of the mitral apparatus.
- The timing of valve replacement is a crucial aspect in managing patients with valve disease.
  - ▸ In general, surgery is indicated once patients become symptomatic or as soon as ventricular dysfunction becomes apparent; otherwise mortality increases significantly.
  - ▸ Because all prosthetic valves are fairly stenotic when placed within the native valve orifice, surgical replacement for valvular stenosis offers benefits only when the original valve is more stenotic than the prosthesis.

Physical therapy recommendations for patients with sternotomy incisions can be found on pages 61 to 62, whereas recommendations for patients with thoracotomy incisions are located on page 34. Patients requiring surgical management of valve disease often experience progressive debilitation before surgery and benefit greatly from exercise training (see Chapter 7 [Cardiovascular and Pulmonary Physical Therapy Treatment], page 298). Clinical monitoring of resting and exercise vital signs is important in patients with prosthetic heart valves, as almost all have mild-to-moderate stenosis and a few have severe stenosis.

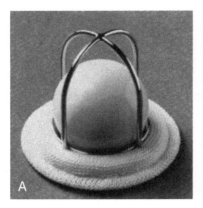
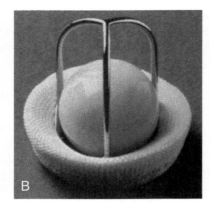
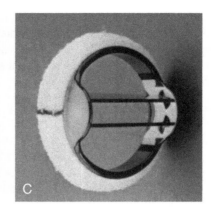
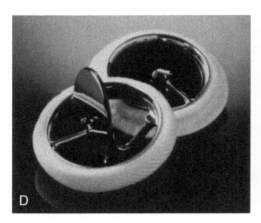
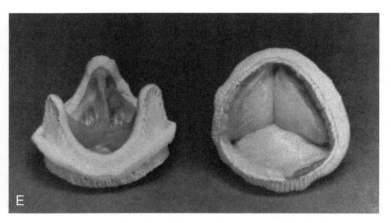

Figure 3-29: Various types of prosthetic heart valves. **A,** Starr-Edwards caged-ball mitral prosthesis. **B,** Starr-Edwards aortic valve. **C,** St. Jude Medical bileaflet valve. **D,** Medtronic-Hall tilting disc valve. **E,** Carpentier-Edwards bioprosthesis. (**A, B,** and **E** courtesy Baxter Healthcare Corporation, Edwards CVS Division; **C** courtesy St. Jude Medical, Inc.; **D** courtesy Medtronic, Inc.)

Ross Procedure

Used primarily for the treatment of severe aortic stenosis, the Ross procedure involves the use of the patient's own pulmonary valve and adjacent pulmonary artery to replace a diseased aortic valve and often the adjacent aorta, in which case reimplantation of the coronary arteries into the graft is required. A human pulmonary or aortic homograft is then inserted into the pulmonary position. The advantages of this procedure include obviation of the need for lifetime anticoagulation therapy, the long-term durability of the graft, and the ability of the graft to grow along with the patient.

Surgical Treatment of the Failed Heart

Surgical treatment of the failing heart is currently receiving a great deal of attention. The goal is to improve the quality of life of patients with refractory heart failure that has not responded to maximal medical therapy, while delaying cardiac transplantation with its limited resources. Some of these treatments are still considered investigational and thus are not widely available.

Intraaortic Balloon Counterpulsation

The intraaortic balloon pump (IABP) uses inflation and deflation of a balloon in the aorta to provide short-term mechanical circulatory assistance for patients with certain types of cardiogenic shock, usually after acute myocardial infarction, as well as for those with postoperative low cardiac output or difficulty weaning from

cardiopulmonary bypass. In addition, IABP can be used for unstable angina refractory to medical treatment and acute myocardial infarction.

- Inflation of the balloon with carbon dioxide or helium during diastole boosts intraaortic pressure and thus restores arterial pressure and improves coronary and systemic perfusion.
- Rapid deflation of the balloon during ventricular systole decreases afterload and therefore assists the emptying of the LV, resulting in enhanced stroke volume and reduced myocardial oxygen consumption.
- Researchers are currently developing an ambulatory IABP and a permanent implantable IABP.

Physical therapists must be careful not to interfere with the tubes running between the patient and the IABP when they are providing any type of treatment for these patients. When a femoral vessel is used as part of the circuit, hip flexion is usually kept to a minimum.

Extracorporeal Life Support

Extracorporeal life support (ECLS) is used for the management of life-threatening cardiac failure when no other form of treatment has been or is likely to be successful (e.g., cardiogenic shock following cardiotomy or heart transplantation and severe heart failure due to cardiomyopathy, myocarditis, and acute coronary syndrome). It is also being used during cardiopulmonary resuscitation and has been shown to improve survival rates. ECLS involves the establishment of temporary percutaneous cardiopulmonary bypass whereby venous blood is diverted from the right atrium and pumped across a membrane oxygenator and heat exchanger and then back to the aortic arch via a catheter in the right carotid artery (thus, it is sometimes referred to as veno-arterial ECLS). It is typically used for days to weeks to support recovery of heart function or as a bridge to a more permanent device or cardiac transplantation. Full systemic heparinization is required, as discussed on page 30.

Ventricular Assist Devices

For longer term treatment of end-stage heart failure, right and left ventricular assist devices (RVAD and LVAD, respectively) and biventricular assist devices (BiVAD) provide mechanical support for the ventricles. With an LVAD, the most commonly used device, a conduit connected to the left atrium sends oxygenated blood to the device, which then pumps the blood through a conduit connected to the aorta to be delivered to the body. With an RVAD, the device is attached to the right atrium and pulmonary artery, thus bypassing the RV; and with a BiVAD, both ventricles are bypassed. The patient's natural heart is unloaded but is available to assist in increasing cardiac output when necessary, as during physical activity.

- VADs are most commonly used as a bridge to either cardiac transplantation or to recovery of myocardial function, which results from the mechanical unloading provided by the device in a small percentage of patients.[10] In addition, some VADs have been approved for use as "destination therapy," or permanent support for end-stage heart failure in patients who are not eligible for cardiac transplantation (Table 3-8).

- In extracorporeal VADs, the pump chamber is outside the body, usually contained in a large portable console. These include the Abiomed BVS 5000 (Abiomed, Danvers, MA) and Thoratec VAD (Thoratec, Pleasanton, CA).

- Implantable VADs consist of an implantable pump, which is usually placed within the abdomen or under the sternum, and an exterior power supply (Figure 3-30). These include the HeartMate VE, XVE, and II LVASs (Thoratec), the Novacor

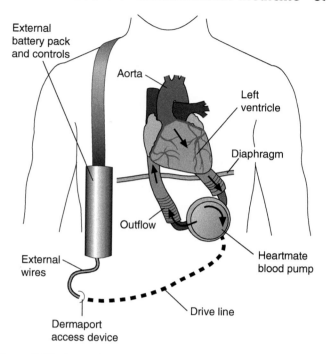

Figure 3-30: Example of a wearable left ventricular assist device and its components. The inflow catheter is inserted into the apex of the left ventricle, and the outflow cannula is anastomosed to the ascending aorta. A transcutaneous cable carries the electrical supply and air vent to the device. (Modified from Goldstein DJ, Oz MC, Rose EA. Implantable left ventricular devices. *N Engl J Med.* 1998;339:1522–1533.)

LVAS (WorldHeart, Oakland, CA), and the DeBakey VAD and the newer HeartAssist 5 pediatric LVASs (MicroMed Cardiovascular, Houston, TX).

- Patients are often referred to physical therapy for general strengthening and endurance training to increase peripheral efficiency while they are using one of these devices and awaiting transplantation. Usually they tolerate gradual, low-level exercise very well, with their progress being limited by peripheral

TABLE 3-8: U.S. FDA-approved Ventricular Assist Devices

Device	Ventricular Support	Indication	Type
Abiomed AB5000	LV, RV, bivent	Bridge to recovery	Extracorporeal
Abiomed BVS 5000	Bivent	Bridge to recovery or transplant	Extracorporeal
HeartAssist5 Pediatric VAD (formerly the DeBakey VAD Child)	LV	Bridge to transplant for pediatric patients, age 5 to 16 yrs	Implantable
HeartMate IP LVAS	LV	Bridge to transplant	Extracorporeal
HeartMate VE and XVE LVASs	LV	Bridge to transplant, destination therapy	Implantable
HeartMate II LVAS	LV	Bridge to transplant	Implantable
Novacor LVAS	LV	Bridge to transplant	Implantable
Thoratec VAD System	LV, RV, bivent	Bridge to transplant	Extracorporeal

Bivent, Biventricular; FDA, Food and Drug Administration; LV, left ventricle; LVAS, left ventricular assist system; RV, right ventricle; VAD, ventricular assist device.

deconditioning rather than cardiac dysfunction. The physician should be consulted regarding specific precautions or guidelines that might be indicated. In addition, it is critical that PTs who treat patients with VADs be trained to handle occasional device power failure, which could spell disaster for the patient unless manual pumping is provided. Furthermore, the physician should be notified if there is any change in a patient's neurologic status, signs of bleeding from the drive line or catheter sites, or an abnormal reduction in either stroke volume or pump flow.

Cardiac Resynchronization Therapy

Cardiac resynchronization therapy (CRT) typically uses biventricular pacing to stimulate the ventricle at multiple sites in order to improve coordination between the septum and the LV free wall, between the left and right ventricles, and between the atria and ventricles and thus improve cardiac performance. It is applied in patients with heart failure and left bundle branch block. Numerous clinical trials have documented improved exercise capacity, NYHA functional class (see Chapter 6, Table 6-2 on page 223), and quality of life, and some have found reductions in filling pressures, LV size, and mitral regurgitation and improved diastolic filling, ejection fraction, and cardiac output, as well as peak oxygen consumption and 6-minute walk test distance.[3,7]

Mitral Valve Annuloplasty

Functional mitral regurgitation (MR) resulting from altered ventricular geometry and distortion of the valve annulus is a common complication seen in patients with severe heart failure. MR leads to increased LV preload, wall tension, and diastolic volume, all of which contribute to a significant decrease in the efficiency of LV contraction and reduced forward cardiac output. Because a number of studies have demonstrated the importance of preserving the annular-ventricular apparatus for maintaining overall LV function and geometry, mitral valve repair with an undersized flexible annuloplasty ring has proven to be more successful than valve replacement in improving LV function in these patients.[6] Documented benefits include improved NYHA functional class, LV ejection fraction, cardiac output, end-diastolic volume, and LV geometry.

Heart and Heart—Lung Transplantation

The surgical implantation of a donor heart or heart and lungs offers the patient with end-stage heart failure an opportunity to return to an active lifestyle.

- Heart transplantation is performed for patients with end-stage cardiomyopathy, coronary artery disease, valvular disease, and congenital heart disease.
  ‣ Heart transplantation is usually orthotopic, where the recipient's heart is removed and replaced with a donor heart. Typically both the donor and recipient hearts are excised by transecting the atria at the midatrial level, leaving the multiple pulmonary venous connections to the left atrium intact in the posterior wall of the LA, and then the aorta and pulmonary artery are transected just above their respective valves (Figure 3-31). Care is taken during anastomosis of the RA to avoid injury to the donor SA node.

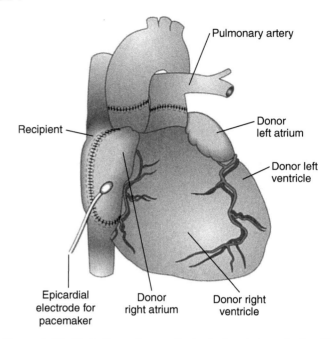

Figure 3-31: Illustration of an orthotopic heart transplant with anastomosis sites indicated by the suture lines. An atrial epicardial pacemaker electrode is in place in the donor right atrium. (From Versluis-Burlis T, Downs A. Thoracic organ transplantation: Heart, heart–lung, and lung. In Hillegass EA, Sadowsky HS, editors. *Essentials of Cardiopulmonary Physical Therapy.* 2nd ed. Philadelphia: Saunders; 2001.)

  ‣ Alternatively, some centers have begun leaving the donor atria intact and making anastomoses at the level of the superior and inferior vena cavae and pulmonary veins, which may reduce the requirement for postoperative pacemaker placement.
- Combined heart-lung (cardiopulmonary) transplantation may be performed in patients with congenital heart disease and irreversible pulmonary vascular occlusive disease (i.e., Eisenmenger's syndrome). In this case, the heart and either one lung or two lungs are transplanted as a unit.
- Immunosuppression after heart and heart-lung transplantation is required to avoid organ rejection. The highest levels of immunosuppression are required immediately after surgery; the doses are then decreased over time until the lowest maintenance levels of suppression necessary to prevent rejection are identified for each patient.
  ‣ Almost half of patients receive induction therapy, which refers to higher dose immunosuppression used in the early posttransplantation period and is aimed at effecting a state of hyporesponsiveness against the allograft.[23,26] The most commonly used agents are anti-interleukin-2 antibodies (daclizumab or basiliximab) or rabbit anti-thymocyte globulin (ATG).
  ‣ Maintenance immunosuppression consists of multiple agents, including a calcineurin inhibitor (either cyclosporine or tacrolimus [FK 506]), an antimetabolite (usually mycophenolate mofetil but occasionally azathioprine) or sirolimus, and a corticosteroid.[13,28a]
  ‣ Episodes of rejection requiring augmentation of immunosuppression, usually corticosteroids, occur in more than one third of patients.[23]

- Newer immunosuppressive agents and modalities are currently under investigation.
- The most common morbidities associated with heart transplantation include allograft vasculopathy (accelerated atherosclerosis is the leading cause of morbidity and mortality after heart transplantation, responsible for the high levels of late graft loss and death),[13] hypertension, hyperlipidemia, renal dysfunction, diabetes, and posttransplant malignancies.[28a]

Because patients are extremely debilitated by the time they qualify for transplantation, they are often referred to physical therapy for general strengthening and physical conditioning exercise during the waiting period before transplantation. The goal is to increase peripheral efficiency through gradually progressive, low-level aerobic exercise and resistance training, and thus aid the patient in returning more quickly to a more functional lifestyle after transplantation.

After transplantation, physical therapy is typically initiated as soon as possible after surgery and consists of breathing exercises, coughing, progressive mobility, light range of motion, calisthenic and postural exercises, and progressive aerobic exercise, usually walking and/or stationary cycling. Patients are often referred to outpatient cardiac rehabilitation programs after discharge.

- Postoperative sternotomy precautions are followed (see pages 61 to 62).
- Physiological monitoring is important in this patient group because of the denervated status of the donor heart and the hypertensive side effects of some of the immunosuppressive drugs, particularly cyclosporine.
  - The denervated heart usually has a higher resting HR than normal (typically 90 to 110 bpm) because of the lack of vagal stimulation, and there is no HR response to the Valsalva maneuver or changes in position from supine to sitting to standing.
  - During exercise, a prolonged warm-up period is recommended because the HR response is delayed and blunted, being stimulated by circulating catecholamines rather than sympathetic nervous system stimulation. However, cardiac output increases normally at the onset of activity because of an immediate augmentation of stroke volume per Table 3-2. The maximal HR is lower than normally expected for age, so the heart rate reserve is diminished, and peak exercise cardiac output is reduced by 30% to 40%.[9,13b,20]
  - After the conclusion of exercise, the HR may continue to rise for a few minutes into the recovery period and then gradually decrease because of the slow uptake of the circulating catecholamines; therefore, a more prolonged cooldown period is advised after exercise.
  - BP responses to progressive aerobic exercise are fairly normal initially, but many patients develop hypertension as a side effect of their immunosuppressive drugs later on. The BP responses to isometric exercise show an increase similar to normal because of a greater increase in total peripheral resistance.
  - Unless the surgery is performed in such a way as to leave the donor heart's atria intact, ECG monitoring reveals two independent P waves (one from the native heart remnant and one from the donor heart); only the P wave from the donor heart will be associated with QRS complexes.
  - Also of importance, patients with denervated hearts are unable to perceive the pain associated with myocardial ischemia, yet grafted hearts are known to develop accelerated atherosclerosis, often within 1 to 2 years of transplantation,[13] so patients should be monitored carefully for the signs and atypical symptoms of myocardial ischemia (i.e., anginal equivalents described on page 103).
- Other medication side effects that should be addressed include hypercholesterolemia, obesity, and osteoporosis and skeletal muscle atrophy due to glucocorticosteroids. Specific resistance training has been shown to restore bone mineral density, increase lean body mass, and reduce body fat.[9,28]

Endoventricular Patch Plasty

Endoventricular patch plasty, also referred to as the Dor procedure, involves the replacement of large dyskinetic or akinetic segments of myocardium with a circular patch (usually Dacron or Gore-Tex) in order to reshape the remaining ventricular wall so that muscle fiber tension is restored toward a normal helical arrangement.[22] Similar to the Dor procedure with some technical modification, the surgical anterior ventricular endocardial restoration (SAVER) procedure is used for the treatment of postinfarction ventricular dilation. In addition, it usually includes revascularization and mitral valve repair or replacement. These procedures produce improved systolic and diastolic ventricular function and NYHA functional class.

Cardiomyoplasty

Dynamic cardiomyoplasty involves the use of the latissimus dorsi muscle (LDM) with its neurovascular bundle still attached; it is brought into the chest through a lateral thoracotomy and wrapped around the heart in order to support and augment ventricular function.[21] Usually, an AV sequential pacemaker is inserted with the atrial electrodes attached to the LV wall and the ventricular electrodes attached to the LDM flap so that synchronized function can be achieved. In addition, patients participate in a 6- to 8-week muscle training program to condition the fast-twitch type IIA skeletal muscle fibers to gradually take on the oxidative characteristics of slow-twitch type I fibers. Although this procedure has been shown to produce some improvement in cardiac function, its application is limited by its complexity and high mortality rate, especially among patients with advanced heart failure.[7]

Left Ventricular Reduction: The Batista Procedure

Partial left ventriculectomy, commonly known as the Batista procedure, may be used to treat dilated cardiomyopathies and entails the excision of a portion of LV free wall between the papillary muscles and, frequently, repair or replacement of the mitral valve.[1] The goal is to decrease the LV radius and thus improve wall tension and overall LV function. However, controlled studies in the United States have failed to demonstrate improved long-term ventricular function or survival for most patients.[8]

New Devices to Improve Mechanical Efficiency

The shortcomings of dynamic cardiomyoplasty and partial left ventriculectomy have led to the development of two new procedures that involve the use of elastic to support the LV.[7] One uses the CorCap (Acorn Cardiovascular, St. Paul, MN), an elastic material placed around the heart to prevent progressive myocardial stretch and adverse remodeling. Because it has differential elastic properties in the longitudinal and circumferential directions, the CorCap encourages a more elliptical shape, which further decreases wall stress. The second procedure uses the Myosplint (Myocor, Maple Grove, MN), in which three elastic cords or splints are place through the LV to bisect it and change its shape from one large sphere to two smaller merged circles with substantially lower wall stress.

Artificial Hearts

The total artificial heart (TAH) is a mechanical replacement for an individual's diseased heart and is used as a temporary bridge to transplantation. These devices are implanted by removing the patient's ventricles and all four valves and attaching the total artificial heart to the remaining atria.

- The CardioWest temporary total artificial heart (SynCardia Systems, Tucson, AZ), which evolved from the Jarvik-7 TAH, became the first device approved by the U.S. Food and Drug Administration in 2004. It is a pneumatic device with a large external console that controls its functions.
- The AbioCor implantable replacement heart (Abiomed) is a self-contained, electrically powered hydraulic heart powered by an internal battery that is charged through the skin from an external battery pack. It includes a controller, implanted in the patient's abdominal wall, that monitors and controls the pumping speed of the device to allow a cardiac output of more than 10 L/min, when needed.

For physical therapy implications, see the section Ventricular Assist Devices (page 67).

Other Surgical Interventions

Aneurysectomy/Myectomy

Aneurysectomy/myectomy involves the surgical resection of a dyskinetic region of the myocardium (i.e., an LV aneurysm) or another segment of cardiac muscle. The primary indications for aneurysectomy are angina pectoris associated with prior myocardial infarction and multivessel coronary artery disease and recurrent hemodynamically significant ventricular arrhythmias; the indications for myectomy are recurrent arrhythmias and outflow tract obstruction.

Septal Myectomy

When patients with hypertrophic cardiomyopathy (HCM) experience obstruction to ventricular ejection of blood because of contact of the anterior mitral valve leaflet with the intraventricular septum during systole, a myotomy and myectomy may be performed to relieve the outflow obstruction. Typically, a surgical incision is made through the aorta and a small amount of muscle tissue is excised from the proximal to mid-interventricular septum at the point where the mitral valve leaflet makes contact. This procedure has proved to be successful in eliminating outflow obstruction, reducing secondary mitral regurgitation, and markedly improving symptoms so that many patients are able to achieve near normal exercise capacity.[21]

REFERENCES

1. Abe T, Fukada J, Morishita K. The Batista procedure: Fact, fiction, and its role in the management of heart failure. *Heart Failure Rev.* 2001;6: 195-199.
2. Abo-Auda W, Benza R. Transmyocardial and percutaneous myocardial revascularization: Current concepts and future directions. *J Heart Lung Transplant.* 2003;22:837-842.
3. Abraham WT. Electrophysiological aids in congestive heart failure: Supporting and synchronizing systole. *Med Clin North Am.* 2003;87:509-521.
4. Ades PA. Cardiac rehabilitation and secondary prevention of coronary heart disease. *N Engl J Med.* 2001;345:892-902.
5. American Association of Cardiovascular and Pulmonary Rehabilitation. *Guidelines for Cardiac Rehabilitation and Secondary Prevention Programs.* 4th ed. Champaign, IL: Human Kinetics; 2004.
6. Bakir I, Casselman FP, Brugada P, et al. Current strategies in the surgical treatment of atrial fibrillation: Review of the literature and Onze Lieve Vrouw Clinic's strategy. *Ann Thorac Surg.* 2007;83:331-340.
7. Boehmer JP. Device therapy for heart failure. *Am. J. Cardiol.* 2003;91 (suppl):53D-59D.
8. Bolling SF, Smolens IA, Pagani FD. Surgical alternatives for heart failure. *J Heart Lung Transplant.* 2001;20:729-733.
9. Braith RW, Edwards DG. Exercise following heart transplantation. *Sports Med.* 2000;30:171-192.
9a. Chen J, Krumholz HM. Screening for coronary artery disease with electron-beam computed tomography is not useful. *Circulation.* 2006;113:135-146.
9b. Clouse ME. Noninvasive screening for coronary artery disease with computed tomography is useful. *Circulation.* 2006;113:125-135.
10. Deng MC, Edwards LB, Hertz MI, et al. Mechanical circulatory support device database of the International Society for Heart and Lung Transplantation: Second annual report—2004. *J Heart Lung Transplant.* 2004; 23:1027-1034.
11. DeSouza CA, Shapiro LF, Clevenger CM, et al. Regular aerobic exercise prevents and restores age-related endothelium-dependent vasodilation in healthy men. *Circulation.* 2000;102:1351-1357.
12. Dor V. The endoventricular circular patch plasty ("Dor procedure") in ischemic akinetic dilated ventricles. *Heart Failure Rev.* 2001;6:187-193.
13. Eisen H, Ross H. Optimizing the immunosuppressive regimen in heart transplantation. *J Heart Lung Transplant.* 2004;23:S207-213.
13a. Elhendy A, Bax JJ, Poldermans D: Dobutamine stress myocardial perfusion imaging in coronary artery disease. *J Nucl Med.* 2002;43:1634-1646.
13b. Fink AW. Exercise responses in the transplant population. *Cardiopulm Rec.* 1986;1(3):7-10.
14. Gerber TC, Kuzo RS, Karstaedt N, et al. Current results and new developments of coronary angiography with use of contrast-enhanced computed tomography of the heart. *Mayo Clin Proc.* 2002;77:55-71.
15. Greenland P, Kizilbash MA. Coronary computed tomography in coronary risk assessment. *J Cardiopulm Rehab.* 2005;25:3-10.
16. Horvath KA. Clinical studies of TMR with the CO_2 laser. *J Clin Laser Med Surg.* 1997;15:281-285.
17. Khargi K, Hutten BA, Lemke B, et al. Surgical treatment of atrial fibrillation: A systematic review. *Eur J Cardiothorac Surg.* 2005;27:258-265.
18. Kobashigawa JA, Leaf DA, Lee N, et al. A controlled trial of exercise rehabilitation after heart transplantation. *N Engl J Med.* 1999;340:272-277.
19. LaFontaine TP, Gordon NF. Comprehensive cardiovascular risk reduction in patients with coronary artery disease. In: *American College of Sports Medicine: ACSM's Resource Manual for Guidelines for Exercise Testing and Prescription.* 4th ed. Philadelphia: Lippincott Williams & Wilkins; 2001.
20. Marconi C, Marzorati M. Exercise after heart transplantation. *Eur J Appl Physiol.* 2003;90:250-259.
21. Maron BJ. Hypertrophic cardiomyopathy: A systematic review. *JAMA.* 2002;287:1308-1320.
22. Moreira LFP, Stolf NAG. Dynamic cardiomyoplasty as a therapeutic alternative: Current status. *Heart Failure Rev.* 2001;6:201-212.
23. Mueller XM. Drug immunosuppression therapy for adult heart transplantation. 2. Clinical applications and results. *Ann Thorac Surg.* 2004;77: 363-371.
24. Pepine CJ, Balaban RS, Bonow RO, et al. Women's Ischemic Syndrome Evaluation: Current status and future research directions. Report of the National, Heart, Lung, and Blood Institute Workshop. October 2-4, 2002. Section 1: Diagnosis of stable ischemia and ischemic heart disease. *Circulation.* 2004;109:44e-46e.
25. Piña IL, Apstein CS, Balady GJ, et al. Exercise and heart failure: A statement from the American Heart Association Committee on exercise, rehabilitation, and prevention. *Circulation.* 2003;107:1210-1225.
26. Shapiro R, Young JB, Milford EL, et al. Immunosuppression: Evolution in practice and trends, 1993-2003. *Am J Transplant.* 2005;5:874-886.
27. Solway S, Brooks D, Lacasse Y, et al. A qualitative systematic overview of the measurement properties of functional tests used in the cardiorespiratory domain. *Chest.* 2001;119:256-270.

28. Stewart KJ, Badenhop D, Brubaker PH, et al. Cardiac rehabilitation following percutaneous revascularization, heart transplant, heart valve surgery, and for chronic heart failure. *Chest.* 2003;123:2104-2111.

28a. Taylor DO, Edwards LB, Boucek MM, et al. The registry of the International Society for Heart and Lung Transplantation: twenty-first official adult heart transplant report – 2004. *J Heart Lung Transplant.* 2004;23:796-803.

29. Tegtbur U, Busse MW, Jung K, et al. Time course of physical reconditioning during exercise rehabilitation late after heart transplantation. *J Heart Lung Transplant.* 2005;24:270-274.

30. Verdeccia P, Schillaci G, Reboldi G, et al. Different prognostic impact of 24-hour mean blood pressure and pulse pressure on stroke and coronary artery disease in essential hypertension. *Circulation.* 2001;103:2579-2584.

31. Verdeccia P, Reboldi G, Porcellati C, et al. Risk of cardiovascular disease in relation to achieved office and ambulatory blood pressure control in treated hypertensive subjects. *J Am Coll Cardiol.* 2002;39:878-885.

ADDITIONAL READINGS

Andreoli TE, Carpenter CCJ, Griggs RC, Loscalzo J, eds. *Cecil Essentials of Medicine.* 6th ed. Philadelphia: Saunders; 2004.

Crawford MH, DiMarco JP, Paulus WJ, et al. *Cardiology.* 2nd ed. Edinburgh: Mosby; 2004.

Ellestad MH. *Stress Testing—Principles and Practice.* 5th ed. New York: Oxford University Press; 2003.

Frownfelter D, Dean E. *Cardiovascular and Pulmonary Physical Therapy – Evidence and Practice.* 4th ed. St. Louis: Mosby; 2006.

Fuster V, Alexander RW, O'Rourke RA, eds. *Hurst's The Heart.* 11th ed. New York: McGraw-Hill; 2004.

Goldman L, Ausiello D, eds. *Cecil Textbook of Medicine.* 22nd ed. Philadelphia: Saunders; 2004.

Guyton AC, Hall JE. *Textbook of Medical Physiology.* 10th ed. Philadelphia: Saunders; 2000.

Hillegass EA, Sadowsky HS, eds. *Essentials of Cardiopulmonary Physical Therapy.* 2nd ed. Philadelphia: Saunders; 2001.

Huff J. *ECG Workout – Exercises in Arrhythmia Interpretation.* 4th ed. Philadelphia: Lippincott Williams & Wilkins; 2002.

Humes HD, ed-in-chief. *Kelley's Textbook of Internal Medicine.* 4th ed. Philadelphia: Lippincott Williams & Wilkins; 2000.

Irwin S, Tecklin JS. *Cardiopulmonary Physical Therapy.* 4th ed. St. Louis: Mosby; 2004.

McArdle WD, Katch FI, Katch VL. *Exercise Physiology—Energy, Nutrition, and Human Performance.* 5th ed. Philadelphia: Lea & Febiger; 2001.

St. John MG, Rutherford JD. *Clinical Cardiovascular Imaging: A Companion to Braunwald's Heart Disease.* Philadelphia: Elsevier; 2004.

Topol EJ, Califf RM, Isner J, et al. *Textbook of Cardiovascular Medicine.* 2nd ed. Philadelphia: Lippincott Williams & Wilkins; 2002.

Wagner GS. *Marriott's Practical Electrocardiography.* 10th ed. Philadelphia: Lippincott Williams & Wilkins; 2001.

Zipes DP, Libby P, Bonow RO, et al. *Heart Disease—A Textbook of Cardiovascular Medicine.* 7th ed. Philadelphia: Elsevier Saunders; 2005.

Cardiopulmonary Pathology

The purpose of this chapter is to describe the more common diseases and disorders that affect the respiratory and cardiovascular systems and the clinical implications for physical therapy interventions. In addition, the cardiopulmonary complications associated with other medical diagnoses are presented, as well as recommendations for physical therapy treatment modifications. To provide optimal treatment, the reader is encouraged to study more detailed descriptions, such as those cited at the end of this chapter.

4.1 PULMONARY DISEASES AND DISORDERS

When injury to the lungs occurs, usually by exposure to toxic substances or pathogens or by autoimmune processes, the lungs respond with an acute inflammatory reaction involving numerous cytokines, cell types, and inflammatory mediators. This is followed by either complete resolution, tissue breakdown with subsequent destruction, or fibrosis. Although the initial physiologic defects vary according to each pathology, most acute and chronic lung diseases share several pathophysiological consequences, particularly as the disease progresses in severity, as shown in Figure 4-1. In all pathologies, the earliest common event is a mismatch between ventilation and perfusion in the area of pathology, which can result in impaired gas exchange as well as increased work of breathing.

With progressive disease or that involving a large volume of lung tissue, impaired gas exchange and increased work of breathing initiate two pathophysiological cascades of events that lead to the major causes of morbidity and mortality associated with pulmonary disease. In the first case, impaired gas exchange produces localized alveolar hypoxia, which induces hypoxic vasoconstriction in an attempt to maintain a normal ventilation–perfusion ($\dot{V}/\dot{Q}$) ratio. If a large area of the lungs is diseased, significant hypoxic vasoconstriction and often pulmonary vascular inflammation and remodeling occur, so that pulmonary arterial pressure rises. Thus, pulmonary vascular resistance and the pressure load on the right ventricle (RV) increase, which stimulates RV hypertrophy and dilation. With progressive pulmonary hypertension, RV dysfunction can develop, followed by RV failure and cor pulmonale. In the second cascade, increased work of breathing leads to recruitment of the accessory muscles of respiration; persistent or progressive disease, as well as acute exacerbations, can lead to respiratory muscle fatigue and eventual respiratory failure.

A brief description of the more common diseases and disorders affecting the respiratory system is presented in this section, including their pathophysiology, clinical manifestations, and treatment options. In addition, the clinical implications for physical therapy are listed for the major categories of obstructive and restrictive lung disease and also some of the specific disorders.

OBSTRUCTIVE LUNG DISEASES

Obstructive lung diseases (OLD) include asthma, chronic bronchitis, emphysema, bronchiectasis, and cystic fibrosis, among others, which are characterized by airflow limitation that is particularly noticeable during forced expiration. Airflow limitation can result from impediments within the airways (e.g., excessive secretions, edema fluid, or foreign material), airway narrowing (e.g., bronchoconstriction, mucous gland hypertrophy, or inflammation), or peribronchial abnormalities (e.g., destruction of lung parenchyma, as in emphysema, or compression by enlarged lymph nodes or tumor).

Because there is a great deal of overlap in the clinical and pathophysiological features of asthma, chronic bronchitis, and emphysema and many patients have features of more than one of these diseases, as demonstrated in Figure 4-2, the generic diagnosis of chronic obstructive pulmonary disease (COPD) is frequently used (sometimes called chronic obstructive lung disease or chronic obstructive airway disease [COLD or COAD, respectively]). Common to all obstructive pathologies is chronic inflammation of the airways and parenchymal and vascular destruction, which occur in highly variable combinations. In most cases, COPD is slowly progressive and only partially reversible with treatment.

Smoking is the principal cause of COPD, with many of its chemical substances inducing proinflammatory, cytotoxic, and carcinogenic effects. In addition, inhibition of ciliary function is associated with recurrent episodes of bronchitis and lower respiratory tract infections. However, only a small minority of smokers actually develop COPD; more commonly they experience serious cardiovascular, cerebrovascular, and peripheral vascular diseases.[127]

A general description of COPD is presented here, followed by the specific characteristics of the more common types of COPD.

Pathophysiology

The general pathophysiological effects of COPD are illustrated in Figure 4-3, and their progression is depicted in the events below the dashed line in Figure 4-1.

- Chronic inflammation of the airways leads to mucosal edema, increased mucus production, ciliary dysfunction, and sometimes bronchoconstriction, all of which increase airway resistance, resulting in expiratory flow limitation. Initially, the disease is asymptomatic, but once the forced expiratory volume in 1 second (FEV_1) falls to approximately 50% of predicted normal, symptoms usually appear.
- As COPD progresses, obstruction of the small airways occurs because of airway thickening (caused by reparative remodeling) and accumulation of inflammatory exudates induced by

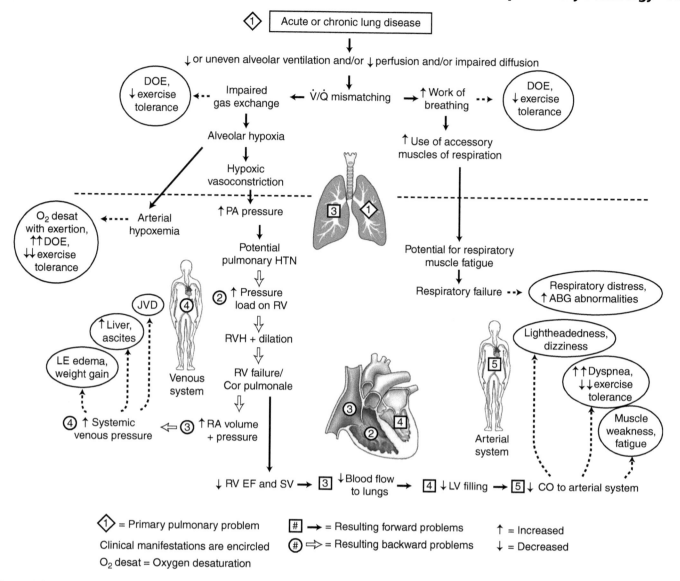

Figure 4-1: Common pathophysiological events occurring in both obstructive and restrictive lung diseases, whether acute or chronic in nature. Events depicted above the *dashed line* are common in mild to moderate disease, whereas those below the line occur as disease progresses to become more severe to very severe, with respiratory failure and/or cor pulmonale usually being the terminal events. Clinical manifestations associated with various events are enclosed in *circles*. ABG, Arterial blood gas; CO, cardiac output; DOE, dyspnea on exertion; EF, ejection fraction; HTN, hypertension; JVD, jugular venous distension; LE, lower extremity; LV, left ventricular; O_2, oxygen; PA, pulmonary arterial; RA, right atrial; RV, right ventricular; $\dot{V}/\dot{Q}$, ventilation-perfusion.

mucociliary dysfunction.[112] Thus, in moderate to severe disease, early airway closure and incomplete alveolar emptying give rise to increased residual volume, air trapping, and lung hyperinflation, which are usually exacerbated by exercise (i.e., dynamic hyperinflation).

- Destruction of alveoli decreases the surface area for gas exchange, while bronchial obstruction and expiratory air trapping produce uneven ventilation. Thus, there is $\dot{V}/\dot{Q}$ mismatching, interference with gas exchange, and increased work of breathing, which initiate the cascade of pathophysiological events detailed in the lower portion of Figure 4-1.
- In addition, increased residual volume and air trapping producing lung hyperinflation result in a barrel-shaped chest, which

alters the mechanics of breathing. The efficiency of the primary respiratory muscles is reduced as the diaphragm becomes flattened (so its pull becomes more horizontal and inhibits chest expansion) and the accessory muscles of respiration are recruited, further increasing the work of breathing.

- Acute exacerbations, which are usually precipitated by respiratory infection or environmental pollutants, occur with greater frequency and severity as the disease processes progress and can be life-threatening.[172]
- Airway resistance suddenly increases because of bronchospasm, mucosal edema, and intensified sputum production, which aggravate expiratory flow limitation and dynamic hyperinflation.

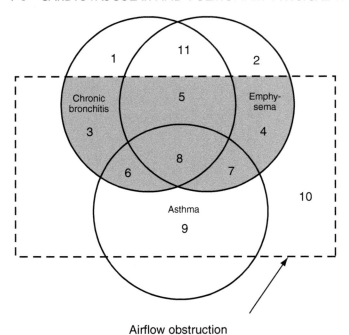

Airflow obstruction

Figure 4-2: Schema of chronic obstructive pulmonary disease (COPD). A Venn diagram shows subsets of patients with chronic bronchitis, emphysema, and asthma in three overlapping circles; the subsets comprising COPD are *shaded*. The areas of the subsets are not proportional to the size of the subset. Most patients with severe disease have features of both chronic bronchitis and emphysema and fall into subset 5; some patients have features of asthma as well and fall into subset 8. Those with features of asthma and chronic bronchitis fall into subset 6. Patients with asthma whose airflow obstruction is completely reversible (subset 9) and those with chronic bronchitis or emphysema without airflow obstruction (subsets 1, 2, and 11) are not classified as having COPD. (From Shapiro SD, Snider GL, Rennard SI. Chronic bronchitis and emphysema. In Mason RJ, Broaddus VC, Murray JF, Nadel JA, editors. *Murray & Nadel's Textbook of Respiratory Medicine.* 4th ed. Philadelphia: Saunders; 2005.)

- The subsequent escalation of $\dot{V}/\dot{Q}$ mismatching and work of breathing increases the potential for ventilatory failure and/or RV failure and cor pulmonale.
- During exercise, pulmonary dysfunction increases and is associated with cardiovascular limitations. Exercise intolerance is the chief clinical complaint and is caused by a number of complex interdependent factors:
  ‣ Ventilatory limitation develops as a result of expiratory flow limitation, abnormal breathing mechanics and dynamic hyperinflation, impaired gas exchange, and increased work of breathing.[171]
  ‣ Excessively increased pulmonary vascular pressures at low workloads, even in individuals with normal pressures and little or no hypoxemia at rest, often result in pulmonary hypertension (PH) even without exercise-induced hypoxemia.[47]
  ‣ RV pump dysfunction induced by PH leads to reduced stroke volume and higher submaximal heart rates.[207]

‣ Impaired skeletal muscle function develops as a result of structural and functional changes arising from hypoxemia, disuse atrophy, cachexia, corticosteroid therapy, and hormonal deficiencies (e.g., testosterone and growth hormone).[11a,15,39,147a]
‣ Dynamic hyperinflation during exercise increases the load on the respiratory muscles, which are already limited by reduced functional inspiratory strength and endurance.[169]
- Finally, COPD, independent of smoking, age, and gender, doubles the risk of cardiovascular morbidity and mortality, possibly as a result of the persistent low-grade systemic inflammation that is present in stable COPD.[149]
- The prognosis for individuals with mild COPD, especially if smoking cessation is achieved, is good, whereas that for patients with severe disease, especially if there is hypercapnia or cor pulmonale, is poor, with a mortality rate of ≈30% at 1 year and 95% at 10 years.[186a] The BODE Index, shown in Table 4-1, is a simple multidimensional grading system that can be used to predict the risk of death for patients with COPD.[40]

General Clinical Manifestations

- Dyspnea, especially on exertion
- Cough, often productive
- Reduced exercise tolerance
- Use of pursed-lip breathing and tripod positioning for relief of dyspnea
- Prolonged expiration, so inspiratory-to-expiratory (I:E) ratio increases to 1:3 or 1:4 (normal, 1:2); with tachypnea expiration is shortened, so I:E ratio decreases to 1:1, leading to increased air trapping in COPD
- Abnormal pulmonary function test (PFT) results with increased total lung capacity (TLC), residual volume, and functional residual capacity (FRC) and normal or decreased vital capacity (VC) (see Figure 2-8 on page 13); reduced flow rates at all lung volumes (see Figures 2-9 and 2-10 on page 16); and impaired diffusing capacity. COPD can be classified on the basis of spirometric data[179]:
  ‣ Stage 0/at risk: normal spirometry with chronic productive cough
  ‣ Stage I/mild COPD: FEV_1/FVC (forced vital capacity) less than 70% and FEV_1 at least 80% predicted normal
  ‣ Stage II/moderate COPD: FEV_1/FVC less than 70% and FEV_1 50% to 79% predicted for stage IIA and 30% to 49% predicted for IIB
  ‣ Stage III/severe COPD: FEV_1/FVC less than 70% and FEV_1 less than 30% predicted
- With more advanced disease:
  ‣ Abnormal chest x-ray findings with hyperinflated lungs and flattened diaphragms and possibly an enlarged right ventricle
  ‣ Signs and symptoms of hypoxemia (see page 241) and hypercapnia (see Box 6-2, page 243)
  ‣ Possible signs and symptoms of respiratory/ventilatory muscle fatigue or failure if severe dysfunction (see page 243)
  ‣ Possible signs and symptoms of PH, right ventricular hypertrophy (RVH), or cor pulmonale if severe dysfunction (see page 93)
- The term *"blue bloaters"* is often used to describe patients who have a stocky body build, bloated abdomen, and cyanosis

Obstructive Lung Disease

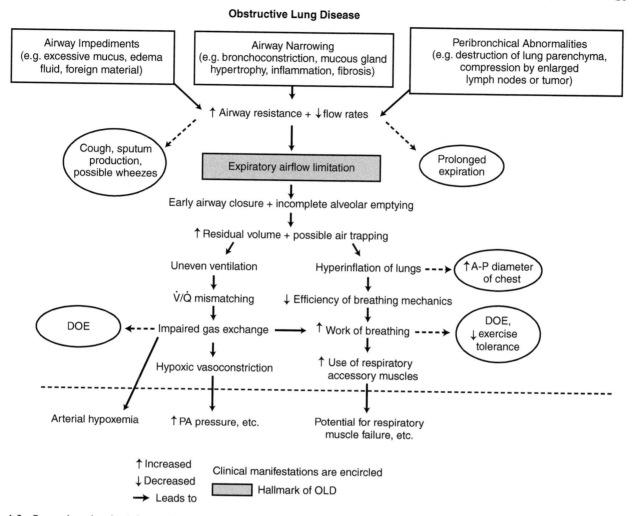

Figure 4-3: General pathophysiology of obstructive lung diseases leading to increased ventilation–perfusion mismatching ($\dot{V}/\dot{Q}$) and increased work of breathing; the resultant clinical manifestations are *encircled*. The pathophysiological events that may be induced by these as disease progresses are depicted in Figure 4-1 as the events below the dashed line. A-P, antero-posterior; DOE, dyspnea on exertion; $\dot{V}/\dot{Q}$, ventilation-perfusion.

(most common in chronic bronchitis), and the term *"pink puffers"* is used to describe patients who increase their work of breathing in order to maintain relatively normal oxygenation (most common in emphysema).

General Treatment

- Health education (symptoms, avoidance of risk factors, smoking cessation, influenza immunization, etc.)
- Medications (e.g., bronchodilators and drugs that prevent bronchoconstriction, antiinflammatory agents, and mucolytic agents) (see Chapter 5 [Pharmacology] and each pathology)
- Physical therapy interventions (see the next section and Chapter 7 [Cardiovascular and Pulmonary Physical Therapy Treatment])
- Pulmonary rehabilitation (see pages 32 and 309)
- Supportive measures
  - ▸ Oxygen therapy for hypoxemic patients and those who exhibit significant desaturation with exertion
  - ▸ Nutritional support
- Management of acute exacerbations
  - ▸ Inhaled bronchodilators

- ▸ Glucocorticosteroids
- ▸ Antibiotics for signs of infection
- ▸ Ventilatory support (e.g., noninvasive positive-pressure ventilation)
- Surgical interventions (see page 34)
  - ▸ Excision or plication of dominant bullae
  - ▸ Lung volume reduction surgery
  - ▸ Lung transplantation

Clinical Implications for Physical Therapy

- Physical therapy evaluation of patients with increased risk for pulmonary disease should include assessment of airway clearance, chest wall and shoulder mobility, respiratory muscle strength, and physiological responses to exercise (e.g., heart rate [HR], blood pressure [BP], respiratory rate, oxygen saturation, and signs and symptoms of activity intolerance), as described in Chapter 6 (Cardiopulmonary Assessment).
- Physiological monitoring is indicated during physical therapy (PT) sessions, at least initially, to avoid adverse reactions and to achieve optimal physiological benefits.

TABLE 4-1: The BODE Index: Predicting Risk of Death in Ambulatory Patients With Chronic Obstructive Pulmonary Disease

Points on BODE Index

Variable	0	1	2	3
FEV_1 (% predicted)	≥ 65	50–64	36–49	≤ 35
Distance walked in 6 min (m)	>350	250–349	150–249	≤ 149
MMRC Dyspnea Scale*	0–1	2	3	4
BMI	>21	≤ 21		

Total Score

BODE Index Score	1-Year Mortality	2-Year Mortality	52-Month Mortality
0–2	2%	6%	19%
3–4	2%	8%	32%
5–6	2%	14%	40%
7–10	5%	31%	80%

*Modified Medical Research Council Dyspnea Scale: 0, no breathlessness except with strenuous exercise; 1, breathlessness when hurrying on the level or walking up a slight hill; 2, walks slower than people of same age on the level because of breathlessness or has to stop for breath when walking at own pace on the level; 3, stops for breath after walking about 100 yards or a few minutes on the level; 4, too breathless to leave the house or breathless when dressing or undressing.
Data from Celli BR, Cote CG, Marin JM, et al. The body-mass index, airflow obstruction, dyspnea, and exercise capacity index in chronic obstructive pulmonary disease. *N. Engl. J. Med.* 2004;350:1005–1012.
BMI, Body mass index; BODE, *b*ody mass index, airflow *o*bstruction, *d*yspnea, and *e*xercise capacity; FEV_1, forced expiratory volume in 1 second; MMRC, Modified Medical Research Council.

- Use of a bronchodilator before PT treatments may enhance exercise tolerance in patients with reversible disease on PFTs.
- Patients should never exercise on less oxygen than they are using at rest. Monitoring of oxygen saturation can assist in identifying patients who need supplemental oxygen, or increased oxygen, during activity (a physician's order is required to use or increase oxygen dose at any time).
- Physical therapists should be able to recognize the signs and symptoms of hypoxemia as well as those of respiratory muscle fatigue (see pages 241 and 242).
- Side effects of medications may affect exercise responses (see Chapter 5, pages 214 and 216).
  - Increased resting and exercise HRs may be seen in patients taking caffeine derivative bronchodilators.
  - Increased arrhythmias, nervousness, confusion, and/or tremors may indicate bronchodilator toxicity.
  - Corticosteroids provoke increased catabolism, so physical therapists must observe for skin breakdown and use caution regarding overstressing bones and musculoskeletal structures.
- Endurance exercise training is extremely valuable for patients with COPD, resulting in improved functional exercise capacity and reduced shortness of breath, probably due to increased skeletal and respiratory muscle strength and improved endurance.[50,169] Exercise training may also improve motivation for exercise, reduce depression, decrease symptoms, enhance cardiovascular function, and improve health-related quality of living.

- Patients should be referred to pulmonary rehabilitation once their FEV_1 falls below 50% to 60% of its predicted value, which corresponds to the transition from mild to moderate disease.[50]
- Before exercise training is initiated, patients should be receiving optimal medical management, including bronchodilator therapy, long-term oxygen therapy, and treatment of comorbidities.
- Exercise prescription typically consists of at least 30 minutes of intermittent or continuous low- to moderate-intensity aerobic exercise performed at least 3 days/wk (see Chapter 7, page 303). Once an individual can perform exercise independently, frequency can increase to at least 5 days/wk, per public health recommendations (see page 301).[166] Interval training with periodic rest periods increases patient tolerance for more vigorous activities. The goal is to gradually increase exercise duration. Exercise intensity is usually guided by symptomatology (typically a Borg score of 4 to 6 for dyspnea or fatigue) or 60% of peak exercise capacity. If tolerated, higher intensity exercise is encouraged, as it provokes greater physiological training effects. Use of supplemental oxygen during exercise increases exercise tolerance in both normoxemic and hypoxemic patients so higher intensity exercise training can be performed.[72,83] Coordination of breathing with activity increases efficiency of effort. Use of dyspnea relief positions is helpful for recovery from shortness of breath.
- Resistance exercise training is also recommended for patients with COPD to improve skeletal muscle strength and endurance and to increase muscle mass (see Chapter 7).[169,212a,223a]

Training sessions generally include 1 to 3 sets of 8 to 10 repetitions at intensities ranging from 50% to 85% of one repetition maximum performed 2 or 3 days/wk.

- Other PT interventions that may benefit patients with COPD are described in Chapter 7 and include the following:
  ▸ Identification of triggers for dyspnea
  ▸ Bronchial hygiene techniques for patients with increased secretions
  ▸ Therapeutic exercise to improve shoulder and chest mobility as well as posture
  ▸ Relaxation techniques
  ▸ Energy conservation and work simplification techniques
  ▸ Creative problem solving to deal with functional limitations
- PTs should also encourage preventive health measures, such as adequate hydration, good nutrition, compliance with medications and other treatments, self-monitoring, early treatment if signs of problems occur, and flu and pneumonia prevention.

Disorders That Result in Obstructive Lung Disease

Chronic Bronchitis

Chronic bronchitis is characterized by a chronic cough with excessive mucus production that is not due to known specific causes, such as bronchiectasis or tuberculosis, and that is present for most days of at least 3 months of the year for two or more consecutive years.

Pathophysiology

Chronic irritation of the airways (due to smoking, air pollution, occupational exposure, or bronchial infection) provokes an inflammatory response that stimulates pathological change in the bronchial walls, as depicted in Figure 4-4, and leads to a chronic productive cough and recurrent pulmonary infections.

- Chronic inflammation of the airways induces mucosal edema, hypersecretion of mucus, and destruction of cilia, all of which increase airway resistance and produce expiratory flow

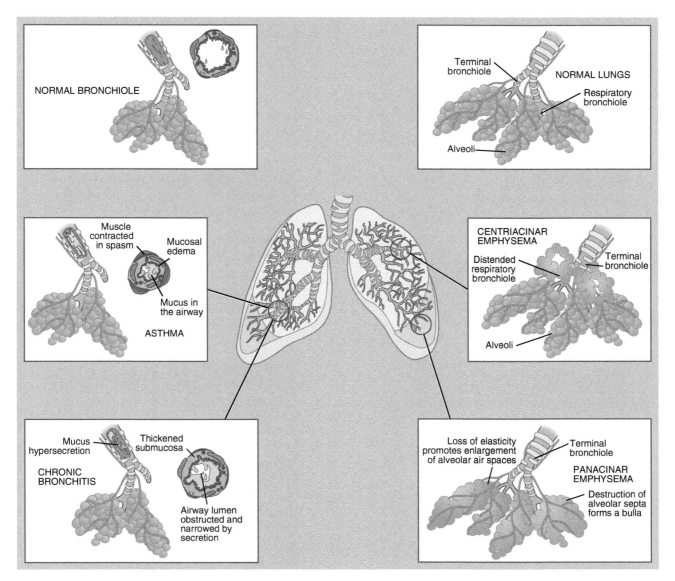

Figure 4-4: Comparisons of normal airways and those affected by asthma, chronic bronchitis, and emphysema, both centriacinar and panacinar. (From Goodman CC, Boisonnault WG, Fuller KS. *Pathology: Implications for the Physical Therapist.* 2nd ed. Philadelphia: Saunders; 2003.)

limitation. Airway obstruction and pulmonary dysfunction develop as previously described (refer to Figures 4-1 and 4-3).

- In addition, irritation of the airways can cause bronchoconstriction, which further increases airway resistance and expiratory flow limitation.
- During acute exacerbations, sputum production escalates and more secretions are retained, resulting in further aggravation of $\dot{V}/\dot{Q}$ mismatching and increased work of breathing, and so on, as presented on pages 72 to 75.
- With severe disease, the excessive work of breathing and deterioration of gas exchange, along with polycythemia, lead to ventilatory failure, cor pulmonale, or both.

Clinical Manifestations

- Insidious onset of smokers' cough, which progresses to chronic productive cough
- Progressive exertional dyspnea, with possible respiratory distress late in the disease
- Increased respiratory symptoms due to irritants, cold, damp or foggy weather, and acute pulmonary infections
- Normal breath sounds with prolonged expiratory time and possible crackles or wheezing (for other physical signs see Chapter 6, page 294)
- With more advanced disease:
  ‣ Hypoxemia and increased arterial carbon dioxide (Pa_{CO_2}) (i.e., hypercapnia), respiratory acidosis
  ‣ Clinical manifestations of cor pulmonale, respiratory failure, or both (see page 95)

Specific Treatment

- Medications include the following:
  ‣ Anticholinergic bronchodilators versus long-acting β-agonists
  ‣ Inhaled corticosteroids?
- Supplemental oxygen
- Pulmonary rehabilitation and other treatment options for COPD (see page 75)

Emphysema

Emphysema consists of several diseases that ultimately result in permanent overdistension of the air spaces distal to the terminal nonrespiratory bronchioles accompanied by destruction of the alveolar walls and without obvious fibrosis. Abnormal air spaces, called *bullae* and *blebs,* may be seen on chest radiograph when the disease is moderately advanced. The most common causes of emphysema include cigarette smoking and occupational exposure (see page 92), which typically produce centriacinar destruction (see Figure 4-4). A rarer cause is α_1-protease inhibitor deficiency (α_1-PI; also called α_1-antitrypsin deficiency), which tends to cause a diffuse panacinar emphysema.

Pathophysiology

Repeated inflammation of the airways produces an imbalance between endogenous proteinases and antiproteinases, which causes progressive lung destruction.

- Loss of elastic recoil due to tissue destruction leads to expiratory collapse of distal, poorly supported airways, resulting in air trapping and alveolar overdistension. The alveolar walls fragment and attenuate so that several alveoli coalesce to form bullae, which can become quite large and compress adjacent lung tissue.
- In addition, the loss of large portions of lung parenchyma reduces the pulmonary vascular bed, which further increases pulmonary vascular resistance and accelerates pulmonary hypertension (PH), and so on, as illustrated in Figure 4-1.
- As the disease progresses, pulmonary hyperinflation decreases the efficiency of the respiratory muscles and increases the work of breathing (see Figure 4-3).
- Loss of functional alveoli results in gross $\dot{V}/\dot{Q}$ mismatching throughout the lungs, hyperventilation of well-ventilated, well-perfused alveoli in order to maintain normal blood gases, increased work of breathing, and greater risk of ventilatory muscle fatigue and failure (see page 94).
- Also, increased $\dot{V}/\dot{Q}$ mismatching with more advanced disease interferes with gas exchange, leading to PH, RV failure, and cor pulmonale (see page 94).

Clinical Manifestations

- Progressive dyspnea, especially on exertion
- Cough, often severe, with variable degrees of productiveness
- Increased symptoms with acute respiratory infections
- Decreased breath sounds with prolonged expiration, possible end-expiratory wheeze on forced expiration (for other physical signs see Chapter 6, page 294)
- With more advanced disease:
  ‣ Diminished nutritional status, weight loss from greater energy used for breathing
  ‣ Hypoxemia and hypercapnia, respiratory acidosis
  ‣ Possible signs and symptoms of cor pulmonale, ventilatory failure, or both when end-stage disease develops

Specific Treatment

- Medications:
  ‣ Anticholinergic bronchodilators versus long-acting β-agonists
  ‣ Inhaled corticosteroids
  ‣ Supplemental oxygen
- Surgical interventions (see page 34)
  ‣ Bullectomy
  ‣ Lung volume reduction
  ‣ Lung transplantation, particularly for α_1-PI deficiency
- Pulmonary rehabilitation and other treatment options for COPD (see page 75)

Asthma

Asthma is a chronic inflammatory condition characterized by airway hyperreactivity to various external and internal stimuli and manifested as recurrent episodes of intermittent reversible airway obstruction.

- When the provocative stimuli are immunologic in origin, sensitized mast cells exposed to specific antigens degranulate and release bronchoactive mediators, causing extrinsic, or atopic, asthma, which is most commonly seen in children.
- When the cause is not clearly related to allergy, as in adult-onset asthma, intrinsic or nonatopic asthma is present; sometimes it is due to sensitivity to aspirin or nonsteroidal antiinflammatory drugs (NSAIDs), nasal polyposis, or sinusitis.[156]

TABLE 4-2: Factors That May Precipitate Acute Asthma

Type of Asthma	Irritant or Inducing Stimulus
Nonatopic (intrinsic)	Inhaled irritants (e.g., smoke, dusts, pollution, sprays)
	Weather (e.g., high humidity, cold air, fog)
	Respiratory infections (e.g., common cold, bronchitis)
	Drugs (e.g., aspirin, other analgesics)
	Emotions (e.g., stress)
	Exercise
Atopic (extrinsic)	Pollens (e.g., tree, grass, ragweed)
	Animal danders
	Feathers
	Mold spores
	Household dust
	Food (e.g., nuts, shellfish)

- Factors that may precipitate acute asthmatic attacks are listed in Table 4-2.

Pathophysiology

- Hyperreactivity of the airways to various stimuli provokes bronchial smooth muscle contraction and hypertrophy, mucosal edema, and overproduction of viscous mucus, as depicted in Figure 4-4.
- Over time, bronchial airway remodeling occurs with increased thickness of all layers of the airways and leads to chronic stable asthma with intermittent acute exacerbations.[228]
- Because ventilation is significantly reduced in numerous alveoli and perfusion is preserved or even increased by increased cardiac output, $\dot{V}/\dot{Q}$ matching is poor to very poor, which impedes gas exchange and increases the work of breathing, as described on pages 72 to 75.
- Usually the individual hyperventilates in order to maintain near-normal oxygenation, resulting in hypocapnia and respiratory alkalosis; however, prolonged or severe attacks may lead to respiratory muscle fatigue with hypercapnia and respiratory acidosis, necessitating ventilatory support.
- If respiratory distress continues without response to treatment, *status asthmaticus* is present and hospitalization is required.
- *Occupational asthma* develops as a result of toxic exposure to various substances in the work place, as described on page 92.
- In *exercise-induced asthma*, acute bronchoconstriction during exercise is thought to be provoked by hyperventilation, change in airway temperature, or water loss. The resultant increase in osmolality is proposed to stimulate activation of mast cells or afferent nerve endings, leading to bronchoconstriction.

Clinical Manifestations

- Recurrent paroxysmal attacks of cough, chest tightness, and difficult breathing, often accompanied by audible wheezing
- Thick, tenacious sputum, which may be difficult to expectorate
- Symptom-free between attacks versus chronic state of mild asthma, with symptoms particularly noticeable during periods of exertion or emotional excitement
- Distant breath sounds, prolonged expiration; high-pitched expiratory and possibly inspiratory wheezes throughout both lungs (for other physical signs see Chapter 6, page 294)
- Tachypnea, possible signs of respiratory distress (e.g., increased use of accessory muscles, intercostal retractions, nasal flaring)
- Markedly reduced FEV_1, forced expiratory flow from 25% to 75% of vital capacity ($FEF_{25\%-75\%}$), and maximal expiratory flow rate at all lung volumes and increased total lung capacity (TLC) during acute attacks; increased airway resistance and reduced maximal expiratory flow rates during remissions (patients often monitor their status via daily peak expiratory flowmeter readings). Table 4-3 differentiates the various classifications of asthma control in patients 12 years of age or older who are taking asthma medication.
- During acute attacks, hypoxemia with hypocapnia is common; normal or increased $Paco_2$ is a serious sign indicating ventilatory insufficiency and possible impending respiratory failure.

Specific Treatment

- Medications (see pages 156 to 162)
  - ▸ Short-acting β_2-agonists as rescue therapy
  - ▸ Inhaled corticosteroids
  - ▸ If unsuccessful, long-acting bronchodilators, leukotriene modifiers, mast cell stabilizers, or anticholinergic drugs
- Avoidance of asthma triggers
- Aerobic conditioning, relaxation techniques, and dyspnea positions

Bronchiectasis

Bronchiectasis is characterized by progressive dilation and destruction of bronchi and bronchioles. It is usually localized to a few lung segments or an entire lobe of one lung, although bilateral diffuse involvement is also common. Before antibiotic therapy and immunizations, bronchiectasis usually developed as a sequela of a chronic necrotizing pulmonary infection, but now it occurs most often in patients with underlying systemic disorders on which airway infection is superimposed, such as primary ciliary dyskinesia, cystic fibrosis, allergic bronchopulmonary aspergillosis, and immune deficiency. Although bronchiectasis can be classified according to the resultant airway deformities (e.g., cylindrical, varicose, or saccular/cystic), there is little clinical or pathophysiological difference between the types. The hallmark of bronchiectasis is a chronic productive cough, often with copious amounts of mucopurulent sputum.

Pathophysiology

- Inflammation of the bronchial walls, due to acute or chronic infection or possibly defective regulation of the inflammatory response caused by congenital syndromes, immune

TABLE 4-3: Classification of Asthma Control for Patients ≥12 Years of Age Who Are Taking Medications

Components of Control		Classification of Asthma Control* (Youths ≥12 yr of age and adults)		
		Well-Controlled	**Not Well-Controlled**	**Very Poorly Controlled**
Impairment	Symptoms	≤2 da/wk	>2 da/wk	Throughout the day
	Nighttime awakening	≤2x/mo	3–4x/mo	≥4x/wk
	Interference with normal activity	None	Some limitation	Extremely limited
	Short-acting β_2-agonist use for symptom control (not prevention of EIB)	≤2 da/wk	>2 da/wk	Several times per day
	FEV_1 or peak flow	>880% predicted/ personal best	60%–80% predicted/ personal best	<60% predicted/ personal best
	Validated questionnaires			
	• ATAQ	0	1–2	3–4
	• ACQ	≤0.75[‡]	≥1.5	N/A
	• ACT	≥20	16–19	≤15
Risk	Exacerbations	0–1 /yr[†]	≥2/yr[†]	
		Consider severity and interval since last exacerbation		
	Progressive loss of lung function	Evaluation requires long-term followup care		
	Treatment-related adverse effects	Medication side effects can vary in intensity from none to very troublesome and worrisome. The level of intensity does not correlate to specific levels of control but should be considered in the overall assessment of risk.		

From National Asthma Education and Prevention Program, National Heart, Lung, and Blood Institute, National Institutes of Health: Expert Panel Report 3: *Guidelines for the Diagnosis and Management of Asthma.* NIH Publication No. 07-4051. Bethesda, MD, 2007, National Institutes of Health. (Available at http://www.nhlbi.nih.gov/guidelines/asthma/asthgdln.pdf)
ACQ, Asthma Control Questionnaire (Juniper et al. 1999b); ACT, Asthma Control Test (Nathan et al. 2004); ATAC, Asthma Therapy Assessment Questionnaire (Vollmer et al. 1999); EIB, exercise-induced bronchospasm; FEV_1, forced expiratory volume in 1 second.
*The level of control is based on the most severe impairment or risk category. Impairment is assessed by patient's recall of previous 2–4 weeks and by spirometry or peak flow measures. Symptom assessment for longer periods should reflect a global assessment, such as inquiring whether the patient's asthma is better or worse since last visit.
†At present, there are inadequate data to correspond frequencies of exacerbations with different levels of asthma control. In general, more frequent and intense exacerbations (e.g., requiring urgent, unscheduled care, hospitalization, or ICU admission) indicate poorer disease control.
‡ACQ values of 0.76–1.4 are indeterminate regarding well-controlled asthma.

deficiencies, and many other disorders, results in mucociliary clearance dysfunction, which leads to a vicious cycle of persistent bacterial colonization, chronic mucosal inflammation, and progressive tissue destruction.[7,17]
- Bronchial dilation and distortion are caused by destruction of the elastic and muscular airway components and hypertrophy and hyperplasia of the surrounding undamaged musculature, as depicted in Figure 4-5.
- With long-standing disease there is damage to the peribronchial alveolar tissue by inflammation followed by fibrosis, squamous metaplasia of the bronchial epithelium with loss of ciliated cells, obliteration of the distal bronchi and bronchioles, and hypertrophy of the bronchial arteries with anastomosis and sometimes considerable shunting of blood to the pulmonary arteries.
- During exacerbations, there is increased obstruction and additional secretion production, causing greater $\dot{V}/\dot{Q}$ mismatching,

which results in impaired gas exchange and increased work of breathing.
- In rare cases in which disease is severe, increased $\dot{V}/\dot{Q}$ mismatching can activate the two cascades of events that ultimately lead to respiratory muscle fatigue or failure and cor pulmonale, as depicted in Figure 4-1 (page 73).

Clinical Manifestations
- Persistent or intermittent productive cough with variable amounts of purulent sputum (often copious)
- Dyspnea, particularly if both lungs are extensively involved; tachypnea
- Possible pleuritic chest pain
- Fever, loss of appetite, weakness, weight loss
- May be asymptomatic between episodes of acute infection
- Possible blood-streaked sputum or frank hemoptysis

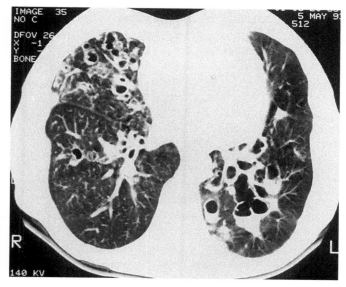

Figure 4-5: High-resolution chest computed tomography (CT) of a patient with bronchiectasis shows dilated and thickened airways in both lungs. The airways on the *left* have grapelike clusters of saccular bronchiectasis. (From Goldman L, Ausiello D. *Cecil Textbook of Medicine,* 23rd ed. Philadelphia: Saunders; 2008.)

- Adventitious breath sounds, including crackles and often wheezes (for other physical signs see Table 6-34 on page 294)
- Possible clubbing of digits
- Expiratory air flow limitation on PFTs, which correlates with the severity of the disease and may be reversible with bronchodilators
- Possible hypoxemia even in mild disease; severe hypoxemia with hypercapnia and acidemia if diffuse disease
- If severe disease, signs and symptoms of pulmonary hypertension and possibly cor pulmonale

Specific Treatment
- Medications:
  ▶ Antibiotics for acute exacerbations
  ▶ Inhaled corticosteroids
  ▶ Mucolytics
  ▶ Possible long-acting β_2-agonists, leukotriene modifiers, oral steroids
- Surgical resection if localized disease
- Pulmonary rehabilitation and other treatment options for COPD (see page 75)

Cystic Fibrosis

Cystic fibrosis (CF) is a genetic disorder characterized by dysfunction of the exocrine glands, especially the lungs, where abnormally thick, tenacious mucus along with impaired mucociliary and cough clearance results in chronic pulmonary infection and progressive lung destruction, which accounts for 90% of morbidity and mortality. Because CF is predominantly a disease affecting children, it is described in detail in Chapter 8 (Pediatrics; see page 352). However, milder cases of CF may not be diagnosed until the late teens or early adulthood. Also, more effective medical management is allowing most patients with classic CF to survive into adulthood, albeit with repeated cycles of infection and inflammation-induced injury, which ultimately cause significant bronchiectasis. In addition, more patients are undergoing lung transplantation.

Bronchiolitis Obliterans

Obliterative bronchiolitis, or bronchiolitis obliterans (BO), is a rare obstructive lung disease that can develop as a consequence of any injury to the bronchiolar epithelium when there is excessive proliferation of granulation tissue during the repair process. It has been observed as a complication of inhalation injury, infection, connective tissue disorders, and of bone marrow, stem cell, lung, and heart–lung transplantation. The clinical course of BO is quite variable, consisting of insidious versus rapid onset and slow versus intermittent (with long periods of stable function) versus rapid progression. There are two distinct pathological forms of the disease:
- Proliferative bronchiolitis is characterized by intralumenal polyps of organizing connective tissue.
- Constrictive bronchiolitis features partial or complete bronchiolar obstruction resulting from chronic inflammation, concentric submucosal or adventitial scarring, and smooth muscle hypertrophy.
- *Bronchiolitis obliterans syndrome (BOS)* provides a clinical, rather than histologic, description of BO and is used to connote persistent airflow obstruction due to graft deterioration in lung transplantation patients.[75]

Pathophysiology
- Inflammation of the bronchiolar walls causes epithelial damage followed by an exaggerated healing response with excessive connective tissue, fibrosis, and/or smooth muscle hypertrophy, resulting in airway obstruction and expiratory flow limitation.
- Some patients develop marked hyperinflation of one or both lungs.
- Refer to pages 72 to 75 for the pathophysiological features of obstructive lung diseases.

Clinical Manifestations
Appearance of symptoms usually 2 to 8 weeks after an acute respiratory illness or toxic exposure or several months to years after lung or heart–lung and bone marrow transplantation[131]
- Nonproductive cough and dyspnea
- Prolonged expiration with possible diffuse expiratory wheezes
- Variable chest x-ray findings: diffuse nodular versus reticulonodular pattern or occasionally normal, possible hyperinflation

Specific Treatment
- Early inhaled corticosteroids
- Prevention of chronic graft-versus-host disease and rejection and augmented immunosuppression for transplant patients

RESTRICTIVE LUNG DYSFUNCTION

An abnormal reduction in lung expansion, and therefore pulmonary ventilation, can be caused by a number of lung parenchymal diseases that interfere with lung expansion, pleural abnormalities, or ventilatory pump dysfunction, as listed in Table 4-4, and result in restrictive lung dysfunction (RLD). Chest x-ray findings are extremely variable in RLD because of the diverse nature of the abnormalities that produce it. Pulmonary function testing typically reveals reductions in almost all volumes and capacities (see Figure 2-8, page 13) with

TABLE 4-4: Causes of Restrictive Lung Dysfunction

Diseases Affecting the Lung Parenchyma	Diseases Affecting the Pleurae	Disorders Affecting Ventilatory Pump Function
Atelectasis	Pleural effusion	Impaired respiratory drive (e.g., CNS depression due to drugs or disease, head injury)
Pneumonia	Pleural fibrosis	
Interstitial lung disease/pulmonary fibrosis	Pneumothorax	Neurologic and neuromuscular disease (e.g., spinal cord injury, CVA, ALS, Guillan-Barré syndrome, Parkinson's disease, myasthenia gravis, paralysis of the diaphragm)
Acute respiratory distress syndrome	Hemothorax	
Pulmonary edema		
Neonatal respiratory distress syndrome		Muscle weakness (e.g., muscular dystrophy, myopathy)
Bronchopulmonary dysplasia		Lung hyperinflation (e.g., COPD)
Occupational lung diseases*		Thoracic deformity or trauma (e.g., kyphoscoliosis, thoracic surgery)
Collagen vascular and connective tissue disorders (e.g., ankylosing spondylitis, RA, SLE, polymyositis, progressive systemic sclerosis, Marfan's disease, osteogenesis imperfecta)		Collagen vascular and connective tissue disorders affecting the thoracic joints
		Extrathoracic conditions (e.g., pregnancy, obesity, ascites, abdominal incision)

ALS, Amyotrophic lateral sclerosis; COPD, chronic obstructive pulmonary disease; CVA, cerebrovascular accident; RA, rheumatoid arthritis; SLE, systemic lupus erythematosus.
*See Table 4-5.

relatively normal flow rates (see Figures 2-9 and 2-10, page 16), as well as reduced diffusing capacity when RLD is due to lung disease. The general characteristics of RLD are presented first, followed by more detailed information about a number of the specific diseases and disorders that result in RLD.

Pathophysiology

The general pathophysiological effects of RLD are illustrated in Figure 4-6, and their progression is depicted by the events below the dashed line in Figure 4-1 (page 73).

- RLD results in limited lung expansion.
  - ▸ If a lung is less compliant, greater transpulmonary pressure is required to expand it to any given volume, which is usually less than normal.
  - ▸ If pleural abnormalities compress the lung, normal expansion is inhibited.
  - ▸ If ventilatory pump dysfunction impairs expansion of the thoracic cage in any direction, lung expansion will be reduced even though lung compliance may be normal.
- Thus, decreased pulmonary compliance results in greater resistance to lung expansion, increased effort of the inspiratory muscles, especially the diaphragm, with recruitment of the accessory muscles of inspiration, and higher respiratory rates; thus the work of breathing is markedly increased.
- The greater the severity of restriction, the more dependent the individual is on respiratory rate as the only means to increase minute ventilation to meet higher demands for oxygen, and the greater the ventilatory limitation.
- In addition, reduced pulmonary compliance produces ventilation–perfusion ($\dot{V}/\dot{Q}$) mismatching and intrapulmonary right-to-left

shunt, which further increases the work of breathing, creating the potential for ventilatory muscle fatigue and ventilatory failure as the disease progresses in severity (see page 94).

- Furthermore, chronic hypoventilation seen in moderately severe disease results in hypoxemia with resultant hypoxic vasoconstriction and increased pulmonary artery (PA) pressures (especially during exertion), as well as polycythemia; this further increases the workload of the RV, leading to RVH and possible eventual cor pulmonale (see page 95).
- During exercise, there is a greater potential for significant pulmonary and hemodynamic impairment, although there is wide variability due to the many different causes of pulmonary restriction.[137,207]
  - ▸ Diffuse interstitial diseases are often associated with more extensive abnormalities of pulmonary vascular structures and therefore greater pulmonary hypertension (PH). Impaired gas exchange can lead to marked arterial desaturation. Cardiac output may also be inappropriately low because of reduced stroke volume resulting from abnormally high submaximal HRs and biventricular dysfunction.
  - ▸ Interstitial diseases secondary to systemic diseases, such as autoimmune rheumatic disorders and sarcoidosis, are often complicated by pulmonary vasculitis and cardiovascular abnormalities, as detailed later on page 136.
- Pneumonectomy, with its resultant loss of pulmonary circulation and total lung volume, is associated with only modest elevation of pulmonary pressures at rest and moderate increases during exercise. However, cardiac output and stroke volume may be reduced and fail to increase appropriately with exercise training.

Restrictive Lung Disorders

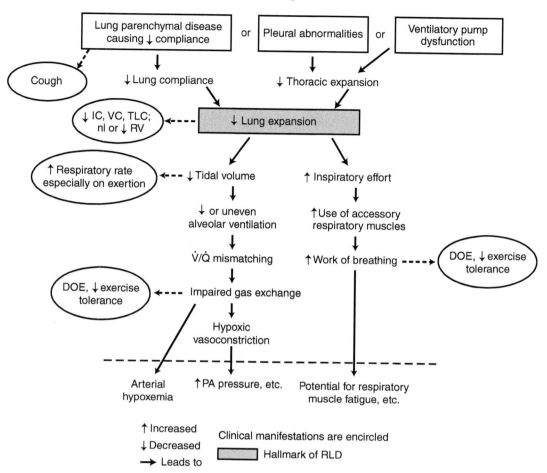

Figure 4-6: General pathophysiology of restrictive lung disorders; severe ventilatory limitation provokes progression to events below the *dashed line* and their sequelae, which are illustrated in Figure 4-1, possibly leading to respiratory failure and/or cor pulmonale. Clinical manifestations of various events are enclosed in *circles.* DOE, Dyspnea on exertion; IC, inspiratory capacity; PA, pulmonary arterial; RV, residual volume; TLC, total lung capacity; VC, vital capacity; V̇/Q̇, ventilation-perfusion.

Clinical Manifestations

- Dyspnea, especially on exertion
- Reduced exercise tolerance
- Cough, usually dry nonproductive
- Tachypnea
- Possible weight loss
- Possible hypoxemia with associated signs and symptoms (see page 241)
- Abnormal PFTs with decreased VC, inspiratory capacity (IC), and TLC, and possible impaired diffusing capacity, but relatively normal expiratory flow rates (see pages 13 to 16)
- Abnormal breath sounds that vary with specific disease (see page 294)
- Abnormal chest x-ray findings according to specific disorder
- Possible signs and symptoms of ventilatory muscle fatigue or failure if severe dysfunction (see page 243)
- Possible signs and symptoms of PH, RVH, or cor pulmonale if severe dysfunction (see pages 94 to 95)

General Treatment

- Specific therapeutic or corrective measures (e.g., appropriate anti-microbial therapy for pneumonia, treatment of pulmonary edema, reversal of drug-induced central nervous system depression)
- Supportive measures
  ▸ Supplemental oxygen
  ▸ Nutritional support
  ▸ Ventilatory support
- Physical therapy interventions to increase ventilation (see page 310)
- Possible pulmonary rehabilitation (see pages 32 and 309)

Clinical Implications for Physical Therapy

- Physiological monitoring during all initial PT evaluations may identify patients with RLD (many of whom will not have been diagnosed). Continued monitoring may be indicated during PT treatment sessions, at least initially, to avoid adverse reactions.
- The more severe the degree of restriction, the more dependent the patient will be on respiratory rate as the only means to increase minute ventilation during exertion.

- Physical therapists should be able to recognize the signs and symptoms of hypoxemia, as well as those of ventilatory muscle fatigue (see pages 241 and 242).
- Side effects of medications may affect exercise responses (see Chapter 5, page 214).
  ‣ Some antimicrobial drugs are known to produce pulmonary toxicity on occasion, including nitrofuantoin (Furadantin), sulfasalazine, tetracycline, and minocycline, and a number of other antibiotics have rare reports of associated pulmonary reactions.
  ‣ Corticosteroids provoke increased catabolism, so physical therapists must observe for skin breakdown and use caution regarding overstressing bones and musculoskeletal structures.
  ‣ Patients with pain that limits activity will tolerate exercise better with effective analgesia; however, excessive sedation can impair ventilation and gas exchange.
- PT interventions that may benefit patients with RLD are described in Chapter 7 and include the following:
  ‣ Airway clearance techniques if poor secretion management
  ‣ Techniques to increase pulmonary compliance (e.g., breathing exercises, thoracic mobility and posture exercises, soft tissue mobilization)
  ‣ Coughing techniques
  ‣ Respiratory muscle training
  ‣ Chest mobility, posture exercises
  ‣ Endurance exercise training with appropriate modifications,[165] such as low-level activity initially with gradual progression, periodic rest periods to increase patient tolerance for more vigorous activities, coordination of breathing with activity, and supplemental oxygen for hypoxemic patients
  ‣ Relaxation training
  ‣ Energy conservation and work simplification techniques
  ‣ Creative problem solving to deal with functional limitations
- Preventive health measures as listed on page 77.

Common Disorders That Result in RLD

As shown in Table 4-4, a wide variety of diseases and abnormalities can lead to restrictive lung dysfunction. Some are common, particularly in postoperative patients and those with impaired mobility (e.g., atelectasis and pneumonia), whereas others are encountered less frequently (e.g., pneumothorax and pulmonary fibrosis).

Atelectasis

Atelectasis is a state of lung tissue characterized by the collapse of alveoli so they become airless. It is associated with many pulmonary abnormalities, both pathological and mechanical, and is caused by obstruction of a bronchial airway (e.g., by mucus or tumor), lung compression (e.g., by pleural effusion, pneumothorax, or marked elevation of the diaphragm), and insufficient surfactant production, as well as inadequate inspiratory volume. Atelectasis is commonly seen in postoperative patients, particularly when there is an abdominal or thoracic incision, and in those with neurologic and musculoskeletal disorders that hinder proper lung expansion.

- Atelectasis occurs only if there is blood flow to the affected alveoli, allowing absorption of gases.

- It can occur as microatelectasis, which involves a diffuse area of terminal lung units, or as segmental or lobar atelectasis, which follows anatomic distribution of a blocked airway.

Pathophysiology
- Complete obstruction of an airway produces entrapment of air within the alveoli distal to the obstruction; the slow absorption of gases into the pulmonary capillary blood results in collapse of the alveoli, allowing absorption of gases.
- Collapsed, airless alveoli reduce lung compliance, which increases the work of breathing, as described on page 81.
- If the atelectasis is localized, hypoxic vasoconstriction usually limits $\dot{V}/\dot{Q}$ mismatching and helps to maintain relatively normal gas exchange; however, if atelectasis is extensive, the increase in pulmonary arterial pressure often overrides the vasoconstriction, creating an intrapulmonary shunt (i.e., blood flows past nonventilated alveoli), and gas exchange deteriorates.

Clinical Manifestations
- Few or no symptoms if atelectasis evolves slowly; possible fever and cough
- If acute collapse of a large section of lung:
  ‣ Profound dyspnea
  ‣ Severe hypoxemia (see page 241)
  ‣ Tracheal and mediastinal shift toward the affected side, with elevated diaphragm, as demonstrated in Figure 4-7.
- Reduced or absent breath sounds, crackles and possible wheezes (for other physical signs see Chapter 6, page 294)
- Chest x-ray showing well-defined area of increased density, volume loss, and tracheal and mediastinal shift toward the affected side

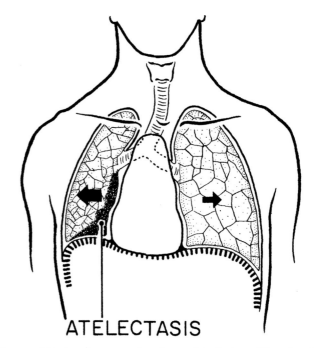

ATELECTASIS

Figure 4-7: A diagram showing atelectasis with elevated hemidiaphragm and mediastinal shift toward the affected side. (From Cherniack RM, Cherniack L. *Respiration in Health and Disease.* 3rd ed. Philadelphia: Saunders; 1983.)

Specific Treatment

- Prevention (e.g., airway clearance techniques, breathing exercises, mobilization)
- Removal of obstruction
  - ▸ Vigorous chest physical therapy techniques to mobilize mucous obstructions
  - ▸ Flexible bronchoscopy with lavage for removal of mucus plugs and retained secretions (see page 25)
  - ▸ Bronchoscopic or surgical removal of aspirated foreign object
  - ▸ Excision of tumor
- Treatment of underlying disorder if not obstructive atelectasis
  - ▸ Chest tube insertion for pneumothorax (see page 32)
  - ▸ Pleurocentesis for drainage of pleural effusion (page 25)

Pneumonia

Pneumonia is an inflammatory process of the lung parenchyma, which results from infection in the lower respiratory tract, inhalation of noxious chemicals, or aspiration of food or fluids into the lungs. It typically leads to consolidation of some or all of the alveoli as they fill with exudate and cellular debris. Many conditions are associated with an increased risk of developing pneumonia, including impaired airway defense mechanisms (e.g., due to cigarette smoking, upper respiratory infection, or dehydration), chronic obstructive lung disease, hospitalization, debilitation, dysphagia, and compromised immune status.

- *Lobar pneumonia* occurs when one or both lungs are involved at the lobar level with nearly homogeneous consolidation (Figure 4-8).

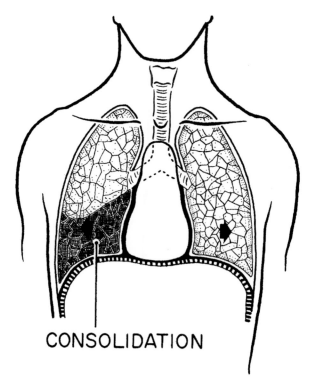

CONSOLIDATION

Figure 4-8: A diagram showing pneumonia with consolidation of the right lower lobe. Because the alveolar air is replaced by exudate, there is little, if any, change in the size of the affected lung. (From Cherniack RM, Cherniack L. *Respiration in Health and Disease.* 3rd ed. Philadelphia: Saunders; 1983.)

- *Bronchopneumonia* results from inflammation at the level of the bronchioles and alveoli with various amounts of pulmonary consolidation.
- *Walking pneumonia* refers to pneumonia that is not so severe that it requires bed rest or hospitalization. It is usually caused by *Mycoplasma pneumoniae,* although sometimes viral pneumonia is mild and also called walking pneumonia.
- *Cryptogenic organizing pneumonia (COP),* sometimes referred to as organizing pneumonia or bronchiolitis obliterans with organizing pneumonia (BOOP), is characterized pathologically by proliferative bronchiolitis with the formation of granulation buds that fill the distal airways. Most cases are idiopathic whereas the others are usually related to other medical conditions, including drug reactions, autoimmune rheumatic diseases, viral pneumonitis, malignancy, bone marrow and organ transplantation, and toxic fume or smoke inhalation. Most patients present with symptoms of pneumonia that progress over several weeks and respond well to corticosteroids, if prescribed early; in rare cases the disease progresses rapidly with death within 2 months of diagnosis.[43,73]

Pathophysiology

Infection with various pathogens (e.g., bacteria, viruses, mycoplasmas, and fungi) produces damage due to the specific tissue and immunologic responses to the microbe as well as the release of toxic inflammatory mediators, such as interleukin-1 and tumor necrosis factor. The specific microorganism responsible for infection is identified in only about half of all cases and varies with the type of pneumonia (e.g., community-acquired versus hospital-acquired or nursing home–acquired pneumonia).

- Bacterial infection (e.g., *Streptococcus pneumoniae, Klebsiella pneumoniae,* and *Haemophilus influenzae*) causes acute inflammation of the airway epithelium and suppuration along with increased porosity of the pulmonary membranes, so that there is accumulation of edema fluid, mucous secretions, and cellular debris in the airways. The result is consolidation, usually of one or two lobes, and often inflammation of the pleurae (i.e., pleurisy). Symptoms of bacterial pneumonia include high fever, chills, dyspnea, tachypnea, productive cough, and pleuritic pain.
- Viral pneumonia is usually mild and self-limiting with typical complaints of moderate fever, dyspnea, nonproductive cough, and myalgia. Viral infection generally results in acute inflammation of the bronchi and bronchioles with destruction of the ciliated epithelium and mucosal surface of the airways and disruption of mucociliary clearance. Hence, secondary bacterial infections are the most common cause of morbidity and mortality. When viral infection reaches the alveoli, which occurs most often in young children, the elderly, and the immunocompromised, it causes diffuse alveolar damage with loss of alveolar cells, edema, and hemorrhage followed by hyaline membrane formation.[31]
- Mycoplasmas are small microorganisms with characteristics of both bacteria and viruses, and are responsible for about 20% of all pneumonias. They generally cause an atypical pneumonia involving mild widespread inflammation.
- Common fungal pneumonias include histoplasmosis, coccidioidomycosis, and blastomycosis. Usually they cause only minor

or no symptoms, but occasionally they develop into serious acute or chronic infections with granuloma formation that may spread to other parts of the body. Certain fungal pneumonias, such as cryptococcosis or aspergillosis, are generally seen only in immunocompromised patients and tend to invade the lung parenchyma. *Pneumocystis jiroveci* pneumonia (formerly called *Pneumocystis carinii* pneumonia, or PCP) is another opportunistic infection that occurs predominantly in immunocompromised patients, particularly those with acquired immunodeficiency syndrome (AIDS). The alveolar spaces become filled with frothy exudates containing alveolar macrophages and large numbers of the organism.[140] Clinical manifestations include progressive dyspnea, fever, nonproductive cough, bilateral interstitial infiltrates with progression to an alveolar pattern, and impaired gas exchange.

- Most pneumonias result in:
  - ▸ Reduced surface area for gas exchange, leading to $\dot{V}/\dot{Q}$ mismatching
  - ▸ Decreased diffusing capacity resulting in hypoxemia and hypercapnia
  - ▸ Increased work of breathing with recruitment of accessory muscles
  - ▸ Resolution via phagocytosis by polymorphonuclear leukocytes, followed by localized deposition of fibrin

Clinical Manifestations
- Pleuritic chest pain or chest discomfort
- Cough, sometimes productive
- Dyspnea
- Fever, possible shaking chills, especially if bacterial
- Other constitutional symptoms (e.g., fatigue, weakness, malaise, headache, pharyngitis, rhinitis)
- Bronchial breath sounds, crackles, or both (for other physical signs see Chapter 6, Table 6-34, page 294)
- Possible signs or symptoms of hypoxemia (see page 241)
- Infiltrate(s) or dense consolidation on chest radiograph
- Possible increased white blood cell count

Specific Treatment
- Appropriate antimicrobial therapy
- Deep breathing exercises and coughing, mobilization, bronchial drainage, and possibly percussion and vibration if patient's cough is productive
- Supportive measures (e.g., oxygen and replacement of fluids)

Diffuse/Interstitial Lung Disease and Pulmonary Fibrosis

Diffuse, or interstitial, lung disease (DLD or ILD) is a term that describes more than 100 heterogeneous disorders of known and unknown etiology, which are characterized by various degrees of inflammatory–fibrotic infiltration of the alveolar walls and alveolar–capillary basement membranes, producing a disease with similar clinical and pathophysiological features. Most forms of pulmonary fibrosis are considered to be a progression of ILD, in which chronic inflammation induces fibrosis, destruction, and distortion of the lung parenchyma. The majority of cases are idiopathic, whereas others have been associated with drug toxicities, environmental exposure, immune-mediated diseases (e.g., autoimmune rheumatic diseases,

extrinsic allergic alveolitis, and sarcoidosis), infection, traumatic injuries, genetic and hormonal abnormalities, and cancer treatments (e.g., chest irradiation and some chemotherapeutic agents).

- Alveolar epithelial and endothelial injury, which results in extravasation of the serum contents into the alveolar spaces, provokes a diffuse inflammatory process that leads to fibroblastic proliferation and excessive collagen deposition in the alveolar structures and sometimes within the distal airways.
- Whether the repair processes result in fibrosis or full resolution with normal anatomy depends on the success of clearing the intraalveolar exudates and on the rapid reepithelialization of the injured alveolar surface. Withdrawal of known environmental or drug triggers along with early treatment with corticosteroids is most likely to effect resolution; otherwise ILD progresses to pulmonary fibrosis.
- The distribution of fibrous tissue in the lungs varies with the different disease processes, and the resulting scar tissue may be confined to a lung segment or lobe or disseminated throughout one or both lungs. The prognosis depends on the etiology of the disease, the response to avoidance of known causes and treatment (e.g., corticosteroids), the host responses to injury, and the rate of disease progression.[216]
- Idiopathic pulmonary fibrosis (IPF, formerly called cryptogenic fibrosing alveolitis) is the most aggressive interstitial lung disease, which may result from a failure of lung repair processes whereby injury leads to excessive fibrosis rather than a controlled inflammatory and healing process.[103] It is characterized by the presence of usual interstitial pneumonia (UIP) on surgical biopsy.
- The clinical course for IPF/UIP is variable, and acute fatal deterioration often occurs in patients with mild to moderate disease.[153] Mean survival is only 3 years, with most patients succumbing to respiratory failure or cor pulmonale.[27]

Pathophysiology
- Intraalveolar exudates and a diffuse inflammatory response lead to reduced lung compliance and uneven ventilation and cause $\dot{V}/\dot{Q}$ mismatching, impaired gas exchange, and increased work of breathing, as depicted in Figure 4-6.
- If excessive fibrosis develops, increased lung elastic recoil and stimulation of mechanoreceptors lead to reduced tidal volume and a faster respiratory rate, which correlates with disease severity and becomes more pronounced during exercise.[137] This increases the work of breathing further, which may induce respiratory muscle fatigue and respiratory failure, as described in Figure 4-1.
- Uneven ventilation increases $\dot{V}/\dot{Q}$ mismatching and leads to impaired gas exchange with hypoxemia and hypoxic vasoconstriction, especially during exercise, which may progress to pulmonary hypertension and provoke eventual cor pulmonale.

Clinical Manifestations
- Rapid, shallow breathing, which becomes more pronounced during exercise
- Dyspnea on exertion (DOE), which may progress to resting dyspnea
- Possible repetitive, nonproductive cough
- Fatigue, loss of appetite, weight loss

- Decreased breath sounds with bibasilar end-inspiratory rales (for other physical signs see Chapter 6, page 294)
- Digital clubbing, possible cyanosis late in disease
- Abnormal chest x-ray with diffuse reticulonodular pattern in involved areas, or it may be normal
- Hypoxemia during exercise initially, later at rest, with further desaturation during exertion; usually normal Pa_{CO_2} until later in disease
- Possible signs and symptoms of cor pulmonale, respiratory failure, or both (see page 95)

Specific Treatment
- Withdrawal of causative agent, if known
- Early corticosteroids
- Pulmonary rehabilitation and other treatment interventions for RLD (see page 84)

Pleural Effusion

The accumulation of excessive fluid within the pleural space leads to pleural effusion, which may affect one or both lungs. Pleural effusions can develop as a result of disorders of the pleura or underlying disease of the adjacent lung, as well as many common extrapulmonary disorders, particularly thromboembolism and diseases of the heart or abdominal organs.
- The fluid may be a transudate, which results from increased hydrostatic pressure within the pleural capillaries (e.g., due to congestive heart failure [CHF], hepatic cirrhosis, renal disease, hypoproteinemia, myxedema, and pulmonary embolus); or
- The fluid may be an exudate, which is caused by increased permeability of the pleural surfaces so that protein and excess fluid move into the pleural space (e.g., due to pulmonary infection, malignancy, pulmonary embolism or infarction, acute pancreatitis, drug toxicity, and immune-mediated diseases, such as rheumatoid arthritis, systemic lupus erythematosus, and sarcoidosis).
- When the pleural fluid is grossly purulent or contains pyogenic organisms, it is called an *empyema*.

Pathophysiology
The degree of functional impairment depends on the size of the pleural effusion.
- Excessive pleural fluid results in compression of the underlying lung tissue, leading to atelectasis, which reduces alveolar ventilation and increases the work of breathing, and so on, as depicted in Figure 4-6.
- The increased pressure caused by the accumulating fluid restricts the expansion of the underlying lung and causes the mediastinum to shift away from the affected side (see Figure 4-9).
- If perfusion is normal, there will be a shuntlike venous admixture and $\dot{V}/\dot{Q}$ mismatching, which causes hypoxemia, but Pa_{CO_2} typically remains normal because of hyperventilation of the remaining alveoli.

Clinical Manifestations
The severity of symptoms depends on the rate of fluid accumulation more than on the size of the pleural effusion.
- Possibly asymptomatic
- Dyspnea

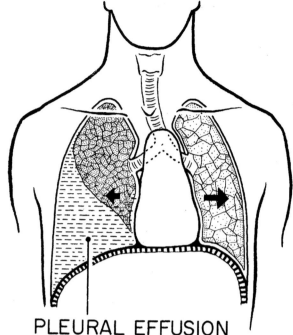

PLEURAL EFFUSION

Figure 4-9: A diagram showing a large right pleural effusion with marked compressive atelectasis and mediastinal shift away from the affected side. (From Cherniack RM, Cherniack L. *Respiration in Health and Disease.* 3rd ed. Philadelphia: Saunders; 1983.)

- Pleuritic chest pain (varying from a dull ache to excruciatingly severe, sharp, stabbing pain), aggravated by deep inspiration or coughing; often no chest pain if effusion is a transudate
- Possible fever, shaking chills, night sweats
- Decreased or absent breath sounds over effusion, possible bronchial breath sounds just above the effusion, possible pleural rub (for other physical signs see Table 6-34, page 294)

Specific Treatment
- Observe for natural reabsorption
- Segmental expansion and diaphragmatic breathing exercises to prevent underlying atelectasis; increased mobilizaton
- Thoracentesis (see page 25)

Chest Trauma

Closed chest trauma can cause injuries to the chest wall and lungs, including rib fractures, flail chest, and lung contusion. Open chest trauma due to penetrating wounds gives rise to pneumothorax, hemothorax, or pulmonary laceration (see the later section, Pneumothorax).

Pathophysiology
- Nondisplaced rib fractures, which commonly involve ribs 5 through 9, can be very painful, especially for the first 2 weeks after injury. To minimize movement of the painful area, the individual uses muscular splinting, restricts inspiration, and inhibits coughing. Individuals with multiple rib fractures, older than 50 years, or with preexisting cardiovascular or pulmonary disease are at greater risk for developing pneumonia subsequent to rib fracture.

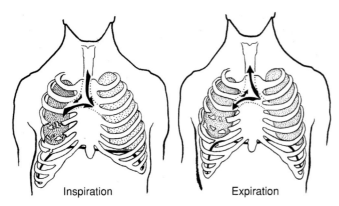

Inspiration   Expiration

Figure 4-10: A diagram showing the paradoxical movements that occur with a flail chest. During inspiration, the flail segment is sucked inward, and on expiration it bulges outward. (From Cherniack RM, Cherniack L. *Respiration in Health and Disease.* 3rd ed. Philadelphia: Saunders; 1983.)

- Fracture of two or more adjacent ribs in at least two places or accompanied by separation of the costosternal cartilages produces a segment of chest wall that is free-floating and results in paradoxical movement of the chest wall in the affected area (i.e., flail chest, as illustrated in Figure 4-10).
  - ‣ The severity of the injury depends on the number of ribs that are fractured, as well as flail, and the presence of any lung injury.
  - ‣ The flail segment will exhibit paradoxical movement during respiration (i.e., the negative pressure created by inspiration causes the flail segment to be sucked inward, while the higher pressure during expiration forces the flail area to bulge outward) and evoke severe pain.
  - ‣ The result is restricted chest expansion, overall hypoventilation, increased $\dot{V}/\dot{Q}$ mismatching, and hypoxemia.
  - ‣ Associated hemothorax and lung contusion further compromise pulmonary function and contribute to possible respiratory distress.
  - ‣ The majority of patients with flail chest have chest wall pain and deformity, dyspnea on exertion, and mild restrictive lung dysfunction for months after injury.
- Lung contusion results in localized edema, hemorrhage into the parenchyma, and increased secretion production.
  - ‣ Parenchymal congestion and additional fluid in the alveoli reduce lung compliance, increase $\dot{V}/\dot{Q}$ mismatching, and lead to hypoxemia, the degree of which is dependent on the extent and severity of the injury.
  - ‣ The inability to maintain adequate oxygenation often necessitates mechanical ventilation.
  - ‣ Common complications of lung contusion include pneumonia, empyema, and occasionally acute respiratory distress syndrome (ARDS).

Clinical Manifestations

- Chest pain, especially on inspiration or movement
- Tachypnea, possible respiratory distress
- Hypoxemia with hypercapnia
- Weak cough
- Tachycardia

Specific Treatment

- Maintain oxygenation (supplemental oxygen, mechanical ventilatory assistance)
- Analgesia
- Breathing exercises, mobilization as able
- Possible surgery for internal fixation of flail segment
- Possible extracorporeal membrane oxygenation (ECMO) if all else fails (see page 30)

Thoracic Deformity

Several forms of thoracic deformity impede the ability of the chest, and therefore, the lungs, to expand fully. The most common are curvatures of the spine, including kyphosis, scoliosis, and kyphoscoliosis, which are often idiopathic, but also can be produced by neuromuscular weakness and paralysis (e.g., muscular dystrophy), trauma, or thoracotomy.

Pathophysiology

Thoracic deformities affect respiratory function and produce restrictive lung dysfunction mainly when they are severe. In addition, marked deformity can lead to compression of the mediastinal structures with displacement and rotation of the heart, which may impair its pumping function.

- Kyphosis induces pulmonary dysfunction only when it is severe and develops in early childhood, affecting the development of the lungs.
- In scoliosis the hemithorax on the side of the concavity of the scoliosis is compressed whereas the hemithorax on the side of the convexity is overinflated, so that the respiratory muscles operate at a mechanical disadvantage.
  - ‣ PFTs typically show reduced VC, TLC, and FRC and normal or slightly increased residual volume.
  - ‣ The degree of dysfunction is proportional to the severity of the angle of scoliosis when it is idiopathic, but not when it is due to neuromuscular disease, in which respiratory muscle weakness is a dominant factor.
- Kyphoscoliosis involves lateral curvature and rotation of the spine, resulting in rib angle prominence in the thoracic spine and lumbar lordosis (Figure 4-11). Pulmonary dysfunction due to compression of one lung and overinflation of the other is more prevalent than with other thoracic deformities.
- Pectus excavatum (funnel chest) and pectus carinatum (pigeon chest) are congenital deformities of the chest that rarely cause impairment of pulmonary function unless they are severe.
- Decreased thoracic compliance due to severe thoracic deformity restricts chest expansion and provokes $\dot{V}/\dot{Q}$ mismatching, which leads to alveolar hypoventilation, increased respiratory rate, and a substantial increase in work of breathing (see Figure 4-6). In extreme cases, usually involving kyphoscoliosis, hypoxemia provokes pulmonary hypertension, which gives rise to RVH and cor pulmonale, and eventually RV failure, as depicted in Figure 4-1.
- Exercise tolerance may be severely reduced due to reduced efficiency of movement and increased oxygen consumption by both the respiratory and postural muscles.

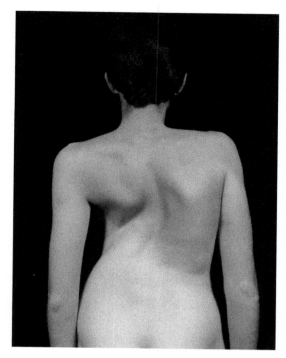

Figure 4-11: A patient with severe kyphoscoliosis. The left lung is compressed, and the right lung is over-expanded. (From Swartz MH. *Textbook of Physical Diagnosis: History and Examination.* 5th ed. Philadelphia: Saunders; 2006.)

Clinical Manifestations

- Symptoms are most prominent in severe disease:
  - ▸ Dyspnea on exertions, tachypnea
  - ▸ Hypoxemia with hypercapnia
  - ▸ Weak cough

Specific Treatment

- Close observation for progression; bracing versus surgical correction
- Supplemental oxygen, mechanical ventilatory assistance when indicated
- Thoracic mobility and breathing exercises

Pneumothorax

The presence of air or gas in the pleural space creates a pneumothorax, which occurs via disruption of either the visceral or parietal pleura. Approximately 40% of pneumothoraces are traumatic (due to chest wall trauma or iatrogenic procedures). Spontaneous pneumothorax occurs without a precipitating event in individuals with preexisting lung disease (e.g., due to bronchopleural fistula, rupture of subpleural bleb, spontaneous rupture of alveoli or an infected abscess, gas-producing anaerobic organisms in the pleural space). Primary spontaneous pneumothorax is said to arise without precipitating event in a person with no clinically apparent lung disease; however, evidence now suggests that most are caused by an obstruction check-valve mechanism due to inflammatory changes of the distal airways in smokers.[202]

Pathophysiology

The degree of functional impairment depends on the size of the pneumothorax.

- Air in the pleural space abolishes negative intrapleural pressure and results in the collapse of the underlying lung, causing decreased TLC, vital capacity, and residual volume and creating a shuntlike venous admixture with $\dot{V}/\dot{Q}$ mismatching and resultant early hypoxemia; later, blood is diverted away from the involved lung, and $\dot{V}/\dot{Q}$ matching is improved so there is less hypoxemia.
- In addition, accumulation of air in a hemithorax increases intrathoracic pressure, causing the mediastinum to shift away from the side with pneumothorax.
- If paradoxical chest movement develops, there is shunting of air back and forth between the normal and collapsed lung, which produces increased physiological dead space.
- In severe cases alveolar hypoventilation leads to hypoxemia and hypercapnia.
- In a *tension pneumothorax,* the pleural defect functions as a one-way valve with air leaking into the pleural space during inspiration but unable to exit on expiration, leading to a progressive increase in positive pleural pressure. Eventually complete collapse of the lung occurs with mediastinal shift to the contralateral side, which interferes with venous return to the heart and causes reduced cardiac output, tachycardia, and shock.
- *Hemothorax* (blood in the pleural space) complicates spontaneous pneumothorax in up to 12% of patients and often causes abrupt deterioration due to blood loss and consequent hemodynamic instability.[168] Hemothorax also occurs in thoracic malignancies, primary vascular events, coagulopathy, and a variety of infectious diseases.
- Refer to page 81 for a description of the general pathophysiological features of RLD.

Clinical Manifestations

The severity of symptoms depends on the size of the pneumothorax and the degree of collapse of the underlying lung. If the pneumothorax is small, it is usually asymptomatic with no abnormal physical findings. When there are symptoms, they are abrupt in onset:
- Unilateral chest pain
- Respiratory distress, marked if pneumothorax is large
- Tachycardia, possible hypotension, and diaphoresis
- Possible deviation of mediastinum toward contralateral side
- Decreased or absent breath sounds with decreased or absent vocal fremitus on the affected side (for other physical signs see Chapter 6, page 294)
- Abnormal chest x-ray showing dense-appearing underlying lung tissue; thin, fine line at periphery; and uniform translucency with complete absence of lung markings in area of pneumothorax; possible overexpansion of the affected rib cage with flattening of the hemidiaphragm if pneumothorax is large

Specific Treatment

- Observation (i.e., allow natural reabsorption) if small and asymptomatic

- Simple manual needle aspiration versus intrapleural small-caliber catheter or chest tube insertion (see page 25)[150a]
- Segmental expansion breathing exercises

Acute Respiratory Distress Syndrome

Acute respiratory distress syndrome (ARDS) is a serious clinical syndrome caused by severe acute lung injury and characterized by inflammatory pulmonary edema, diffuse alveolar damage, and severe hypoxemia. ARDS is also referred to as noncardiogenic pulmonary edema, shock lung, increased permeability pulmonary edema, and posttraumatic pulmonary insufficiency. There are two different forms of the disease:

- Pulmonary ARDS, which is caused by the direct effects of lung injury on the epithelial cells (e.g., aspiration, inhaled toxins, and diffuse pneumonia)
- Extrapulmonary ARDS, in which lung injury is precipitated by a systemic inflammatory response (e.g., severe sepsis [the most common cause of ARDS], trauma, massive blood transfusions, drug overdose, and pancreatitis)

Pathophysiology

In ARDS specific types of inflammation damage the alveolar epithelium and capillary endothelium and provoke a number of pathophysiological events.

- Increased permeability of the alveolar capillary membrane causes leakage of fluid and plasma proteins into the interstitial tissue and then into the alveoli, which results in marked reduction in lung compliance and greatly increased work of breathing, as shown in Figure 4-6.
- Altered production of surfactant along with alveolar fluid and edema in the interstitial spaces gives rise to significant atelectasis, severe $\dot{V}/\dot{Q}$ mismatching, impaired gas exchange, and severe hypoxemia.
- Progression of the pathophysiological events is illustrated in the lower portion of Figure 4-1, with those leading to ventilatory failure being of particular importance in ARDS.

ARDS results in death in 40% to 60% of patients, often due to iatrogenic events, such as ventilator-induced lung injury, pneumonia and other infections, and sepsis.[150] Some survivors will experience complete resolution with normal pulmonary function, whereas others, especially those requiring prolonged mechanical ventilation, enter a subacute phase with alveolar fibrosis and capillary obliteration leading to chronic RLD.[157] Survivors tend to have reduced exercise capacity and health-related quality of life, and are unable to return to employment or normal activities for as long as 12 months after hospital discharge.[70,107]

Clinical Manifestations

- Respiratory distress (see page 241), tachypnea
- Pallor or cyanosis
- Tachycardia, possible arrhythmias
- Decreased breath sounds with crackles, possible wheezing and rhonchi
- Refractory hypoxemia with associated symptoms (see page 241); usually hypocapnia initially, then hypercapnia
- Abnormal chest x-ray with bilateral patchy peripheral infiltrates and often air bronchograms

Specific Treatment

- Treatment of underlying disease
- Supplemental oxygen
- Mechanical ventilation (usually with low tidal volume and high positive end-expiratory pressure [PEEP])
- Nutritional and fluid balance support
- Prevention and treatment of complications (e.g., barotraumas and nosocomial infections)

Other Causes of RLD

There are many other diseases and disorders that affect lung or thoracic expansion to produce RLD:

- Neurologic and neuromuscular disorders (e.g., spinal cord injury, amyotrophic lateral sclerosis, Guillain-Barré syndrome, polio, myasthenia gravis, muscular dystrophy, cerebrovascular accident, and diaphragmatic paralysis; see page 140)
- Connective tissue and autoimmune rheumatic diseases (see page 138)
- Neonatal respiratory distress syndrome, bronchopulmonary dysplasia (see page 347)
- Others (e.g., sarcoidosis, obesity, ascites, diabetes mellitus, CNS depression by drugs, and drug or radiation toxicity)

In addition, several factors associated with surgery can lead to restrictive pulmonary dysfunction.

- *General anesthesia* (GA) has a number of adverse effects on cardiorespiratory function.
  - The loss of muscle tone during GA alters the shape and configuration of the chest and reduces thoracic volumes.
  - GA depresses ventilatory drive, leading to hypoventilation and diminished ventilatory response to hypoxia and hypercapnia.
  - GA hinders ciliary function, impairing secretion clearance.
  - Airway resistance is increased by endotracheal intubation and irritation of the airways by the commonly used anesthetic gases.
  - The pulmonary arterial vasoconstrictive response to hypoxia is also inhibited, resulting in ventilation–perfusion mismatching and impaired gas exchange.
  - Other adverse cardiorespiratory effects include hypotension, decreased cardiac output, and depressed myocardial function and contractility.
- *Thoracic and abdominal incisions* result in significant temporary restrictive impairment.
  - After upper abdominal surgery, vital capacity and functional residual capacity are reduced (by 55% and 30%, respectively) for 24 to 48 hours[88]; lung volumes improve towards normal in 5 days but full recovery may take up to 2 weeks. Also, approximately 50% of patients develop a pulmonary effusion in the first few postoperative days.[143a] The incidence of postoperative complications is reduced when surgery is performed laparoscopically and when thoracic extradural block (or epidural anesthesia) is used.
  - Both thoracic and upper abdominal surgery can result in diaphragmatic dysfunction.
  - Incisional pain often leads to muscle splinting, which decreases thoracic compliance and may reduce ventilatory volumes and increase the work of breathing during the

postoperative period. Ventilation is also inhibited by impaired mobility induced by incisional pain.

▸ A posterolateral thoracotomy incision causes greater pulmonary dysfunction than a median sternotomy.

▸ Excision of lung tissue, as in lobectomy or pneumonectomy, reduces ventilatory volume, which can lead to permanent restrictive impairment, particularly in patients with preexisting lung disease.

▸ In addition, postoperative pain medications can further reduce ventilation through increased somnolence and depression of the respiratory control centers.

• Postoperative atelectasis is the most common pulmonary complication of GA and many types of surgery, resulting from hypoventilation, reduced activity level, and impaired secretion clearance. Other common pulmonary complications include pneumonia and pulmonary emboli.

Finally, more than 300 drugs are known to have adverse effects on the lungs, including pneumonitis, pulmonary edema, acute respiratory insufficiency, bronchospasm, pulmonary hemorrhage, pleural effusion, and pulmonary vascular changes, among others. Chemotherapeutic agents comprise the largest class of drugs that can cause pulmonary toxicity, and these are presented later in this chapter (see page 144). Other drugs include the following:

• Antibiotics: amphotericin B, nitrofurantoin, sulfasalazine
• Antiinflammatory agents: acetylsalicylic acid, gold, methotrexate, nonsteroidal antiinflammatory agents, penicillamine
• Analgesics: cocaine, heroin, methadone, naloxone, Placidyl, propoxyphene, salicylates
• Cardiovascular drugs: amiodarone, angiotensin-converting enzyme (ACE) inhibitors, anticoagulants, β-blockers, dipyridamole, flecainide, protamine, tocainide
• Inhalants: aspirated oils (mineral or neutral oils, animal fats) and oxygen
• Miscellaneous drugs: bromocriptine, dantrolene. hydrochlorothiazide, methysergide, tocolytic agents, tricyclic antidepressants, L-tryptophan

COMBINED RESTRICTIVE AND OBSTRUCTIVE DEFECTS

Patients sometimes have more than one cardiopulmonary disorder, which can result in a clinical picture consistent with both restrictive and obstructive abnormalities (e.g., a patient with emphysema and CHF, a smoker with interstitial lung disease, or an obese patient with asthma). In addition, some pulmonary disorders can produce combined defects, as in pulmonary edema and some interstitial and occupational lung diseases.

Pulmonary Edema

Pathological accumulation of extravascular fluid in the interstitial and alveolar spaces in the lungs is known as *pulmonary edema*. There are two types:

• Increased pressure, hydrostatic, or cardiogenic pulmonary edema (elevated left heart pressures reflected back to the pulmonary microvasculature leads to flooding of the pulmonary interstitial space and alveoli with low-protein transudative fluid); the most

common causes are coronary artery disease, hypertensive heart disease, aortic or mitral valve disease, and cardiomyopathy.

• Increased permeability, or noncardiogenic, pulmonary edema (acute lung injury causing inflammation-induced damage to the alveolar epithelium and endothelium causes fluid and protein leakage into the alveoli, as described in the preceding section on ARDS).

Pathophysiology

Increased permeability pulmonary edema (ARDS) has already been described, so only cardiogenic pulmonary edema is presented here. The consequences of pulmonary edema depend on how much fluid accumulates.

• Elevated left atrial (LA) and left ventricular (LV) pressures are reflected back to the lungs, which impedes blood flow through the pulmonary vasculature, leading to increased intrapulmonary blood volume (i.e., pulmonary congestion) and pulmonary capillary hydrostatic pressure. Mild elevation of LA pressure (i.e., 18 to 25 mm Hg) produces edema in the peribronchovascular interstitial spaces, whereas LA pressure exceeding 25 mm Hg leads to flooding of the alveoli and often the pleural space (producing pleural effusion).[230]

▸ Interstitial edema can increase airway resistance, raising closing volume and reducing expiratory flow rates. With alveolar flooding air trapping can develop as airway closure occurs earlier.

▸ Interstitial edema usually diminishes lung compliance, impeding lung expansion; in addition, chronic interstitial edema can provoke fibrotic changes in the lungs, which further reduce lung compliance. If alveolar flooding occurs, lung compliance is markedly decreased with resultant reductions in many lung volumes, particularly inspiratory capacity and vital capacity.

▸ Impaired alveolar ventilation induces $\dot{V}/\dot{Q}$ mismatching and impaired gas exchange, and increases the work of breathing, and so on, as depicted in Figures 4-6 and 4-1. With more severe pulmonary edema and alveolar flooding, gas exchange is seriously impaired, provoking possible respiratory distress and failure requiring ventilatory assistance.

• When cardiac output is significantly reduced, the resultant decrement in peripheral tissue perfusion produces significant tissue hypoxia and lactic acidosis.

Clinical Manifestations

The clinical features of cardiogenic and noncardiogenic pulmonary edema are similar:

• Dyspnea, respiratory distress
• Orthopnea (dyspnea when lying flat), paroxysmal nocturnal dyspnea (awakening at night with acute shortness of breath)
• Pallor or cyanosis
• Diaphoresis
• Tachycardia, possible arrhythmias
• Anxiety, agitation
• Bibasilar or diffuse crackles, possible wheezes (see Table 6-15, page 247)
• Abnormal chest x-ray with pulmonary congestion or central infiltrates
• Third heart sound (S_3) (see page 44)

Specific Treatment

Prompt diagnosis of the cause of pulmonary edema is critical to appropriate treatment. The treatment of increased perfusion pulmonary edema is described on the preceding page; the treatment of cardiogenic pulmonary edema consists of:

- Supplemental oxygen, possible assisted ventilation
- Morphine
- Diuretics
- Nitroglycerin and other afterload reducers

Occupational and Environmental Lung Diseases

A variety of lung diseases, including occupational asthma, hypersensitivity pneumonitis, and pneumoconiosis, can be caused by the inhalation of many dusts, fibers, particles, microbes, and fumes. More than 300 causative agents have been identified, some of which are listed in Table 4-5. With the implementation of governmentally regulated protective measures, there has been a substantial decrease in the frequency of occupational lung disease; however, individual cases of lung disease resulting from exposures to ordinary antigens in the home environment (e.g., molds) are

TABLE 4-5: Occupational Lung Diseases and Causative Agents

Occupational Lung Disease	Causative Agents
Occupational asthma	Animal proteins (e.g., hair, dander, and urine of animals, insects, birds, fish)
	Enzymes (e.g., detergents, spices, pharmaceutical manufacturing)
	Plant proteins (e.g., grain dusts, flour, coffee, tea, soybeans, castor bean, latex, wood dusts, flax, cotton, guar gum)
	Metals (e.g., platinum salts, nickel, cadmium, vanadium, tungsten)
	Chemicals and plastics (e.g., isocyanates, formaldehyde, formalin, Freon, piperazine, anhydrides, dyes, henna, psyllium, some antibiotics and other drugs)
Pneumoconiosis	Inorganic dusts (e.g., asbestos, coal, silica), other minerals and metals (e.g., talc, kaolinite, mica, vermiculite, beryllium, barium, tin, cobalt)
Hypersensitivity pneumonitis	Bird and animal proteins, microbial contaminants of moist areas, such as heating, ventilating, and air-conditioning systems (e.g., fungi and fungal spores, bacteria) and low molecular weight chemicals (e.g., isocyanates, anhydrides, pyrethrum insecticide)
Inhalation injuries	Noxious gases and fumes (e.g., ammonia, hydrochloric acid, chlorine, cadmium, zinc chloride, osmium tetroxide, vanadium)

being recognized with greater frequency, and sometimes a specific causative antigen is never identified.

The development of occupational or environmental lung disease depends on the toxicity of the inhaled substance, the intensity and duration of exposure, and the individual's physiological and biological susceptibility. Early intervention with remediation of the causative environment and lifestyle modifications to prevent reexposure are crucial to preventing disability and premature death.

Pathophysiology

Exposure to the agents listed in Table 4-5 can cause obstructive disease (e.g., occupational asthma), restrictive disease (e.g., pneumoconiosis or hypersensitivity pneumonitis), or mixed disease (e.g., exposure to coal dust, silica, or beryllium).

- The most common reaction to toxic exposure is *occupational asthma*, which is characterized by coughing, wheezing, chest tightness, and shortness of breath that occur and often progress during the work week or while at home if that is the locus of exposure; improve during the weekend or while on vacation; and recur on returning to work or home. It can be precipitated by direct airway irritation by substances that trigger preexisting asthma, allergic sensitization by repeated exposure to specific substances, or intrinsic reactions caused by excess release of naturally occurring chemicals in the body, such as histamine and acetylcholine.

- *Hypersensitivity pneumonitis (HP)*, also called extrinsic allergic alveolitis, is an immune-mediated interstitial lung diseases produced by repeated inhalation of and sensitization to antigenic organic particles or chemicals.[136] Chronic inflammation gives rise to multiple nonnecrotizing granulomas, which may progress to severe pulmonary fibrosis. Restrictive changes with impaired diffusion are seen on PFTs.
  - ▸ HP accounts for 12% to 19% of incident cases of ILD (see page 86).[3]
  - ▸ HP can present in three overlapping clinical forms: as an acute disease, with sudden onset of fever, chills, myalgia, dyspnea, and nonproductive cough occurring 2 to 9 hours after a high-level exposure and followed by resolution, usually within 12 to 24 hours after cessation of exposure; as a subacute disease with gradual development of productive cough, dyspnea, fatigue, anorexia, and weight loss, which occur after repeated low-level exposures and often improve rapidly with avoidance of exposure; or a chronic disease with insidious onset of cough, progressive dyspnea, fatigue, and weight loss that is caused by prolonged and continuous exposure to low levels of antigens and shows only partial improvement on removal of exposure.
  - ▸ In subacute/chronic HP, elevated risk of idiopathic pulmonary fibrosis has been noted in workers exposed to metal or wood dusts and in beauticians.[91]

- Inhalation of mineral particles and dusts (e.g., asbestos, coal, and silica) and sensitizing metals (e.g., beryllium and cobalt) causes *pneumoconiosis*, a form of interstitial lung disease in which the prevalence and severity of the disease are related to the intensity and duration of the exposure. Although the imposition of government regulations has decreased exposure to many materials, the mortality rates of some of the pneumoconioses continue to rise because of the long latency periods between exposure and disease manifestation. In addition, exposure to these agents is associated with increased risks for lung cancer, particularly in smokers, and malignant mesothelioma.[60]

▸ *Asbestosis* appears 15 to 40 years after asbestos exposure (e.g., construction trades, building maintenance, production of acoustic ceiling tiles or insulation, and ship building and repair) and features diffuse inflammatory and fibrotic lesions of the small airways, areas of pleural thickening that may calcify into plaques, and benign pleural effusions. Progression of disease with more extensive fibrosis occurs in 20% to 40% of patients.[91]

▸ Inhalation of coal mining dust results in *coal workers' pneumoconiosis,* which is characterized by inflammatory lesions consisting of focal collections of coal mine dust–laden macrophages, which surround the respiratory bronchioles and may extend to the alveoli. More advanced disease is marked by larger lesions, progressive massive fibrosis, and/or emphysema.

▸ *Silicosis* follows the inhalation of crystalline silica or silica dusts (e.g., hard rock mining, tunnel drilling, stone quarrying or crushing, granite/stone work, stone carving and sculpture; silica flour production; manufacture of plastics and resin, paint, glass, and ceramics; road construction and repair; and concrete construction and demolition) and can present as acute, accelerated, or chronic disease, depending on the clinical picture and time course in relation to exposure.

⊙ Chronic or classic silicosis is distinguished by silicotic nodules, consisting of a collagen core surrounded by a capsule of macrophages, lymphocytes, and fibroblasts, that develop 10 to 40 years after exposure; some patients develop progressive massive fibrosis and hilar adenopathy with possible calcification.

⊙ Accelerated disease develops more quickly and progresses more rapidly to progressive massive fibrosis.

⊙ Acute silicosis involves alveolar filling with proteinaceous material with few or no nodules.

⊙ Patients with silicosis are particularly susceptible to a chronic indolent form of pulmonary tuberculosis.

▸ Exposure to certain metals (e.g., cobalt and beryllium) causes lung disease due to sensitization or toxicity rather than cumulative dust exposure, affects only a minority of exposed workers on the basis of individual susceptibility, and manifests itself clinically soon after a relatively brief exposure.[61] Once an individual is sensitized, low levels of exposure can trigger disease, and removal from exposure usually stops or reduces the severity of disease; however, sometimes there is continued progression.

⊙ *Chronic beryllium disease (CBD),* or berylliosis, is a granulomatous disease similar to sarcoidosis that develops in 2% to 10% of persons exposed to beryllium dust and fumes (e.g., nuclear weapons, electronics, aerospace, ceramics, metal recycling, and the defense industry).[61] CBD is characterized by nodular infiltrates in the middle and upper lung zones, with the gradual onset of dyspnea on exertion and dry cough. Later, easy fatigability, weakness, anorexia, and weight loss may develop; and with severe disease, there will be dyspnea at rest, hypoxemia, cor pulmonale, and peripheral edema. PFTs show restrictive impairment and diffusion defects, and often evidence of airflow limitation. In addition, other organ systems, including the skin, liver, spleen, lymph nodes, and bone marrow, are occasionally affected.

⊙ Cobalt exposure can lead to occupational asthma and pneumoconiosis, known as "hard metal disease," which can occur in a subacute form with rapidly progressive cough, fever, and dyspnea, as well as a more chronic form with gradually progressive pulmonary impairment.

▸ Other agents that can give rise to pneumoconioses are talc, kaolinite, mica, and vermiculite, as well as metal dusts such as barium and tin.

• Prolonged or severe exposure to any of the agents listed in Table 4-5 can result in progressive $\dot{V}/\dot{Q}$ mismatching and increasing work of breathing, as per Figure 4-1, with significant disability.

Specific Treatment

• Avoidance of exposure to causative agent
• Corticosteroids
• Supplemental oxygen if hypoxemia is present
• Treatment of intercurrent infections

OTHER PULMONARY ABNORMALITIES

Pulmonary abnormalities other than those that can be classified as obstructive or restrictive, or as combined defects, also deserve description, including pulmonary emboli and infarction, pulmonary hypertension, respiratory failure, cor pulmonale, and lung cancer. The clinical implications for these abnormalities are presented at the end of these descriptions, as there is a great deal of overlap and many of the implications apply to most of them.

Pulmonary Emboli and Infarction

Pulmonary embolism (PE) is a sudden blockage of blood flow through a pulmonary artery, which is most commonly caused by detachment of a venous thrombosis, usually from the lower extremities (see page 124) and therefore referrred to as venous thromboembolism (VTE). PE can also arise from the right side of the heart or be caused by nonthrombotic materials (e.g., amniotic fluid, fat, air, bone spicules, and fragments of organs). VTE is highly prevalent both in the community and in hospitals and is associated with significant morbidity and mortality.

Pathophysiology

The severity of the hemodynamic and respiratory alterations depends on the size of the embolus, underlying cardiopulmonary status, and compensatory neurohumoral adaptations. Occlusion of a small pulmonary artery may go unnoticed, but larger emboli can result in a number of acute and chronic pathophysiological events.

• Acute PE provokes the release of pulmonary artery vasoconstrictors and hypoxemia, both of which increase pulmonary vascular resistance and right ventricular (RV) afterload, which reduce RV output.

• Reduced RV output leads to decreases in left heart volume filling and cardiac output, which sometimes rapidly progress to developing systemic arterial hypotension, cardiogenic shock, and sudden death.

- Impaired gas exchange can result from $\dot{V}/\dot{Q}$ mismatching, increased total dead space, and right-to-left shunting and gives rise to hypoxemia, which is usually accompanied by hyperventilation-induced hypocapnia and respiratory alkalosis.
- Larger and multiple PEs produce severe pulmonary hypertension, RA and RV dilatation and hypokinesis with tricuspid regurgitation, and ultimately RV failure with engorgement of the peripheral veins.
- Most patients undergo gradual resolution of PE and pulmonary hypertension with increasing LV output, although it may take many months (<50% of patients show complete resolution of PE by 6 mo after diagnosis).[170] Mortality rates from PE vary from ≈2.5% to ≈25%.
- Pulmonary infarction occurs in approximately one third of patients with PE, especially if there is CHF, compromised bronchial circulation, alveolar hypoventilation, or pulmonary infection.[106]
- A small percentage of patients go on to develop chronic thromboembolic pulmonary hypertension due to progressive pulmonary vascular remodeling, causing progressive exertional dyspnea and fatigue that respond poorly to medical treatment. Progressive right heart failure eventually develops.[110]

Clinical Manifestations

The signs and symptoms of both deep venous thrombosis (DVT) and PE are often nonspecific, so that many patients who are evaluated with diagnostic tests for the following complaints associated with PE do not end up with the correct diagnosis:

- Acute dyspnea, tachypnea
- Pleuritic chest pain (particularly if pulmonary infarction is present)
- Cough, possible hemoptysis
- Tachycardia with rapid feeble pulse, arrhythmia
- Hypotension, lightheadedness, dizziness (occasionally induced by exercise only)
- Unexplained vascular collapse or syncope
- Accentuated P_2 (pulmonary component of second heart sound) with decreased physiological splitting (see page 44)
- Prominent *a* wave in the jugular pulse (and atrial pressure tracing; see pages 43 to 44)

Specific Treatment

- Supportive therapy:
  - ‣ Supplemental oxygen
  - ‣ Analgesics
  - ‣ Vasoactive drugs
- Anticoagulation
- Pulmonary thromboembolectomy for massive PE and thromboendarterectomy for selected patients with chronic thromboembolic pulmonary HTN

Pulmonary Hypertension

When mean pulmonary arterial pressure exceeds 25 mm Hg at rest or 30 mm Hg during exercise, pulmonary (arterial) hypertension (PH or PAH) is diagnosed. PH is caused by an increase in pulmonary vascular resistance induced by hypoxic vasoconstriction, occlusion of the pulmonary vascular bed, or parenchymal disease with loss of vascular surface area. Persistent pulmonary arterial vasoconstriction induces structural remodeling with arterial smooth muscle hypertrophy and intimal proliferation.[152,209a]

Idiopathic pulmonary arterial hypertension (PAH), formerly known as primary pulmonary hypertension (PPH), occurs without a demonstrable cause or may be inherited, and most often affects young or middle-aged women.

Pathophysiology

- Sustained elevation in pulmonary arterial pressure creates a pressure overload on the RV, which induces RV hypertrophy and later dilation (cor pulmonale); RV dilation without hypertrophy can develop acutely when massive PE obstructs more than 60% to 75% of pulmonary blood flow.
- Initially, compensatory tachycardia and RVH maintain cardiac output at rest but are unable to augment it appropriately during exercise.
- With further sustained increases in RV afterload, RVH progresses and eventually RV failure develops, leading to systemic venous congestion and inadequate cardiac output at rest (see Figure 4-1).
- Most patients with PH die of RV failure, although a small percentage suffer sudden death due to arrhythmias or pulmonary emboli.
- During exercise pulmonary vascular resistance increases further and there is a loss of pulmonary vasodilator response, which increases dead space (due to expanded ventilation of underperfused alveoli), impairing gas exchange and causing dyspnea.[214] In addition, reduced pulmonary blood flow limits LV output, which decreases peripheral oxygen delivery and aggravates exercise intolerance, usually in proportion to disease severity.
- Notably, exercise-induced PH may occur in patients with no or mild hypoxemia at rest and even in many patients without exercise-induced hypoxemia.[47]

Clinical Manifestations

- Dyspnea on exertion initially, later at rest
- Fatigue, weakness
- Exertional chest pain
- Lightheadedness, syncope
- Palpitations
- Possible hemoptysis
- Signs and symptoms of cor pulmonale (see the next section)

Specific Treatment

- Specific therapies for underlying disease
- Supplemental oxygen
- Medications (see Chapter 5)[109a]:
  - ‣ Anticoagulants
  - ‣ Diuretics
  - ‣ Vasodilators
  - ‣ Prostacyclins
  - ‣ Endothelin receptor blockers
  - ‣ Phosphodiesterase-5 inhibitors
- Treatments for cor pulmonale (see the next section)

Cor Pulmonale

Cor pulmonale (i.e., pulmonary heart disease) is a form of secondary heart disease, specifically right ventricular hypertrophy and dilation caused by pulmonary hypertension that results from pulmonary dysfunction. The most common cause is COPD, but it also occurs as a late manifestation of severe RLD, primary pulmonary arterial disease, pulmonary vascular occlusion, high-altitude disease, and congenital pulmonary defects. Acute cor pulmonale can be provoked by massive pulmonary embolism, which leads to dilation of the RV with thinning of its muscular walls.

Pathophysiology

- See the preceding section on PH.
- Increased secretions and acute respiratory infection, which increase $\dot{V}/\dot{Q}$ mismatching, often worsen PH and RV dysfunction and precipitate decompensation into RV failure.

Clinical Manifestations

- Signs and symptoms of underlying disease
- Dyspnea on exertion, tachypnea
- Reduced exercise tolerance
- Digital clubbing, exercise-induced peripheral cyanosis
- Signs and symptoms of low cardiac output (e.g., lightheadedness, dizziness, fatigue, weakness, pallor, hypotension)
- Signs and symptoms of PH (see the preceding section)
- Possible signs and symptoms of right heart failure (e.g., jugular venous distension, hepatomegaly, peripheral edema, nocturia)
- Loud P_2 (pulmonary component of second heart sound) with increased physiological splitting, possible murmur of tricuspid regurgitation (see page 44)
- Chest x-ray findings of RVH, bulging PA, and prominent hilar vessels with normal or increased intrapulmonary vascular markings

Specific Treatment

- Specific treatments for underlying cause and exacerbating factors
- Medications (see the preceding section on PH)
- Atrial septostomy (creation of an intraatrial defect to allow right-to-left shunting to unload the failing RV) as a bridge to transplantation?[152]
- Heart–lung versus single- or double-lung transplantation (see page 35).

Respiratory Failure

When pulmonary gas exchange becomes so impaired that severe hypoxemia with or without hypercapnia develops, respiratory failure is present. It results in deficient oxygen delivery to the tissues, which can be acute, chronic, or acute-on-chronic in nature. Although usually caused by pulmonary disease, acute respiratory failure can also be caused by severe impairment of the musculoskeletal, circulatory, or central nervous systems, as noted subsequently.

- Hypoxemic respiratory failure occurs when there is severe hypoxemia ($Pa_{O_2} \leq 50$ to 59 mm Hg) that is refractory to oxygen therapy despite hyperventilation (with resultant hypocapnia). Failure to achieve adequate oxygenation can result from a number of abnormalities:
  - ▶ Low inspired oxygen level (e.g., altitude >10,000 ft)
  - ▶ Impaired diffusion (e.g., pulmonary edema or fibrosis if marked tachycardia occurs)
  - ▶ Ventilation–perfusion mismatching (e.g., pneumonia, atelectasis, bronchoconstriction, aspiration, pneumothorax, and pulmonary embolus)
  - ▶ Right-to-left shunting (e.g., cyanotic congenital heart disease and pulmonary arteriovenous malformation)
  - ▶ Increased metabolic demands (e.g., septic or cardiogenic shock, severe burns, and pancreatitis)
- Hypercapnic respiratory failure, also called ventilatory failure, arises when true alveolar hypoventilation leads to poor gas exchange, as depicted in Figure 4-1. It is most commonly seen in patients with COPD when acute respiratory dysfunction is superimposed on chronic disease. Causes of ventilatory failure include the following:
  - ▶ Central hypoventilation (e.g., head injury, stroke, drug overdose, sleep-disordered breathing)
  - ▶ Neuromuscular weakness (e.g., cervical spine injury, neuromuscular disease, respiratory muscle fatigue, infections [botulism, tetanus, and poliomyelitis], drug toxicity [paralytic agents, aminoglycoside antibiotics, and organophosphate poisoning]), phrenic nerve palsy [thoracic surgery and mediastinal tumor infiltration], metabolic disorders [malnutrition, and low levels of phosphate, potassium, magnesium, or calcium])
  - ▶ Airway obstruction (e.g., obstructive sleep apnea, vocal cord paralysis, and endobronchial tumor)
  - ▶ Chest wall deformities (e.g., kyphoscoliosis and flail chest)
  - ▶ Marked abdominal interference with diaphragm descent (e.g., massive ascites and obesity)

Pathophysiology

- Hypoxemia results in the activation of numerous compensatory mechanisms in an attempt to improve tissue oxygenation (e.g., hypoxic vasoconstriction, use of accessory muscles of respiration, elevated HR, and increased arteriovenous oxygen extraction); when these fail, respiratory failure develops.
- Hypercapnia induces hyperventilation in an attempt to eliminate excess carbon dioxide; when either respiratory chemoreceptor insensitivity to hypercapnia or respiratory muscle fatigue develops, Pa_{CO_2} will progressively rise, producing severe dyspnea and then lethargy, followed by semicoma, anesthesia, and death.
- Respiratory acidemia associated with hypercapnia decreases cardiac contractility and respiratory muscle contractility and endurance, promotes arterial vasodilation, increases cerebral blood flow, induces loss of consciousness, and raises the seizure threshold. However, compensatory sympathetic nervous system (SNS) stimulation counters some of these effects, increasing vascular tone, myocardial contractility, and CNS arousal.

Clinical Manifestations

- Signs and symptoms of respiratory distress (see page 241)
- Signs and symptoms of hypoxemia (see page 241)
- Signs and symptoms of respiratory muscle fatigue (see page 243)
- Signs and symptoms of underlying pulmonary disease

Specific Treatment

- Supplemental oxygen or heliox (20% oxygen, 80% helium)
- Ventilatory support (invasive or noninvasive; see page 28)
- Treatment of primary cause if acute

Sleep Apnea/Sleep-disordered Breathing

Sleep apnea, also called sleep-disordered breathing, is a common disorder characterized by episodes of breathing cessation lasting 10 to 30 seconds, which occur repeatedly throughout sleep. The vast majority of cases are caused by complete obstruction of the oropharynx as the tongue and palate relax during sleep (obstructive sleep apnea, OSA); more rarely it results from reduced ventilatory drive (central sleep apnea, CSA). Sleep apnea is more common in men than women and in overweight and obese individuals. It is also a common finding in many chronic diseases, such as COPD and heart failure.

Pathophysiology

Significant periods of apnea may occur more than 100 times per hour in severe cases, provoking serious cardiorespiratory and neuropsychiatric consequences.[69]

- Asphyxia, arousal from sleep, and higher negative intrathoracic pressure stimulate the SNS, inducing a rise in systemic BP, which becomes sustained HTN in more than 50% of patients.
- Exaggerated negative intrathoracic pressures generated during OSA reduce ventricular preload and increase afterload, causing reductions in stroke volume and cardiac output, especially in individuals with underlying LV dysfunction.
- Apnea-induced hypoxia can also adversely affect preload, afterload, and contractility, further impairing ventricular performance, and intensifies SNS stimulation.
- Higher LV afterload and augmented SNS stimulation act to increase myocardial oxygen demands, which can precipitate myocardial ischemia, nocturnal angina, and cardiac arrhythmias in individuals with coronary artery disease.
- Individuals with sleep apnea have an increased risk of myocardial infarction (MI), CHF, arrhythmias, and stroke, which may be due in part to coexistent obesity and HTN.[187]
- Ten percent to 15% of patients with OSA develop severe nocturnal oxygen desaturation, daytime hypoxemia, and hypercapnia, leading to sustained pulmonary hypertension and right-sided heart failure. These patients are usually obese and have diffuse airway obstruction and impaired respiratory drive.
- Frequent arousals to lighter sleep or full awakening in order to terminate apneic episodes, which the individual is often not aware of, lead to poor sleep quality and neuropsychiatric symptoms when awake. Daytime somnolence can be life-threatening, particularly when driving.

Clinical Manifestations

- Alternating episodes of silence, loud snoring, and gasps during sleep
- Daytime somnolence
- Neuropsychiatric symptoms: intellectual impairment, memory loss, poor judgment, personality changes
- Cardiorespiratory manifestations: systemic HTN, signs and symptoms of myocardial ischemia, arrhythmias, dyspnea on exertion, reduced exercise tolerance

Specific Treatment

- Weight reduction, as appropriate
- Avoidance of alcohol and sedatives
- Avoidance of supine sleep position
- Continuous positive airway pressure (CPAP), usually nasal
- Intraoral appliances to maintain forward position of mandible and tongue
- Surgery to remove redundant soft tissue

Lung Cancer

Lung cancer, the most common and lethal form of cancer in the United States, arises in the respiratory epithelium (thus it is also called *bronchogenic carcinoma*). Bronchogenic carcinoma accounts for more than 90% of all lung cancers; other pulmonary tumors include lymphomas, sarcomas, blastomas, mesotheliomas, and more. In addition, malignant tumors in the lungs can occur as a result of metastatic disease from cancers affecting other organs. There are two main types of bronchogenic carcinoma:

- Small cell lung cancer (SCLC, ≈20% of all lung cancers), which includes small cell, or oat cell, carcinoma, is highly associated with cigarette smoking or exposure and usually presents as a large central tumor with mediastinal involvement. It responds reasonably well to chemotherapy and radiation.
- Non–small cell lung cancer (NSCLC, ≈75% of all lung cancers), which includes squamous cell carcinoma, adenocarcinoma (the most common type of lung cancer seen in nonsmokers), and large cell (undifferentiated) carcinoma, is best treated with surgical excision if detected early and exhibits a low response to chemotherapy and radiation.

Pathophysiology

- Obstruction or compression of bronchi results in atelectasis, pneumonia, and/or lung abscess.
- Obstruction or compression of blood vessels causes $\dot{V}/\dot{Q}$ abnormalities and sometimes a superior vena cava syndrome.
- Direct extension of the tumor to the chest wall leads to pain and resultant hypoventilation.
- Involvement of the pleura produces pleural effusion.
- Early spread via the vascular and lymph systems is common, leading to metastasis to the lymph nodes, adrenal glands, brain, bone, and liver.
- Paraneoplastic syndromes occur in approximately 10% to 20% of patients, particularly those with SCLC, and may include digital clubbing and hypertrophic osteopathy, hyponatremia, hypercalcemia, Cushing's syndrome, neuromyopathic disorders, and thrombophlebitis.

Clinical Manifestations

Most patients with lung cancer experience a prolonged asymptomatic period. When symptoms do develop, they are frequently nonspecific and vary depending on location, size, rapidity of growth, cell type, and presence of underlying pulmonary disease. They may include the following:

- Cough
- Hemoptysis
- Chest pain
- Systemic symptoms (e.g., anorexia, weakness, fatigue, and weight loss)
- Symptoms due to local tumor invasion (e.g., wheezing, hoarseness, dysphagia, and edema of the face and upper extremities)
- Metastatic symptoms (e.g., bone pain and neurologic problems)
- Chest x-ray showing a mass or pneumonia

Specific Treatment

Treatment for lung cancer is often successful in achieving cure if detected early (i.e., stage I or IIA). Otherwise, treatment can extend survival or provide palliation of severe symptoms (e.g., relief of obstruction of major bronchi or blood vessels, and reduction of pain).

- Surgical resection for early-stage NSCLC and occasionally SCLC
- Combination chemotherapy
- Radiation therapy
- Novel treatments using monoclonal antibodies, inhibitors, angiogenic substances, and gene transfer and alteration are under investigation.

Clinical Implications for Physical Therapy

- Refer to the clinical implications for COPD and RLD, which are listed on pages 75 and 83, respectively, for relevant information that may be applicable to the disorders presented in this section.
- Physiological monitoring is essential during PT evaluation and treatment sessions, particularly in acute care patients, who are at high risk for adverse reactions.
- Patients with large PEs, PH, cor pulmonale, and respiratory failure usually have markedly compromised cardiopulmonary function and extremely impaired exercise tolerance.
  - ▸ Exercise is contraindicated until the patient's cardiopulmonary status has stabilized.
  - ▸ When exercise is initiated, it is likely to be low level (concentrating on functional skills), require modifications, and progress slowly.
  - ▸ For patients with respiratory failure, a balance must be achieved between providing rest through assisted ventilation to relieve respiratory muscle fatigue and performing exercise to prevent further respiratory muscle deconditioning.
    - ⊙ Breathing exercises and inspiratory muscle training are used to improve respiratory muscle strength and endurance.
    - ⊙ Therapeutic exercises and functional mobility training are used to provide general conditioning to assist in weaning patients from mechanical ventilation and to improve functional status and exercise tolerance during recovery.
- Patients with chronic disease and stable cardiovascular and pulmonary status may benefit from a number of PT interventions already listed.

- ▸ Patients with chronic stable cor pulmonale benefit from exercise training and pulmonary rehabilitation, as described in Chapter 7 (see page 308).
- ▸ There is also evidence that it is safe to ambulate patients with acute DVT and submassive PE.[218]
- ▸ Although it is commonly believed that physical activity or training may hasten the evolution and progression of PH, a study by Mereles and colleagues has demonstrated that exercise and respiratory training is well tolerated and results in improvements in exercise capacity, quality of life, and World Health Organization (WHO, Geneva, Switzerland) functional class.[161]
- ▸ For patients with cancer, physical activity provides many benefits, (as described on page 149), and has been shown to have positive effects on patients after lung resection for cancer, improving dyspnea, exercise capacity, and quality of life.

4.2 CARDIOVASCULAR DISEASES AND DISORDERS

Approximately 40% of American adults aged 40 to 59 years and 70% to 75% of those aged 60 to 79 years have one or more types of cardiovascular disease (CVD), including hypertension, coronary heart disease, cerebrovascular disease, heart failure, and others, and CVD is the number one cause of death of both men and women.[11] The essential elements, including pathophysiology, clinical manifestations, and treatment, of the most common diseases and disorders affecting the heart and blood vessels in adults are described in this section. The clinical implications for physical therapy are offered for the more common diagnoses. Congenital heart disease is covered in Chapter 8.

HYPERTENSION

Hypertension (HTN) is defined as a persistent elevation of arterial blood pressure above 140 mm Hg systolic or 90 mm Hg diastolic, as described in Table 4-6, and is the most common cardiovascular condition in the world. According to the National Health and Nutrition Examination Survey (NHANES) data, in 1999 to 2004, the prevalence of HTN among Americans 40 to 59 years of age was 33% and for those 60 years of age or older it was 66%, being highest in non-Hispanic blacks and lowest in Mexican Americans.[174] Approximately 76% of all participants were aware of their HTN, and 65% of them were being treated.[50a] BP was controlled in 57% of those taking medications and in only 37% of all hypertensive participants. Diastolic HTN, usually isolated or sometimes combined with systolic HTN, is the most common finding in hypertensives less than 50 years of age, whereas isolated systolic HTN becomes more common in those more than 50 years old and is associated with greater cardiovascular morbidity and mortality.[46]

- *Primary, or essential, HTN* is diagnosed when no known cause can be identified (about 90% to 95% of cases). Risk factors associated with the development of HTN include age,

TABLE 4-6: Classification of Blood Pressure in Adults 18 Years of Age and Older*

Classification[†]	Systolic (mm Hg)	Diastolic (mm Hg)
Normal	<120	<80
Prehypertension	120–139	80–89
Stage 1 hypertension[†]	140–159	90–99
Stage 2 hypertension	≥160	≥100

From Chobanian AV, Bakris GL, Black HR, et al. The seventh report of the Joint National Committee on Prevention, Detection, Evaluation, and Treatment of High Blood Pressure. *Hypertension.* 2003; 42:1206–1252.
*Classification is based on the average of two or more readings on two or more occasions.
[†]A classification of systolic hypertension takes precedence over a normal or prehypertensive diastolic blood pressure.

ethnicity, obesity, glucose intolerance, smoking, stress, excess sodium or alcohol intake, decreased intake of potassium, calcium, and magnesium, and lack of exercise.

- On rarer occasions, HTN can be directly attributed to a specific cause, such as renal, endocrine, vascular, and neurologic disorders and various drugs and toxins (e.g., cyclosporine, erythropoietin, cocaine, and nonsteroidal antiinflammatory drugs), and therefore it is referred to as *secondary HTN.*
- *Labile HTN* occurs when BP is sometimes elevated and other times normal.
- *White-coat HTN,* which is defined as elevated BP that occurs in the clinic but not during normal daily life, accounts for about 25% of patients with HTN.[8]
- *Masked HTN* exists when an individual has a normal clinic BP but high ambulatory BPs, which may occur in up to 10% of the general population and is associated with an increased rate of target organ damage and increased mortality.[184]
- *Malignant HTN* involves markedly elevated BP (usually >160/110 mm Hg) causing retinal hemorrhages, exudates, or papilledema.

BP is determined by cardiac output and total peripheral resistance (TPR), or systemic vascular resistance (SVR), each of which are affected by a number of other factors. Cardiac output is a factor of HR and stroke volume (SV); their determinants are listed in Table 3–2 on page 42. TPR is affected by the caliber of the arteriolar bed (i.e. peripheral vascular resistance, PVR), the viscosity of the blood, and the elasticity of the arterial walls. BP rises when cardiac output, TPR, or both are increased.

HTN develops when an imbalance occurs among the various systems that regulate BP: the SNS, the renin–angiotensin–aldosterone system (RAAS), vasopressin, nitric oxide, and a number of vasoactive peptides (e.g., endothelin and adrenomedullin). Hyperactivity of the SNS, in which an increase in cardiac output predominates, may create HTN early in the disease process, particularly in the young, but established HTN is characterized by increased PVR.

Regardless of cause, without effective treatment and control, HTN begets more HTN due to arteriolar remodeling, which leads to target organ damage (e.g., retinopathy, left ventricular

hypertrophy [LVH], renal insufficiency, and encephalopathy), organ failure, and premature death. In addition, patients with HTN are more likely to be obese and to have insulin resistance, type 2 diabetes mellitus (DM), and dyslipidemia (high triglycerides and low levels of high-density lipoprotein cholesterol).

Pathophysiology

Alterations in endothelial and arteriolar structure, mechanical properties, and function lead to HTN, which creates a pressure load on the left ventricle (LV) followed by compensatory LVH that reduces wall stress. In addition, stiffening of the large systemic arteries with age increases LV afterload and widens the pulse pressure, leading to greater LVH.[101] Concomitant activation of the RAAS leads to further adverse ventricular remodeling and eventual heart failure.

- Initially, normal LV systolic function is maintained by the hypertrophied LV, but *diastolic dysfunction* develops early in the disease process (Figure 4-12)[114a,115]:
  ‣ LVH and associated myocardial fibrosis results in prolonged relaxation time as well as a stiffer (less compliant) LV, both of which produce higher LV end-diastolic, left atrial, and pulmonary venous pressures, which leads to pulmonary congestion.
  ‣ To achieve adequate filling, the stiffer LV becomes more dependent on active atrial contraction and is adversely affected by tachycardia and arrhythmias where active atrial contraction is absent (e.g., atrial fibrillation, nodal rhythms, and frequent premature ventricular contractions).
  ‣ When filling volume is inadequate, SV is reduced and symptoms of pulmonary congestion and inadequate cardiac output may develop (i.e., diastolic heart failure; see page 108).[114a]
  ‣ Higher filling pressures inhibit coronary flow and reduce coronary reserve, increasing the risk of myocardial ischemia and arrhythmias.
- As HTN becomes more severe and/or prolonged *systolic dysfunction,* defined as an LV ejection fraction (EF) of 40% to 50%, develops.[115]
  ‣ LVH, although initially adaptive and desirable, has long-term deleterious effects on cardiac energy balance and contractile function. Adverse neurohumoral activation (SNS and the RAAS) perpetuates the vicious cycle of ventricular remodeling, and LV systolic function becomes impaired with resultant decrease in SV and increases in end-systolic and end-diastolic volumes (ESV and EDV, respectively), as illustrated in Figure 4-13.
  ‣ In the presence of LVH with its reduced compliance, this increase in EDV causes a rise in end-diastolic pressure (EDP), which is reflected back to the LA and pulmonary vessels, resulting in pulmonary edema if the pressure rises high enough to produce transudation of fluid from the capillaries into the interstitial spaces.
  ‣ Initially systolic dysfunction is manifested as reduced LV functional reserve during exercise, but later symptoms can develop even at rest (i.e., CHF). However, systolic dysfunction is asymptomatic in up to one half of patients.[115,143,160]
- HTN is associated with an increased incidence of all-cause and CVD mortality, stroke, coronary artery disease, peripheral arterial disease, and renal insufficiency.[8,101,189] Both increased systolic blood pressure (SBP) and pulse pressure (the difference

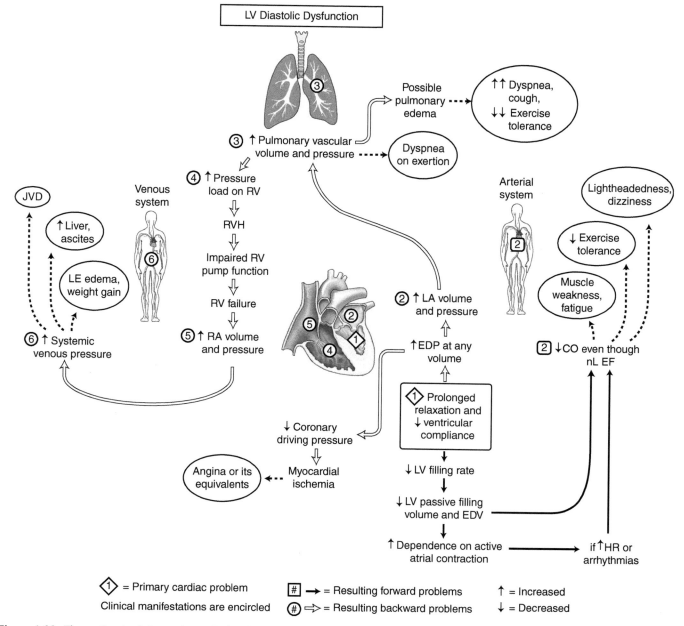

Figure 4-12: The pathophysiology of ventricular diastolic dysfunction, which develops early in the process of hypertensive heart disease and also occurs during myocardial ischemia and in other causes of ventricular hypertrophy. The initial pathophysiological effect is prolongation of ventricular relaxation, which results in a less compliant (stiffer) ventricle. As LV dysfunction progresses, its effects on the lungs and RV, as well as on cardiac output, become more apparent. The clinical manifestations associated with various events are *encircled.* CO, Cardiac output; EDP, end-diastolic pressure; EDV, end-diastolic volume; ESV, end-systolic volume; HR, heart rate; JVD, jugular venous distension; LA, left atrial; LE, lower extremity; LV, left ventricular; RA, right atrial; RV, right ventricular; RVH, right ventricular hypertrophy.

between SBP and diastolic blood pressure [DBP]) if ≥60 mm Hg are strong predictors of CVD risk.[49,80]

Clinical Manifestations

HTN is generally asymptomatic until complications develop in target organs, resulting in:

- An accelerated, malignant course
- Cerebral vascular accident
- Hypertensive heart disease
- Atherosclerotic heart disease
- Renal insufficiency or failure, nephrosclerosis
- Aortic aneurysm, simple or dissecting
- Peripheral vascular disease
- Retinopathy

The clinical manifestations of *hypertensive heart disease* include the following:

- Exertional dyspnea
- Fatigue

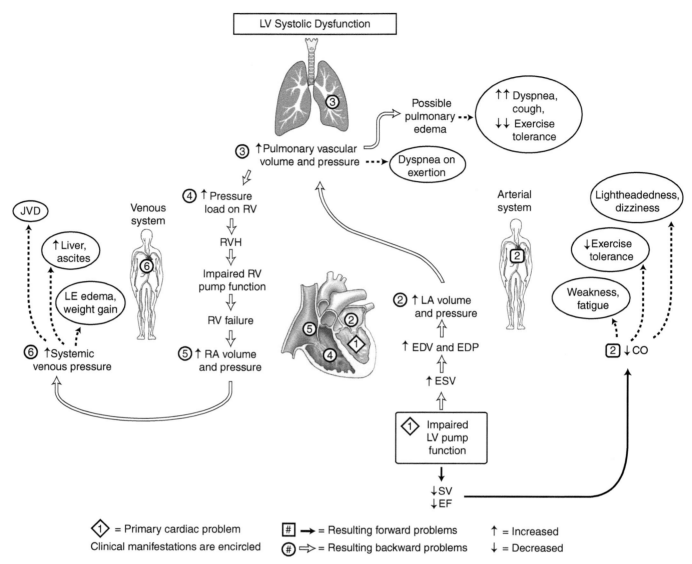

Figure 4-13: The pathophysiology of ventricular systolic dysfunction, which is induced by many pathologies that eventually lead to impairment of pump function. The results include reductions in ejection fraction (EF) and stroke volume (SV) with consequently increased end-systolic volume (ESV), as well as increases in end-diatolic volume and pressure (EDV and EDP, respectively). The elevated filling pressures are transmitted back to the pulmonary vasculature. As LV dysfunction progresses, its effects on the pulmonary vessels and RV, as well as on cardiac output, become important. CO, Cardiac output; JVD, jugular venous pressure; LA, left atrial; LE, lower extremity; LV, left ventricular; RA, right atrial; RV, right ventricular; RVH, right ventricular hypertrophy.

- Impaired exercise tolerance
- Increased symptoms with tachycardia and loss of active atrial contraction
- Exertional chest discomfort
- Possible signs and symptoms of heart failure (see page 109)

Specific Treatment

Successful treatment of HTN usually requires two or more medications along with lifestyle modifications. For most patients the goal is to achieve a BP less than 140/90 mm Hg; however, lower levels (<125–130/75–85 mm Hg) are recommended for patients with comorbidities, such as diabetes mellitus, renal disease, and possibly heart failure.[51] Lowering SBP by 20 mm Hg reduces cardiovascular risk by half.

- Pharmacologic therapy (see Chapter 5, page 168):
  ‣ Diuretics
  ‣ β-Blockers
  ‣ α-Blockers
  ‣ Calcium channel blockers (CCBs)
  ‣ Angiotensin-converting enzyme (ACE) inhibitors
  ‣ Angiotensin receptor blockers (ARBs)
  ‣ Vasopeptidase inhibitors (VPIs)
- Lifestyle modifications:
  ‣ Weight reduction (SBP and DBP decrease ≈1 mm Hg for every kilogram of weight loss)[167]
  ‣ Avoidance of tobacco
  ‣ Diet modifications (e.g., low salt, higher potassium and magnesium, high in fruits and vegetables and nonfat dairy products, moderation of alcohol intake)[101a]

▸ Physical activity

▸ Stress management

▸ Complementary/alternative medicine, including garlic, autogenic training, biofeedback, and yoga[74]

Clinical Implications for Physical Therapy

- Because a significant number of individuals with HTN do not know they have it and almost half of those taking medications are not adequately treated, clinical monitoring should be included as part of the physical therapy evaluation for most adults and children with CV risk factors:
  ▸ Resting BP values should be obtained in all patients older than 35 years and younger patients who are obese, have a history of glucose intolerance or diabetes mellitus or renal disease, or are African American.[81,87,92,181,187]
  ▸ Clinical monitoring should also be performed during activity in these same individuals. The BP responses to activity may be normal or abnormal:
    ⊙ Although a patient may have normal BP at rest, his/her medications may not maintain their effectiveness in controlling BP during exercise.
    ⊙ In moderate HTN, there is often an exaggerated BP response to isometric and sometimes dynamic exercise because of a blunted reduction in total peripheral resistance (TPR).
    ⊙ In more severe HTN, TPR may increase and cardiac output may remain normal or decrease so that the SBP response may appear normal, hypertensive, blunted, flat, or hypotensive, depending on the balance between these two determinants. Therefore, monitoring of BP as well as other signs and symptoms of exercise intolerance is essential.
    ⊙ Normotensive individuals who exhibit an exaggerated BP response to exercise are more likely to develop future HTN.[8]
    ⊙ Patients may develop angina or dyspnea with exertion.
- If a patient is found to have HTN either at rest or during exercise, s/he should be questioned about prior knowledge of the problem, any medications that have been prescribed, and whether medications are being taken as prescribed, and the patient's physician should be notified.
- Precautions and contraindications:
  ▸ If a patient has a resting SBP greater than 200 mm Hg or DBP greater than 110, medical clearance should be obtained before initiating physical therapy or performing any exercise.[9] *Note:* The patient may exhibit an auscultatory gap (see page 277).
  ▸ If the patient has a history of retinopathy, renal failure, or LVH, BP must be controlled at rest (<125–130/75–85) and during exercise (≤10-mm Hg/metabolic equivalent [MET] rise in SBP during dynamic exercise and ≤10-mm Hg rise in DBP) to avoid increased morbidity.
  ▸ If a patient exhibits HTN at rest or during exercise, the physician should be contacted for guidance before the next exercise session (the patient's medications may need adjustment).
  ▸ If SBP rises to more than 250 mm Hg or if DBP exceeds 115 mm Hg, exercise should be terminated.[9]

▸ Higher HRs or arrhythmias lacking active atrial contraction (see page 113) may increase symptoms caused by diastolic dysfunction.

- Exercise training is beneficial for individuals with hypertension:
  ▸ After a bout of dynamic exercise, there is an immediate reduction in BP (i.e., *postexercise hypotension, PEH*), which is greatest in those with the highest baseline BPs and typically lasts for 4 to 10 hours and sometimes up to 22 hours after exercise cessation, with more prolonged duration induced by consecutive sessions.[8,180]
  ▸ Aerobic exercise training decreases resting BP in the large majority of patients with HTN, with reductions averaging 7 to 11 mm Hg for SBP and 6 to 8 mm Hg for DBP, due to a reduction in systemic vascular resistance.[8,77,100]
  ▸ There are conflicting data regarding the optimal exercise dose when prescribing exercise to optimize the blood pressure–lowering effects:
    ⊙ Most studies conclude that moderate-intensity exercise (40% to <65%–70% of $\dot{V}_{O_2}$ reserve, i.e., the difference between resting oxygen consumption [$\dot{V}_{O_2}$] and maximal oxygen consumption [$\dot{V}_{O_2 \, max}$]) is effective in achieving antihypertensive benefit.[77,100] However, some data show that vigorous exercise (≥85% of $\dot{V}_{O_2}$ reserve) is more effective.[215] The American College of Sports Medicine (ACSM, Indianapolis, IN) recommends intensities of 40% to less than 60% of $\dot{V}_{O_2}$ reserve to maximize benefits, minimize the risk of CV and musculoskeletal complications, and improve adherence.[8]
    ⊙ The benefits appear to be similar for frequencies between 3 and 5 days/wk; however, because of PEH, daily or near-daily exercise is recommended, which is also in keeping with the latest public health recommendations (see page 301).[104]
    ⊙ Duration of exercise is recommended to be 30 to 60 minutes of continuous or intermittent exercise per day (numerous bouts of moderate intensity exercise of at least 10 minutes in duration accumulated throughout the day to total 30 to 60 minutes of exercise).
  ▸ Training HR ranges can be calculated according to the standard formulas (see page 305) unless the client is taking medications that affect HR (e.g., β-blockers; see Table 5-10 on page 176; also refer to Table 5-22 on page 216 for other medications that affect resting and exercise HRs); alternatively, a rating of perceived exertion (RPE) scale can be used to guide exercise intensity (see page 281).
  ▸ Resistance exercise of moderate intensity has also been shown to produce small reductions in resting SBP and DBP in adults without causing adverse effects and is encouraged as a supplement to aerobic exercise.[8,52,104,130,166]
- The side effects of medications and any exercise interactions should be recognized and explained to the patient (see Chapter 5, page 214):
  ▸ Most antihypertensive drugs are associated with orthostatic and postexercise hypotension, so caution is required when making quick changes to upright positions and an extended cooldown is recommended after exercise. The application of heat modalities can also induce hypotension.

▸ Diuretic therapy may result in dehydration and electrolyte imbalance, including hypokalemia (thiazide and loop diuretics) or hyperkalemia (potassium-sparing diuretics), both of which can trigger ventricular arrhythmias, which can be serious and life-threatening. Hypokalemia can also cause muscle weakness, fatigue, and cramps.

▸ β-Blockers reduce HR and myocardial contractility, especially during exercise, blunting HR and BP responses. Other common side effects that can limit tolerance for exercise are muscle weakness, fatigue, and cramps, and sometimes bronchospasm (with nonselective drugs or high doses of selective drugs). A major concern related to β-blockers is the hazard associated with abrupt withdrawal, which can trigger serious arrhythmias, angina, and MI.

▸ ACE inhibitors and angiotensin II receptor blockers attenuate the BP response to exercise. Some patients taking ACE inhibitors develop a persistent dry cough that is annoying but relatively harmless.

▸ Short-acting α_1-adrenergic blockers and vasodilators often trigger reflex tachycardia unless they are used in combination with β-blockers. Patients taking vasodilators may also complain of weakness.

▸ Calcium channel blockers tend to decrease HR (although short-acting nifedipine induces reflex tachycardia) and blunt HR and BP responses to exercise.

▸ β-Blockers and thiazide diuretics can produce hyperglycemia and glucose intolerance. In addition, β-blockers can mask the adrenergic symptoms of and delay recovery from hypoglycemia; diabetics, therefore, should become skilled in self-monitoring and preventive measures.

▸ β-Blockers and diuretics may impair thermoregulation during exercise in environments that are hot and/or humid, so people taking these medications should be taught to recognize the signs and symptoms of heat illness and the importance of adequate hydration, proper clothing to facilitate cooling, exercising during the cooler times of the day, and reducing exercise dosage when exercising in heat and humidity.

▸ Some NSAIDs can raise BP in hypertensive individuals and antagonize the BP-lowering effects of antihypertensive medications.[29,82]

• Other physical therapy treatment modifications may be indicated:

▸ Use caution with isokinetic, high-intensity isometric, and high-resistance exercises, because they result in marked increases in BP, particularly if associated with breath holding.

▸ Breath holding and the Valsalva maneuver should be avoided because of the BP elevations they induce; instead, coordination of breathing with effort should be encouraged.

▸ Because many individuals with HTN are overweight or obese, exercise programs should also be designed to promote weight loss (see page 129).

▸ Other treatment modifications, described in Chapter 7, may be indicated.

• Finally, physical therapists should encourage compliance with antihypertensive treatments, both pharmacologic and nonpharmacologic. In addition, better BP control is achieved when home BP monitoring is performed.

CORONARY ARTERY DISEASE

Coronary artery disease (CAD), also known as atherosclerotic heart disease or coronary heart disease (ASHD and CHD, respectively), is a progressive disease process that begins in childhood and becomes clinically apparent in mid- to late adulthood. Although the mechanisms of atherogenesis are not fully understood, several risk factors, listed in Table 4-7, are associated with an increased likelihood of developing CAD. In addition, some relatively new risk factors have been identified to play a role in the development and progression of atherosclerosis: homocysteine, infection or inflammation, hypertriglyceridemia, and fibrinogen. It is now believed that endothelial damage related to these risk factors and with oxidative stress induces local inflammation and activates vascular repair processes that lead to the formation of intimal lesions, which may progress to atheromatous plaques.[102,190] Ultimately, it may be that it is the balance between endothelial cell injury and repair processes that directs the progression of cardiovascular disease.

During the early phases of the disease, outward expansion of the external vessel wall compensates for plaque growth so that normal lumen size is maintained. Later, plaque accumulation overcomes vessel remodeling and irregularly distributed, focal obstructions are found. The distribution of lipid and connective tissue in the lesions determines whether they are stable, with increasing fibrosis and calcification (i.e., calcified plaques), or vulnerable to erosion, ulceration, or rupture and thrombosis (i.e., noncalcified plaques). With repeated episodes of myocardial ischemia, collateral circulation may develop via growth of small auxiliary blood vessels to maintain coronary blood flow, at least at rest and during low-level activities, and these vessels help to minimize damage and improve survival in acute myocardial infarction.[33]

CAD leads to more than half of all cardiovascular events in men and women under age 75 years, producing an estimated 565,000 new MIs each year and 300,000 recurrent attacks.[11] It is the single greatest cause of death in American men and women, although women lag behind men by about 10 years for total CAD and by 20 years for more serious events such as MI and sudden death.

The clinical spectrum of CAD ranges from silent (asymptomatic) myocardial ischemia to chronic stable angina, unstable angina or acute coronary syndrome (ACS), acute MI, chronic ischemic cardiomyopathy, CHF, and sudden death.

Women and CAD

Data derived from the Women's Ischemia Syndrome Evaluation (WISE) Study necessitate mention of some issues related to women and CAD that have been revealed:

• There are substantial differences between women and men in the type, frequency, and quality of symptoms for myocardial ischemia. Women, and also some men, tend to have variable activity thresholds for ischemia and symptoms that are often atypical for angina pectoris, such as fatigue, sleep disturbance, and dyspnea. A classification of "typical" angina misses 65% of women who actually have CAD.[182] However, the presence of typical symptoms is significantly associated with acute coronary syndromes in women.

• In women the compilation of traditional risk factors underestimates cardiovascular risk. The metabolic syndrome, but not body

TABLE 4-7: Cardiovascular Risk Factors

Major Risk Factors	Defining Criteria*
Family history	MI, coronary revascularization, or sudden death before age 55 yr in father or other male first-degree relative, or before age 65 yr in mother or other female first-degree relative
Cigarette smoking	Current cigarette smoker or those who quit within previous 6 mo
Hypertension	SBP ≥140 mm Hg or DBP ≥90 mm Hg or taking antihypertensive medication
Dyslipidemia	LDL cholesterol >130 mg/dL or HDL cholesterol <40 mg/dL or taking lipid-lowering medication, or total cholesterol >200 mg/dL if LDL not available
Impaired fasting glucose or DM	Fasting blood glucose ≥100 mg/dL
Obesity and overweight	BMI ≥30 or waist circumference >40 in. (102 cm) for males, >35 in. (88 cm) for females[†]
Sedentary lifestyle	Persons not participating in a regular exercise program or not accumulating ≥30 minutes of moderate physical activity on most days of the week
CV disease	History of angina, MI, peripheral arterial disease, TIA, ischemic stroke
Other Factors	
↑ Triglycerides	≥150 mg/dL
Thrombogenic/hemostatic factors	↑ Levels of fibrinogen, plasminogen activator inhibitor-1, tissue factor, tissue plasminogen activator antigen
Infection/inflammation	High-sensitivity CRP >3
Ethnicity, socioeconomic class	African Americans, non-Hispanic whites, Hispanic Americans, lower socioeconomic class
Psychosocial factors	Depression, mental stress, chronic hostility, social isolation, perceived lack of social support
Exogenous estrogens	Hormone replacement therapy started >10 yr after onset of menopause[‡]
Alcohol consumption	No consumption or >1 drink per day for females, >2 drinks per day for males
Other medical conditions	Examples: rheumatoid arthritis, systemic lupus

↑, Increased; BMI, body mass index; CRP, C-reactive protein; CV, cardiovascular; DBP, diastolic blood pressure; DM, diabetes mellitus; HDL, high-density lipoprotein; LDL, low-density lipoprotein; MI, myocardial infarction; SBP, systolic blood pressure; TIA, transient ischemic attack.
*Unless otherwise noted, all data is compiled from American College of Sports Medicine: *ASCM's Resource Manual for Guidelines for Exercise Testing and Prescription*. 4th ed. Philadelphia: Lippincott Williams & Wilkins; 2001; and Zipes DP, Libby P, Bonow PO, Braunwald E, editors. *Braunwald's Heart Disease*. 7th ed. Philadelphia: Saunders; 2005.
[†]Refer to Table 6-31 on page 287.
[‡]Based on data from references 149a,149b,164, and 198a.

mass index (BMI) or abdominal obesity, is a leading risk factor for major cardiovascular morbidity and death in women. In addition, clustering of traditional and novel risk factors (e.g., metabolic syndrome plus inflammation, as indicated by high levels of high-sensitivity C-reactive protein) further intensifies the risk in women.[141]

- The role of hormone replacement therapy (HRT) in relation to risk for CAD has been controversial. For years HRT was prescribed to protect against the increase in CVD that occurs after menopause. However, major research studies have failed to document CV benefits despite desirable changes in lipid levels, and in fact, one study found an increased risk of CVD in some women taking HRT, mainly during the first year of treatment.[149b,163c] Further analyses of the data reveal that HRT, when started early in menopause, does offer cardioprotective effects and is associated with a reduction in all-cause mortality.[149a,198a]
- Despite equivalent risk profiles, women are much more likely to be classified as lower risk and less likely to receive appropriate evidence-based care.
- Standard stress testing evaluating inducible electrocardiographic (ECG) changes, myocardial perfusion defects, and regional wall motion abnormalities is of limited value in the assessment of women with chest pain.[182] Newer techniques using magnetic resonance spectroscopy appear to be more useful.[141]

- The majority of women (and some men) who undergo coronary angiography for evaluation of chest pain do not show significant obstructive coronary disease, but are more likely to exhibit abnormal microvascular coronary flow reserve and macrovascular endothelial dysfunction.[123,190]
- Women with persistent chest pain despite normal coronary angiograms and those who demonstrate endothelial dysfunction experience significantly more adverse cardiovascular events, including acute myocardial infarction, CHF, stroke, and death.[32,123]
- After suffering a cardiac event, women tend to play down the impact of their health situation, avoid burdening their social contacts, and have greater psychosocial distress and lower self-efficacy and self-esteem.[23]

Myocardial Ischemia

Myocardial ischemia is a relative condition that results from insufficient oxygen supply to meet the metabolic demands of a region of myocardium, which can be induced by excessive myocardial demand, reduced level of oxygenation of the blood, or insufficient blood supply. It is usually caused by reduced blood supply due to fixed atherosclerotic stenoses in the epicardial coronary arteries or occasionally by coronary vasospasm or small-vessel disease superimposed on increasing demand provoked by activity. The various factors that affect the balance between myocardial oxygen supply and demand are illustrated in Figure 4-14, as are the clinical consequences. Because the myocardium relies almost entirely on aerobic metabolism to provide its energy, ventricular dysfunction develops quickly when there is insufficient coronary blood flow. Notably, many patients experience symptoms of myocardial ischemia immediately after activity because of the postexercise rise in plasma catecholamine levels.[9]

Pathophysiology

An imbalance between myocardial oxygen supply relative to demand, which typically occurs during exertion or emotional stress with luminal narrowing of more than 65% to 70% in an epicardial coronary artery, leads to:

- Impaired diastolic function (i.e., impaired relaxation), as detailed in Figure 4-12, resulting in increased LV EDP
- Impaired systolic ventricular function (i.e., diminished force of contraction) leading to reduced SV, as described in Figure 4-13

- In addition, higher LV EDP due to either diastolic or systolic dysfunction further reduces coronary driving pressure and thus blood flow (which occurs during diastole only), thereby inducing more ischemia.
- Myocardial irritability producing arrhythmias
- *Myocardial stunning:* When the balance between myocardial oxygen supply and demand is restored, myocardial function usually returns to normal; however, reperfusion injury (flow compromise with impairment of coronary vasodilation) sometimes delays recovery of contractile function, producing *myocardial stunning,* until blood flow is restored and glycogen stores are replenished.
- *Myocardial hibernation:* Repeated episodes of ischemia–reperfusion can induce a state of depressed function, or *myocardial hibernation,* with noncontractile but viable myocardium that may regain function after revascularization.

Clinical Manifestations

- Angina pectoris (ischemic chest discomfort): classic characteristics include the following:
  - Pain type: Pressure, heaviness, squeezing, tightness, burning
  - Location: Substernal, jaw, shoulder, epigastrium, back or arm
  - Precipitated by: Exertion, stress, emotions, meals
  - Duration: 3 to 15 minutes

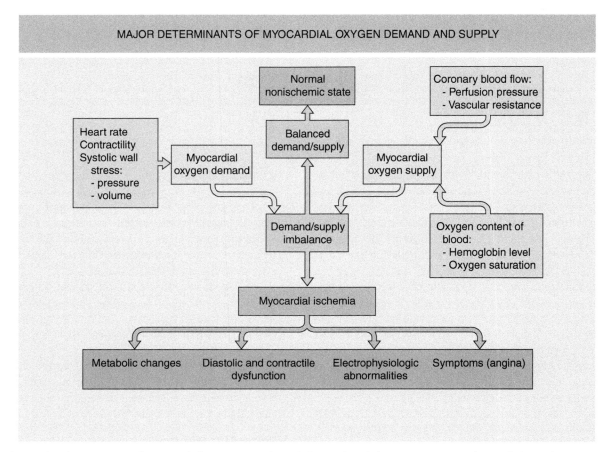

Figure 4-14: Major determinants of myocardial oxygen supply and demand and the consequences of an imbalance between them (i.e., ischemia). (From Shah PK, Falk E. Pathophysiology of myocardial ischemia. In Crawford MH, DiMarco JP, Paulus WJ, editors. *Cardiology,* 2nd ed. St. Louis: Mosby; 2004.)

▶ Relieved by: Rest or mitigation of stress, nitroglycerin

▶ Pain free: Between bouts

- Anginal equivalents: Other symptoms (e.g., dyspnea, fatigue, lightheadedness, or belching) that are brought on by exertion or stress and relieved by rest or nitroglycerin
- Arrhythmias resulting from myocardial irritability
- Characteristic ECG changes: ST-segment depression with possible T-wave inversion (see Figure 6-4, page 233), although significant transmural ischemia may produce transient ST-segment elevation
- Hypotension caused by reduced cardiac output

Note: Most patients with known myocardial ischemia have at least some episodes of *silent ischemia* (i.e., without any symptoms), up to one third of patients experience the vast majority of episodes as silent, and some patients have only silent ischemia (particularly those with diabetes and elderly males). Only 18% of heart attacks are preceded by long-standing angina.[11]

Stable or chronic stable angina describes the presence of episodic chest discomfort that is generally predictable, as described previously.

Unstable angina is defined as chest pain or other anginal equivalent that occurs at rest or with minimal exertion and usually lasts at least 20 minutes (unless interrupted by nitroglycerin), or severe chest pain of new onset, or anginal discomfort occurring with increasing frequency, duration, and/or severity. It is usually a warning sign of impending MI.

Prinzmetal's or *variant angina* (also called *atypical angina*) is chest pain, often severe, that typically occurs at rest or at night rather than with exertion or emotional stress and is associated with ST elevation and often arrhythmias. It is caused by coronary vasospasm, which usually occurs adjacent to or at the site of at least minimal atherosclerotic changes, if not severe atherosclerosis, and can be intense enough to cause acute MI.

Chest pain with normal coronary arteries (sometimes called *cardiac syndrome X*) is a clinical entity that describe patients with many of the common features of angina-like chest pain, normal epicardial coronary arteries, and no evidence of large-vessel spasm. The etiology of this syndrome is likely heterogeneous, including microvascular dysfunction with an exaggerated response of the small coronary arteries to vasoconstrictor stimuli, myocardial metabolic abnormalities, and enhanced pain perception or sensitivity (sensitive heart syndrome). Some patients demonstrate evidence of myocardial ischemia, particularly of the subendocardium.

Acute Coronary Syndromes

The term *acute coronary syndrome (ACS)* is used to describe patients who present to the emergency room with either acute MI or unstable angina. This diagnostic term is designed to expedite the triage and management of these patients in hopes of reducing myocardial damage and associated morbidity and mortality.

- The most common cause of ACS is rupture of a noncalcified atheromatous plaque that is less than 50% occlusive, followed by formation of a superimposed thrombus.
- Current research is investigating the role of various biomarkers, including troponin, B-type natriuretic peptide (BNP), and a number of inflammatory biomarkers, as a means of stratifying risk and guiding management of patients with ACS, particularly those without ST elevation.[90]

Myocardial Infarction

Myocardial infarction (MI) occurs as a result of interruption of blood supply to an area of myocardium for 20 minutes or more, causing tissue necrosis. In more than 80% of cases, MI is precipitated by thrombosis due to disruption of the fibrous cap (see the previous section) or superficial erosion of the endothelium of a atheromatous plaque; less often it is produced by coronary spasm, embolism, and thrombosis in a normal coronary artery.[33] Acute MI is usually classified according to the presence or absence of ST-segment elevation.

- *ST elevation MI* (STEMI) is the most lethal form of ACS and results from total occlusion of a coronary artery, leading to cessation of blood flow to a zone of myocardium. They are usually associated with Q-wave formation and full or nearly full-thickness myocardial necrosis and thus produce marked increases in specific serum cardiac markers (e.g., troponins, creatine kinase MB; see page 407).
- *Non-ST elevation MI* (NSTEMI) is diagnosed in patients with ST depression or other ST- or T-wave changes accompanied by a rise and fall in serum cardiac markers.
- Other diagnostic criteria include the clinical history and presenting signs and symptoms, evolution of the ECG changes over time, and cardiac imaging showing reduced or absent tissue perfusion or wall motion abnormalities.

Pathophysiology

- Acute MI creates three concentric pathological zones: the central area of myocardial necrosis and the surrounding areas of injury and ischemia (Figure 4-15), which can give rise to:
  ▶ Diastolic and systolic dysfunction, which may lead to ventricular dilation and CHF or cardiogenic shock, depending on the size of the infarct (see Figures 4-10 and 4-11)
  ▶ Increased myocardial irritability, causing arrhythmias and possible sudden death
  ▶ Rupture of infarcted tissue producing a ventricular septal defect, cardiac rupture, or acute mitral regurgitation
  ▶ Extension of infarction with expanded area of necrosis
  ▶ Pericarditis; pulmonary or systemic emboli
- Hyperkinesis of the remaining noninfarcted myocardium occurs during the first 2 weeks after acute MI, although there may also be some areas of hypokinesis.
- β-Adrenergic antagonists (β-blockers) are known to limit the extent of myocardial damage and increase survival after acute MI, apparently by reducing myocardial oxygen demand.
- Over time, ventricular remodeling occurs, leading to changes in ventricular size, shape, and thickness of both the infarcted and noninfarcted areas.
  ▶ Myocardial wall motion may appear normal, as in a small MI or a subendocardial MI with scarring of only the innermost layer of the heart; or
  ▶ It may be abnormal, as in a transmural MI with full-thickness scar, as shown in Figure 4-16:
    ⊙ Hypokinesis occurs when an area of the myocardium contracts less than normal
    ⊙ Akinesis is depicted by lack of motion of an area of myocardium
    ⊙ Dyskinesis is characterized by paradoxical systolic expansion of an area of myocardium

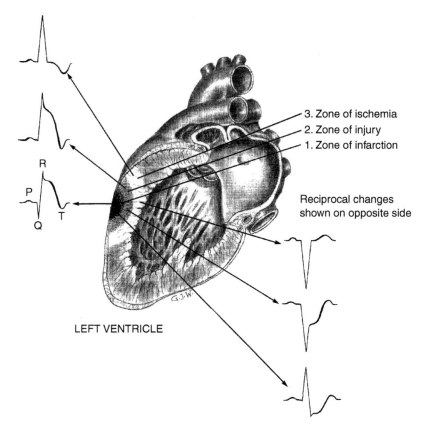

Figure 4-15: The zones of infarction and the electrocardiographic changes that correspond to them. *1,* The innermost zone of infarction causes permanent Q waves along with acute ST elevation. *2,* The surrounding zone of injury causes acute ST-segment elevation and some T-wave inversion. *3,* The outermost zone of ischemia causes acute inversion of the T wave. (From Aehlert B. *ECGs Made Easy.* 3rd ed. St. Louis: Mosby; 2005.)

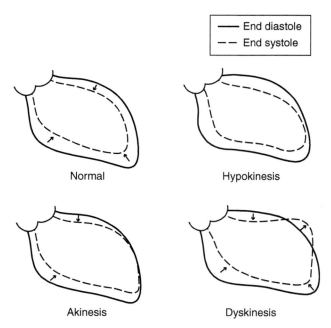

Figure 4-16: Regional wall motion abnormalities observed after myocardial infarction (MI): Reduced motion of a myocardial wall segment is called *hypokinesis,* lack of motion of a segment of myocardium is termed *akinesis,* and paradoxic motion of a segment is known as *dyskinesis,* which produces a ventricular aneurysm. (Redrawn from Kennedy JW. *Cardiovasc. Nurs.* 1976;12:23–27.)

Clinical Manifestations

- Classic symptoms of acute MI:
  ▸ Severe crushing chest pain, with or without radiation to the arm(s), neck, jaw, teeth, or back
  ▸ Diaphoresis
  ▸ Dyspnea
  ▸ Nausea, vomiting
  ▸ Lightheadedness, dizziness, syncope
  ▸ Apprehension or sense of impending doom
  ▸ Weakness
  ▸ Denial
- Sudden death
- *Note:* 20% to 25% of MIs occur without any symptoms ("silent" MIs).[9]
- ECG changes (ST elevation or depression), which evolve over time, as illustrated in Figure 4-17.
- Elevation of specific serum enzymes or isoenzymes: troponins and creatine kinase or phosphokinase (CK or CPK, particularly the myocardial band isoenzyme, MB) (see page 407)

Ischemic Cardiomyopathy

Some patients with severe coronary artery disease develop diffuse myocardial dilation with reduced contractility, even without any evidence of previous myocardial infarction. This ischemic cardiomyopathy can be induced by frequent recurrent episodes of

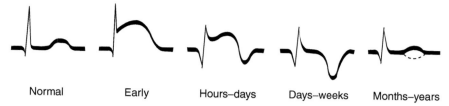

Normal   Early   Hours–days   Days–weeks   Months–years

Figure 4-17: Sequential electrocardiogram (ECG) changes following acute MI. Initially, there is a Q wave with marked ST elevation. Over the next few days the Q wave becomes deeper and wider, the ST segment moves toward the baseline, and the T wave becomes inverted. Within weeks of an acute MI, the ST segment is near the baseline and the T wave is deeply inverted. Finally, within months the T wave returns to a less inverted or somewhat upright position.

myocardial ischemia–reperfusion, especially if the patient has myocardial stunning or large segments of hibernating myocardium or diffuse fibrosis, or by multiple infarctions, or by a combination of these.

Congestive Heart Failure

CHF can develop as an acute or chronic manifestation of CAD. Acute onset of CHF is most commonly precipitated by MI, particularly with a large, transmural anterior infarction or papillary muscle dysfunction. On occasion, CAD is first diagnosed when a patient exhibits the signs and symptoms of acute CHF (see page 110) resulting from LV systolic dysfunction. Chronic CHF due to CHD is usually related to loss of at least 20% of the myocardium or ventricular septal defect or severe mitral regurgitation caused by acute MI. With improved disease management, patients with CAD are living longer, and the prevalence of associated CHF is increasing.

Sudden Death

Not infrequently, a patient is discovered to have CAD during autopsy for unexplained sudden death. In the majority of these cases, lethal arrhythmias associated with acute MI are the cause of death.

Treatment of CAD

- Pharmacologic therapy (see pages 176 to 201):
  ▸ Antianginal medications (β-blockers, calcium channel blockers, and nitrates)
  ▸ Antiarrhythmic agents (several classes of drugs that target specific phases of the action potential)
  ▸ Antithrombin or antiplatelet therapy (e.g., aspirin, clopidogrel and related drugs, dipyridamole [Persantine], abciximab, and tirofiban)
  ▸ Anticoagulants (e.g., heparin, low molecular weight heparin, and warfarin)
  ▸ Thrombolytics (e.g., streptokinase, urokinase, tissue plasminogen activator, anistreplase, and reteplase)
  ▸ Medications for reduction of coronary risk factors (e.g., HTN, dyslipidemia, diabetes)
  ▸ Medications for the treatment of heart failure
- Surgical interventions (see pages 60 to 64)
  ▸ Percutaneous transluminal coronary angioplasty
  ▸ Intracoronary stents
  ▸ Atherectomy
  ▸ Coronary artery bypass graft (CABG)

  ▸ Transmyocardial revascularization
  ▸ Pacemaker insertion
  ▸ Automatic implantable cardiac defibrillator (AICD)
- Other
  ▸ Lifestyle modifications for risk factor reduction (see page 59)
  ▸ Cardiac rehabilitation (see pages 59 and 309)

Clinical Implications for Physical Therapy

- Because of the deleterious effects of bedrest, early mobilization, including therapeutic exercise and ambulation, is beneficial for patients after acute MI and cardiac surgery.
- Individuals with cardiac disease are at increased risk of having a cardiac event during exercise and rehabilitation activities, which can be stratified according to several clinical factors (see page 238). The risk is greatest in patients with poor LV function (EF <40%), significant ventricular arrhythmias, or a non–Q-wave MI (because of increased risk for subsequent ischemic events), as well as those who exceed prescribed exercise intensity.
- Because many PT activities increase myocardial oxygen demand and thus can disturb the balance between it and myocardial oxygen supply, patients with known CAD should always have with them their short-acting nitroglycerin (NTG), which comes in the form of sublingual or buccal tablets or as a sublingual spray.
  ▸ Patients should be encouraged to report any chest discomfort and take NTG exactly as directed. If symptoms persist 5 minutes after taking NTG, the dose can be repeated an additional two times with 5 minutes between doses. If chest pain continues, prompt medical attention is indicated.
  ▸ NTG has a short half-life, so patients should be instructed to immediately replace it after its expiration date.
  ▸ NTG can be used prophylactically 5 to 10 minutes before activities that are likely to induce angina and thereby increase exercise tolerance.
  ▸ Every PT department or home health service should have an established policy on how to manage ischemic events when a patient does not have a prescription for NTG or fails to have it on hand.
- The physiological responses to activity should be monitored during PT in order to detect any signs or symptoms of myocardial ischemia:
  ▸ Patients may exhibit normal physiological responses with low-level activities.

- ▸ Patients usually exhibit abnormal HR and/or BP responses during episodes of myocardial ischemia (see pages 260 and 274). The HR and BP should be recorded at the onset of angina for calculation of the rate–pressure product (see page 279).
- ▸ Patients with CAD may develop angina or other signs and symptoms of exercise intolerance during or immediately after PT activities (see page 281).
  - ⊙ If a patient develops any signs or symptoms of myocardial ischemia, s/he should reduce the intensity of activity or, if necessary, sit and take NTG and rest for a few minutes.
  - ⊙ When activity is resumed, it should be at a lower intensity than that which induced the ischemic symptoms.
  - ⊙ The occurrence of angina after an acute MI is abnormal and should be reported to the physician immediately.
- Exercise training is extremely beneficial for individuals with CAD and those with increased risk for its development. It improves functional status, reduces risk factors associated with cardiovascular disease and its progression (plasma lipid abnormalities, endothelial dysfunction, impaired insulin sensitivity, inflammation, and HTN) and contributes to a 20% to 25% reduction in total and CV-related mortality.[78,114,197,234] To obtain the greatest effect, exercise training should be combined with other positive lifestyle modifications and in many cases with appropriate medical therapy to reduce CV risk factors.
  - ▸ Traditionally, exercise training has focused on aerobic exercise of moderate intensity performed for 30 to 45 minutes at least 3 days/wk. However, some studies indicate that vigorous intensity exercise may elicit greater cardioprotective benefits,[215] and public health recommendations advise a frequency of at least 5 days/wk when moderate-intensity exercise is performed (see page 301).[104,166]
  - ▸ Resistance exercise of low to moderate intensity is also recommended as an adjunct to aerobic exercise for individuals with stable CAD (see page 308) to enhance muscular strength and endurance, increase lean body mass, reduce body fat, and improve functional performance and independence, and quality of life.[166,235]
  - ▸ Because isometric exercise produces higher DBPs than dynamic exercise, nonsustained static exercise may increase subendocardial perfusion and reduce the incidence of myocardial ischemia and angina.[9]
  - ▸ Clinical monitoring is required, at least initially, to identify adverse responses and guide exercise intensity and progression in order to avoid complications.
  - ▸ The cardiovascular risks associated with exercise, both aerobic and resistance, are largely determined by the age of the individual, his/her habitual level of physical activity and fitness level, underlying CVD and other comorbidities, and the intensity of exercise.
- Side effects of medications and any exercise interactions should be recognized (see Chapter 5):
  - ▸ Refer to page 102 for side effects of β-blockers and calcium channel blockers.
  - ▸ Nitrates and vasodilators are associated with higher resting and sometimes exercise HR, as well as hypotension, especially orthostatic and postexercise hypotension. The application of heat modalities can also induce hypotension.

- ▸ NTG commonly produces headache, dizziness, and orthostatic hypotension, so the patient should be seated when taking a dose.
- Physical therapy treatment modifications may be indicated, such as reduced exercise intensity or inclusion of frequent rest breaks, to reduce the energy cost of more strenuous rehabilitation activities (see page 309).
- Patients recovering from CABG or transmyocardial revascularization surgery via median sternotomy incision require consideration of precautions related to the incision and any chest tubes that are in place (see pages 61 and 32).

HEART FAILURE

Heart failure is a clinical syndrome that arises from ventricular dysfunction (acute or chronic), in which venous return to the heart is normal but the heart is unable to pump sufficient cardiac output to meet the body's metabolic demands, or can do so only at abnormally elevated diastolic pressures or volumes. It is the final pathway for many diverse diseases that affect the heart through structural and functional abnormalities, as well as through biological alterations (e.g., the RAAS and the SNS) and circulating substances (e.g., vasodilators, such as bradykinin, nitric oxide, and prostaglandins; natriuretic peptides; cytokines; and vasopressin).

Congestive, or chronic, heart failure (CHF) is characterized by pulmonary congestion due to the "backup" of blood from the left ventricle to the left atrium and pulmonary vasculature. It is the most common diagnosis leading to hospitalization of patients, accounting for at least 20% of all hospitalizations in patients over age 65 years. Persistent symptomatic CHF has a poor prognosis, with a 1-year mortality rate of approximately 45%.[121]

Heart failure may develop as a result of right or left ventricular systolic dysfunction or diastolic dysfunction, or a combination of both, as shown in Table 4-8.[13,121,241]

- *Systolic heart failure* is characterized by impaired myocardial contractility and reduced ejection fraction, leading to a large dilated heart.
  - ▸ Systolic dysfunction is depicted on page 100.
  - ▸ Increased ventricular volumes and pressures are reflected back to the atria and antecedent vasculature, resulting in congestion and edema.
  - ▸ Significant ventricular dilatation often causes functional mitral regurgitation, tricuspid regurgitation, or both, as valvular structures are pulled farther apart.
- *Diastolic heart failure,* also referred to as *heart failure with normal ejection fraction (HFNEF),* occurs in 20% to 50% of patients with HF, particularly women, hypertensives, and older individuals, and is characterized by impaired ventricular relaxation and increased passive stiffness (decreased compliance) with normal systolic function and a normal ejection fraction.[222a]
  - ▸ Diastolic dysfunction is illustrated and described on page 99.
  - ▸ Abnormal ventricular filling can reduce cardiac output, especially during exertion when faster HRs reduce the filling time.
  - ▸ Ventricular filling and cardiac output are also affected adversely by arrhythmias in which active atrial contraction is absent (e.g., atrial fibrillation, nodal rhythms, and frequent premature ventricular complexes)

TABLE 4-8: Relative Roles of Left Ventricular Systolic and Diastolic Dysfunction in the Development of Congestive Heart Failure for a Number of More Common Diseases

Disease	Frequency of Occurrence	Systolic Dysfunction	Diastolic Dysfunction
Ischemic heart disease	+++++	++++	+++*
Hypertensive heart disease	++++	+++	+++
Dilated cardiomyopathy	++	++++	++
Hypertrophic cardiomyopathy	+	0	++++
Restrictive cardiomyopathy	+	+	+++
Aortic stenosis	++	+++	+++
Aortic regurgitation	+	++	++
Mitral regurgitation	++	+	+
Mitral stenosis	+	0, ++†	++++
Constrictive pericarditis	+	0	++++
Pericardial tamponade	+	0	++++

*During episodes of myocardial ischemia.
†Right ventricle is affected, not left.

▸ At any given volume, ventricular pressures are elevated and reflected back to the atria and antecedent vasculature, resulting in congestion and edema, similar to systolic HF.

• A combination of systolic and diastolic dysfunction exists in many patients, particularly those with CAD and hypertensive heart disease.

Classification systems have been created to describe the severity of HF symptoms and the disease process. The New York Heart Association (NYHA) functional classification describes the severity of a patient's HF symptoms and the functional impact (see Figure 6-2). However, it is important to note that concordance between NYHA classification and peak oxygen consumption is less than 50%, so it is not a good predictor of exercise performance.[198b] The American College of Cardiology (Washington, DC) and American Heart Association (Dallas, TX) have developed another staging classification for HF, which emphasizes the evolution and progression of the disease, similar to those for cancer, denoting patients who are at risk for developing HF, patients with in situ disease, and those with established or widespread disease (Table 4-9).[113,121]

Left Ventricular Failure (Congestive Heart Failure)

Intrinsic myocardial disease (e.g., atherosclerotic heart disease and cardiomyopathy), excessive workload on the heart (e.g., hypertension, valvular disease, and congenital defects), cardiac arrhythmias, or iatrogenic damage (e.g., alcohol, drug toxicity, and chest irradiation) can lead to left ventricular dysfunction (systolic, diastolic, or the two combined) and eventual failure, commonly referred to as CHF.

Pathophysiology

LV failure is characterized by pulmonary congestion and edema and low cardiac output:

• In the case of systolic dysfunction, poor LV contractile function results in an increase in EDV and a decrease in SV, with a resultant drop in ejection fraction (EF, which equals SV/EDV) (see Figure 3-5, page 43).

▸ As shown in Figure 4-13, reduced EF further increases LV EDV, which is reflected back to the LA, leading to LA dilatation, and then to the pulmonary vasculature, causing pulmonary congestion.

TABLE 4-9: ACC/AHA Stages of Heart Failure

Stage	Description	Examples
A	Patients at high risk for the development of HF, but with no apparent structural abnormality of the heart	Systemic HTN, CAD, DM, h/o cardiotoxic drug therapy or alcohol abuse, h/o rheumatic fever, family h/o cardiomyopathy
B	Patients with structural abnormality of the heart, but who have never had symptoms of HF	LV hypertrophy or fibrosis, LV dilatation or hypocontractility, asymptomatic valvular heart disease, previous MI
C	Patients with structural abnormality of the heart and current or previous symptoms of HF	Dyspnea or fatigue due to LV systolic dysfunction, asymptomatic patients who are undergoing treatment for prior symptoms of HF
D	Patients with end-stage symptoms of HF that are refractory to standard treatment	Frequent hospitalizations for HF or cannot be safely discharged home, intravenous inotropic support, VADs, heart transplantation candidates

Adapted from American College of Cardiology/American Heart Association guidelines for the evaluation and management of chronic heart failure in the adult (2001).[113]
CAD, Coronary artery disease; DM, diabetes mellitus; HF, heart failure; h/o, history of; HTN, hypertension; LV, left ventricular; MI, myocardial infarction; VAD, ventricular assist device.

- ▸ Rising pulmonary pressures lead to transudation of intravascular fluid from the capillaries into the interstitial space, which may progress to alveolar flooding.
- ▸ Marked LV dilatation can result in functional mitral regurgitation, which increases during exercise.
- When diastolic dysfunction is present (e.g., due to LVH or CAD), impaired ventricular relaxation and increased passive stiffness lead to decreased ventricular filling and elevated ventricular and pulmonary vascular pressures, as illustrated in Figure 4-12.
  - ▸ Reduced ventricular filling will cause a drop in SV, according to the Frank-Starling mechanism, which cannot be compensated for by an increase in HR, as higher HRs reduce filling time and further compromise EDV.
  - ▸ If pulmonary vascular pressures rise high enough to cause transudation of intravascular fluid from the capillaries, gas exchange will be impaired and pulmonary edema may develop, causing dyspnea.
- Compensatory mechanisms are activated to maintain pump function, as listed in Table 4-10. When they become exhausted, cardiac output will fall.
- In addition, higher LV EDP due to either diastolic or systolic dysfuncion impedes coronary blood flow to the endocardium (which occurs during diastole only), thus increasing the risk of subendocardial ischemia.
- CHF is associated with a reduction in renal blood flow and glomerular filtration rate, producing renal ischemia and proteinuria. Activation of angiotensin, aldosterone, and the sympathetic nervous system causes further damage to the kidneys and frequently leads to chronic kidney disease and renal failure.[209] Furthermore, chronic kidney disease, as well as the resultant anemia, can worsen CHF.

TABLE 4-10: Compensatory Mechanisms Activated in Heart Failure

Compensatory Mechanism	Effects
SNS stimulation	↑ HR, ↑ contractility, ↑ rate of ventricular relaxation, arterial and venous constriction
Activation of the renin–angiotensin–aldosterone system	Arterial vasoconstriction, ↑ sodium and water retention, ↑ myocardial contractility
Frank-Starling effect (cardiac dilatation)	↑ Preload and thus stroke volume
Ventricular remodeling (LV hypertrophy)	↓ Myocardial wall stress
↑ Peripheral oxygen extraction	↑ Oxygen available for aerobic energy production
Anaerobic metabolism	Continued energy production despite insufficient oxygen for aerobic metabolism

↑, Increased; ↓, decreased; HR, heart rate; LV, left ventricular; SNS, sympathetic nervous system.

- Reduced peripheral blood flow leads to skeletal muscle abnormalities, including predominance of glycolytic over oxidative metabolism and ultrastructural modifications in muscle composition.[185] Resultant stimulation of the SNS likely contributes to the vicious cycle of chronic HF.
- Inspiratory muscle weakness and deconditioning contribute to the typical symptoms of fatigue and dyspnea seen in patients with stable HF, who often exhibit reduced maximal inspiratory pressure ($P_{I_{max}}$) and inspiratory muscle endurance.[57,162] In fact, $P_{I_{max}}$ has been found to decrease with NYHA functional class and is an independent predictor of prognosis.[162]
- Exercise-limiting changes in every step of the oxygen transport system are found in patients with HF and are exhibited as abnormal physiological responses to physical activity:
  - ▸ Augmented venous return increases preload on a poorly functioning heart, further raising pulmonary pressures and reducing cardiac output.
  - ▸ Increasing pulmonary pressure during exercise provokes dyspnea and sometimes pulmonary edema.
  - ▸ β-Receptor down-regulation and/or myocardial β-adrenergic receptor desensitization in the presence of the compensatory increase in circulating catecholamines leads to chronotropic incompetence in more than 20% of patients with systolic HF and may contribute to exercise intolerance.[30,201]
  - ▸ Redistribution of blood flow due to low cardiac output reduces flow to the kidneys and skin initially and later to the brain, gut, and skeletal muscle.
  - ▸ Peripheral muscle abnormalities lead to lower anaerobic threshold, early acidosis, and depletion of high-energy compounds, which increase ventilation and stimulation of the SNS, further impairing LV function.[185]
  - ▸ Peripheral arteriovenous oxygen extraction increases to compensate for reduced peripheral blood flow.
- Not infrequently, patients with CHF also have sleep apnea, which adds to LV dysfunction due to the increased afterload provoked by the resultant HTN.

Clinical Manifestations
- Signs and symptoms of pulmonary congestion:
  - ▸ Dyspnea, dry cough
  - ▸ Orthopnea
  - ▸ Paroxysmal nocturnal dyspnea (PND)
  - ▸ Pulmonary rales, wheezing ("cardiac asthma")
  - ▸ Signs and symptoms of acute pulmonary edema (marked dyspnea, pallor or cyanosis, diaphoresis, tachycardia, anxiety, and agitation)
- Signs and symptoms of low cardiac output:
  - ▸ Hypotension
  - ▸ Tachycardia
  - ▸ Lightheadedness, dizziness
  - ▸ Fatigue, weakness
  - ▸ Signs and symptoms of peripheral hypoperfusion (e.g., weak, thready pulse; vasoconstriction)
  - ▸ Poor exercise tolerance
- S_3 (third heart sound or ventricular gallop), and sometimes S_4 (fourth heart sound or atrial gallop) (see page 44)

- Enlarged heart, increased vasculature on chest x-ray examination
- Possible functional mitral and tricuspid regurgitation

Right Ventricular Failure

The most common cause of RV failure is LV failure, and it can also result from mitral valve disease or acute and chronic lung disease (i.e., cor pulmonale; see page 95).

Pathophysiology

Increased pressure or volume load on the left atrium (induced by LV failure or mitral valve disease) leads to pulmonary congestion and increases pulmonary vascular pressures. Pulmonary hypertension (PH) can also be caused by a number of acute and chronic lung diseases, as described on page 94.

- Increased pressure load on the right ventricle (RV) induced by higher pulmonary vascular pressures leads to RV dilatation with or without hypertrophy (i.e., RVH), depending on the acuteness and severity of the pressure load:
  ▸ If the pressure rises acutely (e.g., massive pulmonary embolism or acute mitral regurgitation), RV dilatation and failure will occur without RVH.
  ▸ If pulmonary pressures are chronically elevated (e.g., COPD and CHF), the RV will hypertrophy to decrease wall stress.
- Prolonged PH causes irreversible anatomic changes in the small pulmonary arteries so that PH becomes fixed, with resultant RV dilatation and RVH.
- Hypoxia, hypercapnia, and/or acidosis cause further pulmonary vasoconstriction with an even greater degree of PH, which again increases the workload on the RV.
- Eventually RV EDP increases, which will be reflected back to the right atrium (RA) and the venous system with subsequent jugular venous distension (JVD), liver engorgement, ascites, and peripheral edema.
- Also, RVH reduces RV compliance, which may interfere with RV filling and reduce cardiac output.
- If the pulmonary vascular bed is reduced or there is an increase in cardiac output, HR, or blood volume (e.g., exercise), PH will worsen, producing increased signs and symptoms of RV failure.

Clinical Manifestations

- Dependent edema
- JVD
- Weight gain
- Liver engorgement (hepatomegaly), abdominal pain
- Ascites
- Anorexia, nausea, bloating
- Cyanosis
- Right-sided S_3 (see page 44)
- Accentuated P_2 (pulmonary component of the second heart sound)
- RV lift of sternum
- Possible murmurs of pulmonary or tricuspid valve insufficiency

Biventricular Failure

As discussed previously, the elevated pulmonary pressures caused by LV failure can eventually cause RV failure. Therefore, the pathophysiological effects and clinical manifestations are those associated with both LV and RV failure.

Compensated Heart Failure

When a patient experiences heart failure, and through activation of the various compensatory mechanisms (see Table 4-10) or therapeutic interventions the heart is able to return to a functional, albeit reduced, cardiac output, heart failure is described as *compensated*. Cardiac reserve and exercise tolerance are usually markedly limited. With greater demands or progression of disease, the patient's status often decompensates again and the clinical manifestations of acute CHF reappear.

Treatment of Heart Failure

The treatment for HF depends on whether it is acute or chronic.
- Correction of the underlying cause if possible (e.g., valve disease and arrhythmias)
- Aggressive management of HTN and CAD
- Pharmacologic therapies (see Chapter 5)[113]
  ▸ ACE inhibitors or angiotensin II receptor blockers*
  ▸ β-Blockers*
  ▸ Aldosterone antagonists
  ▸ Diuretics
  ▸ Vasodilators
  ▸ Diltiazem for microvascular circulatory abnormalities
  ▸ Inotropic agents
  ▸ Nitrates
  ▸ Digoxin
  ▸ Antiarrhythmic agents, as indicated
  ▸ Relief of hypoxia (e.g., oxygen therapy, corticosteroids, bronchial hygiene, and mechanical ventilation)
- Other[113]
  ▸ Rest, if unstable
  ▸ Low-salt diet
  ▸ Exercise training (see following section)
  ▸ Phlebotomy for hematocrit exceeding 55% to 60% in cor pulmonale
  ▸ Pleurocentesis for pleural effusions (see page 25)
  ▸ Continuous positive airway pressure for obstructive sleep apnea (see page 30)
- Surgical interventions (refer to pages 63 to 69)
  ▸ Intraaortic balloon counterpulsation
  ▸ Ventricular assist device (left [LVAD] or right [RVAD]) or biventricular assist device (BiVAD)
  ▸ Organ transplantation (i.e., heart transplant for LV failure, lung transplant for cor pulmonale or interstitial lung disease, and heart–lung transplant for congenital heart disease or Eisenmenger's syndrome)
  ▸ Pacemaker for bradyarrhythmias and some tachyarrhythmias
  ▸ Cardiac resynchronization therapy (i.e., biventricular pacing)

---

*These medications have been proven to retard or reverse the myocardial remodeling that is responsible for disease progression and are recommended for the majority of individuals with systolic HF.

▶ Implantable cardioverter defibrillators
▶ Pulmonary embolectomy for unresolved PE

Clinical Implications for Physical Therapy

- Patients with CHF should be assessed for signs of decompensation at each visit: sudden weight gain, increased shortness of breath, more lower extremity edema or abdominal swelling or pain, more pronounced cough, increased fatigue, or lightheadedness or dizziness.
- Clinical monitoring should be performed at rest and during exercise and rehabilitation activities at each patient visit, at least until the patient is proficient at identifying symptoms of decompensation and exercise intolerance:
  ▶ Patients with HF often have elevated HRs and low BP at rest, and many exhibit chronotropic incompetence (i.e., failure to adequately increase HR during exertion).[30]
  ▶ Individuals with an EF less than 40% are more likely to exhibit abnormal responses to exercise; however, there is a poor correlation between EF and exercise tolerance. Therefore, clinical monitoring is essential to identify those most at risk for adverse reactions during exertion.
  ▶ PTs should recognize the signs and symptoms of exercise intolerance (see page 295) and use them to avoid excessive patient exertion. Exercise should be terminated if any of the following are observed: an acute decrease in BP, onset of angina, significant dyspnea or fatigue, a feeling of exhaustion, and/or serious exercise-induced arrhythmias.
- Treatment modifications are frequently indicated (see page 310):
  ▶ Exercise and rehabilitation activities should be low-level initially and progress slowly. Isokinetic, high-intensity isometric, and high-resistance exercises are usually not tolerated.
  ▶ Frequent 1- to 2-minute rests interspersed with activity will reduce the cost of more demanding activities (e.g., upper extremity exercise and quadruped activities).
  ▶ Caution should be employed when exercising patients with HF in the supine or prone positions, as orthopnea is a common complaint.
  ▶ Breath holding and the Valsalva maneuver should be avoided because they reduce cardiac output; coordination of breathing with effort should be encouraged.
  ▶ Rating of perceived exertion and clinical signs and symptoms can be used to monitor exercise/activity intensity.
- PTs must be familiar with the side effects of medications that may affect patients at rest and during exercise (see Chapter 5):
  ▶ Acute CHF may develop because of either inadequate or toxic drug levels; digoxin toxicity can cause arrhythmias, dizziness, confusion, and/or nausea.
  ▶ Refer to pages 172 to 177 for side effects of β-blockers, diuretics, calcium channel blockers, ACE inhibitors and angiotensin II receptor blockers, and vasodilators.
  ▶ Many of the drugs used to treat CHF are associated with orthostatic and postexercise hypotension, so individuals should be cautioned against making quick changes to upright positions and about the need to perform an extended cooldown after exercise.
- Exercise training is extremely valuable for patients with HF:
  ▶ Low-level, gradually progressive aerobic exercise training improves exercise capacity (through increased maximal cardiac output and peripheral efficiency), psychosocial status, quality of life, and functional status.[184a,186] In addition, data show that it can reduce both morbidity and mortality in patients with stable class I to III CHF, most likely due to reversal of ventricular remodeling.[105,185]

  ⊙ Exercise intensity is often based on symptomatology, such as dyspnea, which typically allows low- to moderate-intensity exercise at 40% to 75% of peak oxygen consumption.

  ⊙ Because many patients are taking β-blockers, which blunt the HR response to exercise, and others have chronotropic incompetence, RPE may be a more reliable indicator of exercise intensity, with ratings of 12 to 13 being well tolerated by most stable patients.

  ⊙ Interval training with brief rest periods as needed may be beneficial in allowing persons with CHF to accumulate a greater volume of exercise. The goal is to work toward an exercise duration of at least 30 minutes of continuous exercise.

  ⊙ Warm-up and cooldown periods are extremely important for patients with HF and may need to be longer than the usual 5 to 10 minutes in patients with advanced disease.

  ▶ Low- to moderate-intensity resistance training is often beneficial for patients with stable HF because of its effects on skeletal muscle abnormalities. Benefits include increases in muscle strength and cardiorespiratory endurance, as well as improved functional ability and quality of life.[35,142,225]

  ▶ Inspiratory muscle training is also advantageous for patients with CHF and inspiratory muscle weakness, as it produces marked improvement in inspiratory muscle strength and endurance, leading to enhanced ventilatory efficiency, functional capacity, and quality of life.[57,162]

- Education should be provided regarding the individual's disease process, the need to measure body weight first thing in the morning every day, and action to take if weight increases by 3 lb or more, the symptoms of decompensation and exercise intolerance, and the side effects of medications and symptoms of toxicity. In addition, instruction about energy conservation techniques is beneficial (see page 311).

CARDIAC ARRHYTHMIAS

Cardiac arrhythmias, or dysrhythmias, result from disturbances of heart rate, rhythm, or impulse conduction. Refer to pages 264 to 275 for descriptions of the various arrhythmias.

Types

Arrhythmias are classified according to the following:
- Site of origin (sinoatrial [SA] node, atria, atrioventricular [AV] node, or ventricles)
- Type of cardiac activity (bradycardia, tachycardia, flutter, or fibrillation)
- Presence of conduction block (SA node, AV node, or bundle branches)

Pathophysiology

Abnormal impulse generation (due to myocardial irritability or damage, drug toxicity, or electrolyte disturbances; or idiopathic) and abnormal impulse conduction (due to conduction blocks or

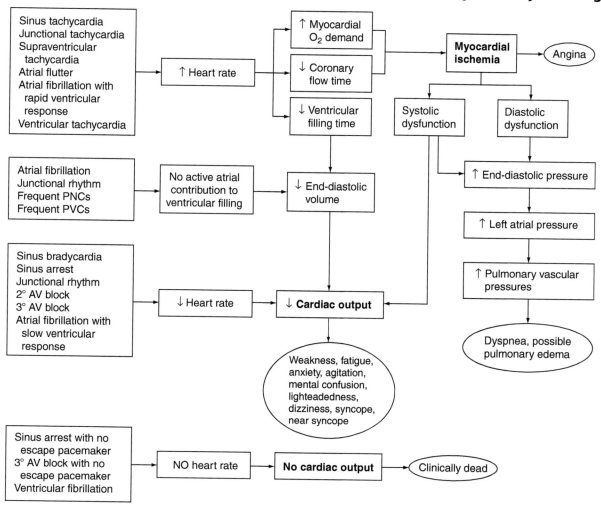

Figure 4-18: The possible pathophysiologic effects of various arrhythmias. The major problems that can develop include myocardial ischemia, diminished cardiac output, or absolutely no cardiac output with clinical death. Clinical manifestations of various events are *encircled.* AV, Atrioventricular; O_2, oxygen; PNCs, premature nodal complexes or contractions; PVCs, premature ventricular complexes or contractions.

accessory pathways) can result in a number of pathophysiological outcomes, as illustrated in Figure 4-18.

- Tachycardia increases myocardial oxygen demands and reduces ventricular filling and coronary flow times, which increase the risk of inadequate cardiac output, myocardial ischemia, and pulmonary congestion.
- Although HRs of less than 120 bpm usually cause few problems, because ventricular filling time is maintained and SV is preserved, individuals with heart disease who suddenly develop slower HRs and subsequently increased EDV, may experience pulmonary congestion. In addition, these individuals and those with severe bradycardias often exhibit decreased cardiac output and hemodynamic compromise.
- Arrhythmias associated with the loss of active atrial contraction (e.g., atrial fibrillation [A-fib or less specific AF], second-degree or third-degree AV block, frequent premature nodal contractions [PNCs] or premature ventricular contractions [PVCs], and ventricular tachycardia [VT or V-tach]) can reduce EDV up to 20% to 30%. Although this is usually not problematic

for healthy individuals, it can lead to low cardiac output and pulmonary congestion or edema in those with impaired cardiac function, particularly if they have tachycardia or diastolic dysfunction.

- A-fib can produce several adverse effects in addition to those created by the loss of atrial contribution to ventricular filling (described previously).
  - ▸ Rapid ventricular rates shorten ventricular filling time, further impairing filling volume. In addition, CHF may be precipitated.
  - ▸ The characteristic irregular rhythm of A-fib worsens the reductions in cardiac output and coronary blood flow.
  - ▸ A-fib often leads to thrombosis formation within the atria, particularly the left atrial appendage, which can give rise to emboli causing stroke.
- Some arrhythmias are characterized by a total loss of cardiac output, as in ventricular fibrillation (VF or V-fib) and sinus arrest without escape pacemaker activity, and the patient will be clinically dead (i.e., without a HR or BP).

Clinical Manifestations

Patient perception of arrhythmias varies widely; some patients feel every irregular heart beat, whereas others are not aware of them at all. The signs and symptoms that may be associated with arrhythmias include the following:

- None
- Palpitations, skipped beats, fluttering
- Lightheadedness, dizziness
- Syncope or near-syncope
- Chest discomfort
- Weakness, fatigue
- Dyspnea, possible pulmonary edema
- Mental confusion, anxiety, agitation
- Hypotension
- Irregular and/or weak pulse
- Sudden death

Specific Treatment

- Treatment of identifiable causes of arrhythmias (e.g., electrolyte disturbances, drug toxicity, and hemorrhage) and avoidance of known cardiac irritants (e.g., caffeine, nicotine, alcohol, and cocaine)
- Antiarrhythmic agents (several classes of drugs that target specific phases of the action potential; see page 187)
- Cardioversion, defibrillation (see page 60)
- Surgical interventions (see pages 60 to 64)
  ‣ Pacemaker
  ‣ Catheter ablation
  ‣ Automatic implantable cardioverter/defibrillator (AICD)
  ‣ Surgical excision (aneurysectomy, myectomy)
  ‣ Maze procedure

Clinical Implications for Physical Therapy

- The clinical significance of an arrhythmia depends on its hemodynamic effects, which is revealed by monitoring the patient's HR and BP, as well as signs and symptoms. Hemodynamically signficant arrhythmias are associated with chest pain, shortness of breath, level of consciousness, low BP, shock, pulmonary congestion, congestive heart failure, and acute myocardial infarction.
  ‣ The hemodynamic significance of an arrhythmia depends on its effects on cardiac output, BP, organ perfusion (e.g., cerebral, coronary, and renal), and ventricular function.
    ⊙ Many arrhythmias have little effect on cardiac output and BP and result in few if any symptoms (e.g., sinus arrhythmia; infrequent atrial, nodal, or ventricular premature beats).
    ⊙ Arrhythmias that cause moderate to severe reductions in cardiac output or are associated with ventricular dysfunction (e.g., sinus exit block, A-fib, paroxysmal supraventricular tachycardia, second-degree heart block, and V-tach) can interfere with organ perfusion and result in significant symptomatology.
    ⊙ A few arrhythmias are life-threatening and require immediate resuscitation (sinus arrest and VF) and some may progress to life-threatening arrhythmias (e.g., frequent PVCs can lead to V-tach, which can progress to VF).
  ‣ The clinical significance of an arrhythmia is also influenced by the duration of the arrhythmia as well as its cause and

the presence or absence of underlying heart disease or other comorbidities.
    ⊙ Occasional irregular beats or brief runs of arrhythmias are usually not troublesome, whereas those that persist for several minutes to hours or longer are more likely to induce discomfort and hemodynamic compromise.
    ⊙ Some arrhythmias are worrisome because they tend to deteriorate into more serious or life-threatening arrhythmias.
    ⊙ Arrhythmias cause more concern in patients with known cardiac disease, especially ischemic heart disease and heart failure. In patients with diastolic dysfunction, higher HRs and arrhythmias with loss of active atrial contraction can reduce ventricular filling and thus cardiac output.
    ⊙ Arrhythmias are also more disturbing in patients taking diuretics and certain medications, as they may indicate electrolyte abnormalities or drug toxicity (e.g., digitalis, theophylline, aminophylline, dyphylline, and oxitriphylline).
    ⊙ Tolerance of arrhythmias can be adversely affected by older age, anemia, cerebrovascular disease, chronic kidney disease, traumatic brain injury, and other comorbidities.

- The physiological responses to activity should be monitored in all patients with a personal or family history of arrhythmias because of the risk of exercise-induced arrhythmias provoked by enhanced sympathetic tone and increased myocardial oxygen demand:
  ‣ Pulse should be monitored for rate and regularity versus irregularity.
    ⊙ Arrhythmias may increase, decrease, or remain the same during exercise; all antiarrhythmics have the tendency to induce arrhythmias.
    ⊙ Increasing arrhythmias during exercise are a cause for concern, as they may indicate myocardial irritability due to ischemia.
  ‣ BP monitoring reveals the hemodynamic significance of arrhythmias.
  ‣ ECG monitoring is helpful in identifying arrhythmias that are provoked by physical activity. PT departments may be able to obtain discarded ECG monitoring equipment from hospitals as they upgrade to newer models.
  ‣ Patients taking antiarrhythmic drugs may be well-controlled at rest, but this control may not hold during exercise, so that arrhythmias appear. A graded exercise test is valuable for identifying this problem.
  ‣ Clinical monitoring should be continued during recovery, as arrhythmias often manifest at this time. Cooldown activity to prevent venous pooling is recommended.

- The referring physician should be notified if a patient exhibits increasing arrhythmias during activity, as further evaluation may be indicated.

- PTs should be familiar with the side effects of antiarrhythmic medications, because they may affect exercise responses or tolerance (see Chapter 5, page 187):
  ‣ All antiarrhythmic agents have the potential to increase arrhythmias.
  ‣ Class I drugs may result in elevated resting and exercise heart rates, quinidine may mask ischemic ECG changes, and procainamide may cause a false-positive exercise test.
  ‣ See pages 172 and 174 for information related to β-blockers and calcium channel blockers.

- Amiodarone lowers resting and exercise heart rates. In addition, a small percentage of patients develop pulmonary toxicity caused by amiodarone.
- Treatment modifications may be indicated:
  - ▶ Be cautious if a patient is taking drugs that cause hypotension or orthostatic intolerance; avoid sudden changes to upright postures.
  - ▶ Activity/exercise intensity may need to be restricted to avoid arrhythmias; frequent 1- to 2-minute rests during activity will reduce exercise intensity.
  - ▶ It is important to assess balance and risk of falls for all patients with a personal or family history of arrhythmias. A falling prevention program may be indicated for some patients.
- Exercise training may be beneficial for individuals with arrhythmias because of improvement in ischemic threshold and/or reduction in sympathetic tone. They should follow the public health recommendations regarding regular physical activity (see page 302).[104,166]
- All PT departments should possess a portable automatic external defibrillator (AED) and all staff should be skilled in its operation.

VALVULAR HEART DISEASE

Malfunction of the heart valves, which can be caused by infection, congenital abnormalities, aging, or disease, is much more common on the left side of the heart than on the right and often involves more than one valve. Valvular abnormalities are often asymptomatic for years to decades, but eventually cardiac function may become impaired, resulting in diastolic dysfunction, systolic dysfunction, or both, with consequent pulmonary or systemic vascular congestion, as well as decreased cardiac output (see Table 4-8, page 109 and Figures 4-12 and 4-13, pages 99 to 100). When valve disease is severe, heart failure and sudden death may occur.

- Abnormal valvular structures create turbulent blood flow, which increases the hemodynamic stress on these structures and leads to progressive damage and dysfunction.
- Compensatory mechanisms, including ventricular hypertrophy, chamber dilatation, and peripheral adaptations, can help maintain the overall performance of the heart for may years, often decades, even when there is malfunction of more than one valve.
- Eventually, however, these compensatory mechanisms may become exhausted so that heart failure develops.

Patients with congenital or acquired valvular heart disease have traditionally received prophylactic antibiotics for infective endocarditis (IE) or subacute bacterial endocarditis (SBE) before dental, genitourinary, or gastrointestinal tract procedures. However, more recent guidelines from the American Heart Association have concluded that only an extremely small number of cases of IE might be prevented by antibiotic prophylaxis and therefore its use is reasonable only for patients with underlying cardiac conditions associated with the highest risk of adverse outcome from IE.[236] For isolated valvular defects, only patients who have undergone valve repair with prosthetic valves or material and those with previous IE require antibiotic prophylaxis (see Box 8-2, page 362). Good dental hygiene continues to play a critical role in preventing IE in all patients.

Pathophysiology and Clinical Manifestations

The pathophysiology and clinical manifestations of specific valvular abnormalities are described in Table 4-11.

- Valvular stenosis (restricted valvular opening) creates an obstruction to forward flow through the valve and thus a pressure and volume load on the chamber preceding it and generates a pressure gradient across the valve that is proportional to the severity of stenosis. Concentric hypertrophy develops in response to the pressure load and attempts to normalize the SV that is pumped through the narrow valve.

TABLE 4-11: Valvular Heart Disease: Pathophysiology and Clinical Manifestations

	Abnormality	
Etiology	**Pathophysiology**	**Clinical Manifestations**
	Aortic Stenosis	
Congenital; senile calcification; inflammatory valvulitis; RF; severe atherosclerosis	Restricted opening of the AoV → ↑ pressure load on LV → ↑ LV systolic pressure, prolongation of ejection, + LVH → ↓ compliance → ↑ LV filling pressures Dependence of adequate LV filling on atrial contraction ↑ Risk of subendocardial ischemia Initially, even with severe AS, there is normal cardiac output at rest but failure to ↑ on exertion Prolonged severe AS → LV systolic dysfunction + LV dilation → ↑ pressures in pulmonary vessels + RV	May be asymptomatic, even with significant AS, for many years Once symptoms develop, prognosis is poor: Dyspnea, especially on exertion Angina pectoris Lightheadedness, syncope on exertion Sudden death Possible systemic emboli Harsh SEM at second ICS radiating to the neck, ↓ A$_2$ (aortic closure sound)

Continued

TABLE 4-11: Valvular Heart Disease: Pathophysiology and Clinical Manifestations—Cont'd

	Abnormality	
Etiology	**Pathophysiology**	**Clinical Manifestations**
	Aortic Insufficiency/Regurgitation	
Congenital, RF, infective endocarditis, aortic root disease, other (e.g., rheumatic arthritis, SLE)	Incomplete closure of the AoV → regurgitation of blood from the Ao to the LV during diastole → ↑ volume load on the LV during both systole and diastole	If chronic AI, gradual ↑ LV dilatation allows asymptomatic status for decades, then similar to AS (see above), except for less angina and syncope
	If chronic AI, LV dilation + compensatory eccentric LVH → ↑ total SV + possible ↑ forward SV if compensatory peripheral vasodilation	If acute AI, LV cannot adapt to sudden ↑ volume → S & S of LV failure
	If severe acute AI, ↑ total SV but ↓ forward SV → ↑ LV end-diastolic volume + ↑↑ LV end-diastolic pressure	Diastolic decrescendo murmur at LSB or sometimes RSB
	If significant LVH, ↓ LV compliance → dependence of adequate LV filling on atrial systole	
	Mitral Stenosis	
RF, congenital, other	Restricted opening of the MV →	Often asymptomatic for 20–25 yr, then gradually ↑ symptoms over 5 yr:
	↑ pressure and volume load on the LA → LA dilation + ↑ LA pressure → ↑ pulmonary vascular pressure → ↑ workload on RV → RVH	Dyspnea Fatigue Chest pain Chronic bronchitis
	↑ HR (e.g., uncontrolled a-fib, pregnancy, exercise, emotional stress, general anesthesia) → ↓ diastolic flow time across tight MV → ↑↑ LA pulmonary pressures → possible pulmonary edema	Orthopnea Hemoptysis Palpitations Systemic emboli
	Adequate LV filling is dependent on atrial systole	S & S of pulmonary HTN S & S of RV failure
	Over time, ↑ pulmonary HTN → possible RV failure + TR (see below) + sometimes PR (see below).	Diastolic rumble, loud S_1 (first heart sound) unless there is severe calcification
	Mitral Regurgitation	
LV dilatation, calcification, RF, infective endocarditis, papillary muscle dysfunction, chordal rupture, MVP	Regurgitation of blood from the LV into the LA during early systole → ↑ volume load on LA + ↓ impedance to LV emptying	If chronic, usually asymptomatic for decades (until LV fails) or for life if mild MR; then S & S of low cardiac output (e.g., chronic weakness, fatigue, lightheadedness, dizziness) and those of MS (see above), although less hemoptysis, systemic emboli, pulmonary HTN, and RV failure
	If acute, small LA cannot handle regurgitant flow → ↑↑ LA pressure → pulmonary HTN + acute pulmonary edema	
	If chronic, ↑ LA absorbs regurgitant flow in most patients → normal or only slightly ↑ LA and pulmonary pressures at rest; if inadequate LA dilatation → ↑ LA and pulmonary pressures	If acute, S & S of LV failure
		Loud, high-pitched pansystolic murmur transmitted to axilla; S_3 (third heart sound) is common
	Mitral Valve Prolapse	
Hereditary, congenital, acquired	Ballooning of the MV leaflets into the LA during systole → possible MR (see above) though usually normal hemodynamics	Frequently asymptomatic
		Otherwise, atypical chest pain, fatigue, palpitations, and/or dyspnea
		Late systolic crescendo murmur, which is often preceded by one or more mid-systolic clicks

Continued

TABLE 4-11: Valvular Heart Disease: Pathophysiology and Clinical Manifestations—Cont'd

Etiology	Abnormality	
	Pathophysiology	**Clinical Manifestations**
	Pulmonary/Pulmonic Stenosis	
Congenital, RF	Restricted opening of the PV →	May be asymptomatic if good RV function, sinus rhythm, and no other lesions.
	↑ pressure load on RV → RVH + dilatation:	
	↓ Compliance → ↑ RV end-diastolic pressure → ↑ RA and systemic venous pressures + dependence of adequate RV filling on atrial systole	Otherwise: Dyspnea, especially on exertion Fatigue, weakness Possible cyanosis S & S of RV failure Growth retardation in children Pulsations in throat Possible angina or syncope on exertion
	Once RV systolic dysfunction develops, then ↓ cardiac output + eventual RV failure	
	If other lesions coexist, there will be additional problems:	
	If ASD or PFO, there may be L → R or R → L shunting	Harsh, diamond-shaped SEM at upper LSB, opening sound, S_4 (fourth heart sound) if severe PS
	If VSD, there is usually L → R shunting*	
	If TR, ↓ forward output from RV	
	Pulmonary/Pulmonic Regurgitation	
Dilation of PA (from pulmonary HTN) endocarditis, RF, congenital, other	Regurgitation of blood from the PA into the RV during diastole → ↑ volume load on RV	Tolerated well for decades unless pulmonary HTN is present
	If coexistent pulmonary HTN, then ↑ RV failure	Otherwise, S & S of pulmonary HTN and/or RV failure
	If infective endocarditis, then septic pulmonary emboli, pulmonary HTN, + severe RV failure	Diamond-shaped diastolic murmur along left parasternal border with ↑ on inspiration, possible ↑ P_2 (pulmonary closure sound)
	Tricuspid Stenosis	
RF, congenital, carcinoid	Restricted opening of the TV → ↑ RA volume and pressure → A-fib → further ↑ RA and systemic venous pressures	Dyspnea
	↓↓ Resting cardiac output with failure to ↑ during exercise	S & S of ↓ cardiac output, c/o prominent pulsations in neck
		Systemic venous congestion (e.g., JVD, ascites, edema)
	If TS + coexisting MS (not uncommon), then ↓ RV flow → ↓ severity of pulmonary HTN	Diamond-shaped diastolic murmur along lower left parasternal border at fourth ICS
	Tricuspid Regurgitation	
Secondary to pulmonary HTN, congenital, RF, other	TR implies, as well as aggravates, severe RV failure	Well tolerated if no pulmonary HTN; otherwise, similar to TS
	Systolic regurgitation into RA → ↑ volume load on RA → RA dilatation + ↑ RA pressure with reflection to venous system → prominent venous c–v wave	Possible S & S of biventricular failure if due to left heart dysfunction
		Holosystolic murmur at LSB with ↑ on inspiration
	If A-fib →↑ RA volume and pressure + RV dilatation →↑ TR	A-fib is common on ECG

↑, Increased; ↑↑, more markedly increased; ↓, decreased; ↓↓, more markedly decreased; →, results in; A-fib, atrial fibrillation; AI, aortic insufficiency; Ao, aortic/aorta; AoV, aortic valve; AS, aortic stenosis; ASD, atrial septal defect; c/o, complaints of; ECG, electrocardiography; HR, heart rate; HTN, hypertension; ICS, intercostal space; JVD, jugular venous distension; LA, left atria/atrial; L → R, left to right; LSB, left sternal border; LV, left ventricle/ventricular; LVH, left ventricular hypertrophy; MV, mitral valve; MVP, mitral valve prolapse; PA, pulmonary artery; PFO, patent foramen ovale; PR, pulmonary regurgitation; PS, pulmonary stenosis; PV, pulmonary valve; RA, right atrium; RF, rheumatic fever; R → L, right to left; RSB, right sternal border; RV, right ventricle/ventricular; RVH, right ventricular hypertrophy; SEM, systolic ejection murmur; SLE, systemic lupus erythematosus; S & S, signs and symptoms; SV, stroke volume; TR, tricuspid regurgitation; TV, tricuspid valve; VSD, ventricular septal defect.
*See Chapter 7.

- Valvular insufficiency (incompetent valve closure) results in backward flow (regurgitation) of blood from the receiving chamber or vessel to the antecedent chamber or vessel. This creates a volume load (normal filling volume plus regurgitant volume) on the chambers or vessels on both sides of the affected valve, leading to dilatation and often hypertrophy.

Specific Treatment

- Pharmacologic therapy is used for mild symptomatology or when surgical correction is impossible.
  - Diuretics
  - Afterload-reducing drugs
  - ACE inhibitors
  - Anticoagulation and antiarrhythmic drugs for atrial fibrillation
  - Treatment for CHF
  - Treatment for pulmonary edema and shock if acute
  - Antiarrhythmic agents, as indicated
  - β-Blockers and aspirin therapy for mitral valve prolapse
- Other
  - Regular monitoring of cardiac function to determine necessity of surgical interventions before irreversible deterioration develops or risk of sudden death becomes significant
  - Lifestyle modifications (e.g., salt restriction; avoidance of caffeine, alcohol, and nicotine)
  - Prophylactic antibiotics to prevent endocarditis
  - Cardioversion for new atrial fibrillation (if patient is anticoagulated)
- Surgical interventions once symptomatic (see pages 64 to 66)
  - Balloon valvuloplasty or valvulotomy/commissurotomy for valvular stenosis
  - Valvuloplasty or annuloplasty for valvular incompetence
  - Valve replacement, Ross procedure
  - Heart transplantation for extremely high-risk individuals

Clinical Implications for Physical Therapy

- The physiological responses to activity should be monitored in all patients with a history of heart murmurs or valvular disease to determine whether the defect will affect tolerance for rehabilitation activities and exercise.
  - HR and BP responses will indicate hemodynamic significance, which may vary with different activities (e.g., BP may drop during upper extremity [UE] exercise but not lower extremity [LE] exercise, indicating increased regurgitation of blood with an incompetent valve).
  - Attention to any symptoms of exercise intolerance is important.
  - Pulse should be monitored, as patients may experience arrhythmias during or after exercise.
  - Exercise is contraindicated in patients with severe aortic stenosis, because they are at high risk for syncope or sudden death during activity.
  - Breath holding and the Valsalva maneuver should be avoided because they reduce venous return and cardiac output, which may contribute to adverse reactions; coordination of breathing with effort should be encouraged.
  - Symptoms of exercise intolerance should be reported to the patient's cardiologist, so the patient can be evaluated for increasing valvular dysfunction that may require immediate treatment.
  - PTs should be familiar with the side effects of any medications the patient is taking, as they may affect exercise responses or tolerance (see Chapter 5).
  - Patients recovering from valve repair or replacement surgery via median sternotomy or thoracotomy incision require consideration of precautions related to the incision and any chest tubes (see pages 32 to 34 and 61 to 62).
  - PTs need to be aware that there are a growing number of persons with congenital heart defects, including valvular and complex defects, who had surgical repairs as children and are now reaching adulthood. Fewer than half of them are thought to be receiving any regular cardiac follow-up now that they have outgrown their pediatric cardiologist and are no longer being covered by their parents' health insurance. Unfortunately, it appears that these childhood treatments are wearing out with age, and these individuals are now at increasing risk for serious problems, including arrhythmias, cardiomegaly, heart failure, and even sudden death on occasion.

CARDIOMYOPATHIES

The cardiomyopathies consist of a diverse group of disorders that originate in the myocardium. Technically they do not include myocardial dysfunction resulting from other cardiovascular disease, such as hypertension, CAD, valvular disease, and congenital defects, although the term *ischemic cardiomyopathy* is commonly used to describe the diffuse dilation and hypocontractility that sometimes results from severe coronary disease with or without documented myocardial infarction. Cardiomyopathies are classified according to the type of abnormal myocardial structure and function: dilated, hypertrophic, and restrictive, as illustrated in Figure 4-19. The features of the three types of cardiomyopathy are compared in Table 4-12. However, there is considerable overlap, as some disorders have characteristics of more than one type of cardiomyopathy (e.g., HCM has some restrictive elements) or change from one category to another during disease progression (e.g., cardiac amyloidosis). The clinical implications for PT are presented later in this chapter.

Dilated Cardiomyopathy

Dilated cardiomyopathy (DCM), the most common type, is characterized by cardiac enlargement, impaired systolic function of one or both ventricles, and often symptoms of congestive heart failure (formerly called congestive CM). DCM accounts for about 25% of cases of CHF in the United States, and more than half of them have no identifiable etiology and thus are called *idiopathic DCM*.

Pathophysiology

Infectious and noninfectious inflammatory processes, toxins (e.g., alcohol and drugs), pregnancy/postpartum, metabolic disorders (e.g., endocrine and nutritional disorders, and altered metabolism), or hereditary diseases (e.g., glycogen storage diseases and muscular dystrophies) may cause DCM with the same pathophysiological features described for LV failure, RV failure, or both (see page 111).

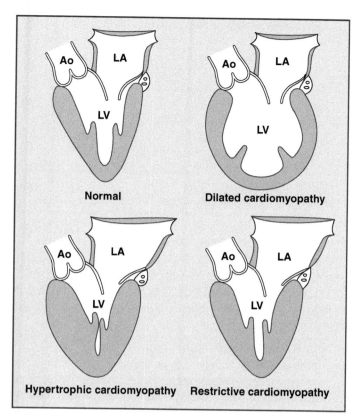

Figure 4-19: A diagram showing three morphologic types of cardiomyopathies. Ao, aorta; LA, left atrial; LV, left ventricular. (From Waller BF. Pathology of the cardiomyopathies. *J Am Soc Echocardiogr.* 1988;1:4.)

Clinical Manifestations

- Dyspnea initially on exertion and then at rest
- Nocturnal dry cough
- Signs and symptoms of LV failure
- Possible signs and symptoms of RV failure
- Chest pain on exertion
- LV impulse displaced lateral to the mid-clavicular line
- S_3–S_4 summation gallop rhythm (see page 44)
- Systolic murmurs of mitral and/or tricuspid regurgitation caused by ventricular dilatation (see Table 4-11)
- Atrial enlargement, decreased QRS, nonspecific ST–T changes on ECG
- Considerable cardiomegaly, possible LA and RA enlargement, and redistribution of blood flow on chest x-ray examination

Specific Treatment

As listed for heart failure on page 111.

Hypertrophic Cardiomyopathy

Hypertrophic cardiomyopathy (HCM) is characterized by a considerable unexplained increase in cardiac mass (hypertrophy), which can be symmetrical or asymmetrical, without cavity dilatation, and normal or hyperdynamic systolic function. In addition, some individuals exhibit subaortic LV outflow obstruction (hypertrophic obstructive cardiomyopathy [HOCM], formerly called idiopathic hypertrophic subaortic stenosis [IHSS]).

Pathophysiology

- LVH results in diastolic dysfunction due to abnormal LV relaxation and distensibility (see Table 4-8), which results in

---

TABLE 4-12: Comparison of the Three Types of Cardiomyopathy

	Dilated	Hypertrophic	Restrictive
Ventricular volume			
End-diastolic	↑	nl	↓–nl
End-systolic	↑↑	↓	nl
Ventricular mass	↑	↑↑↑	nl–↑
Mass-to-volume ratio	↓	↑↑	nl–↑
Systolic function			
Ejection fraction	↓–↓↓	nl–↑–↓	nl
Myocardial shortening	↓–↓↓	↑–↓	nl
Wall stress	↑	↓	↓
Diastolic function			
Chamber stiffness	↓	↑↑	↑↑
Filling pressure	↑↑	nl–↑	↑
Symptoms	CHF, fatigue, weakness	Dyspnea, angina, fatigue, syncope or presyncope	Dyspnea, fatigue, RV failure

↑, Mildly increased; ↑↑, moderately increased; ↑↑↑, markedly increased; ↓, mildly decreased; ↓↓, moderately decreased; CHF, congestive heart failure; nl, normal; RV, right ventricular.

decreased LV compliance and increased LV filling pressures, as illustrated in Figure 4-12.

- Decreased LV compliance increases the dependence of LV filling on atrial systole and so on, as described for diastolic dysfunction on page 99.
- Hyperdynamic LV function produces rapid ejection of blood and increased ejection fraction early in systole.
- Systolic anterior motion (SAM) of the mitral valve apparatus can cause contact with the intraventricular septum and outflow obstruction.
- Myocardial ischemia is common and may result from:
  ‣ Impaired vasodilator reserve
  ‣ Increased oxygen demands, especially if HOCM develops
  ‣ Increased filling pressures with resultant subendocardial ischemia

Clinical Manifestations

The signs and symptoms of HCM vary widely, even on a day-to-day or hour-to-hour basis for the same individual, and are partially dependent on the extent and severity of morphologic abnormalities, rate of progression, and presence and degree of obstruction. Many patients are asymptomatic or only mildly symptomatic, whereas others suffer disabling symptoms at times.

- Dyspnea
- Angina pectoris
- Fatigue and weakness
- Presyncope and syncope
- Palpitations
- On occasion, paroxysmal nocturnal dyspnea and symptoms of CHF
- LV lift; point of maximal impulse displaced laterally, abnormally forceful and enlarged; possible prominent presystolic apical impulse, systolic apical thrill
- Loud S_4 (fourth heart sound); harsh diamond-shaped systolic murmur if HOCM develops, which may radiate to lower sternal border, axillae, and base of heart; possible murmur of mitral regurgitation
- Briskly rising carotid pulse, which may decline in mid-systole as outflow obstruction develops
- ST–T abnormalities and sometimes LVH on ECG; there may also be prominent abnormal Q waves in inferior and/or lateral leads
- Supraventricular tachycardia; ventricular arrhythmias, including tachycardia and fibrillation causing sudden death; occasional atrial fibrillation

Specific Treatment

The majority of symptomatic patients require only medical management, which aims to improve diastolic filling and thus alleviate symptoms, prevent complications, and reduce the risk of sudden death. Invasive interventions are usually reserved for patients with outflow obstruction who remain severely symptomatic despite optimal drug therapy.

- Pharmacologic agents (see Chapter 5)
  ‣ β-Adrenergic blockers
  ‣ Calcium channel blockers
  ‣ Diuretics if fluid retention
  ‣ Antiarrhythmic agents for atrial fibrillation
  ‣ Prophylactic antibiotics

- Surgical interventions (see page 70)
  ‣ Left ventricular septal myotomy–myectomy (LVMM) to relieve obstruction in HOCM
  ‣ Mitral valve replacement to eliminate SAM in HOCM or to relieve severe mitral regurgitation
  ‣ Alcohol septal ablation
  ‣ Laser myoplasty (under investigation)
  ‣ Dual-chamber pacing to alter the pattern of depolarization so that outflow obstruction is prevented
  ‣ Implantable cardioverter/defibrillator for high-risk patients
- Other
  ‣ Avoidance of strenuous exercise because of increased risk of sudden death

Restrictive Cardiomyopathy

Endomyocardial or myocardial disease (infiltrative and noninfiltrative) can lead to restrictive cardiomyopathy (RCM), which is characterized by diastolic dysfunction and associated reduction in ventricular filling caused by excessively rigid ventricular walls.

Pathophysiology

- Decreased compliance results in impaired ventricular filling and elevated end-diastolic pressures (i.e., diastolic dysfunction; see Table 4-8), which are reflected back to the atria (causing atrial enlargement) and then to the lungs or systemic venous system (causing congestion). Restricted ventricular filling reduces cardiac output (see diastolic dysfunction on page 99).
- Distortion of the ventricular cavity and involvement of the papillary muscles and chordae tendineae can cause mitral or tricuspid regurgitation.
- Partial obliteration of the ventricle by fibrous tissue and thrombus results in reduced SV and often compensatory tachycardia.
- Eventually systolic function becomes impaired.
- When the LV is involved, pulmonary HTN is common.

Clinical Manifestations

- Impaired exercise intolerance
- Weakness and fatigue
- Dyspnea
- Increased central venous pressure leading to jugular venous distension, peripheral edema, enlarged liver, ascites
- S_3, S_4, or both (see page 44)
- Possible inspiratory increase in venous pressure (Kussmaul's sign)
- Symptoms of CHF (see page 111)
- Diastolic dip and plateau (square root sign) in ventricular pressure pulse; prominent a wave, often of same amplitude as the v wave
- Conduction disturbances, arrhythmias, and ST–T abnormalities on ECG

Specific Treatment

- Same as for diastolic HF, except as contraindicated in amyloidosis (see Chapter 5)
  ‣ Diuretics
  ‣ Vasodilators, with caution
  ‣ Calcium channel blockers?

- Antiarrhythmic drugs, pacemaker; AICD if at high risk for sudden death
- Antiarrhythmics and anticoagulation for atrial fibrillation
- Possible heart transplantation
- Other specific treatments, depending on etiology
  - Corticosteroids for sarcoidosis, hypereosinophilia
  - Hydroxyurea and interferon-α for hypereosinophilia and endomyocardial fibrosis
  - Immunosuppressive therapy for amyloidosis
  - Repeated phlebotomy for hemochromatosis

Clinical Implications for Physical Therapy

- Refer to clinical implications listed for HF on page 112.
- The physiological responses to activity should be monitored in all patients with CM to determine whether there are adverse effects on tolerance for rehabilitation activities and exercise.
  - HR and BP responses will indicate hemodynamic significance, which may vary with different activities and different treatment session in HCM.
  - Attention to any symptoms of exercise intolerance is important.
  - Pulse should be monitored for regularity, as patients may experience arrhythmias during or after exercise, which sometimes provoke decompensation and other adverse reactions.
  - ECG monitoring may be indicated for patients with arrhythmias or HCM.
  - Patients with HCM have an increased risk of syncope or sudden death; close monitoring is recommended.
- Treatment modifications may be indicated:
  - Activity/exercise intensity may need to be moderated to avoid adverse reactions; frequent 1- to 2-minute rests during activity will reduce intensity.
  - Be cautious if a patient is taking drugs that cause hypotension or orthostatic intolerance; avoid sudden changes to upright postures.
  - Instruction in energy conservation techniques may be helpful.
- Breath holding and the Valsalva maneuver should be avoided because they reduce venous return and cardiac output, which may contribute to adverse reactions; coordination of breathing with effort should be encouraged.
- PTs should be familiar with the side effects of any medications the patient is taking, as they may affect exercise responses or tolerance (see Chapter 5).

VASCULAR DISEASES

The arteries and veins can be affected by a number of diseases as a result of infection or inflammation, trauma, or involvement by other systemic diseases. Moreover, arterial disease caused by atherosclerosis frequently involves the peripheral and cerebral vessels.

Occlusive Peripheral Arterial Disease

Atherosclerosis of the peripheral arteries, which creates occlusive plaques and obstruction of the medium to large peripheral arteries, particularly in the lower extremities, affects approximately 12% to 20% of adults over the age of 70 years. It is particularly common in smokers and those with diabetes and the metabolic syndrome.[19] Progressive occlusion results in diminished blood supply to the affected extremities, inducing ischemia. Disruption of proximal plaques can result in distal thrombosis.

Occlusion can also be caused by acute embolization of a blood clot located in the left ventricle, vasculitis induced by autoimmune diseases (e.g., polyarteritis nodosa; Takayasu's arteritis; giant cell, or temporal, arteritis; or thromboangiitis obliterans, also called Buerger's disease), or vasospastic disease, such as Raynaud's phenomenon.

Aneurysms typically form when arterial degeneration due to aging is superimposed on atherosclerotic vessels, resulting in localized dilatation, as described in section on aortic aneurysm (see page 122).

Clinical Manifestations

The clinical manifestations of peripheral arterial disease (PAD) are related to the severity of obstruction (symptoms rarely occur until there is 70% occlusion) and the resultant reduction in blood flow to the skeletal muscles and skin.

- Intermittent claudication is the classic symptom of lower extremity disease, which is typically described as a painful, aching, cramping, or tired feeling in the muscles of the leg(s), as illustrated in Figure 4-20. It occurs regularly and predictably during ambulation and is relieved promptly by rest.
- Chronic severe disease is associated with hair loss, muscle atrophy, cool feet, and skin and nail changes; pallor occurs on elevation.
- Critical stenosis is evidenced by resting or nocturnal pain and skin ulcers or gangrene.

Specific Treatment

- Lifestyle modifications and secondary prevention
  - Aggressive risk factor reduction, especially smoking cessation and control of hyperglycemia
  - Exercise training, which is as effective as surgery in treating PAD[19,170a,212]
- Pharmacologic agents
  - Antihypertensive therapy, regardless of baseline BP
  - Lipid-lowering treatment with statins, even if cholesterol level is normal
  - Antithrombotic therapy
  - Cilostazol for symptom relief
  - Prostaglandins to relieve pain and promote healing of ulcers
- Revascularization procedures
  - Catheter-based (percutaneous transluminal angioplasty, with or without stent placement; thromboembolectomy; and endovascular brachytherapy)
  - Surgical (endarterectomy, bypass grafting)[216a]

Clinical Implications for Physical Therapy

Because the same disease process is involved, the vast majority of patients with PAD also have CAD and possibly cerebrovascular disease, although they are often not diagnosed.[94] Therefore, the recommendations listed on page 107 apply to these patients as well. In addition, there are some other concerns specific to these individuals:

- Individuals who have an increased risk of PAD should be examined for the status of their peripheral pulses and the possibility of an abdominal aortic aneurysm, as described on page 253.

RELATIONSHIP BETWEEN LOCATION OF ARTERIAL OBSTRUCTIONS AND SYMPTOMS IN PAOD

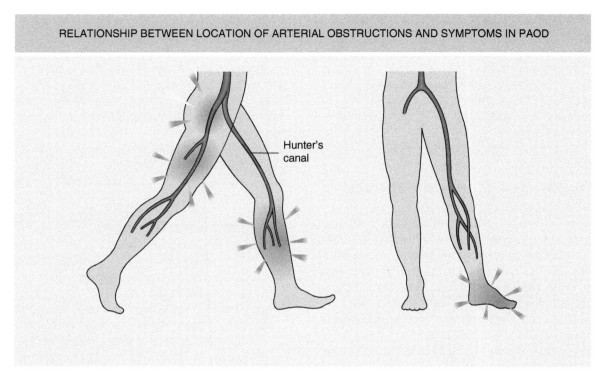

Hunter's canal

Figure 4-20: Relationship between location of arterial obstructions and symptoms in peripheral arterial disease (PAD). Obstructions in the iliac artery give rise to pain in the buttock and thigh, femoral lesions provoke pain in the calf muscles, and lower leg arterial obstructions most often induce rest pain and skin necrosis. (From Crawford MH, DiMarco JP, Paulus WJ, editors *Cardiology.* 2nd ed. St. Louis: Mosby; 2004.)

- Clinical monitoring of vital signs and rate–pressure product during exercise is important for patients with PAD because of the likelihood of concomitant CAD, HTN, and DM, as well as COPD due to smoking; these patients are therefore predisposed to abnormal physiological responses to exercise. They often exhibit a precipitous rise in BP during exercise because of atherosclerosis and a diminished vascular bed.
- Patients with intermittent claudication have moderate to severe impairment in walking ability, which is significantly improved with exercise training because of its beneficial effects on endothelial vasodilator function, skeletal muscle structure and function, blood viscosity, and inflammatory response.[212] Because exercise training has been shown to be as effective as surgical interventions in reducing symptoms and improving walking distances, it is recommended as the best practice treatment of PAD.[19,109,170a,212]
- A subjective scale for expressing the discomfort of claudication can be useful (see page 283). It is generally recommended that patients exercise at an intensity that elicits claudication symptoms but avoids pain above grade 2 to 3 (more stressful exercise elicits anaerobic metabolism, which exacerbates the claudication pain); however, one meta-analysis revealed that the greatest improvement in walking distance occurred with training to near-maximal pain.[88]
- The time and/or distance walked to onset of pain and to grades 2 and 3 claudication pain can be used as criteria for assessing the functional severity of disease, as well as for documenting improvement in status.

- Exercise training in the form of interval training with short rest periods as needed for relief of moderate claudication is most effective. The goal is to work up to 30 to 50 minutes of intermittent or continuous walking at a normal speed of 3.0 mph, performed at least 3 to 5 days/wk (see page 303 for information related to exercise prescription). *Note:* Public health recommendations for physical activity state that a frequency of at least 5 days/wk is advisable (see page 302).[166]
- Lower exercise intensities are often suggested because they maximize the potential duration of the training sessions.
- Patients should be instructed in proper foot care, including good footwear, careful hygiene, and daily inspection.

Aortic Aneurysm

As stated previously, *aneurysms* typically form when arterial degeneration due to aging is superimposed on atherosclerotic vessels, resulting in localized dilatation. With increasing shear stress (as caused by HTN or obstructive lesions), destruction of the media and elastic tissue, and weakness of the arterial wall lead to the formation of aneurysms, which occur most commonly in the abdominal aorta (abdominal aortic aneurysm, AAA) below the level of the renal arteries. They can also develop in the thoracic or thoracoabdominal aorta and in the iliac, femoral, popliteal, and cerebral arteries. In addition, aneurysms can result from trauma, infection, inflammation, cystic medial necrosis, or congenital vascular disease.

- When a tear takes place in the arterial intima, allowing blood to flow in a channel between the medial layers of the vessel, *dissection* has occurred (e.g., dissecting aortic aneurysm) and rupture is likely.

- Aneurysms of the ascending aorta, which happen most often in Marfan's syndrome, may involve the aortic root, producing aortic regurgitation, as well as the sinuses of Valsalva and the proximal coronary arteries.

Clinical Manifestations

Most individuals with aortic aneurysms are asymptomatic and the defect is detected on routine physical examination or on rupture. When symptoms are present, they vary with the level of the defect.

- Abdominal aortic aneurysms, which occur two to five times more often in men than in women, may be manifested as a pulsatile mass and sometimes abdominal discomfort or back pain. Expansion of the aneurysm can cause compression of neighboring structures with increasing pain and radiation to the groin, buttocks, or legs. Aneurysm dissection or impending rupture usually provokes sudden, excruciating pain and distress, with hypotension, tachycardia, pallor, diaphoresis, or shock.
- Thoracic aortic aneurysms, which can occur in the ascending or descending aorta, occasionally produce symptoms, which vary with the size and location of the defect.
  - ▸ Symptoms of CHF may develop in ascending aortic aneurysm due to aortic valve regurgitation or rupture of an aneurysm of the sinuses of Valsalva directly into the RV cavity, RA, or PA.
  - ▸ Involvement of the sinuses of Valsalva with direct compression or thromboembolism of the coronary arteries can lead to myocardial ischemia or infarction.
  - ▸ Chest pain can be induced by compression of surrounding structures, erosion into adjacent ribs, sternum, or vertebrae, or aneurysm dissection or rupture.
  - ▸ An aortic aneurysm can produce dyspnea or cough due to compression of the trachea or mainstem bronchi, dysphagia by compression of the esophagus, or hoarseness due to left vocal cord paralysis.
  - ▸ Compression of blood vessels can lead to superior vena cava syndrome (with head and neck fullness, headache with signs involving the neck and face, prominent superficial veins across the chest, and sometimes upper extremity swelling), or pulmonary artery stenosis.
- Thoracoabdominal aortic aneurysms sometimes cause epigastric or left upper quadrant discomfort, back or flank pain when the individual lies in the left lateral decubitus position, radiculopathy due to erosion of the vertebral bodies, and peripheral atheroembolism. Rupture of the thoracic portion of the aneurysm usually occurs into the left pleural space, producing hemothorax and chest pain, whereas rupture of the abdominal portion leads to severe abdominal or back pain.

Specific Treatment

- Risk factor reduction to minimize risk of progressive atherosclerotic vascular damage
- Regular surveillance by ultrasonography or computed tomography (CT) scanning every 6 months for asymptomatic aneurysms: 4.0 to 5.5 cm in diameter for men and probably smaller size for women (aneurysm rupture occurs at smaller diameters in women)

- Surgical repair consisting of synthetic aortic graft, which often must be extended down to include one or both iliac arteries versus percutaneously implanted, expanding endovascular stent-grafts for aneurysms 5.5 cm or more in diameter or rapidly expanding aneurysms (≥ 0.5 cm/yr) for men and probably smaller diameter for women, although no specific guidelines exist
- More frequent monitoring of patients with Marfan's syndrome because the aneurysms of these patients are at higher risk of dissection and rupture; surgical repair when the aneurysms reach 5 cm in diameter

Clinical Implications for Physical Therapy

- Careful screening is indicated for individuals with significant cardiovascular risk factors and complaints of neck, back, or abdominal pain that may radiate (see Clinical Manifestations).
- Referral to a physician for further evaluation is indicated for individuals with questionable findings.
- Because most patients with known abdominal and thoracoabdominal aortic aneurysms have diffuse atherosclerosis, they should be assumed to have coronary artery disease and monitored accordingly during PT evaluation and treatment.
- Interventions aimed at reducing cardiovascular risk factors should be incorporated in the PT treatment plan whenever possible and encouragement and support should be offered for other interventions, such as treatment for HTN and smoking cessation.
- Patients who are recovering from surgical repair of an aortic aneurysm should receive instructions and interventions directed at reducing their high risk of postoperative pulmonary complications (see pages 314 to 317 and 323 to 324).

Cerebrovascular Disease

Most vascular diseases affect both the heart and the brain; the most common is atherosclerosis, which can cause ischemia, occlusion, or hemorrhage. The cerebral arteries can also be affected by emboli that originate in the heart or as complications of cardiac diagnostic or surgical procedures or by hypoperfusion resulting from cardiopulmonary arrest and resuscitation.

Cerebral Ischemia

In patients with occlusive cerebrovascular lesions, ischemia can be induced by embolism or hypoperfusion. In slowly forming disease, collateral circulation develops and helps to maintain cerebral blood flow, forestalling damage.

- Patients are usually asymptomatic for a prolonged time.
- Some patients experience headache and transient ischemic attacks (TIA), or "mini" strokes. Symptoms of a TIA are similar to those of a stroke but resolve within minutes to a few hours, always within 24 hours.
- Approximately 30% of Americans who have a TIA go on to have an ischemic stroke if they are not treated, and 10% will have a stroke within 90 days, even with standard treatment.[231] Up to one quarter of individuals die within 1 year of a TIA.[11]

Cerebrovascular Accident

Approximately 80% to 87% of all cerebrovascular accidents (CVAs), strokes, or "brain attacks" are ischemic in origin (i.e., due to local thrombosis, embolism, or hypotension).[11,231] Other CVAs occur as a result of intracerebral hemorrhage, arterial dissection, subarachnoid hemorrhage, and other causes. The end result is an interruption in blood flow and delivery of oxygen and glucose to the brain, leading to irreversible brain damage. Approximately 20% to 25% of patients die within 1 year of their stroke, 50% die within 5 years, and 15% to 30% suffer another stroke; 15% to 30% of survivors are permanently disabled.[11]

Risk factors for stroke include age greater than 60 years, diabetes mellitus, atrial fibrillation, HTN, and cigarette smoking (especially >2 packs per day).

Specific Treatment

- Pharmacologic
  - ▸ Antiplatelet drugs (aspirin, clopidogrel, and dipyridamole)
  - ▸ Glycoprotein IIb/IIIa inhibitors for acute CVA
- Thrombolysis for acute CVA in highly selected patients
- Risk factor reduction (e.g., HTN, cholesterol, and hyperglycemia/DM)
- Lifestyle modification (e.g., smoking cessation, diet modification, weight reduction, and exercise)
- Surgical prevention of repeat CVA (e.g., carotid endarterectomy)[216a]
- Stroke rehabilitation
- Other specific treatments (e.g., surgical evacuation or removal of hematomas, clipping of aneurysm)

Clinical Implications for Physical Therapy

- In the acute care setting, PT should be initiated only after the patient's cardiovascular status has stabilized.
- Because most strokes occur in the elderly, patients are likely to be affected by a number of comorbidities, including arthritic, orthopedic, and cardiovascular problems, which may require appropriate treatment plan modifications.
- Because the same disease process is involved, it should be assumed that the vast majority of patients with cerebrovascular disease have CAD, although most will not be diagnosed.[45,108] Therefore, the clinical implications listed on page 107 apply to these patients as they participate in rehabilitation activities.
- Months to years after their stroke, patients with hemiparetic stroke have a low level of ambulatory activity, which is related to the severity of their mobility deficits, especially balance, and very low cardiovascular fitness levels, even those who are level I/II according to the American Heart Association Stroke Outcome Classification (AHA.SOC).[11,131a,163,177] These factors increase the risk of further deconditioning and decline in functional level, as well as subsequent cardiovascular events or stroke, and should be addressed during and after rehabilitation efforts.

Thrombophlebitis and Deep Venous Thrombosis

Thrombosis of a vein usually results in inflammation of the vessel wall (i.e., thrombophlebitis), leading to infiltration of the thrombus with fibroblasts and eventual scarring of the vein wall and destruction of the valves. About half of patients with DVT are asymptomatic or have nonspecific signs and symptoms, yet have an increased risk of morbidity and mortality. The important risk factors for DVT are listed in Table 4-13.

DVT leads to serious complications in many patients, including nonfatal venous thromboembolism (VTE), fatal pulmonary emboli

TABLE 4-13: Important Risk Factors for Deep Venous Thrombosis

Risk Factor	Causes
Immobility, venous stasis	Prolonged bedrest (>3 d) or sitting (e.g., air travel)
	Neurologic disorders (e.g., spinal cord injury and stroke)
	Limb immobilization or paresis
Trauma, venous damage	Varicose veins
	Fracture of hip, pelvis, or leg
	Major surgery, total hip or knee replacement, and arthroscopic knee surgery
	Local trauma
	Intravenous injections and central venous lines
	Certain medications and chemotherapeutic agents
Hypercoagulability	Thrombophilic disorders (e.g., antiphospholipid syndrome; myeloproliferative disorders; elevated levels of coagulation factors VIII, IX, and XI; deficiencies of antithrombin III, protein S, or protein C; resistance to activated protein C; prothrombin gene mutation; and hyperhomocysteinemia)
	Malignancy (e.g., lung, pancreas, liver, gastric, colon, genitorurinary, and brain)
Other	Previous history of DVT
	Age >60 yr
	Obesity
	Acute medical disorders (e.g., myocardial infarction, acute heart or respiratory failure, and acute infections)
	Oral contraceptives, hormone replacement therapy, pregnancy, and puerperium

DVT, Deep venous thrombosis.

(PE), postthrombotic syndrome (PTS), and occasionally nonhemorrhagic stroke (in the presence of patent foramen ovale, which exists in 25% to 30% of individuals).[37] Most patients with symptomatic proximal DVT have evidence of PE, even though the vast majority do not exhibit any symptoms.[148,178] Approximately 20% to 50% of patients with DVT later experience PTS, which is characterized by leg pain, edema, venous distension, skin induration, and ulceration that usually develops within 2 years of the acute thrombotic episode.[126]

DVT typically originates in the calf, and when confined there, poses low risk for serious PE. However, approximately 10% to 20% of these DVTs extend into the more proximal veins, creating a 50% risk of PE with a 10% mortality rate.[148] Likewise, DVT occurring in the popliteal, femoral, and iliac veins, and the inferior vena cava, presents a higher risk of life-threatening complications. On occasion, VTE develops in the axillary and subclavian system, usually as a result of central venous catheter placement for chemotherapy, bone marrow transplantation, dialysis, or parenteral nutrition. Thrombosis of the superficial veins also occurs, most commonly in varicose veins, but rarely causes serious complications.

Clinical Manifestations

- Patients with DVT are often asymptomatic or have nonspecific signs and symptoms, so pulmonary embolism may be the initial manifestation.
- When present in the legs, symptoms may include dull ache, tightness, or pain in the calf, tenderness to palpation, swelling, and/or palpable cord and are usually associated with proximal vein thrombosis; DVT of the arms may produce pain, swelling, and cyanosis of the involved limb.
- Discoloration, venous distension, and/or prominence of the superficial veins sometimes occur; cyanosis may be present if the obstruction is severe.

Note: A positive Homans' sign (discomfort in upper calf during gentle, forced dorsiflexion of foot while knee is extended) is an extremely unreliable finding, as it is present in less than 30% of cases of documented DVT, and more than half of those with the sign do not exhibit any evidence of DVT (positive findings also occur with calf muscle strain or contusion, Achilles tendinitis, and superficial thrombophlebitis).

Specific Treatment

- Primary prevention
  - ▶ Early ambulation whenever possible
  - ▶ Intermittent pneumatic compression
  - ▶ Graduated compression stockings
  - ▶ Anticoagulant drugs for those with moderate to high risk for DVT (e.g., low molecular weight heparin [LMWH], oral anticoagulants, and antithrombin agents)
- Treatment of DVT
  - ▶ Anticoagulation (e.g., heparin, LMWH, and warfarin)
  - ▶ Thrombolytic therapy
  - ▶ Thrombectomy
  - ▶ Vena cava filter placement

Clinical Implications for Physical Therapy

- Prevention of DVT or embolization of an existing thrombus is extremely important and can be facilitated by:
  - ▶ Active and passive range of motion exercises
  - ▶ Frequent early ambulation
  - ▶ Deep breathing and coughing exercises
  - ▶ Instruction in proper positioning for moderate- to high-risk patients with avoidance of pillows under legs postoperatively or prolonged maintenance of any position, especially sitting in chair; elevation of the feet to promote venous return and prevent venous stasis
  - ▶ Encouraging the patient with a DVT to continue wearing elastic support stockings for at least 6 to 8 weeks
- Because research has shown that individual clinical features are of limited value in diagnosing DVT[23a,95] and that physical therapists grossly underestimate the probability of DVT,[196] a risk assessment scale, such as the Autar DVT Scale[14] (Figure 4-21) or Wells' Simplified Clinical Model for Assessment of DVT[233] (Table 4-14), should be used routinely by PTs to assess clinical probability of DVT.

TABLE 4-14: Simplified Clinical Model for Assessment of DVT

Clinical Variable	Score*
Active cancer (treatment ongoing or within previous 6 mo or palliative care)	1
Paralysis, paresis, or recent plaster immobilization of LE	1
Recently bedridden for 3 days or more, or major surgery within past 12 wk requiring general or regional anesthesia	1
Localized tenderness along the distribution of the deep venous system[†]	1
Entire LE swelling	1
Calf swelling at least 3 cm larger than the asymptomatic LE[‡]	1
Pitting edema confined to the symptomatic LE	1
Collateral superficial veins (non-varicose)	1
Previously documented DVT	1
Alternative diagnosis at least as likely as DVT[§]	−2
Total score	

DVT, Deep venous thrombosis; LE, lower extremity.
*Score interpretation: >2, high probability with incidence of 53% (95% confidence interval [CI] f= 44–61%); 1 or 2, probability of DVT is moderate with incidence of 17% (95% CI = 13–23%); and ≤1, probability of DVT is low with incidence of 5% (95% CI = 4.0–8.0%) Data based on reference #233.
[†]Tenderness along the deep venous system is assessed by firm palpation in the center of the posterior calf, the popliteal space, and along the area of the femoral vein in the anterior thigh and groin.
[‡]Measured 10 cm below the tibial tuberosity.
[§]Most common alternative diagnoses are cellulitis, calf strain, and postoperative swelling.

- Any suspicion of DVT, or moderate to high risk using one of the aforementioned scales, should be reported to the referring physician because of the increased risk for morbidity and mortality.
- Once anticoagulation has been instituted, early ambulation, usually with firm compression garments or wraps, appears to be safe for patients with DVT who have adequate cardiopulmonary reserve and no evidence of PE and may lead to more rapid resolution of pain and swelling.[5,178] Some clinicians state that patients with DVT should be placed on bedrest for 48 to 72 hours after beginning medical treatment,[132] whereas others have documented lower risk of thrombus propagation when ambulation begins within 24 hours of treatment initiation.[178] Until this issue is addressed through a large prospective cohort study, it is left to the clinical judgment of the treating physician and PT.
- To counteract the development of PTS, it is recommended that patients wear elastic support stockings with compressive pressure of 30 to 40 mm Hg for 1 to 2 years after the first DVT.[151]

Chronic Venous Stasis/Incompetence

Chronic venous stasis, or incompetence, may develop after DVT or other problems that cause valvular damage, persistent occlusion of

Name: Unit No: Ward:	Age: Type of admission: Diagnosis:
AGE SPECIFIC GROUP (years) score 10-30 0 31-40 1 41-50 2 51-60 3 61-70 4 71+ 5	**BUILD / BODY MASS INDEX (BMI)** Wt (kg/ Ht (m)^2 Build BMI score Underweight 16-18 0 Average/ Desirable 20-25 1 Overweight 26-30 2 Obese 31-40 3 Very obese (morbid) 41+ 4
MOBILITY score Ambulant 0 Limited (used aids, self) 1 Very limited (needs help) 2 Chairbound 3 Complete bedrest 4	**SPECIAL RISK CATEGORY** score Oral Contraceptives: 20-35 years 1 35+ years 2 Hormone replacement therapy 2 Pregnancy/ puerperium 3 Thrombophilia 4
TRAUMA RISK CATEGORY Score item(s) *only preoperatively*. score Head injury 1 Chest injury 1 Spinal injury 2 Pelvic injury 3 Lower limb injury 4	**SURGICAL INTERVENTION:** Score only one appropriate surgical intervention. score Minor surgery <30 mins 1 Planned major surgery 2 Emergency major surgery 3 Thoracic 3 Gynaecological 3 Abdominal 3 Urological 3 Neurosurgical 3 Orthopaedic (below waist) 4
CURRENT HIGH RISK DISEASES: Score the appropriate item(s) score Ulcerative colitis 1 Polycythaemia 2 Varicose veins 3 Chronic heart disease 3 Acute myocardial infarction 4 Malignancy (active cancer) 5 Cerebrovascular accident 6 Previous DVT 7	**ASSESSMENT INSTRUCTION** Complete within 24 hours of admission. Scoring: Ring out the appropriate item(s) from each box, add score, and record total below: Total score: Assessor: Date:
ASSESSMENT PROTOCOL Score range Risk categories ≤10 Low risk 11-14 Moderate risk 15≥ High risk Please record any other clinical observations that may supplement this DVT risk assessment.	**VENOUS THROMBOPROPHYLAXIS** Low risk: Ambulation + Graduated Compression Stockings. Moderate risk: Graduated Compression stockings + Heparin + Intermittent Pneumatic Compression Stockings. High risk: Graduated Compression Stockings + Heparin + Intermittent Pneumatic Compresssion. International Consensus Group recommendation, 2001. ® R Autar 2002

Figure 4-21: The Autar deep venous thrombosis (DVT) scale is composed of seven distinct categories of risk factors designed to assess the risk of a patient developing DVT. [From Autar R. Advancing Clinical Practice in the Management of Deep Vein Thrombosis (DVT). The Autar Scale Revalidated. PhD thesis. Leicester, UK: De Montfort University; 2002.]

the veins, or both. The main symptoms are chronic leg edema, stasis skin changes (reddish brown pigmentation, scaly appearance, and itchiness), and skin ulceration. Sometimes patients complain of a sensation of fullness, aching, or tiredness on standing and walking, which is relieved by rest and elevation.

Varicose Veins

Varicose veins are elongated, dilated, tortuous superficial veins that are caused by incompetent valves in saphenous veins. They can result from any condition that is associated with increased intraabdominal pressure (e.g., pregnancy and ascites) or interference with venous drainage from the lower extremities (e.g., intraabdominal tumors and pelvic vein thrombosis). Varicose veins are often asymptomatic, although many individuals are troubled by local discomfort, especially after prolonged standing. Thrombophlebitis with edema and chronic venous stasis is a possible complication.

OTHER CARDIOVASCULAR DISORDERS

Cardiovascular disease sometimes results from infection or inflammation involving the cardiac structures or blood vessels, trauma, drug toxicity, or involvement by other systemic diseases. Cardiomyopathy may result from these disorders and has already been discussed.

Myocarditis

Inflammation of the myocardium usually results from infectious organisms, most often viral (particularly coxsackievirus B), but can also be caused by hypersensitivity reactions (predominantly due to drugs), toxic agents (e.g., alcohol, cocaine, and chemotherapeutic agents), chest irradiation, and some systemic diseases. Myocardial injury occurs through direct invasion, production of toxin, and induction of nonspecific or specific inflammatory responses. It can be an acute or chronic process, may involve a limited area of myocardium or may be diffuse, and is often accompanied by pericarditis (see the next section).

- The clinical manifestations of myocarditis are quite variable, ranging from asymptomatic (majority of patients) to fulminant CHF; most symptomatic patients have nonspecific complaints, including fever, fatigue, dyspnea, palpitations, and chest discomfort.
- Patient management includes supportive care, pharmacologic agents (diuretics, ACE inhibitors, β-blockers, and aldosterone antagonists) as indicated for specific pathophysiological findings, immunosuppressive therapy for certain subgroups of patients, and limited physical activity with avoidance of strenuous activity for at least 6 months.
- Most patients recover completely, although some develop a chronic dilated cardiomyopathy, as described on page 118, and a small number die.

Pericarditis

Inflammation of the pericardium can be precipitated by a wide variety of diseases, but the majority of cases are idiopathic and presumed to be viral in etiology. Known causes include other infectious organisms, acute myocardial infarction, pericardiotomy associated with cardiac surgery, malignancy, trauma, autoimmune disorders (e.g., rheumatoid arthritis and systemic lupus erythematosus), other inflammatory disorders (e.g., sarcoidosis, amyloidosis, and inflammatory bowel disease), renal failure, drug toxicity, and chest irradiation.

- Clinically, acute pericarditis is demonstrated by a range of signs and symptoms as it progresses from a simple inflammatory response with no cardiovascular compromise to cardiac tamponade (very low cardiac output induced by fluid filling the pericardial sac, causing cardiac compression and interference with diastolic ventricular filling) and constrictive pericarditis (fibrotic, thickened, and adherent pericardium that restricts diastolic filling). Typically, there is chest pain, dyspnea, a pericardial friction rub, and serial ECG abnormalities. Pericardial effusion (fluid within the pericardial sac) may be present and is often asymptomatic.

- Treatment of acute pericarditis consists of NSAIDs for symptom management, which is successful in most cases. For those who require further treatment, narcotic analgesics, corticosteroids, or both, can be used. Less than 5% of patients develop complications requiring additional interventions: Pericardiocentesis or pericardial drainage may be indicated for significant pericardial effusion and tamponade, or occasionally for diagnostic purposes; and surgical stripping of the pericardium (i.e., pericardiectomy) may be required for constrictive pericarditis (see below).

- Some patients with acute, apparently idiopathic pericarditis develop unexplained recurrent or relapsing acute pericarditis after successful treatment and resolution of their first episode. Again, NSAIDs are usually effective. Sometimes colchicine is added for acute management and to prevent other recurrences.

- Constrictive pericarditis, or pericardial scarring with dense fibrosis, often calcification, and adhesions of the parietal and visceral pericardium, can develop years after a bout of acute pericarditis. Abrupt cessation of ventricular filling during early to mid-diastole creates a clinical presentation similar to that of right-sided heart failure (see page 111).

Infective Endocarditis

Bacterial or other microbial infection of the endothelial surface of the heart, particularly the valves, results in the formation of vegetations along the valve cusps (with interference in proper opening and closing), septal defects, chordae tendineae, or mural endocardium. Predisposing conditions that increase the risk of developing infective endocarditis (IE) include structural cardiac abnormalities (e.g., mitral valve prolapse, congenital defects, rheumatic heart disease, and valvular degeneration) and intravenous (IV) drug abuse.

- The clinical manifestations of IE are highly variable and depend on the involvement of other organ systems, due to embolization of valvular vegetation fragments, bacterial seeding of distant foci, or the development of immune complex–associated disease. In general, there are symptoms suggestive of a "flulike illness" and sometimes the clinical manifestations of specific valvular lesions, or CHF.

- Intracardiac infection can result in perforation of valve leaflets; rupture of the chordae tendinae, intraventricular septum, or papillary muscle; valve ring abscesses; occlusion of a valve orifice; coronary emboli; burrowing abscesses of the myocardium; and purulent pericardial effusions.

- Treatment is directed against eradicating the specific infecting microorganism. Surgical intervention (e.g., valve replacement or resection) is indicated for refractory heart failure, valvular obstruction, recurrent or fungal IE, ineffective antimicrobial therapy, serious embolic complications, or an unstable prosthetic valve.

- Antibiotic prophylaxis has traditionally been advised for all patients with congenital or acquired valvular dysfunction, prosthetic heart valves, obstructive hypertrophic cardiomyopathy, a number of other congenital cardiac defects or shunt repairs, and for patients with previous endocarditis in order to prevent the development of infective endocarditis. However, more recent guidelines from the American Heart Association have concluded that only an extremely small number of cases of IE might be prevented by antibiotic prophylaxis and therefore its use is reasonable only for patients with underlying cardiac conditions associated with the highest risk of adverse outcome from IE (see Box 8-2, page 362). Good dental hygiene continues to play a critical role in preventing IE in all patients.

Rheumatic Fever

Acute rheumatic fever (ARF) most commonly affects children 5 to 15 years of age and therefore is discussed in Chapter 8 on page 374. Chronic rheumatic heart disease (RHD) may develop in some patients, particularly those with more severe carditis, and usually results in mitral and/or aortic valve disease. There appear to be two different clinical groups: one that shows evidence of significant valvular disease with a higher percentage of death within the first 5 years after ARF, and one that has relatively mild valve disease initially but develops slowly progressive dysfunction due to gradual wear and tear on the valve caused by turbulent flow through its defective structures. The pathophysiological effects and clinical manifestations of RHD are presented under the specific valvular defect(s), as described on pages 115 to 117.

4.3 CARDIOPULMONARY COMPLICATIONS OF OTHER DISEASES AND DISORDERS

Cardiac and pulmonary dysfunction can develop in association with other systemic diseases and various other disorders, producing disorders of the pericardium (e.g., pericarditis and pericardial effusion), myocardium (e.g., cardiomyopathy and myocarditis), endocardium/valves (e.g., valvular inflammation or dysfunction), coronary arteries (e.g., atherosclerosis, coronary ischemia and vasculitis), and electrocardiographic abnormalities (e.g., arrhythmias, conduction disturbances, and ST–T changes). Common pulmonary manifestations include pleural effusion, infection, pneumonitis, vasculitis, and respiratory muscle dysfunction. A brief description of the cardiovascular and pulmonary complications associated with a number of medical diagnoses is presented in this section, along with more detailed discussions of obesity and diabetes, as they are reaching epidemic proportions.

OBESITY AND OVERWEIGHT

Obesity is defined as an excessive accumulation of adipose tissue so that the BMI reaches 30 kg/m^2 or more. Individuals with a BMI of 25 to 29.9 kg/m^2 are considered overweight, although some may not be overfat if their excess weight is due to increased muscle mass. Because abdominal obesity (also called central or truncal obesity, which includes visceral adiposity) is highly related to cardiovascular risk, waist circumference greater than 40 in.

(102 cm) for men and greater than 35 in. (88 cm) for women and a waist-to-hip ratio exceeding 1.0 for men or 0.8 for women (although precise values vary with age) have become popular clinical indicators for risk related to being overweight or obese.

- In the United States, obesity prevalence has doubled in adults and overweight prevalence has tripled in children and adolescents between 1980 and 2002. As of 2003–2004, 70.8% of adult males and 61.8% of adult females are overweight or obese; a greater percentage of women are obese than men (32.2% vs. 31.1%).[173] As for children and adolescents, 17.1% are overweight or obese whereas another 16.5% are at risk of becoming overweight (BMI, ≥85th to <95th percentile for age and sex).

- The severity of obesity can be classified according to BMI, and disease risk is related to BMI, waist circumference, and waist-to-hip ratio such that morbidity and mortality rates rise in proportion to degree of obesity (see Chapter 6, page 285).

- Although there are neither universally accepted norms for body composition nor a consensus regarding the percentage of body fat that is associated with optimal health status, the lowest statistical health risk is associated with a BMI of 19 to 25 and body fat percentages of 12% to 20% for males and 20% to 30% for females.[1,85,165a]

- The causes of obesity are multifactorial and include excessive caloric intake (high-fat, energy-dense foods; larger portions), reduced physical activity (including daily living, work, and leisure activities), genetic/constitutional susceptibility (actual or functional leptin deficiency, dysregulation of appetite neuropeptide synthesis, polygenic susceptibility traits, intrauterine or perinatal environmental influences, etc.), and environmental factors (alterations in food supply and variety, portion sizes, social and cultural influences, etc.). There are also some secondary causes for obesity, such as medications that cause weight gain, underlying diseases (particularly endocrinopathies such as Cushing's syndrome, insulinoma, and hypothyroidism), and psychological consequence of sexual, physical, and emotional abuse, especially if experienced during childhood or adolescence.

- Adipose tissue is an active endocrine organ that secretes a large number of cytokines and bioactive mediators, such as leptin, adiponectin, interleukin-6 (IL-6), tumor necrosis factor-α, and restin, which influence not only body weight but also insulin resistance, diabetes, lipid levels, inflammation, coagulation, fibrinolysis, and atherosclerosis.[222]

- Obesity is associated with a number of complications:
  ▸ Cardiovascular disease (HTN, CAD, and CHF; see below)
  ▸ Osteoarthritis (due to premature degenerative joint disease caused by the mechanics of moving excess weight)
  ▸ Gastrointestinal disorders (gastroesophageal reflux disease, gallstones, fatty liver, and nonalcoholic steatohepatitis, which can progress to cirrhosis)
  ▸ Cancer (increased risk of breast and endometrial cancer in women, increased mortality with prostate and colon cancer in men)
  ▸ Pulmonary disorders (see next page)
  ▸ Truncal obesity independently increases the prevalence of a number of problems, including:

⊙ Several abnormalities of adipose tissue lipolysis, particularly abnormally high FFA concentrations

⊙ Insulin resistance and type 2 diabetes mellitus (see page 130)

⊙ Dyslipidemia (increased triglycerides, small dense low-density lipoprotein [LDL] particles, and very low density lipoprotein [VLDL]; and decreased high-density lipoprotein [HDL] cholesterol)

⊙ CAD

⊙ Metabolic syndrome (obesity plus glucose intolerance, hypertension, and dyslipidemia; see page 130)

• In addition, obesity in older persons can exacerbate the age-related decline in physical function and lead to frailty.[223]

Cardiovascular and Pulmonary Complications

The major complications associated with obesity are related to cardiovascular disease (CVD), the risk of which is related to the BMI.[136a,187] In addition, there may also be pulmonary dysfunction.

• Cardiovascular complications are common in obese individuals:

  ▸ HTN, which may be caused by increased circulating blood volume, abnormal vasoconstriction, impaired vascular relaxation, and increased cardiac output, is highly prevalent in overweight and obese individuals. A weight gain of 10 kg is associated with an increase in SBP of 3 mm Hg and an increase in DBP of 2.3 mm Hg, which translate into an estimated 12% increased risk for CAD and 24% increased risk for stroke.[187]

  ▸ Obesity, particularly abdominal obesity, is a major risk factor for CAD, because of its association with HTN, dyslipidemia, insulin resistance, diabetes, and systemic inflammation. In addition, factors secreted by adipose tissue may directly impair endothelial function and increase oxidative stress, key factors in the pathogenesis of atherosclerosis and in triggering acute ischemic events.

  ▸ CHF is caused by LVH, which results from the increment in blood volume, SV, cardiac output, and filling pressures induced by excessive adipose tissue, as well as obstructive sleep apnea and hypertension.

  ▸ Arrhythmias and conduction abnormalities induced by LVH and sleep apnea, increase the risk of sudden death in obese individuals.

  ▸ There is also a distinct cardiomyopathy of obesity, which is characterized by the accumulation of fat within the myocardium.

  ▸ Weight loss of 10% of initial body weight significantly improves many of the obesity-related CVD risk factors, producing a 20% decrease in the risk of CVD.[155,186b] More significant weight loss achieved through bariatric surgery results in marked reductions in CVD morbidity and mortality.[155]

  ▸ In addition, a high level of physical fitness has been shown to reduce CVD morbidity and mortality in obese individuals independent of weight loss.[139]

• Pulmonary disorders may also occur in obese individuals:

  ▸ Obese individuals have an increased demand for ventilation and work of breathing, respiratory muscle inefficiency and weakness, reduced functional reserve capacity and expiratory reserve volume, and earlier closure of peripheral lung units.

  ▸ Obesity, especially if massive, can lead to restrictive lung dysfunction (RLD) due to restriction of thoracic expansion caused by the additional weight loading the chest wall and resisting diaphragmatic descent during inspiration.

  ▸ The systemic inflammation that accompanies obesity can elevate levels of C-reactive protein, tumor necrosis factor, and IL-6, which can affect airway reactivity and contribute to the increased incidence of asthma.

  ▸ Obstructive sleep apnea may be exhibited, particularly in moderately to severely obese males, aged 40 to 60 years, causing hypoxemia, hypercapnia, and a stress response due to high catecholamine and endothelin levels (see page 96). It is associated with several cardiovascular complications.

  ▸ About 5% of massively obese individuals develop the obesity hypoventilation syndrome with characteristic hypoxemia, hypercapnia, cyanosis, polycythemia, and somnolence. The resulting biventricular hypertrophy eventually progresses to pulmonary and systemic congestion.

  ▸ Patients who undergo bariatric surgery have an increased risk of postoperative pulmonary complications, including atelectasis, pneumonia, and venous thromboembolism and PE. However, the resultant weight loss induced by successful surgery has been shown to greatly improve or, in some cases, eradicate obesity-related pulmonary dysfunction.[59]

Specific Treatment

Obesity is best viewed as a chronic disease and thus requires life-long treatment, including:

• Dietary changes (500- to 1000-kcal/d reduction in intake with <30% from fats)

• Increased physical activity (lifestyle activity and structured exercise)

• Behavior modification (portion control, self-monitoring of eating and exercise behaviors, and cognitive restructuring)

• Medications (appetite suppressants and intestinal lipase inhibitors)

• Bariatric surgery (Roux-en-Y gastric bypass, gastroplasty, vertical stapling, vertical banded gastroplasty, and gastric banding)

Scientific evidence suggests that the combination of diet modification and exercise is the most effective behavioral approach for achieving weight loss, and continued exercise participation appears to be one of the best predictors of long-term weight maintenance.[10,56,165a] Importantly, even modest reductions in weight (5% to 10%) will significantly improve health, while long-term health benefits may be maximized with sustained weight loss of at least 10% of initial body weight.[187]

Clinical Implications for Physical Therapy

When prescribing exercise for obese individuals, physical therapists consider some specific factors to maximize safety and effectiveness:

• The primary objective when prescribing exercise for obese individuals is to maximize reductions in body fat and weight while preserving lean body mass.

- Many forms of exercise, when used in combination with dietary modification, have been shown to effect weight loss and improve cardiorespiratory fitness, including continuous and intermittent aerobic exercise, lifestyle activities, and resistance exercise.
  - ‣ Aerobic exercise should be prescribed for the vast majority of patients to increase energy expenditure, reduce cardiovascular risk factors, and improve respiratory muscle and functional efficiency.
    - ⊙ Moderate intensity (55% to 69% of HR_{max} or 40% to 59% of HRR or $\dot{V}O_{2\,max}$) is usually recommended, especially initially, although the inclusion of some sessions with more vigorous exercise ($\geq$70% HR_{max} or $\geq$60% of HRR or $\dot{V}O_{2\,max}$) may be more effective for maintaining weight loss.[134] It is important to realize that $\dot{V}O_{2\,max}$ and HR during brisk walking are higher in obese individuals (up to 64% to 98% of maximum in some individuals) than in normal-weight subjects and therefore are often too intense to maintain for more than a short duration.
    - ⊙ Exercise duration should be emphasized over intensity, allowing for gradual increases in duration to targeted levels before advancing to more vigorous activities. To achieve and maintain long-term weight loss, 60 to 90 min/day of at least moderate exercise totaling at least 280 min/wk may be required.[117] Lower durations of moderate intensity physical activity ($\geq$150 min/wk) reduce the health risks of obesity but are not as effective for long-term weight loss.
    - ⊙ Intermittent exercise (several 10- to 15-min bouts per day) that achieves these targets appears to be just as effective as continuous exercise.[68,118]
  - ‣ However, many obese individuals have difficulty with walking for prolonged periods of time because of abnormal gait pattern, joint pain, friction of clothing, and skin problems, all of which may increase the relative oxygen cost and make walking uncomfortable.
  - ‣ Leisure-time, or lifestyle, activities of at least 2000 kcal/wk are as efficacious at increasing fitness and reducing body weight as structured exercise.[10]
  - ‣ Resistance exercise improves muscular strength and endurance and therefore the performance of functional tasks and also offers comparable benefits for weight loss as endurance exercise.
  - ‣ It is important to inform patients about realistic expectations concerning the amount of weight loss that can be achieved through their prescribed exercise program so as to avoid disappointment and discouragement.
- Because of the increased prevalence of HTN and CAD, physiological monitoring of exercise response is indicated, at least initially.
  - ‣ HR is best monitored at the wrist because the carotid pulse may be difficult to palpate in obese individuals.
  - ‣ Obese individuals may exhibit a hypertensive response to exercise even when resting BP is normal. Those with impaired ventricular function may show a drop in BP with exercise due to reduced cardiac output.
  - ▸ Obese adults are more likely to develop myocardial ischemia during exercise.
- Because obese individuals often have cardiovascular disease, they may be taking a variety of medications that may have adverse effects on exercise responses and tolerance (see pages 101, 107, 112, and 114 and Chapter 5, page 214).
- Injury prevention is extremely important when exercising obese individuals, as physical injury is often the primary reason for discontinuation of exercise.
- Low-impact exercise (e.g., walking, elliptical machine) and non–weight-bearing exercise (e.g., swimming, cycling, rowing, and water aerobics) are recommended to minimize the stress placed on joints affected by osteoarthritis.
- Because thermoregulation may be impaired by excess body fat, exercising in a controlled environment with neutral temperature and humidity may be more comfortable than being outdoors.
- Access to home exercise equipment seems to improve adherence and therefore improves long-term weight loss.[118]

METABOLIC SYNDROME

The metabolic syndrome (MetS) refers to a cluster of interrelated risk factors found in one third of American adults and a growing number of children, and associated with increased risk of CVD events and death (which occurs three times as often in men as in women), type 2 DM, and chronic kidney disease.[87,135,193] Although various definitions of the MetS have been created, all agree on the essential components of glucose intolerance, obesity (particularly abdominal obesity), hypertension, and dyslipidemia, which are thought to have a multiplicative effect on CV risk greater than that predicted by their sum.

Even minimal elevations in the defined risk factors significantly increase morbidity and mortality, and appropriate treatment is recommended to delay or prevent the development of type 2 DM and to reduce CV risk[4,6,18,99,138]:

- Treatment of insulin resistance and hyperglycemia
- Diet and exercise, which are essential to reduce obesity and prevent diabetes. Exercise training has beneficial effects on all aspects of the metabolic syndrome, increasing insulin sensitivity, enhancing muscle contraction–induced glucose uptake in muscle, ameliorating endothelial dysfunction, reducing BP, and reducing lipid abnormalities[180]
- Antihypertensive drugs for BP $\geq$130/$\geq$80, particularly using angiotensin-converting enzyme (ACE) inhibitors and angiotensin II receptor blockers[119]
- Lipid-lowering therapy using statins to target LDL cholesterol, regardless of initial cholesterol concentrations and fibrates to treat hypertriglyceridemia
- Management of other cardiovascular risk factors (e.g., smoking, sedentary lifestyle, and proinflammatory state)

DIABETES MELLITUS

Diabetes mellitus (DM) is a group of chronic metabolic diseases characterized by hyperglycemia, which results from defects in insulin production, insulin action, or both. The major functions of insulin serve to control the rise in blood sugar after meals: it inhibits glucose production by the liver and promotes the uptake of glucose from the blood into the muscle and liver. A deficiency of insulin or resistance to its action results in derangements in carbohydrate, fat, and protein metabolism, so that the efficiency of glucose uptake by most cells of the body is impaired. As a result, blood glucose increases while its cellular utilization is hindered, and the use of fats and proteins increases. The elevated levels of blood sugar result in damage to the blood vessels, heart, kidneys, eyes, and peripheral nerves, as well as increased susceptibility to infections, particularly of the skin and gums.

Type 1 DM (formerly insulin-dependent diabetes, IDDM) is caused by autoimmune destruction of the beta cells in the pancreas, resulting in little or no insulin secretion, usually by the age of 10 to 25 years, although it can occur at any age.

- Classic symptoms include polyuria, polydipsia, weight loss, and sometimes polyphagia.
- *Diabetic ketoacidosis (DKA)* is an acute, life-threatening metabolic complication of uncontrolled DM (usually type 1) caused by the production of ketones from the catabolism of triglycerides for cellular fuel; it can develop quickly and without treatment can progress to coma and death within a few hours.

Type 2 DM (formerly non–insulin-dependent diabetes, NIDDM), which accounts for more than 90% of all cases of DM, results from a combination of tissue insulin resistance (which triggers increased insulin production) and insulin deficiency (relative to ambient glucose levels or absolute, which develops as beta cell function deteriorates). Previously, type 2 DM was typically diagnosed after the age of 40 years, but with the surge in obesity, it is now seen in some children and adolescents. The chief risk factors for developing type 2 DM are obesity, age, sedentary lifestyle, and genetic predisposition.

- Symptoms are often insidious and mild, consisting of fatigue, weakness, dizziness, blurred vision, and other nonspecific complaints.
- Before fulfilling the criteria for the diagnosis of type 2 DM, most individuals progress from insulin resistance to *impaired glucose tolerance (IGT)* (2-h oral glucose tolerance test [OGTT] values >120 mg/dL but <200 mg/dL after the ingestion of 75 g of glucose) to *impaired fasting glucose (IFG)* (fasting blood glucose level of 100 to 125 mg/dL).
- CV complications are directly related to the level of blood glucose control, with increasing risk as an individual progresses from insulin resistance to IGT to IFG to DM.[62,191]
- Because patients with type 2 DM retain some endogenous insulin secretion, they rarely develop DKA, except when stressed by a severe intercurrent illness (e.g., acute MI). Instead, uncontrolled hyperglycemia leads to dehydration and a *hyperosmolar hyperglycemic nonketotic (HHNK) syndrome,* which is manifested as postural hypotension, focal neurologic deficits, and hallucinations and is often fatal.

A number of other specific types of diabetes are caused by genetic defects, drug or chemical toxicity, infections, and other immune-mediated and genetic syndromes associated with DM. *Gestational diabetes (GDM)* develops during pregnancy and almost always resolves after parturition; however, women with GDM have a high risk of future DM.

Cardiovascular and Pulmonary Complications

Diabetes is associated with a much higher risk of cardiovascular disease (CVD) than is found in the general population. There is also an increased association with some pulmonary problems, particularly sleep-disordered breathing.

- CVD is the major cause of morbidity and mortality in patients with DM. Abnormalities of the small blood vessels (microangiopathies caused by thickening and/or damage to the basement capillary membrane) result in retinopathy, nephropathy, and neuropathies, whereas those involving the large vessels (macroangiopathies due to atherosclerosis) produce coronary artery, cerebrovascular, and peripheral arterial disease. Pathogenetic mechanisms include insulin resistance, endothelial dysfunction, dyslipidemia, chronic inflammation, procoagulability, and impaired fibrinolysis.[210]
  - ▸ Hypertension (HTN) is 1.5 to 3 times more prevalent in diabetic persons and accelerates both the microvascular and macrovascular complications associated with DM. The goal for BP should be ≤130/≤80 mm Hg.[12,147b]
  - ▸ DM accelerates the development of atherosclerosis, so that CAD, both symptomatic and asymptomatic, is more prevalent. On autopsy almost 75% of diabetics without clinical evidence of CAD were found to have high-grade coronary atherosclerosis and more than 50% had multivessel disease.[97] Thus, DM is considered a risk equivalent to established CAD. Importantly, myocardial ischemia and infarction often present atypically; they may occur "silently" (with little or no discomfort), or ischemia may be manifested as shortness of breath or fatigue that comes on with exertion and resolves immediately with rest (i.e., angina equivalents). Mortality after acute MI is two to three times higher with diabetes and results from arrhythmias or pump failure.
  - ▸ The combination of peripheral neuropathy and atherosclerotic occlusive disease leads to the development of lower extremity tissue necrosis and infection, and sometimes amputation.
- Diabetes is an independent risk factor for CHF, especially in women. Both CHF and DM are believed to share pathophysiological processes, including neurohumoral activation, endothelial dysfunction, and increased oxidative stress.[79] DM predisposes patients to the development of CHF, and CHF predisposes patients to the development of DM. CHF is also related to CAD, HTN, obesity, left ventricular hypertrophy, autonomic dysfunction, and a specific diabetic cardiomyopathy, which is characterized by increased LV wall thickness and cardiac mass and higher heart rates and is related to microangiopathy, metabolic factors, and/or myocardial fibrosis. Diabetic patients who develop CHF have a worse prognosis than those without DM, with increased mortality and hospitalizations.
- Autonomic neuropathy results from damage to vagal and sympathetic neurons as well as their supporting glia. Cardiovascular autonomic neuropathy (CAN) is common in DM (affecting about 50% of patients), appearing early, and its presence is significantly associated with age, duration of DM, microangiopathy, peripheral neuropathy, and with obesity in type 2 DM.[221] It should be suspected in all individuals with type 2 DM and in those with type 1 DM for more than 5 years

(see page 289 for methods of detecting CAN). Once established, CAN is associated with increased morbidity and mortality and a significant deterioration in quality of life.

▸ Clinical manifestations of CAN include exercise intolerance, orthostatic hypotension, intraoperative CV lability, and painless myocardial ischemia and infarction (due to cardiac denervation).[224]

▸ Parasympathetically mediated HR control is affected earlier than sympathetically mediated vasomotor control, causing higher resting HRs and reduced HR variability. When sympathetic dysfunction is added, HRs become slower, and with advanced CAN, HR becomes fixed and does not change with stress, exercise, or postural changes.[154]

▸ Autonomic neuropathy also results in impaired thermoregulation due to reduced blood flow to the skin and sweating, diminished thirst with increased risk of dehydration, impaired night vision due to delayed pupillary reaction, gastroparesis with unpredictable food delivery, and genitourinary dysfunction.[199,224]

- As stated previously, CV complications are directly related to the level of blood glucose control.

▸ Chronic hyperglycemia, even modest levels, and insulin resistance boost CV risk through increased oxidative stress, endothelial dysfunction, coagulation and platelet abnormalities, proinflammatory changes, and dyslipidemia.[154]

▸ There is evidence that insulin resistance is a pivotal causative mechanism of type 2 DM, HTN, and CAD.[16]

▸ Visceral obesity further aggravates the dyslipidemia seen in DM, particularly in men.

▸ Careful glycemic control can reduce the incidence of diabetic complications.[89,210]

- Pulmonary disorders associated with DM include higher incidences of:

▸ Pulmonary infections, particularly fungal infections and tuberculosis

▸ Reduced respiratory muscle strength and endurance in type 1 DM

▸ Sleep-related breathing problems (seen mainly in those with autonomic neuropathy)

▸ Higher mortality in those who develop pneumonia

▸ Hyperventilation, pneumomediastinum, and mucous plugging of the major airways related to diabetic ketoacidosis

Specific Treatment

The treatment of DM is aimed at controlling hyperglycemia, dyslipidemia, and HTN and thus minimizing the resultant long-term damage, dysfunction, and failure of various organs, especially the eyes, kidneys, nerves, heart, and blood vessels.[62,63,191,204a] Individualized according to patient disease and metabolic status, treatment commonly includes education, diet modification, exercise, and insulin and/or oral hypoglycemic agents.

- Primary prevention of type 2 DM through lifestyle changes, including diet and exercise to reduce body weight, is important for patients with prediabetes, especially those with CAD[21]:

- The reduction of other cardiovascular risk factors (e.g., HTN, dyslipidemias, and smoking) in those with prediabetes and DM is crucial to limiting morbidity and mortality.

- Exercise (see the next section) and diet modifications are crucial components in the management of DM. Important diet modifications specific to DM include the following:

▸ Carbohydrate intake before, during, and after exercise may be necessary to prevent exercise-induced hypoglycemia and is dictated by the results of frequent blood glucose monitoring until an individual's responses can be predicted. This is particularly important during prolonged exercise, which requires carbohydrate intake after 40 to 60 minutes of exercise.

▸ Adequate fluid intake is especially important for exercisers with diabetes. Drinks containing no more than 8% carbohydrate are recommended because they provide both needed fluids and carbohydrate.

▸ Greater carbohydrate intake (≈60% of daily calories), particularly complex carbohydrates, is recommended during training with adequate blood glucose control to maintain maximal muscle and liver glycogen stores.

▸ For individuals with type 2 DM, weight loss is an important component of treatment, for it improves glycemic control, reduces insulin resistance, and lowers cardiovascular risk. Modest weight loss of 15 to 30 lb is beneficial and is best accomplished through a combination of exercise, diet, and behavior modification.[199] Diet modifications should include both decreasing overall caloric intake to 1200 to 1500 kcal/day and lowering the amount of dietary fat to 20% to 30% of daily calories.

- Medications (see Chapter 5, page 207)

▸ Individuals with type 1 DM are dependent on insulin therapy for survival. Insulin delivered through either multiple daily injections or continuous subcutaneous insulin infusion (CSII) achieves the tightest metabolic control, but also increases the risk of hypoglycemia with exercise.

▸ Type 2 DM is treated with medications that prevent hyperglycemia by improving peripheral glucose uptake (biguanides and thiazolidinediones), reducing hepatic glucose release (biguanides, incretin potentiators, amylin mimetic, dipeptidyl peptidase [DPP]-4 inhibitor, and insulin), and increasing or replacing insulin secretion (insulin secretogogues [sulfonylureas and glinides] and insulin), as listed in Table 5-21 on page 215.

▸ Early aggressive BP reduction to less than 130/80 mm Hg is critical for protection against nephropathy, retinopathy, and stroke.[12,203] Angiotensin-converting enzyme (ACE) inhibitors and angiotensin receptor blockers (ARBs) are particularly effective.[12,21]

▸ Statins are recommended, even in those with normal cholesterol levels, and can reduce overall cardiovascular events by 30% to 40% in high-risk patients.[124]

- The primary problem associated with insulin therapy, and to a lesser degree the hypoglycemic agents, is hypoglycemia, which may occur during or after exercise or at night.

- Measurement of glycosylated hemoglobin (HbA_{1c}) indicates the average blood glucose level over the preceding 3 to 4 months and thus the level of glycemic control achieved through treatment.

- Newer treatments for type 1 DM include islet cell and pancreas transplantation., which eliminate the need for insulin therapy.

Exercise

Sustained exercise is normally accompanied by a decrease in insulin secretion and increases in the release of glucagon, catecholamines, cortisol, and other hormones, all of which act to ensure an adequate supply of glucose for the exercising muscles. In diabetes, abnormalities in glucose regulation lead to further disturbances in glucose homeostasis.

- Exercise creates both benefits and risks in patients with DM, as listed in Table 4-15, especially if there are comorbid medical conditions. Both aerobic and resistance exercise are routinely recommended because of improved glycemic control and beneficial effects on metabolic risk factors for the development of diabetic complications.
- Glycemic response to exercise depends on the type, intensity, and duration of activity, as well as the circulating insulin and glucose counterregulatory hormone concentrations.
- In type 1 DM, the metabolic responses to activity are influenced by the level of insulin at the onset of exertion.
  - ▸ Commonly, an excess of insulin exists at the onset of exercise (see Figure 5-8 on page 210), which inhibits hepatic glucose production and attenuates the mobilization of other substrates. Thus, hypoglycemia is often induced by exercise, occurring during, immediately after, or several hours after exercise. Risk factors include intensive insulin therapy, inadequate food intake preceding exercise, rapid absorption of depot insulin from an injection site near exercising muscle, exercising at the time of peak insulin effect, and prolonged, high-intensity exercise.
  - ▸ However, when there is an insulin deficiency with marked hyperglycemia at the onset of exercise (as in right after a meal or with poorly controlled DM), glucose uptake by the exercising muscle is impaired, and the release of counterregulatory hormones that is stimulated by exercise causes additional glucose production by the liver. Thus, hyperglycemia is further aggravated, which can last for several hours after intense exercise. In addition, the excessive mobilization of free fatty acids can lead to accelerated ketogenesis and ketoacidosis.
  - ▸ Children with type 1 DM, who exhibit a wide range of glucose levels, and adolescents, who undergo hormonal changes that hamper glycemic control, require even closer monitoring.
- In type 2 DM, increased insulin sensitivity induced by exercise increases glucose uptake by exercising muscle cells and improves glycemic control.[24,208] However, these changes are short-lived, lasting no more than 60 to 72 hours, so that exercise must be repeated at least every 2 to 3 days to sustain the improvements.[26]
  - ▸ Although research has demonstrated that higher intensity aerobic exercise (75% of $\dot{V}O_{2\ max}$) has a greater effect on glycemic control and aerobic fitness than more moderate exercise,[25,195a,208] this intensity may be difficult to sustain or even hazardous for many sedentary individuals with DM.
  - ▸ Greater CVD risk reduction is achieved with at least 4 hrs/wk of moderate to vigorous aerobic and/or resistance exercise.[9,208]
  - ▸ Some oral hypoglycemic agents, particularly the sulfonylureas, have a risk of postexercise hypoglycemia.
- Vigorous aerobic or resistance exercise may be difficult to sustain for many previously sedentary patients and potentially hazardous for those with cardiovascular disease, cardiomyopathy, and autonomic neuropathy. In addition, it may be contraindicated in the presence of proliferative or severe nonproliferative retinopathy because of an increased risk of triggering vitreous hemorrhage or retinal detachment and should probably be avoided for 3 to 6 months after laser photocoagulation.[208] However, high-risk patients usually benefit from lower intensity aerobic training.[145,208]

TABLE 4-15: **Benefits and Risks of Regular Exercise in Diabetes**

Benefits	Risks
Improved glycemic control, as evidenced by lower HbA$_{1c}$	Hypoglycemia
Increased insulin sensitivity	Worsening hyperglycemia, possible ketosis if poor BG control before exercise, especially with high-intensity exercise
Reduced risk of CVD, HTN, obesity, osteoporosis, and colon cancer	Abnormal exercise responses (hypertensive BP response during exercise, postexercise orthostatic hypotension)
Increased exercise tolerance, muscle fitness, and flexibility	
Enhanced sense of well-being, stress reduction	Cardiovascular events (myocardial ischemia or infarction, arrhythmia, sudden death)
Increased overall life expectancy	Possible aggravation of underlying retinopathy or nephropathy
Possible reduction in risk of progression of diabetic retinopathy and nephropathy	Musculoskeletal injury, especially if neuropathy is present

BG, Blood glucose; CVD, cardiovascular disease; HbA$_{1c}$, glycosylated hemoglobin; HTN, hypertension.
Data from Boulé NG, Haddad E, Kenny GP, et al. Effects of exercise on glycemic control and body mass in type 2 diabetes mellitus: A meta-analysis of controlled clinical trials. *JAMA.* 2001;286:1218–1227; Boulé NG, Kenny GP, Haddad E, et al. Meta-analysis of the effect of structured exercise training on cardiorespiratory fitness in type 2 diabetes mellitus. *Diabetologia.* 2003;46:1071–1081; Boulé NG, Weisnagel SJ, Larkka TA, et al. Effects of exercise training on glucose homeostasis. *Diabetes Care.* 2005;28:120–126; Gerich JE. The importance of tight glycemic control. *Am J Med.* 2005;118(9A):7S–11S; Loganathan R, Searls YM, Smirnova IV, et al. Exercise-induced benefits in individuals with type 1 diabetes. *Phys Ther Rev.* 2006;11:77–89; Riddell MC, Perkins BA. Type 1 diabetes and vigorous exercise: Applications of exercise physiology to patient management. *Can J Diabetes.* 2006;30:63–71; and Sigal RJ, Kenny GP, Wasserman DH, et al. Physical activity/exercise and type 2 diabetes. *Diabetes Care.* 2004;27:2518–2539.

Clinical Implications for Physical Therapy

Because of the prevalence of cardiovascular complications in DM and the abnormal metabolic responses to exercise, caution is required when providing physical therapy treatments to patients with DM. The following recommendations are offered:

- Patients should be assessed for the presence of CVD risk factors (dyslipidemia, HTN, smoking, positive family history of premature CAD, and presence of micro- or macroalbuminuria)
- Exercise testing with ECG monitoring is recommended before initiating exercise training at intensities greater than brisk walking in diabetics more than 40 years of age, those more than 30 years of age with known CVD risk factors, and those of any age with known or suspected CVD, autonomic neuropathy, or advanced nephropathy.[89a,208]
- Blood glucose (BG) monitoring is recommended before, after, and several hours after new patterns of exercise are undertaken, at least until the glycemic response can be predicted. BG monitoring may also be indicated during prolonged exercise (≥90 min).
    - When BG levels are elevated before PT, adjustments in treatment may be indicated:[208]
        - ⊙ If BG is ≥250 mg/dL and the patient is on insulin, s/he should check for ketosis (via urine dip stick or BG meter that measures ketones) and, if present, should not perform any exercise, at least until more insulin is administered and hyperglycemia and ketosis resolve.
        - ⊙ If a hyperglycemic patient feels well, is adequately hydrated, and is taking oral medications or urine and/or blood ketones are negative, s/he can perform low- to moderate-intensity exercise for 10 to 15 minutes and then BG should be rechecked. If BG rises exercise should be terminated, and if it drops exercise can be continued with BG monitoring every 15 minutes.
    - If BG levels are low (70 to 100 mg/dL) before therapy, the individual should be given a 10- to 15-g carbohydrate snack and exercise should be postponed until hypoglycemia is corrected (typically about 20 to 30 min). If marked hypoglycemia is present (<70 mg/dL), exercise is contraindicated and a snack should be ingested.
- Exercise prescription should take into consideration safety aspects as well as the mode, frequency, duration, intensity, rate of progression, and timing of physical activity.
    - To improve glycemic control, individuals with impaired glucose tolerance or DM should perform a minimum of 150 min/wk of moderate physical activity (40% to 60% of $\dot{V}_{O_2 max}$ or 50% to 70% of HR_{max}) or 90 minutes of vigorous exercise (>60% of $\dot{V}_{O_2 max}$ or >70% of HR_{max}) at least 3 days/wk, missing no more than two consecutive days.[9,208]
    - In patients with type 2 DM, higher intensity aerobic exercise (75% of $\dot{V}_{O_2 max}$) has a greater effect on glycemic control and aerobic fitness than more moderate exercise but may not be tolerated by many patients.[25,208]
    - Resistance training is valuable for improving glycemic control, especially when high-intensity exercise targeting all major muscle groups is performed for 3 sets of 8 to 10 repetitions at a weight that can be lifted 8 to 10 times to near fatigue 3 times a week.[9,24]
    - Greater CVD risk reduction is achieved with at least 4 hrs/wk of moderate to vigorous aerobic exercise, resistance exercise, or both.[208]

- To achieve and maintain major weight loss, larger volumes of exercise (7 h/wk) are more successful.[117]
- Children with type 1 DM, who exhibit a wide range of glucose levels, and adolescents, who undergo hormonal changes that hamper glycemic control, require close BG monitoring.
- Other exercise precautions are indicated in patients with specific diabetic complications:
    - ⊙ In patients with nephropathy, SBP should be controlled at rest and not exceed 180 mm Hg during exercise.
    - ⊙ For patients with retinopathy, SBP should not rise more than 20 to 30 mm Hg above the resting level (which should be within normal limits [WNL]), the head should be kept at a level above the waist, and head-jarring activities and the Valsalva maneuver should be avoided.
    - ⊙ Patients with autonomic neuropathy require more careful monitoring of BG and exercise responses.
- Because of elevated risk of cardiovascular disease, physiological monitoring of HR, BP, ECG (if available), and signs and symptoms should be included in all physical therapy evaluations and possibly during treatment sessions.
    - Patients with CAN frequently exhibit abnormal responses to exercise (refer to page 289 for methods of assessing CAN).
        - ⊙ A drop in BP of more than 10 mm Hg diastolic or more than 30 mm Hg systolic when a patient quickly moves from supine to standing is indicative of autonomic dysfunction. Thus, their risk for falls is increased and they should be cautioned to avoid quick changes from supine or sitting to standing.
        - ⊙ Resting HRs are often elevated and their responses to standing, deep breathing, and the Valsalva maneuver may be minimal, and responses to exercise are often blunted.[199]
        - ⊙ These patients frequently have severe myocardial ischemia without typical symptoms (i.e., silent ischemia); their risk of sudden death during activity is increased.
    - Patients without autonomic dysfunction often have hypertensive BP responses to exercise but may become hypotensive afterward.
- Therapists should take precautions to avoid exercise-induced hypoglycemia:
    - In individuals taking insulin, avoid scheduling appointments at the time of peak insulin effect, advise that the insulin dose before and sometimes after exercise be reduced (typically by 30% to 50%) unless exercise occurs several hours after a meal when insulin levels are low, and/or have the patient eat a carbohydrate snack 30 minutes before exercising. Also, an injection site should be used that is away from exercising muscle. Patients taking insulin secretagogues (sulfonylureas and glinides) also require a dose reduction of 50% before and sometimes after exercise.[158]
    - Start with moderate workloads and increase intensity gradually.
    - Use a consistent pattern of exercise (time of day, duration, and intensity).
    - Be able to recognize the signs and symptoms of hypoglycemia (Table 4-16).

TABLE 4-16: Signs and Symptoms of Hypoglycemia

Type	Signs and Symptoms
Adrenergic*	Weakness
	Sweating
	Tachycardia
	Palpitations
	Tremor
	Nervousness
	Irritability
	Tingling of mouth and fingers
	Hunger
	Nausea[‡]
	Vomiting[‡]
Neuroglucopenic[†]	Dizziness
	Confusion
	Headache
	Mental dullness
	Difficulty speaking
	Visual disturbances
	Amnesia
	Hypothermia
	Seizures
	Coma

*Caused by increased activity of the autonomic nervous system.
[†]Caused by decreased activity of the central nervous system due to insufficient glucose supply.
[‡]Unusual.

▶ During prolonged physical activity, have the patient consume a 5- to 10-g carbohydrate snack (e.g., fruit, juice or a soft drink) for each 30 minutes of exercise.

▶ Instruct the patient to avoid exercising in the late evening and at night.

• Special attention should be directed toward maintaining adequate fluid replacement, particularly when hyperglycemia is present, and taking proper care of feet, including good footwear, careful hygiene, and daily inspection.

• Individuals with diabetes and peripheral neuropathies and loss of protective sensation should avoid repetitive weight-bearing exercises, such as prolonged walking, treadmill, or jogging, as they may result in blistering, ulceration, infection, and amputation. Instead, non–weight-bearing exercise, such as swimming, bicycling, chair exercises, and arm exercises, are recommended.

• Medications for other comorbidities that are frequently taken by diabetics may have adverse effects on exercise responses and tolerance (see Chapter 5, page 214)

  ▶ The clinical implications of cardiovascular drugs can be found on pages 101, 107, 112, and 114.

  ▶ Statins, especially when combined with fibrates, can produce myositis, which should be reported to the physician immediately.

• Patients should be counseled to always carry identification and some form of DM alert and to *never* exercise alone, because of the potential for hypoglycemia, which can be life-threatening.

CHRONIC KIDNEY DISEASE AND FAILURE

Impairment of glomerular filtration results in renal insufficiency or failure, which can be staged according to severity (see Table 4-17). Chronic kidney disease (CKD) is usually an insidious process that is generally asymptomatic initially (stages 1 and 2) and later presents with symptoms of only vague general malaise and ill health until late in its progression (stages 3 and 4). Only when renal failure becomes marked (stage 5), with the accumulation of water, crystalloid solutes, and waste products, are the symptoms of uremia manifested: altered electrolyte homeostasis and acid–base imbalance, gastrointestinal distress, severe anemia, and multiple other abnormalities involving the skin, respiratory, cardiovascular, neurologic, musculoskeletal, endocrine, genitourinary, and immune systems. Renal failure sometimes develops as an acute problem or more commonly as a progressive and irreversible chronic disease (chronic renal failure, CRF).

Risk factors for CKD include CVD, DM, HTN, and obesity.[232] In approximately 40% of patients undergoing dialysis, the cause is attributable to DM, whereas 25% is due to chronic HTN,[220]

TABLE 4-17: Stages of Chronic Kidney Disease and Corresponding Cardiovascular Risk

Stage	Description	GFR (mL/min per 1.73 m^2)	CV Risk* (Odds Ratio, Univariate)
1[†]	Kidney damage with nl or ↑ GFR	≥90	Depends on degree of proteinuria
2	Kidney damage with mildly ↓ GFR	60–89	1.5
3	Moderately ↓ GFR	30–59	2 to 4
4	Severely ↓ GFR	15–29	4 to 10
5	Kidney failure	<15 or dialysis	10 to 50 to 1000 if ESRD

Data from Schiffrin EL, Lipman ML, Mann JFE. Chronic kidney disease: Effects on the cardiovascular system. *Circulation*. 2007;116:85–97.
↑, Increased; ↓, decreased; CKD, chronic kidney disease; CV, cardiovascular; ESRD, end-stage renal disease (indicating the need for renal replacement therapy); GFR, glomerular filtration rate; nl, normal.
*The increase in CV risk in comparison with people free of CKD depends on the age of the population studied: the younger the person, the higher the relative risk. Microalbuminemia increases the CV risk two- to fourfold.
[†]Stage 1 CKD is typically recognized as either albuminuria or structural renal abnormality (usually identified by ultrasound).

and there is evidence that CHF may be a contributory cause of progressive CKD in many patients.[209,232] Other less common but important etiologies include primary glomerulonephritis, systemic lupus erythematosus, and polycystic kidney disease. The major sequelae of CKD include continued progression of the disease toward CRF, development and progression of CVD (the most common cause of morbidity and mortality), anemia, and bone disease.

Cardiopulmonary Complications

Several cardiovascular and pulmonary complications are seen in CKD.

- CKD increases the risk of major CV events, even when the disease is mild; the risks intensify in proportion to the severity of the disease, as shown in Table 4-17.[92,220] By the time patients start dialysis, 40% have evidence of CAD and 85% of these patients have abnormal LV structure and mass.[204] The annual mortality rate for patients with end-stage renal disease (ESRD) is approximately 20% and about half of these deaths are caused by CVD.[22]
  - ▸ Hypertension is almost invariably present as it is both a cause and a consequence of renal disease and greatly aggravates renal dysfunction in CKD. HTN induces left ventricular hypertrophy (LVH) and as a major CV risk factor contributes to higher incidences of CAD, stroke, and PAD seen in CKD. LVH can also provoke myocardial ischemia, which further impairs LV function.
  - ▸ LVH is also aggravated by anemia, but there is some evidence that treatment of anemia with erythropoietin ameliorates LVH and improves survival.[181]
  - ▸ Accelerated atherosclerosis is related to numerous CV risk factors commonly seen in patients with CKD: DM and insulin resistance, HTN, dyslipidemia, and obesity. Endothelial dysfunction, low-grade inflammation, and hyperhomocysteinuria observed in CKD, as well as enhanced coagulability, contribute to higher prevalences of CAD, CVA and TIA, and PAD. Morbidity and mortality rates are elevated after acute MI and coronary revascularization procedures and are directly related to the degree of renal dysfunction.[22,204]
  - ▸ Accelerated calcifying atherosclerosis and valvular heart disease are common findings in patients with CKD, particularly those with severe uremia and consequent calcium–phosphorus dysregulation, resulting in isolated systolic hypertension, LVH and failure, and reduced myocardial perfusion.
  - ▸ Heart failure is prevalent in CKD, occurring in about 40% of those more than 65 years of age. Causes include HTN, CAD, anemia (leading to hypervolemia and dilated cardiomyopathy), and hypervolemia.
  - ▸ Other abnormalities that occur as complications of CKD and failure include coronary microvascular dysfunction (producing myocardial ischemia), cardiac autonomic neuropathy (≈75% of patients show reduced HR variability),[64] and uremia-induced pericarditis and pericardial effusion (which occasionally produce cardiac tamponade).
- Pulmonary abnormalities are also observed in patients with renal failure.
  - ▸ ESRD is associated with a variety of pulmonary problems.
    - ⊙ Fluid overload, hypoalbuminemia, and possibly increased pulmonary microvascular permeability (in addition to CHF) can result in pulmonary edema.

- ⊙ Fibrinous pleuritis is found in 20% to 40% of patients who die of CRF and is manifested as pleural chest pain with pleural rubs, pleural effusion, or fibrothorax. Pleural effusion also develops on occasion due to uremia.
- ⊙ Pulmonary calcification is common in CRF, possibly due to secondary hyperparathyroidism.
- ⊙ Sleep apnea and periodic limb movements during sleep are prevalent in patients with ESRD treated with hemodialysis.
- ⊙ CRF is also associated with an increased risk of respiratory tract infection, especially tuberculosis and pneumonia, probably due to pathological changes in the respiratory tract and impaired immune function.
- ⊙ There is evidence of respiratory muscle weakness in patients with ESRD, which improves after renal transplantation.
  - ▸ In addition, treatment of ESRD is frequently associated with pulmonary complications.
    - ⊙ The majority of patients develop hypoxemia, the severity of which differs according to the type of dialysis membrane and the chemical nature of the dialysate buffer, but appears to be clinically relevant only in patients with preexisting lung disease.
    - ⊙ Pleural effusions and an elevated diaphragm are common with peritoneal dialysis.
    - ⊙ Pulmonary complications after renal transplantation have been estimated to occur in 18% to 24% of patients, and consist of opportunistic pulmonary infections due to immunosuppression, pulmonary edema, pulmonary thromboembolism, and pulmonary calcification.

Specific Treatment

The treatment options for patients with CKD and failure include preventive measures to limit disease progression and complications, conservative management of symptoms, renal replacement therapy (RRT), and transplantation.

- Interventions to prevent the progression of CKD to ESRD include ACE inhibitors or angiotensin receptor blockers to thwart the renin–angiotensin–aldosterone system and control BP, statins for dyslipidemia, early treatment of anemia to achieve hemoglobin levels of 11 to 12 g/dL, intensive hyperglycemia management, and smoking cessation.
- Because the clearance of metabolic waste products and other substances by the kidneys remains superior to that achieved by dialysis until renal function deteriorates to 10% to 20% of normal, conservative management (e.g., control of diet, fluid balance, BP, mineral metabolism, and symptoms of uremia) is employed as long as possible.
- When the symptoms or complications of CKD become unacceptable, RRT is indicated and is most commonly accomplished by hemodialysis or peritoneal dialysis. However, RRT fails to adequately provide the regulatory and endocrine functions normally afforded by the kidneys and is associated with renal osteodystrophy, anemia, vascular access infections and thromboses, pericarditis, and ascites. Another option is nocturnal hemodialysis performed five or six nights per week at home, which appears to reduce CV injury and improve endothelial function.[147]
- The treatment of choice for ESRD, particularly in younger patients, is kidney transplantation, because it offers the best opportunity for normalization of renal function and lifestyle.

- Medications to reduce risk of CVD and cardiac death through primary and secondary prevention strategies are essential in patients with CKD: aspirin, β-blockers, calcium channel blockers, ACE inhibitors and angiotensin receptor blockers, and statins.

Clinical Implications for Physical Therapy

Patients with CKD exhibit impaired exercise tolerance and reduced muscle strength and endurance as a result of anemia, CVD, physical inactivity, skeletal muscle dysfunction, and metabolic acidosis.[2a] In most patients with ESRD, exercise capacity is so diminished that activities of daily living and lower levels of employment are often difficult.[64] Typically, the limiting symptom is skeletal muscle fatigue. In addition, patients frequently exhibit reduced flexibility and impaired coordination.[84]

Although more randomized clinical trials are needed to identify optimal training regimens according to patient characteristics and the effects on specific outcomes in patients with CKD, there is evidence that monitored exercise training is safe for these patients, increasing exercise capacity, muscle strength, and functional status, and may offer numerous other benefits as well, including improved lipid profiles, enhanced BP control, normalization of insulin sensitivity and glucose metabolism, reduction of inflammation, increased red blood cell mass, and improvements in quality of life, mood, and depression.[122] Benefits appear to be more pronounced in patients with the lowest functional levels.[176] Important considerations are presented here:

- Because patients with CDK tend to be limited by muscle fatigue, are usually unable to reach desired maximal intensity, and are at increased risk for CVD, exercise testing rarely produces meaningful results and therefore is not particularly useful in these patients.[122]
- Laboratory values should be reviewed before each treatment, especially in dialysis patients. Particular attention should be directed to hemoglobin, hematocrit, glucose, potassium, calcium, creatinine and blood urea nitrogen (BUN), white blood cell count (WBC), and platelets (see Chapter 9, Laboratory Medicine), and appropriate treatment modifications should be made if values are abnormal. Treatment of anemia with erythropoietin improves exercise tolerance and quality of life and possibly survival.[22] Fluid status should also be assessed, as hypervolemia may reduce exercise tolerance.
- In predialysis patients with CKD, maximal exercise capacity and muscle strength decrease as renal disease progresses. Exercise training, using both aerobic and resistance exercise, is beneficial for the prevention of physical deterioration as the disease progresses.[48,84]
- For patients with ESRD, aerobic exercise training results in significant increases in exercise capacity and endurance and decreases muscle protein catabolism.[44,93]
  - ▸ Modes of exercise vary according to the exercise setting, which can be at an outpatient rehabilitation center, in a hemodialysis unit, or at home.
    - ☉ For exercise performed during dialysis, aerobic training usually employs cycle ergometers placed in front of dialysis chairs or bed cycles. To avoid complications, exercise is best performed during the first 2 to 3 hours of dialysis.[58] The advantages of exercise during dialysis include improved

dialytic solute removal and phosphate clearance and increased compliance.[175]
    - ☉ Outpatient rehabilitation and home programs use the typical modes of exercise, although non–weight-bearing activities are recommended for patients with renal osteopathy and peripheral neuropathy. Outpatient programs are usually more intense and varied and thus produce the greatest increases in exercise capacity and functional status; however, compliance is a major problem. Poor compliance also limits the effectiveness of home programs.
  - ▸ The recommended frequency of exercise is at least 3 days/wk, with 4 to 6 days/wk advised by some.[76,122]
  - ▸ Exercise intensity is typically 50% to 80% of peak $\dot{V}O_2$, generally starting at the low end of the range initially and often performed at intervals with frequent brief (1- to 2-minute) rests as needed. The exercise dose is increased by increasing the duration and intensity of exercise according to patient tolerance while reducing the number of rest breaks until 30 to 45 minutes of continuous exercise can be performed.
  - ▸ Use of a rating of perceived exertion (RPE) scale (see page 281) is often preferable to HR for monitoring exercise intensity, and patients are encouraged to work at an intensity of "somewhat hard" or 12 to 13 on the 6- to 20-point Borg Scale. After a period of training, more fit individuals may be able to tolerate a perceived intensity of "hard" or 15 points on the 6- to 20-point Borg Scale.
- Exercise training after renal transplantation results in greater improvements in exercise capacity and quality of life.[211]
- Physiological monitoring is critical, especially in dialysis patients, whose fluid volume status and electrolyte balance vary tremendously from day to day, and in transplant patients, who frequently develop HTN and/or a hypertensive response to exercise as a side effect of cyclosporine administration (fortunately, the shift in immunosuppression away from cyclosporine to tacrilimus and other agents has decreased the incidence of posttransplant HTN[238]). Anemia may provoke tachycardia, shortness of breath, increased fatigue, and chest pain, and treatment with erythropoietin may induce hypertension. In addition, patients with DM require monitoring of blood glucose levels before, during, and after exercise.
- Because patients with CKD often have cardiovascular disease, they are often taking multiple medications that may have adverse effects on exercise responses and tolerance (see pages 101, 107, 112, and 114 and Chapter 5, page 214).
- Resistance exercise training is highly beneficial for patient with CKD and usually consists of 1 to 3 sets of 8 to 12 repetitions at low to moderate resistance performed 2 or 3 days/wk, targeting all major muscle groups. Avoidance of breath holding and the Valsalva maneuver is important because of the prevalence of HTN in these patients.
- Therapeutic exercise to increase flexibility and coordination are often indicated.
- Ventilatory muscle training to improve respiratory muscle strength and endurance, as well as training in breathing coordination with activity, are beneficial. In addition, breathing exercises performed during dialysis can promote relaxation, stress reduction, and improved sense of well-being.

- Other forms of exercise may also benefit patients with CKD, including yoga, Feldenkrais movements, Tai Chi, and Qigong, by improving efficiency of movement, sleep quality, pain and fatigue levels, and self-esteem and increasing self-awareness.
- Because of the prevalence of DM in patients with CKD, previously described clinical implications for diabetics should be noted when appropriate (see page 135).

OTHER SPECIFIC DISEASES AND DISORDERS

A wide variety of other medical diagnoses may be associated with cardiovascular and pulmonary complications that can affect patient tolerance of rehabilitation activities; the most common ones encountered by PTs are included in this section. It is beyond the scope of this manual to provide detailed descriptions of these pathologies, and only the most important features are presented. General clinical implications for physical therapy are provided at the end of this section and their applicability to any particular patient is dependent on the specific problems that are identified during PT assessment (see Chapters 6 and 7).

Connective Tissue Diseases

All connective tissue diseases (CTDs) have the potential for cardiovascular and pulmonary involvement, which is often subclinical or found only on autopsy. This may be due, at least in part, to the limitations imposed by the musculoskeletal features of the CTDs, which reduce activity level and thus mask their presence.

The *autoimmune rheumatic diseases (ARDs)* are a diverse group of immune-mediated inflammatory diseases that affect primarily the musculoskeletal system, although other systems are often involved. These diseases are characterized by inflammatory lesions involving the joints, muscles, and connective tissue (CT). Other organs are involved with variable severity and frequency; involvement of the cardiovascular and pulmonary systems is often responsible for increased morbidity and mortality.[54,96,194]

The ARDs can affect all pulmonary and cardiac structures. Pulmonary involvement is frequently manifested as pleuritis, infection, pneumonitis, interstitial disease, and pulmonary vascular disease. Pulmonary disease can also develop as a result of toxic reactions to drugs used to treat ARD (e.g., D-penicillamine, methotrexate, gold, cyclophosphamide, sulfasalazine, and NSAIDs). Pericarditis is the most common cardiac manifestation, and endocardial, myocardial, and coronary involvement also occur. As improved therapies and preventive measures have reduced the incidence and severity of cardiopulmonary complications and extended the longevity of these patients, death and disability from atherosclerotic cardiovascular disease have increased.[205] Inflammatory mechanisms along with physical inactivity are major contributory factors, along with acceleration of atherosclerosis by corticosteroid treatment.[219]

- *Rheumatoid arthritis (RA)* frequently affects other organ systems, including the cardiovascular and pulmonary systems.
  - The most common pulmonary manifestations are pleural effusions (40% to 70% of patients), which are usually small but occasionally are massive, causing shortness of breath, pleural chest pain, or both; interstitial lung disease (80% of cases by lung biopsy), which is typically mild but sometimes evolves into progressive pulmonary fibrosis; bronchiectasis (20% to 35% of cases); and rheumatoid lung nodules (20% to 30% of patients).[54] Chronic airway obstruction and reactive airway disease are common findings on PFTs.
  - Symptomatic cardiac disease is uncommon. Pericarditis can be detected in 30% to 50% of patients and valvular disease is found in 30% to 80% of patients[226]; however, only about 30% of patients have clinically evident valvular disease and less than 10% of patients have signs and symptoms of pericarditis and myocarditis. Increased cardiovascular mortality results from CHF and ischemic heart disease and associated arrhythmias. Cardiomyopathy is noted in 3% to 30% of patients with RA on postmortem studies.
- *Systemic lupus erythematosus (SLE)* is often complicated by pulmonary and cardiac abnormalities.
  - Pleurisy is the most prevalent pulmonary complication, occurring in at least 45% to 60% of patients at some time during the disease.[54] It is often asymptomatic but sometimes causes recurrent or intractable pleuritic chest pain, pleural rub, and effusion. Inflammation of the lung parenchyma sometimes causes diffuse lung disease, with cough, hemoptysis, and pulmonary infiltrates. Restrictive lung dysfunction due to "shrinking lung syndrome" is a well-recognized complication of SLE that is thought to result from reduced thoracic compliance. Uncommon but potentially lethal complications of SLE include pulmonary HTN due to either vasoconstriction or recurrent thromboembolism, diffuse alveolar hemorrhage, and chronic lupus pneumonitis.
  - Cardiovascular disease is the most common cause of death in patients with SLE.[217] Pericarditis (manifested as pericardial effusion or pericardial thickening) can be found in 62% of patients, becoming symptomatic, with chest pain and sometimes a rub, mainly at onset of SLE or during flares. Constriction or tamponade is rare. More than 50% of patients have valvular disease (usually regurgitation or rarely stenosis), which is clinically apparent in about 20% of patients.[96] Another common problem is premature atherosclerotic CAD, which sometimes produces myocardial ischemia or infarction. More uncommon cardiac manifestations include myocarditis, which can lead to dilated cardiomyopathy, and endocarditis (both infective and pseudoinfective), which can result in valvular disease. Cardioembolism from valvular vegetations or left heart thrombi causes ischemic stroke in 10% to 20% of patients.
- *Systemic sclerosis (SSc, or scleroderma)* is known mostly for its pulmonary complications, which are the leading cause of morbidity and mortality, but cardiac involvement also occurs.
  - Accumulation of CT matrix cells and proteins in the lungs leads to interstitial lung disease with progressive fibrosis affecting 75% of patients at autopsy, and subsequent pulmonary HTN in up to 50% of cases.[54] The incidence of lung cancer is increased 4- to 16-fold in patients with SSc and pulmonary fibrosis.
  - Overt heart disease occurs in less than 25% of patients but is found in up to 80% at autopsy.[96] Myocardial fibrosis (resulting from vasospasm and small-vessel disease producing

ischemia–reperfusion damage, as well as occlusive CAD) and pericarditis are common findings.[125] Other cardiac manifestations of SSc include myocarditis and occasionally pericarditis, conduction disturbances, and arrhythmias.

- *Ankylosing spondylitis* is only occasionally associated with significant pulmonary or cardiac manifestations.
  - ▶ Despite thoracic restriction due to severe rib cage immobility and kyphosis, shortness of breath or chest wall pain are uncommon, and restrictive lung dysfunction is usually mild. On rare occasions, patients develop upper lobe fibrobullous lung disease or nonapical interstitial lung disease.
  - ▶ Inflammatory involvement of the aortic cusps, proximal aortic root, and adjacent atrioventricular nodal tissue, which can be identified in up to 100% of patients, leads to aortic regurgitation in 10% of cases and various degrees of junctional conduction disturbances in about 5% of patients.[96] Left ventricular dilatation and diastolic dysfunction are common.
- *Mixed connective tissue disease (MCTD)* is an overlap syndrome with clinical features of SLE, SSc, and myositis. Pulmonary involvement occurs in 20% to 85% of patients according to the most dominant clinical pattern and most often consists of interstitial lung disease and pulmonary fibrosis, pleural effusion, and pulmonary HTN, which is a major cause of morbidity and mortality.[54] The most common cardiac manifestations are pericarditis and mitral valve prolapse.

The *inflammatory myopathies* are often included in the field of CTDs. Two types, *polymyositis (PM)* and *dermatomyositis (DM)*, are particularly likely to be associated with cardiopulmonary complications. Pulmonary involvement, which bears a poor prognosis, includes respiratory muscle dysfunction, interstitial lung disease (one form of which evolves quickly into acute respiratory failure whereas others lead to progressive fibrosis), aspiration pneumonia (due to pharyngolaryngeal muscle weakness), and lung cancer. Death due to respiratory insufficiency occurs in 30% to 66% of patients.[54] The muscle inflammation that is characteristic of the myositic diseases also affects the heart, resulting in myocarditis and cardiomyopathy. The most common clinical manifestations seen in PM and DM are those of CHF and CAD (due to vasculitis, small-vessel disease, and vasospasm, as well as atherosclerosis), which are major causes of mortality.[146]

The *inherited CTDs* are characterized by abnormalities of the connective tissue that affect the great arteries, cardiac valves, skeletal system, and skin.

- *Marfan's syndrome* is characterized by tall stature with long, thin extremities.
  - ▶ Pulmonary manifestations include occasional isolated bulla formation, usually apical, and sometimes generalized emphysema in nonsmoking individuals, which can be fatal in childhood. Pneumothorax occurs in 5% to 10% of patients, most likely as a result of rupture of subpleural bullae, and is often recurrent and bilateral. Pectus excavatum is a common finding and is sometimes severe, but rarely causes significant impairment of lung function. On occasion, kyphoscoliosis is severe enough to cause fatal cor pulmonale. Obstructive sleep apnea is prevalent because of increased upper airway collapsibility.
  - ▶ The most common cardiovascular manifestations are mitral valve prolapse (MVP), which is found in 60% to 80% of patients and often increases in severity with time; sinus of Valsalva and aortic root dilatation leading to aortic regurgitation; and aortic dissection, which can be lethal. Some patients develop serious ventricular or supraventricular arrhythmias.
- The more severe forms of *Ehlers-Danlos syndrome (EDS)* are associated with bullous emphysema and pneumothorax, as well as chest wall defects. Most forms of EDS have an increased prevalence of mitral valve prolapse, and the vascular form of the disease may be complicated by spontaneous rupture of the large- and medium-caliber arteries.
- In *osteogenesis imperfecta* the majority of patients have severe chest wall deformities, particularly kyphoscoliosis, inducing pulmonary compromise, which is the leading cause of death.

Infiltrative Diseases

Some diseases affect the heart, lungs, or both, through the infiltration or deposition of various substances within these organs (and other organs of the body).

- *Amyloidosis* results from the overproduction of certain proteins leading to the deposition of amyloid fibrils in various organs. It can occur as a primary process and also as a complication of some inflammatory processes, as in rheumatoid arthritis, inflammatory bowel disease, and bronchiectasis.
  - ▶ Pulmonary amyloidosis can occur along with systemic disease or as a localized entity, resulting in:
    - ⊙ Progressive diffuse parenchymal infiltrates, RLD, and impaired gas exchange versus localized tracheobronchial plaques or diffuse parenchymal nodules
    - ⊙ Possible pulmonary hypertension
    - ⊙ Obstructive sleep apnea due to massive infiltration of the tongue
    - ⊙ Respiratory failure if infiltration of the diaphragm
  - ▶ Cardiac involvement is manifested as:
    - ⊙ Diastolic dysfunction due to rigid amyloid fibrils (common)
    - ⊙ Systolic dysfunction due to marked amyloid deposition
    - ⊙ Cardiomyopathy (either restrictive or dilated)
    - ⊙ Atrial arrhythmias, especially atrial fibrillation (common, with a high risk of thromboembolism)
    - ⊙ Syncope due to orthostatic hypotension, bradyarrhythmia or tachyarrhythmia (common)
    - ⊙ Sudden death and myocardial infarction due to vascular involvement
- *Sarcoidosis* is a chronic inflammatory disease characterized by the presence of noncaseating granulomas in multiple organ systems with resultant combinations of inflammation and scarring, which can vary from mild and asymptomatic with spontaneous resolution to severe progressive disease leading to organ failure and death.
  - ▶ Pulmonary manifestations occur as:
    - ⊙ Hilar and mediastinal lymph nodes and noncaseating parenchymal granulomas visualized on chest radiography, which are more prominent in the upper than lower lobes (very common)
    - ⊙ Bronchostenosis due to endobronchial granulomas
    - ⊙ Dyspnea and nonproductive cough

▸ Cardiac involvement is noted in up to 50% of patients at autopsy, although clinical manifestations are found in less than 10% of patients:
  ⊙ Ventricular tachyarrhythmias
  ⊙ Cardiomyopathy with impaired LV function or heart failure
- *Hemochromatosis* is a common inherited disorder of iron metabolism that leads to iron deposition in various organs, including the liver, heart, pancreas, joints, skin, and endocrine organs. Complications of chronic liver disease can be fatal but can be prevented by regular therapeutic phlebotomy to reduce circulating iron levels. Excess deposition of iron in the heart can lead to secondary myocardial fibrosis, cardiomyopathy (either restrictive or dilated), and conduction disturbances or arrhythmias.

Neuromuscular Diseases and Neurologic Disorders

A number of disorders affecting the neurologic or neuromuscular systems are associated with cardiac and pulmonary dysfunction. These include spinal cord injury (SCI), cerebrovascular accident (CVA), Parkinson's disease (PD), amyotrophic lateral sclerosis (ALS), Guillain-Barré syndrome (GBS), myasthenia gravis, the muscular dystrophies, Friedreich's ataxia, and many others. The incidence and severity of dysfunction in all of these disorders varies widely.

- Pulmonary complications are common in patients with neuromuscular and neurologic disorders[183]:
  ▸ Respiratory muscle paralysis or weakness, or abnormal tone, restricts chest expansion and ventilation and reduces cough force and effectiveness, leading to retained secretions, atelectasis, and high risk of pneumonia, which is the most common cause of death in SCI.
  ▸ Hypoventilation and microatelectasis can give rise to CO_2 retention and hypoxemia, which may be exacerbated by different positions (e.g., recumbent in high cervical SCI, sitting in lower cervical SCI).
  ▸ Reduced peripheral blood flow, as in SCI, and poor activity level predispose patients to DVT and PE.
  ▸ Bulbar muscle weakness with dysfunction of the pharyngeal and laryngeal muscles increases the risk of aspiration pneumonia and interferes with effective cough force (due to poor glottic closure).
  ▸ Sleep-disordered breathing, including obstructive sleep apnea and nocturnal hypoventilation, is seen in many patients, particularly those with high cervical SCI, ALS, and the muscular dystrophies.
  ▸ Kyphoscoliosis often develops in patients with neuromuscular diseases and results in decreased chest wall compliance, compression of one lung and overdistension of the other, and increased work of breathing.
  ▸ Pulmonary edema can develop because of cardiomyopathy (see below).
  ▸ Respiratory failure due to respiratory muscle fatigue is usually the final morbid event in the neuromuscular disorders, which may be delayed by noninvasive ventilatory assistance (e.g., CPAP or bi-PAP, cuirass, or rocking bed; see page 30) in some patients.[20,183]

- Cardiovascular dysfunction also occurs in many patients with neuromuscular and neurologic disorders, although the typical symptoms of reduced exercise tolerance are difficult to appreciate in nonambulatory patients. Instead these patients may exhibit increased fatigue, difficulty sleeping, impaired concentration, and more subtle variants of poor performance.[65]
  ▸ Cardiomyopathy frequently develops in the muscular dystrophies, myasthenia gravis, and Friedreich's ataxia.
  ▸ Disorders of impulse formation and conduction are common in the muscular dystrophies and arrhythmias occur in almost all diagnoses.
  ▸ Hypertension and CAD affect patients with PD and myasthenia gravis, as they do their same-aged peers.
  ▸ Not surprisingly, the vast majority of patients with ischemic CVA also have CAD, although many have not been diagnosed.[45,108]
  ▸ Autonomic dysfunction (due to disruption of autonomic nerve fibers in SCI with lesions above the T_1 level or nerve involvement by other neurologic pathologies, such as multiple sclerosis, ALS, PD, and GBS) is manifested as orthostatic hypotension and impaired thermoregulation.
  ▸ In persons with SCI above the T_1 level, both preload and afterload are reduced, which results in atrophy of the LV and reduced systolic efficiency.[116]

In addition, abnormal movement patterns due to muscle weakness or abnormal neural input increase the energy cost of mobility and daily activities. And impaired mobility induces a more sedentary lifestyle, which leads to deconditioning (as illustrated in Figure 7-1 on page 300), so that reduced muscular efficiency causes a given level of activity to require greater energy utilization. Both of these factors contribute to more intense physiological demands of mobility and activities of daily life (ADLs) and increase the risk of activity intolerance. Individuals with SCI are particularly affected, and all patients with neuromuscular and neurologic disorders have an increased risk of cardiovascular morbidity and mortality.

Hematologic Disorders

Many hematologic disorders are associated with cardiovascular and/or pulmonary dysfunction because of impaired oxygen-carrying ability, reduced immune function, or coagulopathy.

Anemia

Anemia is defined as a reduced circulating red blood cell (RBC) mass relative to an individual's gender and age and can result from impaired RBC production, excessive destruction of RBCs (hemolysis), loss by hemorrhage, or a combination of these. Anemia has many causes, including dietary deficiency, acute or chronic blood loss, genetic defects of hemoglobin, exposure to toxins or certain drugs, diseases of the bone marrow, and a variety of chronic inflammatory, infectious, or neoplastic diseases.

- The clinical manifestations of anemia depend on its cause, extent, and rapidity of onset, and the presence of other medical problems that compromise an individual's health.
  ▸ Mild anemia is often asymptomatic other than vague fatigue.
  ▸ In chronic anemia, more notable symptoms typically occur only when the hemoglobin concentration falls below 50%

of normal. The most common complaints are fatigue and weakness, diminished exercise tolerance, exertional dyspnea, and palpitations.

▶ Pallor is often observed on physical examination, especially of the hands, fingernails, mucosa, and conjunctiva, and some patients exhibit tachycardia and audible cardiac flow murmurs.

▶ Patients with CAD may experience angina or other manifestations of myocardial ischemia even with mild anemia.

- A number of compensatory mechanisms may be activated to preserve tissue oxygenation.

▶ In acute-onset anemia with severe loss of blood volume, perfusion to vital organs is maintained by peripheral vasoconstriction and central vasodilation.

▶ In persistent anemia, small-vessel vasodilation serves to increase tissue oxygenation by decreasing systemic vascular resistance and increasing cardiac output.

▶ Other reactions include reduced oxygen–hemoglobin affinity, increased plasma volume, slower circulatory time, enhanced oxygen extraction, and stimulation of erythropoietin production.

- CHF can develop in severe anemia even in the absence of cardiac disease, but is usually due to the increased workload being imposed on an unhealthy heart.

- Patients with chronic anemia associated with chronic kidney failure, cancer therapy, HIV therapy, and other chronic diseases, such as CHF, are often treated with erythropoietin (e.g., epoetin-alfa [Epogen, Procrit]), which stimulates the production of RBCs.

Sickle Cell Disease

Sickle cell disease (SCD) is a genetic disease found most commonly in African Americans, and is characterized by structurally abnormal hemoglobin resulting in RBCs that become crescent- or sickle-shaped during deoxygenation. Hemolytic anemia develops because of shortened circulatory survival of damaged RBCs, which are destroyed intravascularly by macrophages and extravascularly in the spleen. Tissue ischemia–reperfusion injury and infarction occur when small capillaries and venules are occluded by the adherence of sickled RBCs to the vascular endothelium followed by cellular aggregation (including RBCs, WBCs, and platelets). Multiple organs are affected, leading to progressive systemic vasculopathy and chronic organ failure. Most patients are anemic but asymptomatic except during painful episodes.

- Acute painful episodes resulting from vaso-occlusion (vaso-occlusive crises) are the most common complication of SCD and typically occur one to six times a year, lasting for a few days up to several weeks. They may be precipitated by cold, dehydration, infection, stress, menses, or alcohol consumption, though the cause is frequently unknown.

- Although nearly all organs are susceptible to damage by SCD, the spleen, kidneys, CNS, bones, liver, lungs, and heart are most often affected.

- Cardiopulmonary dysfunction is common in SCD:

▶ As with anemia, cardiac output and tissue oxygen extraction increase, but in SCD the reduction in oxygen content of the RBCs induces further sickling and compounds the cardiopulmonary complications.

▶ Patients with SCD have a marked increase in susceptibility to bacterial infections, including pneumonia, meningitis, and osteomyelitis, which are a major cause of morbidity and mortality.

▶ The acute chest syndrome, which usually presents with dyspnea, chest pain, fever, tachypnea, hypoxemia, leukocytosis, and a pulmonary infiltrate on chest radiography, but sometimes is insidious with nonspecific signs and symptoms, is the most common cause of hospitalization and death.[20a,222b] It is caused by vaso-occlusion, infection, and pulmonary fat embolism from infarcted bone marrow. Progression to acute respiratory failure has been reported to occur in 10% to 22% of patients, particularly adults.[98]

▶ Episodic symptoms consistent with asthma or reactive airway disease have been reported in several studies.[98]

▶ Veno-occlusion can affect the cardiac and pulmonary vessels, causing pulmonary thromboembolism and infarction and myocardial infarction.

▶ Chronic pulmonary manifestations include abnormal pulmonary function (lower airway obstruction, restriction, and impaired diffusing capacity), hypoxemia, evolving pulmonary hypertension, and exercise intolerance, which likely result from ongoing lung injury related to ischemia–reperfusion, pulmonary vasculopathy, and alterations in nitric oxide metabolism.[98]

▶ Biventricular hypertrophy and dilatation are induced by chronic anemia and the compensatory volume overload that increases cardiac output. Clinical manifestations include diminished exercise tolerance, dyspnea on exertion, and progressive loss of cardiac reserve. Systolic cardiac murmurs are common.[53]

▶ Diastolic dysfunction, most likely due to relative systemic HTN, has been noted in 18% of patients and increases the mortality risk, especially when combined with pulmonary HTN.[200]

▶ Arrhythmias and second-degree AV block may occur during painful episodes and increase the risk of sudden death.

Hematologic Malignancies and Lymphomas

Clonal defects of the hematopoietic stem cells produce a number of preleukemic myelodysplastic or myeloproliferative disorders (which sometimes transform to acute leukemia) and the leukemias (see Table 9-4, page 404). Malignant transformation of lymphocytes, which reside in the lymph system and in blood-forming organs, results in a variety of cancers of lymphoid origin, including the lymphomas, lymphoid leukemias, and plasma cell dyscrasias.

The most common cardiopulmonary complications associated with these malignancies result from impaired immune function (opportunistic infections), anemia, and thrombocytopenia (bleeding complications), or as a side effect of treatment (e.g., chemotherapy, radiation therapy, or stem cell or bone marrow transplantation; see following page). As with patients undergoing treatment for any type of cancer, strict hand-washing precautions and infection control are extremely important.

HIV and AIDS

Patients with human immunodeficiency virus (HIV) are living much longer and suffering less disability than in the 1990s because of highly active antiretroviral therapy (HAART), which aims to preserve immune function and minimize viral replication in order to delay the progression to acquired immune deficiency syndrome (AIDS). Thus, HIV infection has become a chronic illness with episodes of exacerbations and remissions, which often affects the neurologic, cardiopulmonary, integumentary, and musculoskeletal systems.

- Although the success of HAART has sharply reduced the incidence of opportunistic infections, pulmonary complications continue to be a major cause of morbidity and mortality in individuals with HIV/AIDS.[28,128]
  - ▸ Noninfectious pulmonary complications are common in HIV infection and include malignancies (lung, Kaposi's sarcoma, and non-Hodgkin's lymphoma), pulmonary hypertension (possibly through increased production of inflammatory cytokines and chemokines by infected lymphocytes and alveolar macrophages, as well as due to endothelial dysfunction), and lymphoproliferative disorders (lymphocytic interstitial pneumonitis and alveolitis).[128]
  - ▸ HIV infection increases the risk of developing active tuberculosis (TB) and TB recurrence, which are associated with accelerated progression and mortality among patients infected with HIV, partially because of a number of drug–drug interactions between the various medications used to treat the two diseases.[28]
  - ▸ Fungal (e.g., *Pneumocystis* pneumonia, PCP) and bacterial infection (e.g., *Streptococcus pneumoniae, Haemophilus influenzae, Staphylococcus aureus, Pseudomonas,* and *Mycobacterium avium*) also occur more frequently and are a major problem where HAART is not available.[28] In addition, reactivation of cytomegalovirus (CMV) infection may occur in conjunction with PCP and is a marker of poor prognosis.
- Cardiovascular complications also occur in many patients with HIV and are fatal in some patients.[120,195]
  - ▸ The most common CV problem seen in HIV, particularly in children with AIDS, is pericardial effusion, which may be induced by opportunistic infection or malignancy, but more often no definitive cause can be identified. The incidence has decreased in those receiving HAART.
  - ▸ Myocardial abnormalities, including myocarditis, dilated cardiomyopathy, ischemic heart disease, and myocardial involvement with Kaposi's sarcoma or lymphoma, occur in 25% to 75% of patients, according to clinical and autopsy studies.
  - ▸ The prevalence of systemic HTN has been reported by some, but not all, to be much higher in HIV-infected patients than in the general population and to increase the incidence of CAD and MI.[120,195]
  - ▸ Infective endocarditis and nonbacterial thrombotic endocarditis have also been reported with increasing frequency in patients with advanced or terminal HIV (i.e., AIDS).
  - ▸ Other cardiovascular complications include a range of inflammatory vascular diseases and an increased incidence of venous and arterial thrombosis and embolism (due to the presence of a hypercoagulable state), which might be higher in those receiving protease inhibitors and in smokers.

Sequelae to Cancer Treatments

The development of more aggressive treatments for a number of malignancies using chemotherapy, irradiation, and biological agents has yielded higher survival rates and longer survival periods but has also increased the incidence of cardiac and pulmonary toxicity causing acute and late complications. In addition, some of the medications used to support patients during cancer treatments have been associated with cardiopulmonary dysfunction.

Chemotherapy

A number of chemotherapeutic agents are associated with cardiac and pulmonary toxicity, which can occur acutely or may become apparent months to years after the completion of treatment. As with other situations involving cardiopulmonary complications, damage is found on autopsy much more frequently than is clinically apparent. The most notable pulmonary complications are presented here.

- Chemotherapy is often complicated by pulmonary toxicity, as indicated in Table 4-18.[36,38,67,144,198,213] Despite a variety of mechanisms by which chemotherapeutic agents can injure the lungs, the clinical presentations are often similar, with dyspnea, nonproductive cough, and frequently fever that develop weeks to years after treatment.
  - ▸ Bleomycin has the highest incidence of pulmonary toxicity (up to 20% of patients),[144] which is sometimes severe and can be fatal. Acute bleomycin-induced hypersensitivity pneumonitis occurs in a small number of patients even after low doses. More commonly, pneumonitis develops that appears mainly as chronic pulmonary fibrosis; risk factors include higher cumulative dose (especially if >450 to 500 mg), patient age, smoking, renal dysfunction, prior or concomitant thoracic irradiation, and administration of oxygen. Bleomycin can also produce a number of other patterns of interstitial lung disease.
  - ▸ Interstitial pneumonitis can also be induced by busulfan, chlorambucil, cyclophosphamide, methotrexate, mitomycin C, and the nitrosoureas (particularly carmustine and lomustine), and sometimes by fludarabine, irinotecan (Camptosar), paclitaxel (Taxol), and procarbazine (Matulane, Natulan).
  - ▸ A number of other agents can induce other forms of lung damage.
    - ⊙ Busulfan (Myleran) can cause pulmonary fibrosis and sometimes an alveolar–interstitial process with alveolar proteinosis, which often progresses to death.
    - ⊙ Noncardiac pulmonary edema develops in 13% to 28% of patients during the administration of cytosine arabinoside (Cytarabine) and in a few patients months after treatment with mitomycin C.
    - ⊙ Pneumothorax occurs in some patients treated with the nitrosoureas (see above).
    - ⊙ Acute hypersensitivity reactions have occurred with docetaxel (Taxotere), procarbazine, and, as previously mentioned, bleomycin.

TABLE 4-18: Pulmonary Toxicity Associated With Cancer Treatments

Cancer Treatment	Notable Pulmonary Side Effects	Incidence
Chemotherapeutic Agents		
Bleomycin	Acute hypersensitivity pneumonitis, chronic pulmonary fibrosis.	Up to 20%, dose dependent
Busulfan (Myleran)	Interstitial pneumonitis, alveolar–interstitial process with proteinosis	≈4%
Chlorambucil (Leukeran)	Interstitial pneumonitis, pulmonary fibrosis	Rare
Cyclophosphamide, CTX (Cytoxan)	Subacute pneumonitis, late-onset pulmonary fibrosis, ARDS	<5%
Cytosine arabinoside (Cytarabine)	Subacute noncardiogenic pulmonary edema ± pleural effusion	13%–28%
Docetaxel (Taxotere)	Acute hypersensitivity reaction, diffuse alveolar damage	1%–20% (less if premedication), dose related
Fludarabine (Fludara)	Increased risk of opportunistic infections, diffuse pneumonitis, ARDS	Rare–18%
Gemcitabine (Gemzar)	Acute hypersensitivity reaction with bronchospasm, nonspecific interstitial pneumonitis, diffuse alveolar damage/ARDS	<1% up to 10%
Melphalan (Alkeran)	Diffuse pneumonitis 1–48 mo after therapy	Rare
Methotrexate, MTX	Hypersensitivity pneumonitis, respiratory failure	2%–8%
Mitomycin (Mutamycin)	Acute and subacute pneumonitis, chronic pneumonitis; late noncardiac pulmonary edema, ARDS occur with hemolytic uremic syndrome	3%–14%, especially with higher doses
Nitrosoureas (carmustine [BCNU], lomustine [CCNU])	Acute alveolitis/pneumonitis, chronic pulmonary fibrosis, pneumothorax	Up to 20%–30% if preexisting lung disease
Paclitaxel (Taxol)	Anaphylactoid hypersensitivity at or near time of infusion (caused by suspension vehicle, not the drug); hypersensitivity pneumonitis days to weeks after treatment; enhanced XRT-related lung damage?	3% to >10% (less if premedication), dose related
Procarbazine (Matulane)	Acute hypersensitivity pneumonitis, pleural effusion, respiratory muscle weakness	1%–5%
Vinca alkaloids: vinblastine (Velban, Velsar), vincristine (Oncovin, Vincasar, Vincrex) and vindesine (Eldisine, Fildesin), vinorelbine (Navelbine)	Acute interstitial pneumonitis, pulmonary fibrosis; respiratory muscle weakness (vincristine)	Up to 5%, especially if combined treatment with mitomycin or single agent vinorelbine
Biological Agents		
Interferon-α	Severe exacerbation of asthma, granulomatous reaction, interstitial lung disease	Rare
Interleukin-2 (IL-2)	Acute noncardiac pulmonary edema, pleural effusion	≈20%
Monoclonal Antibodies		
Alemtuzumab (Campath)	Dyspnea, neutropenia-associated pneumonia	Up to 15%–28%
Bevacizumab (Avastin)	Hemoptysis in patients with lung cancer	20%
Cetuximab (Erbitux)	Acute dyspnea, which may be severe; delayed dyspnea	5%–13%
Gemtuzumab (Mylotarg)	Acute hypersensitivity pneumonitis, pleural effusion, noncardiac pulmonary edema, ARDS, neutropenia-associated pneumonia	Up to 10%
Ibritumomab (Zevalin)	Acute hypersensitivity pneumonitis	1%–5%
Rituximab (Rituxan, Mabthera)	Interstitial pneumonitis, COP, alveolar hemorrhage	Rare

Continued

TABLE 4-18: Pulmonary Toxicity Associated With Cancer Treatments—Cont'd

Cancer Treatment	Notable Pulmonary Side Effects	Incidence
Tositumomab (Bexxar)	Subacute hypersensitivity pneumonitis, bronchospasm, neutropenia-associated pneumonia	Up to 29%
Trastuzumab (Herceptin)	Bronchospasm, ARDS, pneumonitis, pleural effusion occurring during or after infusion	Rare
Miscellaneous		
Etoposide (VP-16)	Alveolar hemorrhage	Rare
Thalidomide (Thalomid)	Dyspnea, thromboembolic disease, interstitial pneumonitis, pleural effusion	4%–54%
Radiation therapy to chest	Acute radiation pneumonitis developing 4–6 wk after treatment, late radiation fibrosis, COP	Lung, 5%–15%; HD, 3%–11%; breast, >1%
Hematopoietic stem cell transplantation	Pulmonary edema due to fluid overload with infusion, chemotherapy-induced pulmonary toxicity (see above), increased risk of infection, diffuse alveolar hemorrhage, radiation pneumonitis due to total body radiation, idiopathic pneumonia syndrome, bronchiolitis obliterans, delayed pulmonary toxicity syndrome, COP, respiratory muscle weakness	Up to 65%

ARDS, Acute respiratory distress syndrome; COP, cryptogenic organizing pneumonia; HD, Hodgkin's disease; XRT, radiation therapy.

⊙ Gemcitabine (Gemzar) causes dyspnea, which can be severe, in up to 10% of patients.[144] There are reports of pulmonary toxicity occurring as an acute hypersensitivity reaction with bronchospasm, diffuse alveolar damage, and ARDS, and a rare severe idiosyncratic reaction with marked dyspnea and pulmonary infiltrates that may progress to life-threatening respiratory insufficiency.

⊙ Procarbazine and vincristine (and theoretically cytosine arabinoside and chlorambucil) can cause neuropathies that may affect the respiratory muscles, inducing weakness.

⊙ Zinostatin can induce a unique drug reaction involving hypertrophy of the pulmonary vasculature.

▸ Sometimes pulmonary toxicity develops when specific chemotherapeutic agents are combined (e.g., vinblastine [Velban, Velsar] plus mitomycin C, which induces bronchospasm, interstitial pneumonitis, and noncardiac pulmonary edema).

• A number of chemotherapeutic agents also cause cardiovascular dysfunction, as listed in Table 4-19.[38,211a,237,239]

▸ The most well-recognized agents linked with cardiotoxicity are the anthracycline antibiotics (doxorubicin [Adriamycin], daunorubicin [Cerubidine], epirubicin [Ellence, Pharmorubicin], idarubicin [Idamycin], and mitoxantrone [Novantrone]).

⊙ Acute toxicity presents as myocarditis with or without pericarditis, which may cause transient CHF and arrhythmias.

⊙ Late cardiotoxicity occurs in the form of a chronic cardiomyopathy, resulting in LV dysfunction and CHF, which can develop up to 25 years or more after treatment. Survivors of pediatric cancers are particularly vulnerable, and the prognosis is poor.

⊙ Factors that increase the risk of cardiac complications include higher cumulative dose (doxorubicin at ≥ 300 mg/m^2 or epirubicin at ≥ 600 mg/m^2), younger or older age (<18 or >65 yr) at treatment, longer duration of survival, associated HTN, preexisting CAD or LV dysfunction, prior mediastinal irradiation, combination chemotherapy (trastuzumab, cyclophosphamide, etoposide, melphalan, paclitaxel, and mitoxantrone), pregnant or contemplating pregnancy; and participation in extreme/competitive athletics.

⊙ Monitoring of ejection fraction for early detection of deterioration is valuable for preventing cardiac dysfunction. The benefits of cardioprotective agents, such as the free-radical scavenger dexrazoxane, are under investigation.

▸ Myocardial depression and CHF are occasionally noted after treatment with mitoxantrone (Novantrone), cyclophosphamide (Cytoxan), ifosfamide (Ifex), mitomycin (Mutamycin), paclitaxel (Taxol), and all-*trans*-retinoic acid (Tretinoin).

▸ Cisplatin (Platinol) increases the risk of developing HTN and premature atherosclerotic CAD, which appear as long as 10 to 20 years after remission of testicular cancer.

▸ Other agents that have been associated with myocardial ischemia and occasionally infarction include 5-fluorouracil (5-FU, Adrucil), capecitabine (Xeloda), pentostatin (Nipent), the *Vinca* alkaloids, and interleukin-2 (IL-2).

Radiation Therapy

Radiation therapy (XRT) to the chest, as for the treatment of Hodgkin's disease (HD), lymphoma, and lung, breast, esophageal, and head and neck cancers, necessarily exposes the heart and lungs to varying degrees and dosages of radiation, depending on the

TABLE 4-19: Cardiotoxicity Associated With Cancer Treatments

Cancer Treatment	Notable Cardiovascular Side Effects	Incidence
Chemotherapeutic Agents		
Anthracyclines (doxorubicin [Adriamycin, Rubex], daunorubicin [Cerubidine], epirubicin [Ellence, Pharmorubicin], idarubicin [Idamycin, Zavedos], mitoxantrone [Novantrone])	Acute myocarditis ± pericarditis causing CHF, delayed-onset (up to 20+ yr after treatment) cardiomyopathy with chronic CHF. Early detection of falling ejection fraction can prevent dysfunction	6%–57%, dose dependent; <5% with mitoxantrone
Busulfan (Myleran)	Endocardial fibrosis, cardiac tamponade	1%–2%
Capecitabine (Xeloda)	Ischemia, arrhythmias, especially in those with cardiac history	3%–6%
Cisplatin (Platinol)	Ischemia, hypertension, CHF	5%–15%
Cyclophosphamide, CTX (Cytoxan)	Acute myocarditis, acute/subacute CHF; usually transient and reversible	5%–10%
Cytosine arabinoside (Cytarabine, Aca-C, Cytosar)	Pericarditis, CHF	Rare
Fluorouracil, 5-FU (Adrucil)	Ischemia, arrhythmias, MI, cardiogenic shock	1%–8%, ↑ if cardiac history
Ifosfamide (Ifex)	Myocarditis, CHF, arrhythmias; generally transient and reversible	1%–5%
Mitomycin (Mutamycin)	LV dysfunction, CHF	1%–5%
Paclitaxel (Taxol)	Acute or subacute arrhythmias, hypotension, ischemia, hypertension	<1%–5%
Vinca alkaloids: vinblastine (Velban, Velsar), vincristine (Oncovin, Vincasar, Vincrex), and vindesine (Eldisine, Fildesin)	Ischemia, MI, autonomic cardioneuropathy	5%–25%
Biological Agents		
Interferons	Hypotension, arrhythmias, LV dysfunction, ischemia	5%–10%
Interleukins (IL-2, denileukin diftitox [Ontak])	Capillary leak syndrome, hypotension, arrhythmias	1%–15%
Monoclonal Antibodies		
Alemtuzumab (Campath)	Hypotension, CHF	6%–17%
Bevacizumab (Avastin)	Hypertension (may be severe), CHF, DVT	7%–10%
Cetuximab (Erbitux)	Hypotension	Rare
Gemtuzumab (Mylotarg)	Hypertension, hypotension	8%–9% each
Ibritumomab (Zevalin)	Hypotension, chest pain, arrhythmias	1%–5%
Rituximab (Rituxan)	Hypotension, angioedema, arrhythmias, hypertension	1%–5%
Trastuzumab (Herceptin)	LV dysfunction, CHF	3%–5%
Miscellaneous		
All-*trans*-retinoic acid, ATRA (Tretinoin)	Hypotension, CHF	1%–5%
Arsenic trioxide (Trisenox)	Q–T prolongation, tachycardia	8%–55%
Etoposide (VP-16)	Hypotension, especially with rapid infusion	1%–4%
Imatinib (Gleevec)	Pericardial effusion, CHF, edema	6%–10%
Pentostatin (Nipent)	CHF	1%–5%
Thalidomide (Thalomid)	Edema, hypotension, bradycardia, DVT	1%–5%
Radiation therapy to chest		

Continued

TABLE 4-19: Cardiotoxicity Associated With Cancer Treatments—Cont'd

Cancer Treatment	Notable Cardiovascular Side Effects	Incidence
	Pericarditis with effusion, which is usually delayed, possible pericardial tamponade or constriction; premature CAD and MI; valve disease, myocardial disease, arrhythmias and conduction disturbances	2%–12%, volume and dose dependent
Hematopoietic stem cell transplantation	Acute arrhythmias, conduction disturbances, pericardial effusion; late-onset cardiomyopathies; usually related to prior chemotherapy or drugs used to prepare for HSCT	Up to 57%

CAD, Coronary artery disease; CHF, congestive heart failure; DVT, deep venous thrombosis; HSCT, hematopoietic stem cell transplantation; LV, left ventricular; MI, myocardial infarction.

extent of disease. Fortunately, modern treatment techniques instituted in 1985, particularly for HD, have drastically reduced cardiac and pulmonary complications.

- Radiation-induced pulmonary toxicity is usually related to the volume of lung tissue radiated, the total dose of radiation, and the dose per treatment fraction (see Table 4-18).[2,213] The advent of three-dimensional treatment planning has permitted higher radiation doses to be delivered to the tumor while sparing surrounding normal tissue and is associated with a marked reduction in pulmonary toxicity.
  - ▸ Acute radiation pneumonitis, which usually develops 4 to 6 weeks after XRT and is manifested clinically as a nonproductive cough, dyspnea (often at rest), and fever, occurs in 5% to 15% of patients who receive high-dose external beam radiation for lung cancer, 3% of those treated for HD with radiation alone and 11% if combined treatment with chemotherapy, and less than 1% of women treated for breast cancer using breast XRT as part of a breast-conserving approach.[2,38] Most patients require no treatment and show complete resolution within 6 to 8 weeks, but a few patients develop severe pneumonitis requiring hospitalization and aggressive supportive care.
  - ▸ Late radiation fibrosis may develop after radiation pneumonitis and also in patients without prior pneumonitis. It evolves over 6 to 24 months and then usually remains stable after 2 years, being asymptomatic in many patients or manifested as various degrees of dyspnea. On the rare occasions that radiation fibrosis involves a large volume of lung, cor pulmonale and respiratory failure can develop.
  - ▸ Radiation-related cryptogenic organizing pneumonia (COP, formerly called bronchiolitis obliterans with organizing pneumonia, BOOP) sometimes occurs after chest irradiation, most commonly in women treated for breast cancer.
  - ▸ Research regarding medications that can reduce the occurrence of radiation pneumonitis is underway.
- XRT to the chest can damage all structures of the heart (see Table 4-19), with the highest risk occurring in survivors of pediatric HD.[38,237] Late sequelae, which may not become clinically apparent for up to 20 or more years after treatment, often involve more than one cardiac structure in affected individuals,

so that a combination of conditions occurs. An estimate of the aggregate incidence of radiation-induced cardiac dysfunction is between 10% and 30% by 5 to 10 years posttreatment, although asymptomatic abnormalities of the heart muscle, valves, pericardium, and conduction system, and of the vascular system, are detected in up to 88% of patients.[38]

- ▸ Factors that increase the risk of cardiac sequelae after mediastinal irradiation include cotreatment with anthracycline chemotherapy, location of tumor close to the heart border, age less than 18 years at the time of treatment, the presence of cardiac risk factors or preexisting cardiac disease, treatment occurring more than 10 years earlier, and a number of radiation factors (use of orthovoltage radiation [mostly before the 1970s], increased volume of irradiated heart, total dose to the heart exceeding 30 Gy or a daily dose fraction greater than 2 Gy/d, and absence of subcarinal blocking).
- ▸ Cardiotoxicity manifests as pericarditis with pericardial effusion in 2% to 5% of patients receiving modern XRT for HD, which usually has a delayed onset (4 mo to years after treatment). Approximately 10% to 20% of patients with pericardial effusion develop tamponade and require pericardiocentesis.[237] In addition, about 20% of patients progress within 5 to 10 years to develop symptomatic pericardial constriction requiring pericardiectomy.
- ▸ Radiation-induced or accelerated CAD and MI, which may be silent due to radiation-induced nerve damage, are becoming more prevalent as survival times increase, especially in those treated before 1985, when modern XRT techniques were initiated. Current treatment techniques are associated with an incidence of CAD of 12% with a death rate due to MI or sudden death of 4.7%, with those receiving higher doses of XRT being most at risk.[237]
- ▸ Other late cardiac sequelae that are occasionally seen after treatment for HD include valvular abnormalities (usually mild aortic insufficiency), myocardial disease with diastolic and systolic dysfunction, and arrhythmias and conduction disturbances, particularly AV block due to fibrosis of the conduction system.

▸ Patients treated for head and neck cancer have an increased risk of developing carotid artery stenosis and stroke.

Biological Agents

Recombinant technology has stimulated the development of biological response modifiers that enhance the body's defenses against malignant cells; these include monoclonal antibodies, interleukins, interferons, and tumor necrosis factor. Most of these biological agents have some adverse cardiovascular and pulmonary effects.

Interferons

Interferons (IFNs; α, β, and γ) are used in a wide variety of malignant, idiopathic, infectious, and inflammatory conditions.

- Administration of IFNs is associated with a variety of pulmonary reactions[36,67]:
  ▸ Severe exacerbation of bronchospasm in patients with preexisting asthma (IFN-α)
  ▸ A granulomatous reaction similar to sarcoidosis (IFN-α)
  ▸ Interstitial lung disease, possibly cryptogenic organizing pneumonia, developing weeks to months after initiation of treatment
  ▸ Severe radiation pneumonitis with multimodality therapy (IFN-γ)
- Adverse cardiovascular effects are sometimes noted with IFNs.[237,239]
  ▸ Acute toxicity appears as hypotension with compensatory tachycardia or, more rarely, as hypertension. In severe cases, angina and MI have been reported.
  ▸ There are rare reports of cardiomyopathy.

Interleukin-2

Interleukin-2 (IL-2) is used, sometimes in combination with IFN-α, in the treatment of a number of malignancies. Cardiovascular and pulmonary toxicities limit the doses that can be administered.

- Pulmonary toxicity poses a significant risk for patients receiving IL-2, particularly high-dose regimens, which frequently require intensive care unit support.[36,159]
  ▸ Acute toxicity is manifested as noncardiac pulmonary edema resulting from vascular leakage as well as pulmonary edema due to myocardial depression.
  ▸ Approximately 20% of patients receiving high-dose IL-2 develop respiratory distress and 5% to 10% require mechanical ventilation.[159]
- Cardiovascular toxicity is common with IL-2[237,239]:
  ▸ Vascular leak syndrome induces hypotension, which provokes compensatory increases in HR and the cardiac index.
  ▸ Severe acute toxicity can result in arrhythmias, myocardial ischemia and MI, myocarditis, and cardiomyopathy.

Monoclonal Antibodies

Monoclonal antibodies (MAbs) target specific receptors on cancer cells, providing direct cellular effects or carrying substances, such as radioactive isotopes, toxins, and antineoplastic agents, to destroy the cells. MAbs can be formed from mouse cell lines (agents ending in "omab"), human cell lines (agents ending in "zumab"), or genetically combined mouse and human genes (chimeric MAbs ending in "ximab"). They are used as single agents or in combination with chemotherapy. Their value in treating other disorders, such as autoimmune diseases, is also being studied.

- Pulmonary toxicity has been reported for most MAbs (see Table 4-18).[41,42,67,133]
  ▸ Trastuzumab (Herceptin), which is used in the treatment of HER-2–positive metastatic breast cancer, can produce severe pulmonary complications, including pulmonary infiltrates, ARDS, pneumonitis, pulmonary edema, and pleural effusion, occurring during or after infusion.
  ▸ Rituximab (Rituxan) used to treat CD20+ non-Hodgkin's lymphoma, as well as some autoimmune disorders, occasionally causes lung injury, which usually appears as dyspnea, cough, and bronchospasm. More rarely, severe lung toxicity manifests as cryptogenic organizing pneumonia, pneumonitis, and interstitial lung disease, which can be fatal.
  ▸ Gemtuzumab (Mylotarg), indicated for the treatment of CD33+ acute myelogenous (or myeloid) leukemia in first relapse, sometimes results in pulmonary toxicity, with dyspnea and pneumonia, and less frequently pulmonary infiltrates, pleural effusion, noncardiac pulmonary edema, pulmonary insufficiency, ARDS, and death.
  ▸ Bevacizumab (Avastin) is associated with an increased incidence of hemoptysis when used to treat non–small cell lung cancer. Patients treated for other cancers have a higher incidence of hematemesis.
  ▸ Ibritumomab (Zevalin) can induce an acute hypersensitivity pneumonitis, while tositumomab (Bexxar) can cause subacute hypersensitivity pneumonitis and bronchospasm.
  ▸ Some of the MAbs are associated with marked neutropenia (e.g., alemtuzumab, gemtuzumab, ibritumomab, and tositumomab), which increases the risk of pneumonia.
- Cardiotoxicity is often seen with MAbs (Table 4-19).[41,42,133,237,239]
  ▸ Infusion reactions, which typically occur during the initial infusion, are common with MAbs. They are usually mild to moderate, with hypotension, fever and chills, dyspnea, and hypoxia resulting from the massive release of cytokines. On rare occasions, severe reactions occur and can be fatal (gemtuzumab [Mylotarg], ibritumomab [Zevalin], and tositumomab [Bexxar]).
  ▸ Trastuzumab (Herceptin) is associated with myocardial dysfunction, which is usually asymptomatic and reversible, when used as a single agent. Concurrent use with anthracyclines greatly increases the risk of cardiomyopathy and CHF, which may not be reversible. Other risk factors include concurrent or prior treatment with cyclophosphamide and those with a history of cardiac dysfunction.
  ▸ Rituximab (Rituxin) occasionally induces angioedema and arrhythmias
  ▸ Bevacizumab (Avastin) treatment is associated with increased incidences of hypertension, cerebral and cardiac ischemic events, and CHF.
  ▸ Gemtuzumab also provokes hypertension in some patients.
  ▸ Ibritumomab (Zevalin) causes ischemia and arrhythmias in a small percentage of patients.

▸ Because MAb treatment is relatively new, there is concern that an increase in long-term cardiovascular sequelae may be seen over time.

Hematopoietic Stem Cell Transplantation

Hematopoietic stem cell transplantation (HSCT) is used for the treatment of hematologic malignancies, as well as for some solid tumors, nonmalignant hematologic disorders, and autoimmune diseases. Hematopoietic stem cells (HSCs) can be harvested either directly from the bone marrow (i.e., bone marrow transplantation, BMT) or from the peripheral venous system after high-dose treatment with recombinant human granulocyte colony-stimulating factor (rhG-CSF), which results in the mobilization of large numbers of hematopoietic progenitor and stem cells from bone marrow sites into the bloodstream (peripheral blood stem cell transplantation, PBSCT).

For patients with malignancies, HSCT permits the administration of intense myeloablative doses of chemotherapy and radiation therapy capable of eradicating malignant cells. Then, infusion of HSCs obtained earlier from the same patient (autologous HSCT) or from a compatible donor (allogeneic HSCT) "rescues" the patient from the ensuing bone marrow aplasia. Bone marrow– or peripheral blood–derived allogeneic HSCT from an HLA-identical sibling or matched unrelated donor cures more than half of patients with severe aplastic anemia, thalassemia major, congenital immunodeficiency diseases, and genetic metabolic disorders.

For hematologic malignancies, allogeneic HSCT is usually preferred because of the absence of residual malignant cells that could be present in autologous HSCT and the therapeutic immunologic effect mediated by donor lymphocytes and natural killer cells (graft-versus-tumor [GvT] response). Sibling donors have a one-in-four chance of being sufficiently matched with the recipient at the major histocompatibility complex loci to avoid excessive graft-versus-host disease (GvHD) but not so closely matched (as in identical twins) that a GvT response is precluded (in which case the relapse rate is increased). PBSCT is generally preferred over allogeneic BMT because of slightly faster engraftment and less acute GvHD.[103a,163a]

The process of HSCT involves three stages: conditioning of the recipient, infusion of the HSCs, and engraftment. Conditioning, which prepares the patient for transplantation by eradicating as many malignant cells as possible and providing immunosuppression so the allograft will take, usually involves high-dose chemotherapy, often with cyclophosphamide and busulfan, with or without total body irradiation (TBI).

Pulmonary and cardiac toxicity, which are common, significantly limit the short- and long-term success of HSCT. Because the agents used for conditioning are responsible for much of the acute and late cardiopulmonary complications, reduced-intensity conditioning regimens are being investigated, some of which appear to be similarly effective and, it is hoped, will prove to be less toxic.

- Pulmonary toxicity is the major cause of morbidity and mortality after HSC, with specific complications tending to occur within three well-defined periods that correspond with the state of immune reconstitution after transplantation.[47a,143b,227,240]
  - ▸ Neutropenic phase complications occur within the first month of transplantation, before engraftment takes place.
    - ⊙ Pulmonary edema develops in up to 65% of patients because of infusion of large volumes of fluid combined with cardiac and renal impairment caused by chemotherapy and vascular leakage.
    - ⊙ Pulmonary toxicity due to chemotherapy is most commonly manifested as inflammatory or hypersensitivity pneumonitis and noncardiac pulmonary edema.
    - ⊙ Bacterial, fungal, and viral pneumonia are common complications.
    - ⊙ Diffuse alveolar hemorrhage is seen in 5% of patients, particularly those receiving autologous BMT, and has a mortality rate of 80%.[240]
  - ▸ Early-phase complications appear between days 31 and 100 after transplantation, when neutropenia is resolving but humoral and cell-mediated immunity are still impaired.
    - ⊙ Cytomegalovirus (CMV) infection occurs in 10% to 40% of patients after BMT, usually as a result of reactivation of the latent virus from the recipient or the donor.[240] Pneumocystis pneumonia (PCP) is now a rare complication, occurring mainly in patients who are unable to tolerate or are noncompliant with PCP prophylaxis.
    - ⊙ Symptomatic radiation pneumonitis after TBI develops in approximately 7% of patients, typically 1 to 3 months after treatment, and is usually mild.
    - ⊙ Idiopathic pneumonia syndrome is manifested as bilateral diffuse pulmonary infiltrates, fever, dyspnea, and hypoxemia where an infectious agent cannot be identified by bronchoalveolar lavage (BAL). Its estimated incidence is 10% to 17% with an overall mortality of 70% to 90%.[240]
  - ▸ Late pulmonary complications, which appear more than 100 days after transplantation, tend to be noninfectious.
    - ⊙ Bronchiolitis obliterans is an obstructive airway disease (see page 81), which occurs in up to 10% of patients after allogeneic BMT, especially in long-term survivors with GvHD, and carries a poor prognosis, with a mortality rate of about 40%.[47a,227] Delayed pulmonary toxicity syndrome, manifested as dyspnea, cough, and fever, can develop months to years after autologous transplants that involved high-dose chemotherapy. Treatment with corticosteroids is usually effective.
    - ⊙ Cryptogenic organizing pneumonia is a restrictive disease characterized by patchy pulmonary infiltrates due to an inflammatory alveolar-filling process that is occasionally seen after BMT (more often allogeneic and in those with GvHD).
  - ▸ Respiratory muscle weakness has been noted in a significant percentage of patients undergoing pulmonary function testing after HSCT.
- Cardiotoxicity is usually related to previous chemotherapy or that used as part of the HSCT or BMT conditioning regimen.[111,206]
  - ▸ Acute toxicity is usually manifested by ECG abnormalities, such as arrhythmias and conduction disturbances, and pericardial effusion, which are usually asymptomatic but occasionally cause more serious problems.
  - ▸ Some patients develop chemotherapy-induced cardiomyopathies, which may not become clinically apparent for many years to decades after treatment.

▸ A study involving the longitudinal evaluation of cardiopulmonary performance during exercise after BMT in children revealed that maximal cardiac index, oxygen consumption, work performed, and ventilatory threshold were significantly lower than in age-matched, healthy control subjects.[111] Whereas the percentage of predicted $\dot{V}_{O_2\,max}$, maximal work performed, and ventilatory threshold increased over time for most patients, maximal cardiac index did not, providing evidence of subclinical myocardial dysfunction.

Supportive Therapies

Some of the treatments used to support patients with cancer during treatment also have the possibility of inducing cardiovascular and pulmonary complications.

- The *hematopoietic growth factors,* granulocyte and granulocyte-macrophage colony-stimulating factors (G/GM-CSFs) (e.g., Filgrastim), used to facilitate neutropenia recovery and prevent infection after high-dose chemotherapy and stem cell transplantation are associated with some cardiopulmonary toxicity.
  ▸ In patients with pulmonary infiltrates during neutropenia, the prophylactic use of G/GM-CSF to facilitate neutropenia recovery after cytotoxic chemotherapy carries a risk of respiratory deterioration due to acute lung injury or ARDS.[129]
  ▸ Cardiovascular complications include arterial thrombosis and the vascular leak syndrome, which is seen with GM-CSF.
- Platelet and blood transfusions sometimes cause pulmonary edema.

Clinical Implications for Physical Therapy

On the basis of the information presented in this last section, it should be apparent that many patients with a wide variety of primary medical problems can develop cardiopulmonary dysfunction, although most will not be formally diagnosed with it. The symptoms of dysfunction are often nonspecific, such as shortness of breath, lightheadedness, and fatigue, or there may be no symptoms at all, as in hypertension. Furthermore, many patients will not complain of symptoms of exercise intolerance because they have gradually limited their physical activity in order to avoid discomfort.

The general implications of all these diseases are similar to those already presented in this chapter. More specific recommendations can be found under other diagnoses applicable to a particular patient, such as HTN, CAD, or RLD.

- To determine whether an individual has any cardiopulmonary dysfunction, the cardiovascular and pulmonary systems must be assessed, both at rest and during activity, during the PT evaluation for any patient with a history of any of these diseases or disorders, as well as many others not mentioned. In practice, this translates into a need to perform physiological monitoring of all adult and many pediatric patients.
  ▸ Because most patients with chronic illnesses are deconditioned and many of those with diagnoses presented in this section have some degree of cardiopulmonary involvement, exercise responses are often abnormal (see page 294).
  ▸ Patients with autonomic dysfunction are more likely to have elevated resting HR, orthostatic hypotension, blunted BP responses to exercise, and possibly postexercise hypotension.

- PTs should be aware of any medications being taken that may have adverse effects on exercise responses and tolerance (see pages 101, 107, 112, and 114 and Chapter 5, page 214).
- In accordance with public health recommendations (see page 301), endurance and resistance exercise training should be included in the physical therapy treatment plan for every patient who is not already performing regular aerobic exercise, unless they have a condition that would be adversely affected by exercise (e.g., acute illness with cardiovascular or pulmonary system instability, and some debilitating neuromuscular diseases).[104,166] Endurance exercise facilitates the other components of almost every physical therapy program and offers a number of additional health benefits as well (see Chapter 6, page 294).
  ▸ Because of its role in reducing a number of CVD risk factors, aerobic exercise training is recommended for patients with any disease or disorder that is associated with increased risk of atherosclerosis, myocardial ischemia, or MI (e.g., autoimmune rheumatic diseases, the inflammatory myopathies, ischemic CVA, sickle cell disease, and HIV; and also for survivors of cancer).
  ▸ Aerobic exercise training in individuals with CVA,[71,188] SCI,[66,116] MS,[192] or facioscapulohumeral and myotonic muscular dystrophy,[55] results in significant improvements in exercise capacity, workload, and exercise time, among other parameters.
  ▸ Increased levels of physical activity during and after cancer treatment have been shown to reduce fatigue, enhance physical performance, and improve quality of life.[85,158a,231a] Resistance training likely helps to increase muscle function, lean tissue mass, and bone mineral density. There is also evidence that regular physical activity improves survival in patients with breast and colorectal cancers.[229]
- Resistance training is also recommended for all adults to improve muscle strength and endurance, functional status, and quality of life (see Chapter 7, page 308).
- Breathing exercises for improved ventilation, control, and strength and inspiratory muscle training are valuable for patients with many disorders that have associated respiratory muscle dysfunction, unless respiratory muscle fatigue is so severe that rest is required to avoid additional muscle damage.
- Other interventions that can assist patients with neurologic and neuromuscular disorders prevent accumulation of secretions with resultant atelectasis, pneumonia, or bronchiectasis include positioning, assisted cough techniques, an insufflator-exsufflator, glossopharyngeal breathing, inspiratory hold, stacked breathing, and other airway clearance techniques (see Chapter 7, page 311).

REFERENCES

1. Abernathy RP, Black DR. Healthy body weights: an alternative perspective. *Am J Clin Nutr.* 1996;63(suppl):448S-451S.
2. Abratt RP, Morgan GW, Silvestri G, et al. Pulmonary complications of radiation therapy. *Clin Chest Med.* 2004;25:167-177.
2a. Adams GR, Vaziri ND. Skeletal muscle dysfunction in chronic renal failure: effects of exercise. *Am J Physiol Renal Physiol.* 2006;290:F753-F761.
3. Agostino C, Trentin L, Facco M, et al. New aspects of hypersensitivity pneumonitis. *Curr Opin Pulm Med.* 2004;10:378-382.

4. Alberti KGMM, Zimmet P, Shaw J. Metabolic syndrome: a new world-wide definition. A consensus statement from the International Diabetes Federation. *Diabet Med.* 2006;23:469-480.

5. Aldrich D, Hunt DP. When can the patient with deep venous thrombosis begin to ambulate? *Phys Ther.* 2004;84:268-273.

6. Alexander CM, Landsman PB, Teutsch SM, et al. for the Third National Health and Nutrition Survery (NHANES III) and the National Cholesterol Education Program (NCEP): NECP-defined metabolic syndrome, diabetes, and prevalence of coronary heart disease among NHANES III participants age 50 years and older. *Diabetes.* 2003;52:1210-1214.

7. Al-Shirawi N, Al-Jahdali HH, Al Shimemeri A. Pathogenesis, etiology, and treatment of bronchiectasis. *Ann Thorac Med.* 2006;1:41-51.

8. American College of Sports Medicine. Position stand: exercise and hypertension. *Med Sci Sports Exerc.* 2004;36:533-553.

9. American College of Sports Medicine. *ASCM's Guidelines for Exercise Testing and Prescription.* 7th ed. Philadelphia: Lippincott Williams & Wilkins; 2006.

10. American College of Sports Medicine. Position stand: appropriate intervention strategies for weight loss and prevention of weight regain for adults. *Med Sci Sports Exerc.* 2001;33:2145-2156.

11. American Heart Association. Heart Disease and Stroke Statistics—2007 Update. *Circulation.* 2007;115:e69-e171.

11a. American Thoracic Society/European Respiratory Society. Skeletal muscle dysfunction in chronic obstructive pulmonary disease. *Am J Respir Crit Care Med.* 1999;159:S1-S40.

12. Arauz-Pacheco C, Parrott MA, Raskin P. The treatment of hypertension in adult patients with diabetes. *Diabetes Care.* 2002;25:134-147, Technical review.

13. Aurigemma GP, Gaasch WH. Diastolic heart failure. *N Engl J Med.* 2004;351:1097-1105.

14. Autar R. Nursing assessment of clients at risk of deep vein thrombosis (DVT): the Autar DVT Scale. *J Adv Nurs.* 1996;23:763-770.

15. Balasubramanian VP, Varkey B. Chronic obstructive pulmonary disease: effects beyond the lungs. *Curr Opin Pulm Med.* 2006;12:106-112.

16. Bansilal S, Farkouh ME, Fuster V. Role of insulin resistance and hyperglycemia in the development of atherosclerosis. *Am J Cardiol.* 2007;99 (suppl):6B-14B.

17. Barker AF. Bronchiectasis. *N Engl J Med.* 2002;346:1383-1393.

18. Bassuk SS, Manson JE. Epidemiological evidence for the role of physical activity in reducing risk of type 2 diabetes and cardiovascular disease. *J Appl Physiol.* 2005;99:1193-1204.

19. Baumgartner I, Schainfeld R, Graziani L. Management of peripheral vascular disease. *Annu Rev Med.* 2005;56:249-272.

20. Baydur A, Layne E, Aral H, et al. Long-term non-invasive ventilation in the community for patients with musculoskeletal disorders: 46 year experience and review. *Thorax.* 2000;55:4-11.

20a. Bernard AW, Yasin Z, Venkat A. Acute chest syndrome in sickle cell disease. *Hosp Physician.* 2007;43:15-23, 44.

21. Berry C, Tardif J-C, Bourassa MG. Coronary heart disease in patients with diabetes. I. Recent advances in prevention and noninvasive management. *J Am Coll Cardiol.* 2007;49:631-642.

22. Best PJM, Reddan DN, Berger PB, et al. Cardiovascular disease and chronic kidney disease: insights and updates. *Am Heart J.* 2004;148:230-242.

23. Bjarnason-Wehrens B, Grande G, Loewel H, et al. Gender-specific issues in cardiac rehabilitation: do women with ischaemic heart disease need specially tailored programmes? *Eur J Cardiovasc Prev Rehabil.* 2007;14:163-171.

23a. Blann AD, Lip YH. Venous thromboembolism. *BMJ* 2006;332:215-219.

24. Boulé NG, Haddad E, Kenny GP, et al. Effects of exercise on glycemic control and body mass in type 2 diabetes mellitus: a meta-analysis of controlled clinical trials. *JAMA.* 2001;286:1218-1227.

25. Boulé NG, Kenny GP, Haddad E, et al. Meta-analysis of the effect of structured exercise training on cardiorespiratory fitness in type 2 diabetes mellitus. *Diabetologia.* 2003;46:1071-1081.

26. Boulé NG, Weisnagel SJ, Larkka TA, et al. Effects of exercise training on glucose homeostasis. *Diabetes Care.* 2005;28:120-126.

27. Bourke SJ. Interstitial lung disease: progress and problems. Review. *Postgrad Med J.* 2006;82:494-499.

28. Boyton RJ. Infectious lung complications in patients with HIV/AIDS. *Curr Opin Pulm Med.* 2005;11:203-207.

29. Brook RD, Kramer MB, Blaxall BC, et al. Nonsteroidal anti-inflammatory drugs and hypertension. *J Clin Hypertens.* 2000;2:319-323.

30. Brubaker PH, Joo K-C, Stewart KP, et al. Chronotropic incompetence and its contribution to exercise intolerance in older heart failure patients. *J Cardiopulm Rehabil.* 2006;26:86-89.

31. Bruder D, Srikiatkhachorn A, Enelow R. Cellular immunity and lung injury in respiratory virus infection. Review. *Viral Immunol.* 2006;19:147-155.

32. Bugiardini R, Bairey Merz CN. Angina with "normal" coronary arteries: a changing philosophy. *JAMA.* 2005;293:477-484.

33. Burke AP, Virmani R. Pathophysiology of acute myocardial infarction. *Med Clin North Am.* 2007;91:553-572.

34. Deleted in pages.

35. Cahalin LP, Ferreira DC, Yamada S, et al. Review of the effects of resistance training in patients with chronic heart failure: potential effects upon the muscle hypothesis. *Cardiopulm Phys Ther J.* 2006;17(1):15-28.

36. Camus P, Fanton A, Bonniaud P, et al. Interstitial lung disease induced by drugs and radiation. *Respiration.* 2004;71:301-326.

37. Caprini JA. Thrombosis risk assessment as a guide to quality patient care. *Dis Mon.* 2005;51:70-78.

38. Carver JR, Shapiro CL, Ng A, et al. American Society of Clinical Oncology clinical review on the ongoing care of adult cancer survivors: cardiac and pulmonary late effects. *J Clin Oncol.* 2007;25:3391-4008.

39. Casaburi R. Skeletal muscle dysfunction in chronic obstructive pulmonary disease. *Med Sci Sports Exerc.* 2001;33:S662-670.

40. Celli BR, Cote CG, Marin JM, et al. The body-mass index, airflow obstruction, dyspnea, and exercise capacity index in chronic obstructive pulmonary disease. *N Engl J Med.* 2004;350:1005-1012.

41. Cersosimo RJ. Monoclonal antibodies in the treatment of cancer, part 1. *Am J Health Syst Pharm.* 2003;60:1531-1548.

42. Cersosimo RJ. Monoclonal antibodies in the treatment of cancer, part 2. *Am J Health Syst Pharm.* 2003;60:1631-1643.

43. Chang J, Han J, Kim DW, et al. Bronchiolitis obliterans organizing pneumonia: clinicopathologic review of a series of 45 Korean patients including rapidly progressive form. *J Korean Med Sci.* 2002;17:179-186.

44. Cheema BSB, Singh MAF. Exercise training in patients receiving maintenance hemodialysis: a systematic review of clinical trials. *Am J Nephrol.* 2005;25:352-364.

45. Chimowitz MI, Mancini GBJ. Asymptomatic coronary artery disease in patients with stroke: prevalence, prognosis, diagnosis, and treatment. *Curr Conc Cerebrovasc Dis Stroke.* 1991;26:23-27.

46. Chobanian AV, Bakris GL, Black HR, et al. Seventh Report of the Joint National Committee on Prevention, Detection, Evaluation, and Treatment of High Blood Pressure. *Hypertension.* 2003;42:1206-1252.

47. Christensen CC, Ryg MS, Edvardsen A, et al. Relationship between exercise desaturation and pulmonary haemodynamics in COPD patients. *Eur Respir J.* 2004;24:580-586.

47a. Clark JG, Crawford SW, Madtes DK, et al. Obstructive lung disease after allogeneic marrow transplantation: clinical presentation and course. *Ann Intern Med.* 1989;111:368-376.

48. Clyne N. The importance of exercise training in predialysis patients with chronic kidney disease. *Clin Nephrol.* 2004;61(suppl 1):S10-13.

49. Cockcroft JR, Wilkinson IB, Evans M, et al. Pulse pressure predicts cardiovascular risk in patients with type 2 diabetes mellitus. *Am J Hypertens.* 2005;18:1463-1467.

50. Cooper CB. Exercise in chronic pulmonary disease: aerobic exercise prescription. *Med Sci Sports Exerc.* 2001;33(7 suppl):S671-679.

50a. Cooper RS, Durazo-Arvizu R. Hypertension detection and control: population policy implications. *Cardiol Clin.* 2002;20:187-194.

51. Copley JB, Rosario R. Hypertension: a review and rationale of treatment. *Dis Mon.* 2005;51:548-614.

52. Cornelisson VA, Fagard RH. Effect of resistance training on resting blood pressure: a meta-analysis of randomized controlled trials. *J Hypertens.* 2005;23:251-259.

53. Covitz W, Espeland M, Gallagher D, et al. The heart in sickle cell anemia: the Cooperative Study of Sickle Cell Disease (CSSCD). *Chest.* 1995;108:1214-1219.

54. Crestani B. The respiratory system in connective tissue disorders. *Allergy.* 2005;60:715-734.

55. Cup EH, Pieterse AJ, ten Broek-Pastoor JM, et al. Exercise therapy and other types of physical therapy for patients with neuromuscular diseases: a systematic review. *Arch Phys Med.* 2007;88:1452-1464.

56. Curioni CC, Lourenco PM. Long-term weight loss after diet and exercise: a systematic review. *Int J Obesity.* 2005;29:1168-1174.

57. Dall'Ago P, Chiappa GRS, Guths H, et al. Inspiratory muscle training in patients with heart failure and inspiratory muscle weakness: a randomized study. *J Am Coll Cardiol*. 2006;47:757-763.

58. Daul AE, Schäfers RF, Daul K, et al. Exercise during hemodialysis. *Clin Nephrol*. 2004;61(suppl 1):S26-S30.

59. Davis G, Patel JA, Gagne DJ. Pulmonary considerations in obesity and the bariatric surgical patient. *Med Clin North Am*. 2007;91:433-442.

60. Davis GS. Mineral-induced lung disease in modern industry. 1. Pneumoconiosis caused by particles and fibers. *Clin Pulm Med*. 2006;13: 91-102.

61. Davis GS. Mineral-induced lung disease in modern industry. 2. Sensitizing metals. *Clin Pulm Med*. 2006;13:103-110.

62. Deedwania PC, Fonseca VA. Diabetes, prediabetes, and cardiovascular risk: shifting the paradigm. Review. *Am J Med*. 2005;118:939-947.

63. Deeg MA. Basic approach to managing hyperglycemia for the nonendocrinologist. *Am J Cardiol*. 2005;96(suppl):37E-40E.

64. Deligiannis A. Cardiac adaptations following exercise training in hemodialysis patients. *Clin Nephrol*. 2004;61(suppl 1):S39-S45.

65. Dellefave LM, McNally EM. Cardiomyopathy in neuromuscular disorders. *Prog Pediatr Cardiol*. 2007;24:35-46.

66. Devillard X, Rimaud D, Roche F, et al. Effects of training programs for spinal cord injury. *Ann Readapt Med Phys*. 2007;50:490-498.

67. Dimopoulou I, Bamias A, Lyberopoulos P, et al. Pulmonary toxicity from novel antineoplastic agents. *Ann Oncol*. 2006;17:372-379.

68. Donnelly JE, Jacobsen DJ, Heelan KS, et al. The effects of 18 months of intermittent vs continuous exercise on aerobic capacity, body weight and composition, and metabolic fitness in previously sedentary, moderately obese females. *Int J Obesity*. 2000;24:566-572.

69. Dopp JM, Morgan BJ. Cardiovascular consequences of sleep-disordered breathing. *J Cardiopulm Rehabil*. 2006;26:123-130.

70. Dowdy DW, Eid MP, Dennison CR. Quality of life after acute respiratory distress syndrome: a meta-analysis. *Intensive Care Med*. 2006;32:1115-1124.

71. Eldar R, Marincek C. Physical activity for elderly persons with neurological impairment: a review. *Scand J Rehabil Med*. 2000;32:99-103.

72. Emtner M, Porszasz J, Burns M, et al. Benefits of supplemental oxygen in exercise training in nonhypoxemic chronic obstructive pulmonary disease patients. *Am J Respir Crit Care Med*. 2003;168:1034-1042.

73. Epler GR. Bronchiolitis obliterans organizing pneumonia. *Arch Intern Med*. 2001;161:158-164.

74. Ernst E. Complementary/alternative medicine for hypertension: a mini-review. *Wien Med Wochenschr*. 2005;155:386-391.

75. Estenne M, Maurer JR, Boehler A, et al. Bronchiolitis obliterans syndrome 2001: an update of the diagnostic criteria. *J Heart Lung Transplant*. 2002;21:297-310.

76. Evans N, Forsyth E. End-stage renal disease in people with type 2 diabetes: systemic manifestations and exercise implications. *Phys Ther*. 2004;84:454-463.

77. Fagard RH. Exercise characteristics and the blood pressure response to dynamic physical training. *Med Sci Sports Exerc*. 2001;33(suppl 6):S484-S492.

78. Fletcher GF, Balady GJ, Amsterdam ES, et al. Exercise standards for testing and training: a statement for healthcare professionals from the American Heart Association. *Circulation*. 2001;104:1694-1740.

79. Fonarow GC. An approach to heart failure and diabetes mellitus. *Am J Cardiol*. 2005;96(suppl):47E-52E.

80. Franklin SS, Larson MG, Khan SA, et al. Does the relation of blood pressure to coronary heart disease risk change with aging: the Framingham Heart Study. *Circulation*. 2001;103:1245-1249.

81. Freeman V, Rotimi C, Cooper R. Hypertension prevalence, awareness, treatment, and control among African Americans in the 1990s: estimates from the Maywood Cardiovascular Survey. *Prev Med*. 1996;12:177-185.

82. Frishman WH. Effects of nonsteroidal anti-inflammatory drug therapy on blood pressure and peripheral edema. *Am J Cardiol*. 2002;89:18D-25D.

83. Fugimoto K, Matsuzawa Y, Yamaguchi S, et al. Benefits of oxygen on exercise performance and pulmonary hemodynamics in patients with COPD with mild hypoxemia. *Chest*. 2002;122:457-1463.

84. Fuhrman I, Krause R. Principles of exercising in patients with chronic kidney disease, on dialysis, and for kidney transplant recipients. *Clin Nephrol*. 2004;61(suppl 1):S14-S25.

85. Gallagher D, Heymsfield SB, Heo M, et al. Healthy percentage body fat ranges: an approach for developing guidelines based on body mass index. *Am J Clin Nutr*. 2000;72:694-701.

86. Galvão DA, Newton RU. Review of exercise intervention studies in cancer patients. *J Clin Oncol*. 2005;23:899-909.

87. Gami AS, Witt BJ, Howard DE, et al. Metabolic syndrome risk and incident cardiovascular events and death: a systematic review and meta-analysis of longitudinal studies. *J Am Coll Cardiol*. 2007;49:403-414.

88. Gardner AW, Poehlman ET. Exercise rehabilitation programs for the treatment of claudication pain: a meta-analysis. *JAMA*. 1995;274:975-980.

89. Gerich JE. The importance of tight glycemic control. *Am J Med*. 2005;118 (9A):7S-11S.

89a.Gibbons RJ, Balady GJ, Bricker JT, et al. ACC/AHA 2002 guideline update for exercise testing. *Circulation*. 2002;106:1883-1892.

90. Giugliano RP, Braunwald E. The year in non–ST-segment elevation acute coronary syndromes. *J Am Coll Cardiol*. 2006;48:386-395.

91. Glazer CS, Newman LS. Occupational interstitial disease. *Clin Chest Med*. 2004;25:467-478.

92. Go AS, Chertow GM, Fan D, et al. Chronic kidney disease and the risks of death, cardiovascular events, and hospitalization. *N Engl J Med*. 2004;351:1296-1305.

93. Goldberg AP, Geltman EM, Gavin III JR, et al. Exercise training reduces coronary risk and effectively rehabilitates hemodialysis patients. *Nephron*. 1986;42:311-316.

94. Golomb BA, Dang TT, Criqui MH. Peripheral arterial disease: morbidity and mortality implications. *Circulation*. 2006;114:688-699.

95. Goodacre S, Sutton AJ, Sampson FC. Meta-analysis: the value of clinical assessment in the diagnosis of deep venous thrombosis. *Ann Intern Med*. 2005;143:129-139.

96. Goodson NJ, Solomon DH. The cardiovascular manifestations of rheumatic diseases. *Curr Opin Rheumatol*. 2006;18:135-140.

97. Goraya TY, Leibson CL, Palumbo PJ, et al. Coronary atherosclerosis in diabetes mellitus: a population-based autopsy study. *J Am Coll Cardiol*. 2002;40:946-953.

98. Graham LM. The effect of sickle cell disease on the lung. *Clin Pulm Med*. 2004;11:369-378.

99. Hafidh S, Senkottaiyan N, Villarreal D, et al. Management of the metabolic syndrome. *Am J Med Sci*. 2005;330(6):343-351.

100. Hagberg JM, Park J-J, Brown MD. The role of exercise training in the treatment of hypertension. *Sports Med*. 2000;30:193-206.

101. Haider AW, Larson MG, Franklin SS, et al. Systolic blood pressure, diastolic blood pressure, and pulse pressure as predictors of risk for congestive heart failure in the Framingham Heart Study. *Ann Intern Med*. 2003;138:10-16.

101a.Hajjar I, Kotchen JM, Kotchen TA. Hypertension: trends in prevalence, incidence, and control. *Annu Rev Public Health*. 2006;27:465-490.

102. Hansson GK, Nilsson J. Pathogenesis of atherosclerosis. In: Crawford MH, DiMarco JP, Paulus WJ, eds. *Cardiology*. 2nd ed. New York: Mosby; 2004.

103. Harari S, Caminati A. Idiopathic pulmonary fibrosis. *Allergy*. 2005;60: 421-435.

103a.Hart DP, Peggs KS. Current status of allogeneic stem cell transplantation for treatment of hematologic malignancies. *Clin Pharmacol Ther*. 2007;82:325-329.

104. Haskell WL, Lee I-M, Pate RL, et al. Physical activity and public health: updated recommendation for adults from the American College of Sports Medicine and the American Heart Association. *Med Sci Sports Exerc*. 2007;39:1423-1434.

105. Haykowsky MJ, Liang Y, Pechter D, et al. A meta-analysis of the effect of exercise training on left ventricular remodeling in heart failure patients. *J Am Coll Cardiol*. 2007;49:2329-2336.

106. He H, Stein MW, Zalta B, et al. Pulmonary infarction: spectrum of findings on multidetector helical CT. *J Thorac Imaging*. 2006;21:1-7.

107. Herridge MS, Cheung AM, Tansey CM, et al. One-year outcomes in survivors of the acute respiratory distress syndrome. *N Engl J Med*. 2003;348:683-693.

108. Hertser NR, Young JR, Beven EG, et al. Coronary angiography in 506 patients with extracranial cerebrovascular disease. *Arch Intern Med*. 1985;145:849-852.

109. Hirsch AT, Haskal ZJ, Hertzer NR, et al. ACC/AHA 2005 guidelines for the management of patients with peripheral arterial disease (lower extremity, renal, mesenteric, and abdominal aortic). Executive summary: a report of the American College of Cardiology/American Heart Association Task Force on Practice Guidelines) Writing Committee to Develop Guidelines for the Management of Patients with Peripheral Arterial

Disease (Lower Extremity, Renal, Mesenteric, and Abdominal Aortic). *J Am Coll Cardiol.* 2006;47:1239-1312.

109a.Hoeper MM. Drug treatment of pulmonary hypertension. Current and future agents. *Drugs.* 2005;65:1337-1354.

110. Hoeper MM, Mayer E, Simonneau G, et al. Chronic thromboembolic pulmonary hypertension. *Circulation.* 2006;113:2011-2020.

111. Hogarty AN, Leahey A, Zhao H, et al. Longitudinal evaluation of cardiopulmonary performance during exercise after bone marrow transplantation in children. *J Pediatr.* 2000;136:311-317.

112. Hogg JC, Chu F, Utokaparch S, et al. The nature of small-airway obstruction in chronic obstructive pulmonary disease. *N Engl J Med.* 2004;350:2645-2653.

113. Hunt SA, Baker DW, Chin MH, et al. ACC/AHA guidelines for the evaluation and management of chronic heart failure in the adult: executive summary. A report of the American College of Cardiology/American Heart Association Task Force on Practice Guidelines. *Circulation.* 2001;104:2996-3007.

114. Iestra JA, Kromhout D, van der Schouw YT, et al. Effect size estimates of lifestyle and dietary changes on all-cause mortality in coronary artery disease patients: a systematic review. *Circulation.* 2005;112:924-934.

114a.Iriarte M, Muraga N, Sagastagoitia D, et al. Congestive heart failure from left ventricular diastolic dysfunction in systemic hypertension. *Am J Cardiol.* 2001;71:308-312.

115. Izzo JL, Gradman AH. Mechanisms and management of hypertensive heart disease: from left ventricular hypertrophy to heart failure. *Med Clin North Am.* 2004;88:1257-1271.

116. Jacobs PL, Nash MS. Exercise recommendations for individuals with spinal cord injury. *Sports Med.* 2004;34:727-751.

117. Jakicic JM, Otto AD. Treatment and prevention of obesity: what is the role of exercise? *Nutr Rev.* 2006;64:S57-S61.

118. Jakicic JM, Winters C, Lang W, et al. Effects of intermittent exercise and use of home exercise equipment on adherence, weight loss, and fitness in overweight women: a randomized trial. *JAMA.* 1999;282:1554-1560.

119. Jandeleit-Dahm KAM, Tikellis C, Reid CM, et al. Why blockade of the renin–angiotensin system reduces the incidence of new-onset diabetes. *J Hypertens.* 2005;23(3):463-473.

120. Jericó C, Knobel H, Montero M, et al. Hypertension in HIV-infected patients: prevalence and related factors. *Am J Hypertens.* 2005;18:1396-1401.

121. Jessup M, Brozena S. Heart failure. *N Engl J Med.* 2003;348:2007-2018.

122. Johansen KL. Exercise and chronic kidney disease: current recommendations. *Sports Med.* 2005;35:485-499.

123. Johnson BD, Shaw LJ, Pepine CJ. Persistent chest pain predicts cardiovascular events in women without obstructive coronary artery disease: results from the NIH-NHLBI-sponsored Women's Ischaemia Syndrome Evaluation (WISE) Study. *Eur Heart J.* 2006;27:1408-1415.

124. Jones PH. Clinical significance of recent lipid trials on reducing risk in patients with type 2 diabetes mellitus. *Am J Cardiol.* 2007;99(suppl):113B-140B.

125. Kahan A, Allanore Y. Primary myocardial involvement in systemic sclerosis. *Rheumatology.* 2006;45:iv14-iv17.

126. Kahn SR, Azoulay L, Hirsch A, et al. Acute effects of exercise in patients with previous deep venous thrombosis: impact of the postthrombotic syndrome. *Chest.* 2003;123:399-405.

127. Kamholz SL. Pulmonary and cardiovascular consequences of smoking. *Med Clin North Am.* 2004;88:1415-1430.

128. Kanmogne GD. Noninfectious pulmonary complications of HIV/AIDS. *Curr Opin Pulm Med.* 2005;11:208-212.

129. Karlin L, Darmon M, Thiéry G, et al. Respiratory status deterioration during G-CSF–induced neutropenia. *Bone Marrow Transplant.* 2005;36:245-250.

130. Kelley GA, Kelley KS. Progressive resistance exercise and resting blood pressure: a meta-analysis of randomized controlled trials. *Hypertension.* 2000;35:838-843.

131. Kelly K, Hertz MI. Obliterative bronchiolitis. *Clin Chest Med.* 1997;18:319-338.

131a.Kelly-Hayes M, Robertson JT, Broderick JP, et al. The American Heart Association stroke outcome classification. *Stroke.* 1998;29:1274-1280.

132. Kiser TS, Stefans VA. Pulmonary embolism in rehabilitation patients: relation to time before return to physical therapy after diagnosis of deep vein thrombosis. *Arch Phys Med Rehabil.* 1997;78:942-945.

133. Klastersky J. Adverse effects of the humanized antibodies used as cancer therapeutics. *Curr Opin Oncol.* 2006;18:316-320.

134. Klem ML, Wing RR, McGuire MT, et al. A descriptive study of individuals successful at long-term maintenance of substantial weight loss. *Am J Clin Nutr.* 1997;66:239-246.

135. Kurella M, Lo JC, Chertow GM. Metabolic syndrome and the risk for chronic kidney disease among nondiabetic adults. *J Am Soc Nephrol.* 2005;16:2134-2140.

136. Kurup VP, Zacharisen MC, Fink JN. Hypersensitivity pneumonitis. *Indian J Chest Dis Allied Sci.* 2006;48:115-128.

136a.Kushner RF, Blatner DJ. Risk assessment of the overweight and obese. *J Am Diet Assoc.* 2005;105:S53-S62.

137. Lama VN, Martinez FJ. Resting and exercise physiology in interstitial lung disease. *Clin Chest Med.* 2004;25:435-453.

138. LaMonte MJ, Blair SN, Church TS. Physical activity and diabetes prevention. *J Appl Physiol.* 2005;99:1205-1213.

139. Lee CD, Blair SN, Jackson AS. Cardiorespiratory fitness, body composition, and all-cause and cardiovascular disease mortality in men. *Am J Clin Nutr.* 1999;69:373-380.

140. Lee SA. A review of pneumocystis pneumonia. *J Pharm Practice.* 2006;19:5-9.

141. Lerman A, Sopko G. Women and cardiovascular heart disease: clinical implications from the Women's Ischemia Syndrome Evaluation (WISE) Study. *J Am Coll Cardiol.* 2006;47:59S-62S.

142. Levinger I, Bronks R, Cody DV, et al. The effect of resistance training on left ventricular function and structure of patients with chronic heart failure. *Int J Cardiol.* 2005;105:159-163.

143. Levy D, Larson MG, Vasan RS, et al. The progression from hypertension to congestive heart failure. *JAMA.* 1996;275:1557-1562.

143a.Light RW, Broaddus VC. Pleural effusion. Murray JF, Nadel JA, eds. *Textbook of Respiratory Medicine.* 3rd ed. Philadelphia: Saunders, 2000.

143b.Lim DH, Lee J, Lee HG, et al. Pulmonary complications after hematopoietic stem cell transplantation. *J Korean Med Sci.* 2006;21:406-411.

144. Limper AH. Chemotherapy-induced lung disease. *Clin Chest Med.* 2004;25:53-64.

145. Loganathan R, Searls YM, Smirnova IV, et al. Exercise-induced benefits in individuals with type 1 diabetes. *Phys Ther Rev.* 2006;11:77-89.

146. Lundberg LE. The heart in dermatomyositis and polymyositis. *Rheumatology.* 2006;45:iv18-iv21.

147. Ly J, Chan CT. Impact of augmenting dialysis frequency and duration on cardiovascular function. *ASAIO J.* 2006;52(6):e11-e14.

147a.Maltais F, LeBlanc P, Jobin J, et al. Peripheral muscle dysfunction in chronic obstructive pulmonary disease. *Clin Chest Med.* 2000;21:665-677.

147b.Mancia G. The association of hypertension and diabetes: prevalence, cardiovascular risk, and protection by blood pressure reduction. *Acta Diabetol.* 2005;42:S17-S25.

148. Mangat KS, Mehra A, Yunas I, et al. Venous thromboprophylaxis in trauma: a review, *Trauma.* 2006;8:233-247.

149. Mannino DM, Watt G, Hole D, et al. The natural history of chronic obstructive pulmonary disease. *Eur Respir J.* 2006;27:627-643.

149a.Manson JE, Allison MA, Rossouw JE, et al. Estrogen therapy and coronary-artery calcification. *N Engl J Med.* 2007; 356:2591-2602.

149b.Manson JE, Hsia J, Johnson KC, et al. Estrogen plus progesterone and the risk of coronary heart disease. *N Engl J Med.* 2003; 349:523-534.

150. Manthous CA. ARDS redux. *Clin Pulm Med.* 2006;13:121-127.

150a.Marquette C-H, Marx A, Leroy S, et al. Simplified stepwise management of primary spontaneous pneumothorax: a pilot study. *Eur Respir J.* 2006;27:470-476.

151. Marr WL. Deep venous thrombosis recommendations. *J Vasc Nurs.* 2006;24:91-93.

152. Martin KB, Klinger JR, Rounds SIS. Pulmonary arterial hypertension: new insights and new hope. *Respirology.* 2006;11:6-17.

153. Martinez FJ, Safrin S, Weycker D, et al. The clinical course of patients with idiopathic pulmonary fibrosis. *Ann Intern Med.* 2005;142:963-967.

154. Maser RE, Lenhard MJ. Review: cardiovascular autonomic neuropathy due to diabetes mellitus: clinical manifestations, consequences, and treatment. *J Clin Endocrinol Metab.* 2005;90:5896-5903.

155. Mathier MA, Ramanathan RC. Impact of obesity and bariatric surgery on cardiovascular disease. *Med Clin North Am.* 2007;91:415-431.

156. Mathur SK, Busse WW. Asthma: diagnosis and management. *Med Clin North Am.* 2006;90:39-60.

157. Matthay MA, Zimmerman GA. Acute lung injury and the acute respiratory distress syndrome - four decades of inquiry into pathogenesis and rational management. *Am J Respir Cell Mol Biol.* 2005; 33:319-327.

158. McDonnell ME. Combination therapy with new targets in type 2 diabetes: a review of available agents with a focus on pre-exercise adjustment. *J Cardiopulm Rehabil Prevent.* 2007;27:193-201.

158a. McTiernan A. Physical activity after cancer: physiologic outcomes. *Cancer Investig.* 2004;22:68-81.

159. Mekhail T, Wood L, Bukowski R. Interleukin-2 in cancer therapy: uses and optimal management of adverse effects. *BioDrugs.* 2000;14: 299-318.

160. Mensah GA, Croft JB, Giles WH. The heart, kidney, and brain as target organs in hypertension. *Cardiol Clin.* 2002;20:225-247.

161. Mereles D, Ehlken N, Kruescher S, et al. Exercise and respiratory training improve exercise capacity and quality of life in patients with severe chronic pulmonary hypertension. *Circulation.* 2006;114:1482-1489.

162. Meyer FJ, Borst MM, Zugck C, et al. Respiratory muscle dysfunction in congestive heart failure: clinical correlation and prognostic significance. *Circulation.* 2001;103:2153-2158.

163. Michael KM, Allen JK, Macko RF. Reduced ambulatory activity after stroke: the role of balance, gait, and cardiovascular fitness. *Arch Phys Med Rehabil.* 2005;86:1552-1556.

163a. Mimeault M, Hauke R, Batra SK. Stem cells: a revolution in therapeutics – recent advances in stem cell biology and their therapeutic applications in regenerative medicine and cancer therapies. *Clin Pharmacol Therapeut.* 2007;82:252-264.

164. Mosca L, Banka CL, Benjamin EJ, et al. Evidence-based guidelines for cardiovascular disease prevention in women: 2007 update. *Circulation.* 2007;115:1481-1501.

165. Naji NA, Connor MC, Donnelly S, et al. Effectiveness of pulmonary rehabilitation in restrictive lung disease. *J Cardiopulm Rehabil.* 2006;26:237-243.

165a. National Heart, Lung, and Blood Institute. Clinical guidelines on the identification, evaluation and treatment of overweight and obesity in adults: the evidence report. National Institutes of Health. *Obesity Res.* 1998;6 (suppl 2):51-209S.

166. Nelson ME, Rejeski WJ, Blair SN, et al. Physical activity and public health in older adults: recommendation from the American College of Sports Medicine and the American Heart Association. *Med Sci Sports Exerc.* 2007;39:1435-1445.

167. Neter JE, Stam BE, Kok FJ, et al. Influence of weight reduction on blood pressure: a meta-analysis of randomized controlled trials. *Hypertension.* 2003;42:878-884.

168. Ng CSH, Yim APC. Spontaneous hemopneumothorax. *Curr Opin Pulm Med.* 2006;12:273-277.

169. Nici L, Donner C, Wouters E, et al. American Thoracic Society/European Respiratory Society statement on pulmonary rehabilitation. *Am J Respir Crit Care Med.* 2006;173:1390-1413.

170. Nijkeuter M, Hovens MMC, Davidson BL, et al. Resolution of thromboemboli in patients with acute pulmonary embolism. A systematic review. *Chest.* 2006;129:192-197.

170a. Norgren L, Hiatt W, Nehler M, et al. Inter-Society consensus for the management of peripheral arterial disease (TASC II). *Eur J Vasc Endovasc Surg.* 2007;33(1):S1-S75.

171. O'Donnell DE. Ventilatory limitations in chronic obstructive pulmonary disease. *Med. Sci. Sports Exerc.* 2001;33:S647-655.

172. O'Donnell DE, Parker CM. COPD exacerbations. 3. Pathophysiology. *Thorax.* 2006;61:354-361.

173. Ogden CL, Carroll MD, Curtin LR, et al. Prevalence of overweight and obesity in the United States, 1999–2004. *JAMA.* 2006;295:1549-1555.

174. Ong KL, Cheung BMY, Man YB, et al. Prevalence, awareness, treatment and control of hypertension among United States adults 1999–2004. *Hypertension.* 2007;49:69-75.

175. Painter P. Physical functioning in end-stage renal disease patients: update 2005. *Hemodial Int.* 2005;9:218-235.

176. Painter P, Carlson L, Carey S, et al. Physical functioning and health-related quality of life changes with exercise training in hemodialysis patients. *Am J Kidney Dis.* 2000;35:482-492.

177. Pang MYC, Eng JJ, Dawson AS. Relationship between ambulatory capacity and cardiorespiratory fitness in chronic stroke: influence on stroke-specific impairments. *Chest.* 2005;127:495-501.

178. Partsch H. Immediate ambulation and leg compression in the treatment of deep vein thrombosis. *Dis Mon.* 2005;51:135-140.

179. Pauwels RA, Buist AS, Calverley PMA, et al. Global strategy for the diagnosis, management, and prevention of chronic obstructive pulmonary disease. NHLBI/WHO global initiative for chronic obstructive lung disease (GOLD) workshop summary. *Am J Respir Crit Care Med.* 2001;163: 1256-1276.

180. Pedersen BK, Saltin B. Evidence for prescribing exercise as therapy in chronic disease [review]. *Scand J Med Sci Sports.* 2006;16(suppl 1):3-63.

181. Pendse S, Singh AK. Complications of chronic kidney disease: anemia, mineral metabolism, and cardiovascular disease. *Med Clin North Am.* 2005;89:549-561.

182. Pepine CJ, Balaban RS, Bonow RO, et al. Women's Ischemic Syndrome Evaluation: current status and future research directions. Report of the National, Heart, Lung, and Blood Institute Workshop: October 2–4, 2002: Section 1: Diagnosis of stable ischemia and ischemic heart disease. *Circulation.* 2004;109:44e-46e.

183. Perrin C, Unterborn JN, D'Ambrosio C, et al. Pulmonary complications of chronic neuromuscular diseases and their management. *Muscle Nerve.* 2004;29:5-27.

184. Pickering TG, Phil D, Shimbo D, et al. Ambulatory blood-pressure monitoring. *N Engl J Med.* 2006;354:2368-2374.

184a. Piepoli MF, Davos C, Francis DP, et al. Exercise training meta-analysis of trials in patients with chonic heart failure (ExTraMATCH). *BMJ.* 2004;328(7433):189-194.

185. Piepoli MF, Kaczmarek A, Francis DP, et al. Reduced peripheral skeletal muscle mass and abnormal reflex physiology in chronic heart failure. *Circulation.* 2006;114:126-134.

186. Piña IL, Apstein CS, Balady GJ, et al. Exercise and heart failure: a statement from the American Heart Association Committee on Exercise, Rehabilitation, and Prevention. *Circulation.* 2003;107:1210-1225.

186a. Piquette CA, Rennard SI, Snider GL. Chronic bronchitis and emphysema. In Murray JF, Nadel JA, eds. *Textbook of Respiratory Medicine.* 3rd ed. Philadelphia: Saunders; 2000.

186b. Pi-Sunyer FX. Use of lifestyle changes treatment plus drug therapy in controlling cardiovascular and metabolic risk factors. *Obesity.* 2006;14 (suppl 3):135S-42S.

187. Poirier P, Giles TD, Bray GA, et al. Obesity and cardiovascular disease: pathophysiology, evaluation, and effect of weight loss: an update of the 1997 American Heart Association Scientific Statement on Obesity and Heart Disease from the Obesity Committee of the Council on Nutrition, Physical Activity, and Metabolism. *Circulation.* 2006;113:898-918.

188. Potempa K, Lopez M, Braun LT, et al. Physiologic outcomes of aerobic exercise training in hemiparetic stroke patients. *Stroke.* 1995;26: 101-105.

189. Prospective Studies Collaboration. Age-specific relevance of usual blood pressure to vascular mortality: a meta-analysis of individual data for one million adults in 61 prospective studies. *Lancet.* 2002;360:1903-1913.

190. Quyyumi AA. Women and ischemic heart disease: pathophysiologic implications from the Women's Ischemic Syndrome Evaluation (WISE) Study and future research steps. *J Am Coll Cardiol.* 2006;47:66S-71S.

191. Rader DJ. Effect of insulin resistance, dyslipidemia, and intra-abdominal adiposity on the development of cardiovascular disease and diabetes mellitus. *Am J Med.* 2007;120:S12-S18.

192. Rampello A, Franceschini M, Piepoli M, et al. Effect of aerobic training on walking capacity and maximal exercise tolerance in patients with multiple sclerosis: a randomized crossover controlled study. *Phys Ther.* 2007;87:545-555.

193. Rashidi A, Ghanbarian A, Azizi F. Are patients who have metabolic syndrome without diabetes at risk for developing chronic kidney disease? Evidence based on data from a large cohort screening population. *Clin J Am Soc Nephrol.* 2007;2:976-983.

194. Rayner CFJ, Grubnic S. Pulmonary manifestations of systemic autoimmune disease. *Best Pract Res Clin Rheumatol.* 2004;18:381-410.

195. Restrepo CS, Diethelm L, Lemos JA, et al. Cardiovascular complications of human immunodeficiency virus infection. *Radiographics.* 2006;26: 213-231.

195a. Riddell MC, Perkins BA. Type 1 diabetes and vigorous exercise: applications of exercise physiology to patient management. *Can J Diabetes.* 2006;30:63-71.

196. Riddle DL, Hillner BE, Wells PS, et al. Diagnosis of lower-extremity deep vein thrombosis in outpatients with musculoskeletal disorders: a national survey of physical therapists. *Phys Ther.* 2004;84:717-728.

197. Roberts CK, Barnard RJ. Effects of exercise and diet on chronic disease. *J Appl Physiol.* 2005;98:3-30.

198. Roig J, Domingo C, Gea E. Pulmonary toxicity caused by cytotoxic drugs. *Clin Pulm Med.* 2006;13:53-62.

198a. Rossouw JE, Prentice RL, Manson JE, et al. Postmenopausal hormone therapy and risk of cardiovascular disease by age and years since menopause. *JAMA.* 2007;297:1465-1477.

198b. Rostagno C, Galanti G, Comeglio M, et al. Comparison of different methods of functional evaluation in patients with chronic heart failure. *Eur J Heart Fail.* 2000;2:273-280.

199. Ruderman N, Devlin JT, Schneider SH, Kriska A, eds. *Handbook of Exercise in Diabetes.* 2nd ed. Alexandria, VA: American Diabetes Association; 2002.

200. Sachdev V, Machado RF, Shizukuda Y, et al. Diastolic dysfunction is an independent risk factor for death in patients with sickle cell disease. *J Am Coll Cardiol.* 2007;49:472-479.

200a. Saetta M, Turato G, Maestrelli P, et al. Cellular and structural bases of chronic obstructive pulmonary disease. *Am J Respir Crit Care Med.* 2001;163:1304-1309.

201. Samejima H, Omiya K, Uno M, et al. Relationship between impaired chronotropic response, cardiac output during exercise, and exercise intolerance in patients with chronic heart failure. *Jpn Heart J.* 2003; 44:515-525.

202. Schramel FM, Postmus PE, Vanderschueren RG. Current aspects of spontaneous pneumothorax. *Eur Respir J.* 1997;10:1372-1379.

203. Schrier RW, Estacio RO, Esler A, et al. Effects of aggressive blood pressure control in normotensive type 2 diabetic patients on albuminuria, retinopathy, and strokes. *Kidney Int.* 2002;61:1086-1097.

204. Schiffrin EL, Lipman ML, Mann JFE. Chronic kidney disease: effects on the cardiovascular system. *Circulation.* 2007;116:85-97.

204a. Shankar A, Klein R, Klein BEK, et al. Relationship between low-normal blood pressure and kidney disease in type 1 diabetes. *Hypertension.* 2007;49:48-54.

205. Shoenfeld Y, Gerli R, Doria A, et al. Accelerated atherosclerosis in autoimmune rheumatic diseases. *Circulation.* 2005;112:3337-3347.

206. Shusterman S, Meadows AT. Long-term survivors of childhood leukemia. *Curr Opin Hematol.* 2000;7:217-222.

207. Sietsema K. Cardiovascular limitations in chronic pulmonary disease. *Med Sci Sports Exerc.* 2001;33:S656-661.

208. Sigal RJ, Kenny GP, Wasserman DH, et al. Physical activity/exercise and type 2 diabetes. *Diabetes Care.* 2004;27:2518-2539.

209. Silverberg D, Wexler D, Blum M, et al. The association between congestive heart failure and chronic renal disease. *Curr Opin Nephrol Hypertens.* 2004;13:163-170.

209a. Simonneau G, Galie N, Rubin LJ, et al. Clinical classification of pulmonary hypertension. *J Am Coll Cardiol.* 2004;43(suppl 12):5S-12S.

210. Sobel BE. Optimizing cardiovascular outcomes in diabetes mellitus. *Am J Med.* 2007;120(9B):S3-S11.

211. Stefonović V, Milojković M. Effects of physical exercise in patients with end-stage renal failure, on dialysis and renal transplantation: current status and recommendations. *Int J Artif Organs.* 2005;28:8-15.

211a. Steinherz LJ, Steinherz PG, Tan CTC, et al. Cardiac toxicity 4 to 20 years after completing anthracycline therapy. *JAMA.* 1991;266:1672-1677.

212. Stewart KJ, Regensteiner JG, Hirsch AT. Exercise training for claudication. *N Engl J Med.* 2002;347:1941-1951.

212a. Storer TW. Exercise in chronic pulmonary disease: resistance exercise prescription. *Med Sci Sports Exerc.* 2001;33(7 suppl):S680-S686.

213. Stover DE, Kaner RJ. Pulmonary toxicity. In: DeVita VT, Hellman S, Rosenberg SA, eds. *Cancer: Principles & Practice of Oncology.* 7th ed. Philadelphia: Lippincott Williams & Wilkins; 2005.

214. Sun X-G, Hansen JE, Oudiz RJ, et al. Exercise pathophysiology in patients with primary pulmonary hypertension. *Circulation.* 2001;104: 429-435.

215. Swain DP, Franklin BA. Comparison of cardioprotective benefits of vigorous versus moderate intensity aerobic exercise. *Am J Cardiol.* 2006;97:141-147.

216. Thannickal VJ, Toews GB, White ES, et al. Mechanisms of pulmonary fibrosis. *Annu Rev Med.* 2004;55:395-417.

216a. Thistlethwaite PA, Kaneko K, Madani MM, et al. Technique and outcome of pulmonary endarterectomy surgery. *Ann Thorac Cardiovasc Surg.* 2008; 14:274-282.

217. Tincani A, Rebaioli CB, Taglietti M, et al. Heart involvement in systemic lupus erythematosus, anti-phospholipid syndrome, and neonatal lupus. *Rheumatology.* 2006;45:iv8-iv13.

218. Trujillo-Santos J, Perea-Milla E, Jiminez-Puente A, et al. Bed rest or ambulation in the initial treatment of patients with acute deep vein thrombosis or pulmonary embolism: findings from the RIETE Registry. *Chest.* 2005;127:1631-1636.

219. Turesson C, Matteson EL. Cardiovascular risk factors, fitness, and physical activity in rheumatic diseases. *Curr Opin Rheumatol.* 2007;19:190-196.

220. US Renal Data System. *USRDS 2005 Annual Data Report: Atlas of End-Stage Renal Disease in the United States.* Bethesda, MD: National Institutes of Health, National Institute of Diabetes and Digestive and Kidney Diseases; 2005.

221. Valensi P, Pariès J, Attali JR, et al. Cardiac autonomic neuropathy in diabetic patients: influence of diabetes duration, obesity, and microangiopathic complications: the French Multicenter Study. *Metabolism.* 2003;52:815-820.

222. VanGaal LF, Mertens IL, DeBlock CE. Mechanisms linking obesity with cardiovascular disease. *Nature.* 2006;444:875-880.

222a. Vasan RS, Benjamin EJ, Levy D. Prevalence, clinical features and prognosis of diastolic heart failure: an epidemiologic perspective. *J Am Coll Cardiol.* 1995;26:1565-1574.

222b. Vichinsky EP, Neumayr LD, Earles AN, et al. Causes and outcomes of the acute chest syndrome in sickle cell disease. *N Engl J Med.* 2000; 342:1855-1865.

223. Villareal DT, Apovian CM, Kushner RF, et al. Obesity in older adults: technical review and position statement of the American Society for Nutrition and NAASO, The Obesity Society. *Obes Res.* 2005;13:1849-1863.

223a. Vincent KR, Vincent HK. Resistance training for individuals with cardiovascular disease. *J Cardiopulm Rehabil.* 2006;26:207-216.

224. Vinik AI, Mehrabyan A. Diabetic neuropathies. *Med Clin N Am.* 2004;88:947-999.

225. Volaklis KA, Tokmakidis SP. Resistance exercise training in patients with heart failure. *Sports Med.* 2005;35:1085-1103.

226. Voskuyl AE. The heart and cardiovascular manifestations in rheumatoid arthritis. *Rheumatology.* 2006;45:iv4-iv7.

227. Wah TM, Moss HA, Robertson RJH, et al. Pulmonary complications following bone marrow transplantation. *Br J Radiol.* 2003;76:373-379.

228. Wang L, McParland BE, Paré PD. The functional consequences of structural changes in the airways. *Chest.* 2003;123:356S-362S.

229. Warburton DER, Nicol CW, Bredin SSD. Health benefits of physical activity: the evidence. *Can Med Assoc J.* 2006;174:801-809.

230. Ware LB, Matthay MA. Acute pulmonary edema. *N Engl J Med.* 2005;353:2788-2796.

231. Warlow C, Sudlow C, Dennis M, et al. Stroke. *Lancet.* 2003;362: 1211-1224.

231a. Watson T, Mock V. Exercise and cancer-related fatigue: a review of current literature. *Rehabil Oncol.* 2003;21:23-30.

232. Weiner DE. Causes and consequences of chronic kidney disease: implications for managed health care. *J Manag Care Pharm.* 2007;13(3 suppl): S1-S9.

233. Wells PS, Hirsh J, Anderson DR, et al. Value of assessment of pretest probability of deep-vein thrombosis in clinical management. *Lancet.* 1997;350:1795-1798.

234. Williams MA, Ades PA, Hamm LF, et al. Clinical evidence for a health benefit from cardiac rehabilitation: an update. *Am Heart J.* 2006;152:835-841.

235. Williams MA, Haskell WL, Ades PA, et al. Resistance exercise in individuals with and without cardiovascular disease: 2007 update. *Circulation.* 2007;116:572-584.

236. Wilson W, Taubert KA, Gewitz M, et al. Prevention of infective endocarditis. Guidelines from the American Heart Association Rheumatic Fever, Endocarditis and Kawasaki Disease Committee, Council on Cardiovascular Disease in the Young, and the Council on Clinical Cardiology, Quality of Care and Outcomes Research Interdisciplinary Working Group. *Circulation.* 2007;116:1736-1754.

237. Yahalom J, Portlock CS. Cardiac toxicity. In: DeVita VT, Hellman S, Rosenberg SA, eds. *Cancer: Principles & Practice of Oncology.* 7th ed. Philadelphia: Lippincott Williams & Wilkins; 2005.

238. Yang H. Maintenance immunosuppression regimens: conversion, minimization, withdrawal, and avoidance. *Am J Kidney Dis.* 2006;47(suppl 4):S37-S51.

239. Yeh ETH, Tong AT, Lenihan DJ, et al. Cardiovascular complications of cancer treatment. Diagnosis, pathogenesis, and management. *Circulation.* 2004;109:3122-3131.

240. Yen KT, Lee AS, Krowka MJ, et al. Pulmonary complications in bone marrow transplantation: a practical approach to diagnosis and treatment. *Clin Chest Med.* 2004;25:189-201.

241. Zile MR, Baicu CF, Gaasch WH. Diastolic heart failure: abnormalities in active relaxation and passive stiffness of the left ventricle. *N Engl J Med.* 2004;350:1953-1959.

ADDITIONAL READINGS

Andreoli TE, Carpenter CC, Griggs RC. *Cecil Essentials of Medicine.* 7th ed. Philadelphia: Saunders; 2004.

Burton GG, Hodgkin JE, Ward JJ, eds. *Respiratory Care. A Guide to Clinical Practice.* 4th ed. Philadelphia: Lippincott; 1997.

Cherniack RM, Cherniack L. *Respiration in Health and Disease.* 3rd ed. Philadelphia: Saunders; 1983.

Clough P. Restrictive lung dysfunction. In: Hillegass EA, Sadowsky HS, eds. *Essentials of Cardiopulmonary Physical Therapy.* 2nd ed. Philadelphia: Saunders; 2001.

Crawford MH, DiMarco JP, Paulus WJ. eds-in-chief. *Cardiology.* 2nd ed. Philadelphia: Mosby; 2004.

Dequeker E, Dodge JA. Classification of cystic fibrosis and related disorders. WHO Report, 2002.

Durstine JL, Moore GE. *ACSM's Exercise Management for Persons with Chronic Diseases and Disabilities.* 2nd ed. Champaign, IL: Human Kinetics; 2003.

Fink JB, Hunt GE. *Clinical Practice in Respiratory Care.* Philadelphia: Lippincott Williams & Wilkins; 1999.

Fuster V, Alexander RW, O'Rourke RA, eds. *Hurst's The Heart.* 11th ed. New York: McGraw-Hill; 2004.

Garritan SL. In: Chronic obstructive pulmonary disease. In: Hillegass EA, Sadowsky HS, eds. *Essentials of Cardiopulmonary Physical Therapy.* 2nd ed. Philadelphia: Saunders; 2001.

George RB, Light RW, Matthay MA, et al. *Chest Medicine: Essentials of Pulmonary and Critical Care Medicine.* 2nd ed. Baltimore: Williams & Wilkins; 1990.

Gibson GJ, Geddes DM, Costabel U, et al., eds. *Respiratory Medicine.* 3rd ed. Philadelphia: Saunders; 2003.

Goldman L, Ausiello D, eds. *Cecil Textbook of Medicine.* 22nd ed. Philadelphia: Saunders; 2004.

Goodman CC, Boissonnault WG, Fuller KS. *Pathology – Implications for the Physical Therapist.* 2nd ed. Philadelphia: W.B. Saunders; 2003.

Guyton AC, Hall JE. *Textbook of Medical Physiology.* 10th ed. Philadelphia: Saunders; 2000.

Hammon WEIII, Dean E. Cardiopulmonary pathophysiology. In: Frownfelter D, Dean E, eds. *Cardiovascular and Pulmonary Physical Therapy – Evidence and Practice.* 4th ed. St. Louis: Mosby; 2006.

Hess DR, MacIntyre NR, Mishoe SC, et al., eds. *Respiratory Care: Principles & Practice.* Philadelphia: Saunders; 2002.

Humes HD, ed. *Kelley's Textbook of Internal Medicine.* 4th ed. Philadelphia: Lippincott Williams & Wilkins; 2000.

Murray JF, Nadal JA, eds. *Textbook of Respiratory Medicine.* 3rd ed. Philadelphia: Saunders; 2000.

Tecklin JS. Common pulmonary diseases. In: Irwin S, Tecklin JS, eds. *Cardiopulmonary Physical Therapy: A Guide to Practice.* 4th ed. St. Louis: Mosby; 2004.

Zipes DP, Libby P, Bonow PO, Braunwald E, eds. *Braunwald's Heart Disease.* 7th ed. Philadelphia: Saunders; 2005.

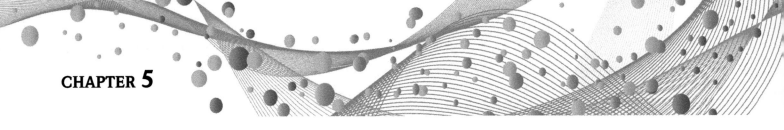

CHAPTER 5

Pharmacology

Patients who are referred to physical therapy are often taking at least one, if not many, medications, which come in the form of prescription drugs and over-the-counter medications. In addition, herbal supplements are increasingly common. It is important for physical therapists (PTs) to recognize the effects and side effects of various medications on their patients and their responses to different physical therapy interventions. Some drugs act synergistically with rehabilitation activities, whereas others may interfere with the patient's responses and progress during treatment.

This chapter introduces the drugs used in the treatment of various pulmonary and cardiovascular conditions and examines to various degrees the mechanisms of action and side effects of these agents. Included are drugs used in the treatment of asthma, chronic obstructive pulmonary diseases, pulmonary hypertension, and some other specific diseases, and general respiratory symptoms. Cardiovascular (CV) medications used to treat hypertension, angina, postmyocardial infarction, chronic heart failure, arrhythmias, hyperlipidemia, shock, and organ transplantation are also presented. Medications used to treat diabetes mellitus are also described because of the increasing prevalence of the disease and implications for cardiovascular disease (CVD) morbidity and mortality.

A comprehensive guide to the medications used in the treatment of the multitude of pulmonary disorders and cardiac conditions is a volume in and of itself. Thus, this chapter provides only an overview of the more important elements of pharmacology of the classes of medications used to manage individuals with CV and pulmonary dysfunction. The manufacturer's current product information or other standard references should be consulted for more detailed information.

Regarding the presentation of adverse reactions, it should be noted that it is not practical to identify all the reactions reported in the literature; therefore, the approach here is limited to (1) very serious reactions, (2) very common reactions, and/or (3) reactions that potentially have a direct impact on the practice of physical therapy in the clinical setting. Note that this is an overview: side effects may arise that are not listed here because they are either uncommon or have not been associated with the particular agent.

5.1 RESPIRATORY DRUGS

Medications used in the management of pulmonary disease aim to maintain optimal airflow and gas exchange in the lungs. A summary of the various respiratory medications is provided in Table 5-1.

- The most commonly used drugs are the bronchodilators, which inhibit the constriction of bronchial smooth muscle that occurs in asthma and in some patients with chronic obstructive pulmonary disease (COPD).
- Antiinflammatory drugs are used to suppress the chronic inflammatory process that promotes bronchospasm in asthma

and sometimes chronic bronchitis. They may also be prescribed for the treatment of other acute inflammatory processes affecting the lungs. Antiinflammatory medications include the glucocorticoids, leukotriene modifiers, and mast cell stabilizers.

- Mucokinetic agents facilitate the clearance of bronchial secretions.
- Oxygen is presented in Chapter 2 (Pulmonology; see page 26).
- A few other medications that are used in the treatment of specific pulmonary pathologies, such as neonatal respiratory distress syndrome (RDS), α_1-protease inhibitor (API) deficiency, and pulmonary hypertension, are also introduced.
- A variety of other medications, including decongestants, antihistamines, and expectorants, are taken for symptomatic relief of pulmonary disease and are discussed briefly.
- Antimicrobial agents that are used to treat respiratory infections are beyond the scope of this chapter and are not included.

Many pulmonary drugs, including bronchodilators, antiinflammatory drugs, mucokinetic agents, and some antimicrobials, are administered directly to the lungs by aerosol inhalation with a pressurized measured, or metered, dose inhaler (pMDI), a dry powder inhaler (DPI), or a nebulizer. Aerosol therapy aims to deposit high concentrations of medications into the lower airways for absorption through the large surface area (so minimal dosing is required), which provides a rapid onset of action and minimizes systemic side effects.

- pMDIs consist of a canister of gaseous medication dissolved or suspended in a liquid and require a propellant. The canister fits into a plastic device with a mouthpiece that releases a set amount of medication; that is, a metered dose. They are convenient to carry and use but require proper technique to achieve optimal drug delivery to the lungs and to minimize oropharyngeal deposition, which can lead to systemic side effects.
  ‣ The recommended technique for open-mouth use of a pMDI is described in Box 5-1 and pictured in Figure 5-1.
  ‣ The closed-mouth technique is the same except that the mouthpiece is inserted in the mouth past the front teeth and the lips are sealed around it. This technique tends to produce greater oropharyngeal deposition of medications and less to the lower airways.
  ‣ A spacer device or holding chamber can be attached to a pMDI to slow the flow of the aerosol, as pictured in Figure 5-2. It improves the effective delivery of medication by improving the deposition of medication in the distal airways rather than in the oropharynx, thus reducing the incidence of systemic side effects. The combination of a pMDI and a large-volume spacer has demonstrated similar effectiveness as nebulized bronchodilator treatments for most cases of moderate to severe asthma.[14] The procedure for using a pMDI with a spacer device is the

TABLE 5-1: Pulmonary Medications

Drug	Trade Name(s)	Method of Delivery	Onset of Action	Time to Peak Effect	Duration of Action	Comments
Short-acting β-Adrenergic Agonists						
Albuterol* (Salbutamol)	Proventil, Ventolin, AccuNeb; ProAir	MDI, neb	5–10 min	1–1.5 h	6–8 h	
Bitolterol	Tornalate	Neb	3–4 min	30–60 min	6–8 h	Disagreeable taste
Epinephrine (Adrenalin)	AsthmaHaler, Bronkaid Mist, Primatene Mist, and many others	Neb, ET	3–5 min	—	1–3 h	Stimulates α_1- + β_2- and β_2-adrenergic receptors
		SC	Variable	—	<1–4 h	
	EpiPen, Epi EZ Pen, Twinjects	IM	6–15 min	15–20 min	<1–4 h	
Isoetharine	Arm-A-Med, Bronchosol	MDI, neb	1–6 min	15–60 min	1–4 h	Used outside of U.S.
Isoproterenol	Medihaler	MDI, neb	2–5 min	—	0.5–2 h	Acts on β_1- and β_2-adrenergic receptors
	Isuprel	IV	5–20 min	—	<1 h	
		SL tabs	15–30 min	—	1–2 h	
Levalbuterol	Xopenex	Neb	10–17 min	1–2 h	5–6 h	Fewer side effects
Metaproterenol*	Alupent	MDI, neb	5–30 min	1–2 h	4–6 h	
Pirbuterol	Maxair	MDI	≤5 min	30–60 min	4–6 h	
Procaterol		Neb	≤5 min	90 min	6–8 h	Used outside of U.S.
Terbutaline	Bricanyl	MDI, neb	15–30 min	1–2 h	3–6 h	
		Injection	≤15 min	≤30–60 min	1.5–4 h	
Long-acting β-Adrenergic Agonists						
Albuterol	VoSpire ER, Volmax Proventil Repetabs	Oral tabs	15–30 min	2–3 h	12 h	Do not chew or crush tabs; Volmax tabs should be stored in refrigerator
Formoterol	Foradil	DPI	≤5 min	≤30 min	12 h	Capsule placed in aerolizer inhaler
Salmeterol	Servent	MDI, DPI	10–20 min	3–4 h	12 h	
Terbutaline	Brethine, Bricanyl, Brethaire	Oral	≤1–2 h	≤2–3 h	4–8 h	
Anticholinergic Agents						
Ipratropium	Atrovent	MDI	15–30 min	1–2 h	6 h	
Tiotropium	Spiriva	DPI	≤5 min	≤30 min	24 h	Unpleasant taste
Xanthine Derivatives						
Aminophylline*	Inophylline, Norphyllin, Phyllocontin	IV	<1 min	<30 min	6–12 h	Absorption is variable, many drug interactions
		Oral	20–30 min	1–2 h	6–12 h	
Dyphylline	Dilor, Lufyllin	Injection Oral				

Continued

TABLE 5-1: Pulmonary Medications—Cont'd

Drug	Trade Name(s)	Method of Delivery	Onset of Action	Time to Peak Effect	Duration of Action	Comments
Oxtriphylline	Choledyl	Oral tabs, ER tabs				
Theophylline*	Slo-Bid, Theo-24, Theo-Dur, Uniphyl	Oral	20–30 min	5–9 h	12 h	Absorption is variable, many drug interactions
Glucocorticoids						
Beclomethasone*	Beclovent, QVAR, Vanceril	MDI, DPI	1–2 d	1–2+ wk	6–8 h	Age ≥5 yr
Betamethasone	Celestone	Injection, Oral				
Budesonide	Pulmicort	Neb	2–8 d	4–6 wk	12–24 h	Disagreeable taste, not tested in children
		MDI	24 h	1–2+ wk	12–24 h	
Cortisone	Cortone	Oral, IM				
Dexamethasone*	Decadron, DexPak	Oral	NA		4–6 h	Many systemic side effects
Flunisolide*	Aerobid	MDI	NA	1–2+ wk	12 h	Age ≥6 yr
Fluticasone	Flonase, Flovent	MDI, DPI	24 h	1–2+ wk	12–24 h	Age ≥12 yr
Hydrocortisone	Cortef	Injection, Oral				Many systemic side effects
Methylprednisolone	Medrol	IV, Oral				Many systemic side effects
Prednisolone	Hydeltrasol	Oral				Many systemic side effects
Prednisone	Deltasone, others	Oral				Many systemic side effects
Triamcinolone	Azmacort	MDI	1 wk	2+ wk	12 h	Age ≥6 yr
Leukotriene Modifiers						
Montelukast	Singulair	Oral tabs, granules	NA	2–4 h	24 h	Age ≥12 mo
Zafirlukast	Accolate	Oral tabs	NA	2–3 h	12+ h	Age ≥5 yr; take on empty stomach
Zileuton	Zyflo	Oral tabs	NA	1–2 h	5–8 h	Age ≥12 yr
Mast Cell Stabilizers						
Cromolyn	Intal	MDI, nebulizer	10–15 min	Up to several weeks	6 h	Age ≥5 yr
Nedocromil	Tilade	MDI	10–15 min	≥1 wk	6 h	Age ≥6 yr
Omalizumab	Xolair	SC	NA	7–8 d	3–4 wk	Age ≥12 yr

DPI, Dry powder inhaler; ER, extended release; ET, endotracheal; IM, intramuscular injection; IV, intravenous; MDI, measured/metered dose inhaler; NA, not available; neb, nebulizer; SC, subcutaneous injection; SL, sublingual; tabs, tablets; U.S., United States.
*β₂-Selective agents provide greatest benefit with minimal side effects.

BOX 5-1: Recommended Technique for Open-mouth Use of Metered Dose Inhalers

1. Shake the inhaler and remove the cap.
2. Exhale completely while keeping the mouth closed.
3. Position the upright inhaler 1 to 2 in. in front of a wide open mouth, as shown in Figure 5-1.
4. Begin to inhale slowly and then activate the inhaler by pressing down once on the canister.
5. Continue to inhale slowly and deeply through the mouth for as long as possible (to total lung capacity).
6. Hold breath for at least 5 to 10 seconds or for as long as possible.
7. Exhale slowly through the nose.
8. If the doctor has prescribed two puffs, wait 1 to 2 minutes, shake the inhaler, and repeat the procedure.
9. Clean the plastic mouthpiece thoroughly with soap and water after each use.

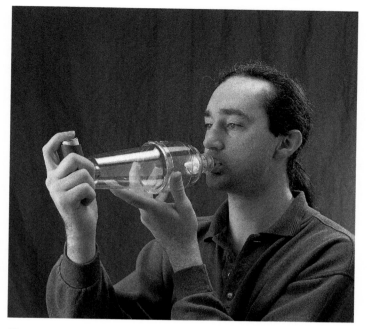

Figure 5-2: A large-volume spacer or extension chamber added to a pressurized metered-dose inhaler. It allows the aerosol cloud to slow down and overcomes problems of patient coordination. (From Forbes CD, Jackson WF. *Color Atlas and Text of Clinical Medicine.* 3rd ed. Edinburgh: Mosby; 2003.)

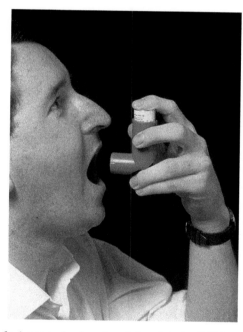

Figure 5-1: A pressurized metered-dose inhaler (MDI), as used for the delivery of bronchodilators, antiinflammatory drugs, and mucokinetic agents. Although convenient and portable, MDIs require good coordination between actuation and inhalation by the patient. (From Forbes CD, Jackson WF. *Color Atlas and Text of Clinical Medicine.* 3rd ed. Edinburgh: Mosby; 2003.)

same as described in Box 5-1, except that the inhaler is connected to the spacer and the spacer's mouthpiece is placed in the mouth with the lips sealed around it, after which the inhaler is squirted into the chamber before beginning a slow inhalation. Of note, static charging on polycarbonate spacers can reduce the delivered dose; regular washing of the device mitigates this problem.

- DPIs are also small, hand-held devices that deliver a precisely measured dose of asthma medicine into the lungs. They are generally easier to use than pMDIs because they are inspiratory flow activated and driven, so good coordination of activation and inspiration is not needed. However, they do require faster inspiratory flow for activation, which may be a problem when inspiratory force is reduced.
  - ▸ There are many types of DPIs and the directions for using them vary for each brand, so patients must read and understand the specific instructions for each device they are using. The general instructions for using a DPI are presented in Box 5-2.
  - ▸ Patients must be instructed to avoid exhaling into a DPI, as moisture interferes with effective drug delivery.
- Rinsing the mouth after using a DPI or a pMDI without a spacer/chamber may reduce oropharyngeal absorption and help alleviate any bad aftertaste.
- Medications are also administered via other routes, including intratracheal instillation (surfactant replacers), oral intake (long-acting bronchodilators [e.g., albuterol, aminophylline, fenoterol, metaproterenol, terbutaline, and theophylline], systemic corticosteroids, and leukotriene modifiers), intravenous or intramuscular injection, and subcutaneous injection (epinephrine).

There is significant interindividual variability in responses to the various medications used to treat asthma and COPD, which

---

BOX 5-2: General Procedure for Using a Dry Powder Inhaler*

---

1. Remove the inhaler cap and check that the mechanism is clean and that the mouthpiece is free of obstruction.
2. Load the dose into the device as directed.
3. Hold the container in the proper position but away from the mouth.
4. Tilt the head back slightly and breathe out slowly and completely. Do not exhale into the inhaler, as this can cause the dry powder to clump together and clog the inhaler.
5. Place the inhaler in the mouth and seal the lips around the mouthpiece, ensuring that the tongue does not block the inhaler.
6. Breathe in quickly and deeply (over 2 to 3 s) through the mouth to activate the flow of the medication.

7. Remove the inhaler from the mouth and hold the breath for at least 5 to 10 seconds (or as long as is comfortable, which allows the medications to get deep into the lungs).
8. Exhale slowly against pursed lips
9. If a second dose is needed, wait 1 to 2 minutes and repeat the procedure.
10. If using an inhaler with corticosteroid medication, gargle and rinse out the mouth with water after using the inhaler to prevent yeast infection in the mouth and to reduce systemic side effects; do not swallow the water.
11. Store inhaler in a clean, sealed plastic bag.

Note: The instructions for using DPIs vary with each brand; the patient must read and understand the specific instructions for each device being used.

---

may be due to genetic differences in receptor function.[22] Pharmacogenetics may play an increasing role in the future in determining which therapies will provide the greatest benefit with the least risk of adverse effects for subsets of patients.

A summary of the effects of various medications on exercise responses is provided later in this chapter (see Table 5-22 on page 216).

BRONCHODILATORS

The major determinant of airway caliber and resistance is the bronchial smooth muscle encircling the airways. Most bronchodilators effect bronchodilation through stimulation of the receptors that cause relaxation of smooth muscle or by blocking the receptors that trigger bronchoconstriction. In general, patients are prescribed a rescue inhaler for quick relief of acute attacks of bronchospasm in patients with asthma or sometimes COPD, and, if their disease requires the use of this inhaler more than twice per week, another drug for long-term control.

β-ADRENERGIC AGONISTS

Normally, the airways experience a constant low level of endogenous β_2-adrenergic stimulation that promotes and maintains airway patency through smooth muscle relaxation and bronchodilation. The administration of β-adrenergic agonists (also called *sympathomimetics*) produces additional bronchodilation and these drugs are used in the treatment of asthma.[22,60]

- β_2-Adrenergic agonists effect relaxation of airway smooth muscle by direct stimulation of β_2-adrenergic receptors. In addition, they may exert other effects on airways, including inhibition of inflammatory cells or substances, reduction of bronchial mucosal edema, improved mucociliary clearance of secretions, and anticholinergic effects (see the next topic).
- Short-acting β_2-agonists are used for all patients with asthma as rescue medications for acute attacks of bronchospasm and may be the only medication used by patients with mild asthma (see

Table 4-3 for classifications of asthma severity and control); they can also be used before exercise to prevent exercise-induced asthma (EIA). Patients should carry their rescue inhaler with them at all times, including to rehabilitation sessions. Increased usage (more than two times per week) is an indicator that the addition of a long-acting β_2-agonist or increased antiinflammatory therapy is needed.

- Long-acting β_2-agonists (LABAs) are used two or more times a day as "controller" medications to prevent bronchoconstriction and are particularly effective in the management of exercise-induced bronchospasm and nocturnal episodic asthma. It is important to recognize that although salmeterol (Serevent) comes as an inhaler, its onset of action is too slow for it to be effective for the treatment of acute asthma attacks. LABAs should not be used as monotherapy in mild persistent asthma, but should be given along with inhaled corticosteroids.[22]
- Short-acting β_2-agonists are also prescribed for patients with COPD who have airway hyperreactivity, although there is inconsistent evidence on the benefits of LABAs in these patients.
- β-Adrenergic agonists may be useful for the treatment of acute lung injury (as in acute respiratory distress syndrome [ARDS]) because of their potential to reduce pulmonary edema by attenuating inflammatory injury to the pulmonary circulation and by accelerating the resolution of alveolar edema.[70,83]
- The side effects of β_2-agonists depend on their mode of administration.
  - Inhaled short-acting β_2-agonists rarely produce side effects at recommended doses.
  - Higher doses or oral or intravenous administration are more likely to cause stimulation of extrapulmonary β-receptors, causing muscle tremors, nervousness, tachycardia and palpitations, hypokalemia, restlessness, insomnia, and, rarely, headaches.
  - There appears to be a small subclass of patients with asthma, especially black patients, who are prone to adverse responses to LABAs, including asthma-related death.[22,76] Specific genetic variations may be responsible.

ANTICHOLINERGIC AGENTS

Anticholinergic agents (also known as parasympatholytic agents) are used to maintain airway patency in patients with COPD and sometimes asthma. These drugs include ipratropium (Atrovent), tiotropium (Spiriva), and oxitropium.

- Anticholinergic agents block the muscarinic receptors in airway smooth muscle, inhibiting vagal cholinergic tone and preventing bronchoconstriction. They may have additive effect with β-agonists, so the two types of medications are usually prescribed together.
- Anticholinergics, along with β-agonists, are the first-line maintenance treatment for patients with COPD.
  - Because they have no significant antiinflammatory effects and little or no effect on mast cells, anticholinergics are less effective in the treatment of asthma. However, they are sometimes prescribed for difficult-to-control asthma (e.g., older patients and those with an element of fixed airway obstruction).
  - The safety and effectiveness of anticholinergic agents have not been established in pediatric patients.
  - Combivent and DuoNeb are combination inhalers containing both ipratropium and albuterol, allowing patients to use only one inhaler to take both medications at the same time.
- Side effects other than dry mouth are uncommon because there is almost no systemic absorption.

METHYLXANTHINES

Methylxanthines, such as aminophylline and theophylline, are systemic bronchodilators that have been largely replaced by inhaled bronchodilators and antiinflammatory drugs because of problems with toxicity. They are less effective than β-adrenergic agonists but when used in combination therapy may have a synergistic effect.

- The mechanism of action of the methylxanthines is uncertain; they reverse bronchoconstriction in patients with asthma, most likely as a result of an antiinflammatory action, and they have a weak bronchodilator effect.
  - Theophylline is proposed to act through antagonism of adenosine receptors, inhibition of the intracellular release of calcium, and/or stimulation of catecholamine release. Theophylline inhibits the late response to allergens, suggesting that it has an antiinflammatory action; however, it does not inhibit the release of mediators from eosinophils.
  - Other beneficial effects of theophylline may include enhanced diaphragmatic function, increased mucociliary clearance, and stimulation of the respiratory drive.
- Methylxanthines are used primarily in patients with acute asthma who fail to respond to β-agonists and anticholinergics; they may also be added to maintenance therapy for patients who continue to experience bronchoconstriction despite optimal doses of other asthma medications. In addition, they may be used in the treatment of patients with COPD with reversible airflow obstruction, especially those with nocturnal symptoms despite optimal doses of β-agonists or anticholinergics.

- The most common side effects include tremor, anxiety, agitation, insomnia, and gastrointestinal upset.
  - Theophylline has a narrow therapeutic window and requires careful monitoring of drug levels to avoid toxicity, which can be fatal.
  - Toxicity is usually dose related but can occur even at low doses; it is manifested by increasing severity of side effects, as listed previously, and most severely by repeated vomiting, tachyarrhythmias, hypotension, and seizures.

ANTIINFLAMMATORY AGENTS

Chronic inflammation appears to sensitize the airways, increasing hyperreactive bronchoconstriction in patients with asthma and other obstructive pulmonary disorders. Therefore, antiinflammatory agents, including glucocorticoids, leukotriene modifiers, and cromones, are frequently prescribed for these patients.

Glucocorticosteroids

Glucocorticosteroids, also called corticosteroids, are taken on a long-term basis to prevent inflammatory-mediated bronchoconstriction.[22,60] The preferred route of administration is via inhaler in order to minimize systemic absorption and thus side effects. Oral glucocorticoids are used in the treatment of some nonobstructive inflammatory lung diseases.

- The effects of these drugs include inhibition of inflammatory cells (e.g., mast cells, eosinophils, neutrophils, macrophages, and lymphocytes), suppression of release of inflammatory mediators (e.g., cytokines, histamine, leukotrienes, prostaglandins, etc.), enhanced production of antiinflammatory proteins, and reversal of enhanced capillary permeability, thus reducing airway edema.
- Inhaled corticosteroids (ICSs) are the first-line treatment for mild persistent to severe asthma (in patients of age ≥5 yr) and other bronchoconstrictive diseases in order to control symptoms, reduce frequency of exacerbations, and improve pulmonary function. Treatment earlier in the course of disease may help delay disease progression.
  - Once-daily dosing may be as effective as the current standard of twice-daily dosing.[71]
  - They are not indicated for the relief of acute bronchospasm.
  - Low-dose ICSs usually have only local side effects resulting from deposition on the posterior pharynx and vocal cords, causing sore throat, hoarseness, and oral thrush (Candida infection). These complications can be minimized by using a spacer device and rinsing the mouth after each inhaler use.
- Combined therapy with low or moderate doses of ICSs with LABAs provides the optimal maintenance treatment for patients with moderate to severe asthma who are not well controlled on ICSs alone.
  - Treatment with budesonide/formoterol is beneficial both as maintenance and reliever therapy, reducing the risk of severe asthma exacerbations and the need for systemic steroids and improving asthma symptoms and nocturnal awakenings; it allows a fourfold lower dose of ICS so it can be used in children as well as adults.[80]

▸ ICSs are also used in combination with anticholinergic bronchodilators or LABAs in patients with COPD to reduce the frequency of exacerbations.[41,87]

- Intravenous and oral glucocorticoids may be prescribed for patients with severe acute asthma attacks who do not respond to inhaled medications. Oral glucocorticoids (e.g., dexamethasone, methylprednisolone, prednisolone, prednisone, and triamcinolone), may be used to treat nonobstructive inflammatory lung diseases, such as sarcoidosis, berylliosis, and aspiration pneumonitis, and sometimes nonresolving ARDS.
  ▸ Side effects of short-term use of systemic corticosteroids include worsening glycemic control, water retention, insomnia and agitation, facial flushing, appetite stimulation, gastrointestinal discomfort, mood changes, and headache.
  ▸ Long-term use of systemic corticosteroids is associated with many serious side effects: osteoporosis, muscle wasting and myopathy, skin breakdown and impaired healing, hyperglycemia and exacerbation of diabetes mellitus, hypertension, cataracts, glaucoma, weight gain, growth retardation, and adrenal gland suppression.

Leukotriene Modifiers

Leukotrienes are inflammatory compounds produced by cells lining the airways, which play a significant role in the pathophysiology of asthma, including constriction of bronchial smooth muscle, swelling, edema, and leakage from bronchial blood vessels, and increased mucus secretion. Leukotriene modifiers reduce airway edema and bronchoconstriction. They are available as oral tablets and include montelukast (Singulair), zileuton (Zyflo), and zafirlukast (Accolate).

- Leukotriene modifiers act through antagonism of the leukotriene receptor (e.g., zafirlukast and montelukast) or inhibition of leukotriene formation through suppression of 5-lipoxygenase (e.g., zileuton).
- They are currently recommended for long-term control of mild persistent asthma in patients 12 years of age or older, although montelukast and zafirlukast may be used in much younger children.
- Systemic side effects are usually minimal although these drugs may interact with other drugs.
  ▸ The side effects of montelukast and zafirlukast include headache, dizziness, nausea, diarrhea, and abdominal pain.
  ▸ Zafirlukast is associated with several drug interactions.
  ▸ The side effects of zileuton include abnormal liver function tests, headache, dizziness, abdominal pain, nausea, pain, and myalgia.

Mast Cell Stabilizers

Mast cell stabilizers are used prophylactically to inhibit the allergic response that triggers airway reactivity, and thus they reduce symptoms and improve lung function in patients with asthma. Currently approved drugs include cromolyn (Intal), nedocromil (Tilade), and omalizumab (Xolair).

- Cromolyn and nedocromil act to stabilize mast cells and possibly other cells, such as eosinophils, macrophages, and neutrophils, and to suppress the release of histamine, leukotrienes, and other inflammatory mediators. Thus, they inhibit the immediate and nonimmediate bronchoconstrictive reactions to inhaled antigens.
  ▸ Cromolyn and nedocromil may be used as the initial antiinflammatory drug for long-term control of asthma in children, as well as adults who do not tolerate the side effects of other antiasthma drugs, and they can be used as pretreatment for exercise-induced asthma and as prophylaxis against exposure to environmental triggers.
  ▸ They are administered by inhaler.
  ▸ The main side effects of these drugs are cough and irritation of the throat.
- Omalizumab is a recombinant DNA–derived humanized monoclonal antibody that blocks the immunoglobulin E (IgE) receptors on the surfaces of the mast cells and basophils, preventing the attachment of antibodies to these cells and consequently the release of inflammatory mediators.
  ▸ Omalizumab is prescribed as adjunctive therapy for allergic adults and adolescents (those with atopy and sensitivity to an aeroallergen) with moderate to severe asthma whose symptoms are inadequately controlled by high-dose ICSs plus LABAs.[75,78]
  ▸ Subcutaneous injections are given every 2 to 4 weeks, with dosage and frequency determined by serum total IgE level.
  ▸ The adverse reactions most commonly observed with omalizumab include injection site reaction, viral infections, upper respiratory infection, sinusitis, headache, and sore throat. However, there have also been rare reports of malignancies and anaphylactic reactions.

Combination Drugs

To facilitate patient compliance, manufacturers have combined some aerosol medications into one inhaler:

- Combivent and DuoNeb contain both albuterol (a short-acting β-agonist) and ipratropium (an anticholinergic) and are used to treat bronchospasm associated with COPD in patients who require more than one bronchodilator.[41]
- Advair contains both salmeterol (a long-acting β-agonist) and fluticasone (a glucocorticoid) and is used for long-term control of asthma.
- Symbicort, containing budesonide (a glucocorticoid) and formoterol (a long-acting β-agonist), is used in the management of asthma and COPD.

MUCOACTIVE AGENTS

Mucoactive agents aim to either facilitate the ease of sputum expectoration or to decrease mucus hypersecretion.

- Hypersecretion of airway mucus, as evidenced by increased production of mucus, excessive mucus in the airways, goblet cell hyperplasia, and submucosal gland hypertrophy, is a feature of a number of serious pulmonary diseases, including asthma, COPD, and cystic fibrosis (CF). However, the characteristics of mucus hypersecretion and the nature of airway obstruction differ in each of these diseases, which means that different treatments may be required for effective control.[92]

- The pathophysiological sequelae of mucus hypersecretion are airway obstruction, airflow limitation, ventilation–perfusion mismatching, and impaired gas exchange. In addition, patients with COPD and CF suffer repeated respiratory infections and exacerbations due to impaired mucociliary function.

The objectives for treatment of mucus hypersecretion are short-term relief of symptoms and prevention of long-term pathophysiological sequelae.[92]

- Short-term symptomatic relief involves enhancing mucus clearance, which can be accomplished by changing the viscoelasticity of mucus, increasing ciliary function, inducing cough, facilitating the release of the gelatinous mucus plugs promoted by tethered goblet cell mucin in asthma, and inhibiting mucin secretion.
  - ▸ Unfortunately, the mucus variables that favor effective mucociliary clearance (thin mucus layer, "ideal" sol depth, increased elasticity, reduced viscosity, and higher adhesivity) are directly opposite to those that favor effective cough (thick mucus layer, excess sol height above the cilia, decreased elasticity, increased viscosity, and low adhesivity).
  - ▸ Thus, it may be reasoned that if mucus obstruction can be cleared by cough (e.g., mucus accumulation in more proximal airways), then drugs that enhance cough effectiveness would be indicated. Conversely, if mucus obstruction is located more distally or if the patient is too weak to produce an effective cough, then drugs that promote mucociliary clearance would be preferred.
  - ▸ The difficulty comes in identifying which situation each patient falls under and which treatment options are appropriate.
- Long-term approaches involve reversal of the hypersecretory phenotype by treating airway inflammation, reducing the number of goblet cells and the size of the submucosal glands, inhibiting plasma exudation in asthma, correcting the increased ratio of gland mucous cells to serous cells in COPD (which may increase the antibacterial enzyme levels), and reversing

the increased ratio of low-charge glycoform MUC5B to MUC5AC seen in COPD.[92]

Numerous mucoactive agents are available, but few are recommended in the various guidelines developed for the clinical management of COPD, asthma, or CF. Medications that act as mucoactive agents are classified as expectorants, mucolytics, mucokinetics, or mucoregulators, according to their characteristics and putative mechanism(s) of action, which are listed in Table 5-2, although the various terms are often confused with each other.

Expectorants

Expectorants increase the production of a thin, watery sputum in the respiratory tract, probably by increasing the secretion of mucins, increasing mucus hydration, or both to such a degree that the volume of secretions produced is sufficient to allow patients to cough them up more easily. These drugs may also be irritants that promote coughing to dislodge mucus.

- The most commonly used expectorant is guaifenesin, which is found in several prescription forms and also in over-the-counter cough medicines, often in combination with other products, such as mucolytics and antitussives. It is the only expectorant that has documented ability to increase the production of secretions and thus aid in expectoration.
- An expectorant that is found in children's cough syrups is ammonium chloride.
- There are no major side effects. On occasion, nausea and vomiting or diarrhea will occur, particularly with excessive doses or intake on an empty stomach. Sometimes, bradycardia occurs due to excess vagal stimulation induced by coughing.

Mucolytics

Mucolytic agents break up the mucoprotein molecules that increase the viscosity of mucus, thus increasing the ease of expectoration. Treatment with oral mucolytics is associated with a modest but significant reduction in acute exacerbations and days of illness in patients with chronic bronchitis and COPD.[86]

TABLE 5-2: Mucoactive Agents and Their Putative Mechanisms of Action

Mucoactive Agent	Putative Mechanism of Action
Expectorants	Increase volume and/or hydration of secretions.
	May also induce cough (e.g., guaifenesin and hypertonic saline)
Mucolytics	Reduce viscosity of mucus
	Nonpeptide ("classical") mucolytics cleave disulfide bonds ("free" or "blocked" sulfhydryl groups)
	Low molecular weight saccharide agents interfere with noncovalent interactions in mucus, and may osmotically pull water into airway lumen
	Peptide mucolytics degrade DNA or actin
Mucokinetic agents	Increase "kinesis" of mucus and facilitate cough "transportability" of mucus
	β_2-Adrenergic antagonists increase airflow, ciliary beat, Cl^-/water secretion, and mucin secretion (small effect)
	Surfactant reduces adherence of mucus to epithelium
Mucoregulatory drugs	Reduce process of chronic hypersecretion (e.g., glucocorticoids, anticholinergics, and macrolide antibiotics)

(From Rogers DF. Mucoactive agents for airway mucus hypersecretory diseases. *Respir Care* 2007;52:1176–1193.)

- Nonpeptide ("classical") mucolytics, such as *N*-acetylcysteine (Mucomyst, Mucosil), carbocysteine, and mecysteine cleave disulfide bonds. The beneficial clinical effects of acetylcysteine may not be due to its mucolytic or antioxidant activity but rather to a reduction in bacterial load.[92] The most common side effect of these agents is mild nausea, and sometimes fever or drowsiness. However, acetylcysteine is sometimes associated with nausea/vomiting, inflammation of the oral mucosa (stomatitis), and rhinorrhea and occasionally induces serious bronchospasm.
- Dornase alfa (Pulmozyme) is a genetically engineered form of the human enzyme deoxyribonuclease (DNase), which breaks down the highly polymerized DNA that is released in large amounts into the airways from necrotic neutrophils; thus, it reduces mucus viscosity, facilitating expectoration. It is approved for use in the long-term maintenance of patients with CF and is administered once per day by nebulizer. It has been shown to improve pulmonary function and to reduce the incidence of pulmonary infection requiring antibiotics.[6a,59]
- Inhaled hypertonic saline likely works by reducing the entanglements in airway mucus gel, and it may also draw liquid osmotically through the airway epithelium, producing greater hydration of secretions so they are easier to mobilize.

Mucokinetics

Mucokinetic agents reduce mucus adhesiveness to the underlying epithelium and thus increase the efficiency of mucociliary function or cough. Surfactant falls into this category.
- Surfactant is not only produced by the type II pneumocytes, it is also secreted in other parts of the upper respiratory tract and in the bronchi by submucous glands in the proximal airways and Clara cells in the distal airways.[5]
- Surfactant production is increased by glucocorticoids, epidermal growth factor, and cyclic adenosine monophosphate (cAMP) and inhibited by tumor necrosis factor-α (TNF-α), transforming growth factor-β (TGF-β), and insulin.[5]
- Surfactant can reduce mucus adhesiveness and increase energy transfer from the cilia to the mucus layer.
- Surfactant also has the important function of maintaining airway stability and patency.

MUCOREGULATORY AGENTS

Mucoregulatory medications reduce the volume of airway mucus production and appear to be especially effective in hypersecretory states, such as bronchorrhea, diffuse panbronchiolitis, and some forms of asthma. These agents include the antiinflammatory agents and anticholinergic drugs already presented, and some macrolide antibiotics.[95]
- Anticholinergic medications reduce the volume of stimulated secretions without increasing viscosity.
- Many inflammatory mediators are potent secretagogues, and chronic inflammation leads to mucous gland hyperplasia. Corticosteroids are known to reduce the volume of secretions, and ibuprofen has been shown to have specific activity against neutrophils. Inhaled indomethacin is used for the treatment of diffuse panbronchiolitis.

- Some of the macrolide antibiotics, particularly erythromycin, clarithromycin, and azithromycin, appear to be able to reduce mucus secretion and improve mucus clearance.[40,95]

SUMMARY OF ASTHMA AND COPD TREATMENT

To facilitate assimilation of the previous information, the following summaries are provided for the medications used to treat asthma and COPD.

Asthma

Pharmacologic therapy of asthma aims to provide rapid relief of acute asthma symptoms and to establish long-term control of underlying inflammation and bronchoconstriction.
- Short-acting β_2-agonist rescue inhalers are prescribed for all patients for acute attacks and may be the only medication required by patients with mild asthma.
- Inhaled corticosteroids are also a first-line treatment for asthma because of their role in directly inhibiting the underlying inflammatory disease process.
- Patients who are not successfully controlled with inhaled corticosteroids are treated with additional drugs, such as LABAs, leukotriene modifiers, mast cell stabilizers, or anticholinergic drugs.
- In addition, asthma triggers should be identified and avoided whenever possible.
- Aerobic conditioning may help reduce the incidence of asthmatic attacks and allow for lower doses of medications in certain patients.

COPD

The primary goals of drug treatment of COPD are the maintenance of airway patency and the prevention of airflow restriction.
- Anticholinergic bronchodilators are usually the treatment of choice in patients with airflow restriction in COPD.
- Alternatively, long-acting β_2-agonists may be prescribed, which have also demonstrated efficacy in reducing COPD exacerbations.
- Inhaled corticosteroids (ICSs) are also beneficial in reducing the incidence of exacerbations, and the combination of LABAs and ICSs seems to be even more effective.
- In addition, participation in a pulmonary rehabilitation program is valuable. Physical therapy interventions that may offer particular benefit include aerobic conditioning, breathing retraining, and others, as described in Chapter 7 (Cardiovascular and Pulmonary Physical Therapy Treatment).

OTHER PULMONARY MEDICATIONS

Some medications are used to treat specific pulmonary disorders, such as neonatal respiratory distress syndrome and severe meconium aspiration syndrome, α_1-protease inhibitor deficiency, and pulmonary arterial hypertension. Some of these are presented here.

Exogenous Surfactant Therapy

Surfactant replacement therapy is used in the treatment of neonatal respiratory disease. These agents are usually administered via endotracheal tube and therefore require intubation and stabilization with mechanical ventilation.[105]

- Natural surfactants derived from animal lungs (Curosurf, Infasurf, and Survanta) are used in the treatment and prevention of neonatal respiratory distress syndrome (RDS) to lower alveolar surface tension and to stabilize them against collapse.
- They also have proven benefit in the treatment of severe meconium aspiration syndrome.
- In addition, evidence suggests that they may be of value in the treatment of ARDS in the pediatric population. However, they have not shown survival benefit in the treatment of ARDS in adults, except possibily for ARDS due to pneumonia or aspiration.[105a]
- A synthetic surfactant, Surfaxin, has been granted orphan drug status for the treatment of bronchopulmonary dysplasia, and final U.S. Food and Drug Administration (FDA) approval for the prevention of RDS in high-risk neonates is pending.

α_1-Proteinase Inhibitor

α_1-Proteinase inhibitors (α_1-PIs) are used for chronic augmentation and maintenance therapy for individuals with α_1-PI deficiency (a hereditary disorder characterized by low serum and lung levels of α_1-PI, which causes a diffuse panacinar emphysema; see page 78) who have clinical evidence of emphysema with initial FEV_1 (forced expiratory volume in 1 s) values of 30% to 65%.[63]

- Three agents have received FDA approval as orphan drugs for the treatment of α_1-PI deficiency: Aralast, Prolastin, and Zemaira. They are derived from human plasma and are administered intravenously at 60 mg/kg once per week. Evidence of their efficacy is limited, but prospective studies with end points of mortality, quality of life, exercise capacity, and density of lung tissue are currently underway.
- Adverse side effects generally occur in less than 3% of patients and include headache, dizziness, light-headedness, pharyngitis and sinusitis, fever, somnolence, cough, pain at the infusion site, and pruritus. However, most patients who receive Aralast develop upper respiratory infection, and some show elevations of liver enzymes.

Treatment of Pulmonary Arterial Hypertension

The primary therapies for pulmonary arterial hypertension (PAH) include treatment of any underlying cause (e.g., hypoxic lung disease, thromboembolism, connective tissue disease, HIV infection, thyroid dysfunction, left-to-right shunts, and left ventricular dysfunction) as well as treatment of the PAH itself. The therapies that treat PAH directly produce pulmonary vasodilation. They consist of the calcium channel blockers, prostanoids, endothelin antagonists, and phosphodiesterase-5 inhibitors, which are detailed in Table 5-3.[7,16,94] In addition, all these agents except the calcium channel blockers have antiproliferative properties. Other medications are also used to manage the clinical sequelae of PAH: anticoagulants, diuretics, and digoxin, all of which are described later in this chapter. In addition, chronic oxygen therapy is important for hypoxemic patients (see Chapter 2, page 26).

Prostacyclins

Patients with PAH exhibit deficient production of prostacyclin, a substance that promotes vasodilation and inhibits vascular proliferation and platelet aggregation. Synthetic prostacyclin analogs (prostanoids) aim to ameliorate all these abnormalities.[7,16,39,94]

- Epoprostenol (Flolan) is a prostanoid used as the treatment of choice for patients with advanced PAH (New York Heart Association [NYHA] classes III and IV; see page 223). It is administered through a continuous portable infusion pump and an indwelling central venous catheter.

TABLE 5-3: **Vasodilators Used to Treat Pulmonary Arterial Hypertension**

Type of Medication	Drugs	Route of Administration	Mode of Action
Calcium channel blockers	Amlodipine	Oral	Vasodilation of pulmonary arterioles, producing a reduction in pulmonary vascular resistance
	Diltiazem	Oral	
	Nifedipine	Oral	
Prostanoids	Epoprostenol (Flolan)	Continuous IV infusion	Vasodilation of pulmonary arterioles, inhibition of vascular proliferation and platelet aggregation
	Trepostinil (Remodulin)	Continuous SC or IV infusion	
	Iloprost (Ventavis)	Inhaled 6–9×/d	
	Beraprost	Oral	
Endothelin receptor antagonists	Bosentan (Tracleer)	Oral	Inhibition of vasoconstriction through antagonism of ET_A and ET_B receptors
	Sitaxsentan (Thelin)	Oral	Inhibition of vasoconstriction through selective antagonism of ET_A receptors
	Ambrisentan (Letairis)	Oral	
Phosphodiesterase-5 inhibitors	Sildenafil (Revatio)	Oral	Prevention of cGMP breakdown, resulting in pulmonary vasodilation and inhibition of smooth muscle proliferation

cGMP, Cyclic guanosine monophosphate; IV, intravenous; SC, subcutaneous.

- Longer acting prostanoids have been developed for intravenous, inhaled, and/or oral use: trepostinil (Remodulin), iloprost (Ventavis), and beraprost (approved in Japan).
- Side effects common to all prostanoids include flushing, jaw pain, and body aches; they can become severe enough to limit the achievable medication dose.

Calcium Channel Blockers

Calcium channel blockers (CCBs) are used predominantly for the small percentage of patients with primary, or idiopathic, PAH who have a favorable response to a vasodilator challenge (defined as a decrease in mean pulmonary artery pressure of ≥ 10 mm Hg to a value ≤ 40 mm Hg) with increased or unchanged cardiac output.[7,94] High doses of amlodipine, nifedipine, or diltiazem are used. Close follow-up is required because of high long-term CCB treatment failure rates. CCBs are described in more detail later in this chapter (see page 172).

Endothelin Antagonists

Endothelin-1 (ET-1) is an amino acid peptide that is produced by vascular endothelium and promotes the release of calcium by the sarcoplasmic reticulum, which causes smooth muscle contraction. ET-1 induces potent vasoconstriction and proliferation of fibroblasts and vascular smooth muscle cells and stimulates the heart, increasing contractility and heart rate (HR); it also stimulates aldosterone secretion, decreases renal blood flow and the glomerular filtration rate, and releases atrial natriuretic peptide (ANP), which indirectly affect CV function. Circulating levels of ET-1 are increased in PAH and correlate with disease severity.[16]

There are two types of naturally occurring endothelin receptors: ET_A and ET_B. When ET-1 binds with ET_A receptors, it causes vasoconstriction, and when it binds with ET_B receptors, it produces nitric oxide (NO) and prostacyclin, which result in vascular smooth muscle relaxation and vasodilation. The ET_B receptors exist to counteract the ET_A receptors and protect against vasoconstriction, but they play a smaller role in vascular hemodynamics than the ET_A receptors.

Endothelin receptor antagonists (ERAs) can be nonspecific, blocking both the ET_A and ET_B receptors, or specific, blocking only the ET_A receptors. They are taken orally.

- Bosentan (Tracleer) is a nonspecific ET antagonist that is approved for the treatment of PAH.
- Sitaxsentan (Thelin) is an ET_A-selective compound that is approved in Canada, Europe, and Australia. It has been granted orphan drug status by the FDA and is awaiting full approval.
- Ambrisentan (Letairis) is another ET_A-selective antagonist that is awaiting FDA approval.
- All these ERAs have been associated with reversible, dose-related increases in liver enzymes, and therefore require monthly liver function testing; excessive increases in transaminases (three to eight times normal) necessitate dose reduction or treatment interruption. The highest incidence of liver dysfunction has been noted with bosentan, occurring in approximately 10% of patients.
- The most common side effect is headache. Other side effects include edema, constipation, nasal congestion, upper respiratory infection, dizziness, and insomnia.

Phosphodiesterase-5 Inhibitors

The inhibition of phosphodiesterase-5 (PDE5) prevents the breakdown of cyclic guanosine monophosphate (cGMP), which is a mediator of nitric oxide (NO) and atrial natriuretic peptide (ANP) action. This results in pulmonary vasodilation and inhibition of smooth muscle cell growth.

- During research into the CV effects of PDE5 inhibition, the side effect of penile erection was noted, which led to the development of sildenafil (Viagra). Nearly a decade later its effects on pulmonary vascular tone, growth, and structure won its approval for the treatment of PAH (as Revatio) with World Health Organization (WHO) functional class II/III symptoms. Sildenafil decreases pulmonary vascular resistance in adult and neonatal patients with positive effects on cardiac indices,[7,58] and has potential use in the treatment of PAH due to pulmonary fibrosis.[68]
- There is also evidence that PDE5 inhibition provides cardioprotection against ischemia–reperfusion injury and anthracycline toxicity, blunts acute adrenergic contractile stimulation, and suppresses chronic hypertrophic stress remodeling to pressure overload.[58]
- Common adverse effects include headache, dyspepsia, flushing, diarrhea, and back ache.

Combination Therapy

An increasing number of patients are being treated with combinations of the previously cited drug classes because of the complementary pathogenic mechanisms targeted by each. Synergistic effects have been demonstrated for all possible combinations in small studies while maintaining safety.[94] A randomized trial evaluating the combination of inhaled iloprost (a prostanoid) and bosentan (an endothelin antagonist) revealed significant improvements in the 6-minute walk test, functional class, time to clinical worsening, and hemodynamic parameters compared with bosentan monotherapy.[73] A number of other studies investigating the safety and efficacy of various other drug combinations for the treatment of PAH are currently under way.

DRUGS USED TO CONTROL AIRWAY IRRITATION AND SECRETIONS

A number of ancillary agents are frequently used to control airway irritation and excess secretions; these include decongestants, antihistamines, antitussives, and expectorants. In addition, antibiotics are also prescribed for exacerbations accompanied by infections.

Antibiotics

As there are many classes of antibiotics, it is beyond the scope of this book to present them. Instead, it is sufficient to say that the primary classes used at this time for the treatment of respiratory ailments are the macrolides (erythromycin, clarithromycin,and azithromycin) and the fluoroquinolones (ciprofloxacin, levofloxacin, gatafloxacin, etc.). Other antibiotics that are sometimes prescribed include penicillins, cephalosporins, and co-trimoxazole. Antibiotic resistance patterns change over time, so the antibiotics of choice in one area may not be effective in another area, as resistance has rendered them impotent. To avoid resistance, antibiotics should be used only when significant infection is present or highly suspected and should not be used for routine maintenance or for all exacerbations.

Decongestants

Decongestants are used to treat upper airway mucosal edema and discharge that produce the typical runny nose and stuffy head of the common cold and seasonal allergies.

- The most common agents are α-sympathetic agonists (e.g., pseudoephedrine hydrochloride and phenylpropanolamine), which stimulate vasoconstriction of the blood vessels in the mucosal lining of the upper airway, reducing congestion.
- Because of their sympathetic activity, their primary side effects consist of headache, dizziness, nervousness, nausea, elevated blood pressure (BP), and palpitations.
- Their mechanism of action and side effects make decongestants, particularly pseudoephedrine hydrochloride, generally contraindicated in patients suffering from hypertension.

Antihistamines

Antihistamines are used to block histamine-mediated reactions associated with seasonal allergies. They reduce mucosal congestion, irritation, and discharge caused by inhaled allergens, and they also reduce coughing and sneezing associated with the common cold. They are often combined with decongestants.

- The "first-generation" antihistamines readily crossed the blood–brain barrier to enter the brain, causing the common side effects of sedation, fatigue, dizziness, and blurred vision. In addition, their anticholinergic effects may cause drying of secretions and lead to further airway obstruction in some patients.
- Newer, "second-generation" antihistamines include astemizole (Hismanal), loratadine (Claritin), terfenadine (Seldane), and fexofenadine (Allegra). They do not easily cross the blood–brain barrier, so they are far less likely to cause sedation or other CNS side effects. However, some may produce cardiotoxicity with serious arrhythmias.

Antitussives

Antitussives suppress the cough reflex and are used to treat the irritating, dry, hacking cough associated with minor throat irritations and the common cold. They are not indicated for productive coughs.

- Two main classifications of drugs provide antitussive effects: nonnarcotic, over-the-counter, cough suppressants (e.g., dextromethorphan and benzonate) and narcotics (e.g., codeine).
- The most common side effect is sedation, although some may also cause dizziness and gastrointestinal distress. Alternatively, some patients become stimulated by some codeine antitussives and have difficulty sleeping.

SMOKING CESSATION

Because smoking is the leading cause of preventable death in the United States and worldwide, a primary goal for health management is smoking cessation. As discussed in Chapter 2 (see page 31), there are many techniques with wide variability in success rates that are used to assist patients in smoking cessation, including patient education programs, group or individual counseling, hypnosis, acupuncture, aversive conditioning, behavior modification, nicotine replacement therapy (NRT), nicotine receptor partial agonists, and some other medications.[35,66] However, the vast majority of individuals who attempt to quit smoking do so on their own, which has a success rate of only 3% to 5% at 1 year but translates into a huge number of people due to the sheer volume of cessations attempted.

Nicotine withdrawal can be uncomfortable for individuals trying to quit smoking; symptoms include craving, nervousness, emotional lability, restlessness, sleep disturbances, impaired concentration, increased appetite, weight gain, fatigue, drowsiness, and headache. Nicotine replacement therapy, which comes in a variety of forms, aims to assist individuals wean from the chemical addiction.

- Nicotine gum and lozenges are available over-the-counter and are absorbed through the mucous membrane of the mouth for fast-acting help in countering nicotine cravings. The gum can be used on a regular schedule, such as 1 or 2 pieces every hour or as needed, with a maximum of 20 pieces per day. Treatment is typically continued for a period of 1 to 3 months and not more than 6 months, with the frequency of use being tapered to facilitate withdrawal. Long-term dependence may develop.
- Nicotine patches are available over-the-counter, convenient to use, and are applied only once per day. They provide a measured dose of transcutaneous nicotine, which is reduced by using different dose patches over a course of weeks, so the tobacco user is gradually weaned off nicotine. Side effects of the patch are related to the dose of nicotine, brand of patch, individual sensitivity, method of application, and length of use. Side effects include skin irritation (e.g., redness and itching), dizziness, tachycardia, insomnia, headache, nausea and vomiting, and muscle aches and stiffness.
- Combination treatment using the patch and gum together may offer improved success. The patch is used routinely and up to four pieces of gum can be chewed per day to control cravings.
- Nicotine nasal spray, which is available only by prescription, works quickly to help control nicotine cravings. Its use is recommended for 3 months and not more than 6 months. Users may develop drug dependence. The most common side effects, which usually fade over the first 1 to 2 weeks of use, include nasal irritation, runny nose, watery eyes, sneezing, throat irritation, and coughing.
- The nicotine inhaler consists of a plastic tube containing a nicotine cartridge that mimics the use of cigarettes by holding the inhaler and puffing, which many smokers find helpful. Nicotine inhalers require a doctor's prescription. Common side effects include throat irritation, coughing, and stomach upset, which tend to occur during early treatment.
- Nicotine replacement therapy is not without toxicity! Symptoms of nicotine overdose consist of nausea, vomiting, diarrhea, abdominal pain, diaphoresis, flushing, dizziness, hypotension, palpitations, weakness, confusion, altered respirations, and visual and auditory disturbances.

Other prescription medications used to treat smoking addiction are bupropion (Zyban) and varenicline (Chantix, Champix).

- Originally developed as an antidepressant, many smokers taking bupropion as Wellbutrin noticed a lessening of the desire for cigarettes. Through further testing, the drug was found to be effective in treating smoking addiction, largely due to its adrenergic and dopaminergic actions, which essentially replace nicotine's neurochemical effects, and the drug was repackaged as Zyban. It is used to address the psychological need for smoking.
  - ‣ Zyban reduces the severity of nicotine withdrawal symptoms such as irritability, frustration, anger, anxiety, difficulty in concentrating, restlessness, and depressed mood or negative affect. Most studies show success rates of 15% to 25%.
  - ‣ Side effects of Zyban include dry mouth, nausea, and difficulty sleeping. There is also an increased risk of seizures in some patients.
- Varenicline is a selective $\alpha_4\beta_2$ nicotinic receptor partial agonist, which mimics (up to 60%) the dopamine agonist effects of nicotine, reducing cravings after cessation.[82] In addition, it decreases the pleasurable effects of cigarettes and other tobacco products.
  - ‣ With quit rates of 45% to 50% with twice-daily use, it appears that it will be more effective in clinical practice than bupropion.[82]
  - ‣ The most frequent side effects of varenicline were nausea, which was usually mild to moderate and tended to fade within 2 weeks; headache; insomnia; abnormal dreams; and taste perversion.
- Cytisine is a strong $\alpha_4\beta_2$ nicotinic receptor agonist that has been used to treat tobacco dependence in Eastern Europe for 40 years, but studies have not been published in English.[30] Adverse effects, which are typically noted at the beginning of treatment, include changes in both taste and appetite, dryness of the mouth, headache, irritability, nausea, constipation, tachycardia, and possible BP elevation, although this not been a consistent finding. In addition, cytisine is a poison that has the potential to cause toxicity similar to nicotine.
- Other pharmacologic approaches to treating nicotine dependence are being investigated and the National Institute on Drug Abuse (Rockville, MD) has been pioneering the development of a vaccine, NicVAX, that promotes the production of nicotine-specific antibodies.

◖ 5.2 CARDIOVASCULAR MEDICATIONS

A vast number of pharmacologic agents are available to treat the pathophysiological and clinical manifestations of diseases and disorders that affect the CV system. Medications used to treat the most common ones are described in this chapter, both in text and in several tables that list the specific pharmacologic effects that are most relevant to each disease. The effects of various cardiovascular medications on exercise responses is provided later in this chapter (see Table 5-22 on page 216).

MEDICATIONS THAT TREAT MULTIPLE DISORDERS

Many of the classes of medications used to treat CV disease have multiple effects and can be used to treat a number of different CV disorders, such as hypertension (HTN), myocardial ischemia and infarction, chronic heart failure (CHF), and arrhythmias. The drugs that can be used for more than one of these disorders include diuretics, β-blockers, angiotensin-converting enzyme (ACE) inhibitors, angiotensin II receptor blockers (ARBs), and calcium channel blockers (CCBs). These agents are described in more detail the first time they appear, and later only the information relevant to other specific disorders will be presented.

ANTIHYPERTENSIVE AGENTS

Arterial blood pressure (BP) is the product of cardiac output and peripheral vascular resistance (PVR), as described on page 97. Medications used to treat HTN exert their effect by reducing cardiac output (by decreasing ventricular filling volume [through moderation of venous tone or blood volume via renal effects] or inhibiting myocardial contractility) or peripheral resistance (by promoting relaxation of vascular smooth muscle or inhibiting vasoconstriction).

The goal of antihypertensive therapy is to achieve effective 24-h/day BP control (<140/90 mm Hg, or <130/80 mm Hg for those with comorbidities, such as diabetes mellitus [DM], renal disease, and CV complications) in order to reduce CV mortality and morbidity. Effective antihypertensive therapy protects against the development of left ventricular hypertrophy (LVH) and markedly reduces the risk of stroke, CHF, and renal insufficiency due to HTN.[1a]

- The first approach to reducing BP consists of lifestyle modification, which includes weight reduction, sodium and alcohol restriction, smoking cessation, regular exercise, and a diet low in saturated fat.
- Several classes of drugs can be used to treat HTN (listed in Table 5-4); pharmacologic therapy is indicated when[46]:
  - ‣ Lifestyle modifications are not successful in normalizing BP
  - ‣ BP is high enough that immediate treatment is indicated (≥160/100 mm Hg)
  - ‣ Cardiovascular disease (CVD) risk is elevated (10-yr risk ≥20% or existing CVD or target organ damage) with persistent BP >140/90 mm Hg
- Joint National Committee (JNC) 7 recommended that pharmacotherapy for stage 1 HTN (see Table 4-6) begin with prescription of a diuretic, or if the patient is diabetic, an ACE inhibitor (ACEI).[17] Some guidelines recommend that treatment begin with ACEIs for patients less than 55 years of age.[46] Alternative step 1 medications include ARBs, CCBs, and β-blockers, particularly if the individual suffers from other comorbidities that would benefit from one of these agents. In addition, the initial medication may need to be changed if a patient experiences adverse side effects.
- If step 1 therapy is not effective or if monotherapy is unlikely to be successful, a second medication is added to rapidly

TABLE 5-4: Drugs Used in the Treatment of Hypertension

Drug	Mode of Action	Pharmacologic Effects*					Specific Indications	Precautions and Contraindications
		HR	CO	PVR	Plasma Volume	Plasma Renin Activity		
Diuretics	Initially, ↑ urinary Na+ excretion → ↓ plasma volume, extracellular fluid volume, and CO. Later, these return toward normal, then (decreased) PVR rules	↓	↓	→	↓↔	↑	Heart failure, advanced age, systolic HTN, osteoporosis (thiazides)	Gout, DM if high doses given, dyslipidemia if high doses given. Avoid K+ salt substitutes if taking K+-sparing diuretics
Calcium channel blockers	↓ Entry of calcium into cardiovascular tissues → vasodilation of peripheral blood vessels → ↓ PVR	↓ or ↑	↓ or ↑	→	↔↑	↔↑	Advanced age, isolated systolic HTN, previous stroke, cyclosporine-induced HTN	Bradyarrhythmias, SA node or AV node conduction disturbances, hypotension, CHF
ACE inhibitors	Inhibition of the enzyme that converts angiotensin I to angiotensin II → prevention of vasoconstriction → ↓ PVR	↕	↕	→	↕	↑	Heart failure or LV dysfn, previous MI, diabetic or other nephropathy or proteinuria	Pregnancy, renal artery stenosis, hyperkalemia
Angiotensin II receptor blockers	Binding to angiotensin II receptors → prevention of vasoconstriction → ↓ PVR	↕	↕	↕	↕	↑	ACE inhibitor-associated cough, diabetic or other nephropathy, heart failure	Pregnancy, renal artery stenosis, hyperkalemia
β-Adrenergic receptor blockers (β-blockers)	Blocking β-adrenergic receptors in heart → ↓ HR and ↓ contractility → ↓ CO; slow conduction in atria and AV node; general ↓ SNS tone	↓ or ↔†	↓ or ↔†	↔→ or ↓†	↓↕	↓ or ↓↔†	Angina or previous MI, heart failure, hyperkinetic HTN, tachyarrhythmias, HOCM, migraine, hyperthyroidism, panic attacks, substance abuse withdrawal, variceal bleeding in portal HTN	Asthma or reactive airway disease, SA or AV nodal dysfunction, DM, depression

Continued

TABLE 5-4: **Drugs Used in the Treatment of Hypertension—Cont'd**

Drug	Mode of Action	Pharmacologic Effects*					Specific Indications	Precautions and Contraindications
		HR	**CO**	**PVR**	**Plasma Volume**	**Plasma Renin Activity**		
α₁-Adrenergic antagonists	Inhibition of α_1-adrenergic receptors → arterial dilation → ↓ PVR	↔↑	↔↑	→	↔↑	↔	Prostatic hypertrophy, peripheral vascular disease	Pregnancy
Central adrenergic inhibitors	Inhibition of SNS discharge from CNS to heart and blood vessels → ↓ CO and PVR	↓↔	↓↔	→	↔↑	↓↔		Sedation, depression; possible rebound HTN on abrupt discontinuation if dose is not tapered
Peripheral adrenergic inhibitors	Inhibition of norepinephrine release from peripheral adrenergic neurons → ↓ SNS stimulation of heart and blood vessels → ↓ CO	↓↔	→	→	↑	↔↑		Depression (reserpine); tricyclic antidepressants (guanadrel)
Direct-acting vasodilators	↓ PVR	↑	↑	→	↑	↑	Heart failure	Tachycardia, myocardial ischemia

↓, Decreased; ↑, increased; ↔, no change; →, resulting in; ACE, angiotensin-converting enzyme; AV, atrioventricular; CHF, chronic heart failure; CO, cardiac output; DM, diabetes mellitus; dysfn, dysfunction; HOCM, hypertrophic obstructive cardiomyopathy; HR, heart rate; HTN, hypertension; K^+, potassium; LV, left ventricular; MI, myocardial infarction; Na^+, sodium; PVR, peripheral vascular resistance; SA, sinoatrial; SNS, sympathetic nervous system.
*With long-term administration.
†β-Blockers with intrinsic sympathomimetic activity.

normalize BP. Two or more antihypertensive drugs are required to achieve and maintain good BP control in the majority of patients.[29] The decision to increase one agent, "max out" on an agent, or to combine agents is generally made by considering a number of factors, including side effects, concomitant diseases, drug interactions, patient tolerance, and patient's willingness to take more than one medication.

- In addition to diuretics, ACEIs, ARBs, CCBs, and β-blockers, other drugs can be used to manage HTN, including α-1 ($α_1$)-blockers, central $α_2$-agonists, direct vasodilators, and other centrally acting drugs.

- Of note, some classes of antihypertensive drugs are more or less effective in controlling BP in certain ethnic groups (e.g., thiazide diuretics are more effective in black patients than in white patients, whereas ACEIs, ARBs, and β-blockers are more effective in lower doses in whites than in blacks; Hispanics show intermediate responses between those of whites and blacks; and East Asians often need lower doses than whites).[36]

- In addition, the elderly often respond differently to different agents (e.g., they respond best to diuretics and calcium channel blockers and tend to have less favorable responses to β-blockers). Furthermore, the side effects of many drugs increase the risk of problems in the elderly (e.g., postural hypotension with vasodilators, and aggravation of left ventricular dysfunction with dihydropyridine calcium channel blockers and β-blockers).

- The effects of antihypertensive agents on resting and exercise vital signs are offered later in this chapter (see Table 5-22 on page 216).

Diuretics

Diuretics are the first-line treatment for HTN, particularly for patients 55 years of age and older and for black patients,[46,76a] and can be divided into three general categories comprised of thiazides and related drugs, loop diuretics, and potassium-sparing agents. Various agents are used to treat HTN, CHF, and edema associated with other disease states, as shown in Table 5-5.

- The pharmacologic effects of the different types of diuretics are depicted in Table 5-6. All the diuretics lower BP initially by increasing urinary sodium excretion and reducing plasma

TABLE 5-5: Diuretics: Indications for Use

Generic Name	Trade Name	HTN	CHF	Edema
Thiazides and Derivatives				
Bendroflumethiazide	Naturetin	✓		
Benzthiazide	Exna	✓		
Chlorthalidone*	Hygroton, Thalitone	✓		
Chlorothiazide	Diuril	✓		
Hydrochlorothiazide	HydroDiuril, Oretic, Esidrix	✓		
Hydroflumethiazide	Diucardin	✓		
Indapamide*	Lozol	✓		
Methyclothiazide	Enduron, Aquatensin	✓		
Metolazone*	Zaroxolyn, Mykrox	✓		
Polythiazide	Renese	✓		
Quinethazone*	Hydromox	✓		
Trichlormethiazide	Metahydrin, Naqua, Diurese	✓		
Potassium-sparing Diuretics				
Amiloride	Midamor	✓–	✓–	
Eplerenone	Inspra	✓	✓†	
Spironolactone	Aldactone	✓		✓
Triamterene	Dyrenium	✓–		✓
Loop Diuretics				
Bumetanide	Bumex		✓	✓
Ethacrynic acid	Edecrin		✓	✓
Furosemide	Lasix		✓	✓
Torsemide	Demadex	✓	✓	✓

*Chlorthalidone (phthalimide derivative), indapamide (indoline), metolazone, and quinethazone (quinazolin derivatives) are included here because of structural and pharmacologic similarities to the thiazides.
†Postmyocardial infarction.
✓–, Weaker indication.

TABLE 5-6: Diuretics: Modes of Action and Adverse Reactions

Drug	Mode of Action	Adverse Reactions
Thiazides and derivatives*†	Increase excretion and inhibit reabsorption of Na^+ so ↓ body Na^+ and plasma fluid volume	Fluid/electrolyte imbalance, erectile dysfunction, ↑ uric acid levels; hyperglycemia, lipid abnormalities
Loop diuretics†‡	Inhibit reabsorption of Na^+ and Cl^- in ascending loop of Henle	Fluid and electrolyte imbalance, hypotension, anorexia, vertigo, hearing loss, and weakness
Potassium-sparing Diuretics§		
Amiloride (Midamor)	Inhibits Na^+ reabsorption in distal tubule and decreases K^+ and H^+ secretion/excretion	Hyperkalemia, GI disturbances (nausea, abdominal discomfort, flatulence, diarrhea), skin rash
Triamterene¶ (Dyrenium)	Inhibits reabsorption of Na^+ in exchange for K^+ and H^+ in distal tubule	Hyperglycemia, ataxia, dizziness, and weakness
Spironolactone (Aldactone)	Binds receptors at aldosterone-dependent Na^+-K^+ exchange site in distal tubule, increases Na^+ and water excretion and retains K^+	Hyperkalemia, GI upset, diarrhea, and possible cardiac irregularities
Eplerenone (Inspra)	Blocks binding of aldosterone, inhibits Na^+ reabsorption in exchange for K^+	Hyperkalemia, renal dysfunction, jaundice, GI upset, diarrhea, and weakness or fatigue

↓, Decreased; ↑, increased; GI, gastrointestinal.
*Indapamide exerts little or no effect on cardiac output.
†See Table 5-5.
‡Torsemide may induce less potassium loss compared with other loop diuretics.
§Effective in patients with renal impairment.
¶Pharmacologic effects of triamterene are not reported directly but are probably similar to those of other diuretics.

volume and cardiac output. However, the reductions in plasma volume and cardiac output are short-lived, returning toward normal within 2 months, at which point the major mechanism of BP control is related to modulation of peripheral resistance.

- Diuretic therapy alone may control BP in about 30% of patients with mild HTN. Diuretics (and dihydropyridine calcium channel blockers) are more effective in lowering BP in African Americans than other classes of medications.[28,33]
  - ▸ Thiazide diuretics are typically the first prescribed drugs. The mechanism by which they lower BP is probably independent of their diuretic effect. Although diuresis initially occurs, plasma and extracellular fluid volume return to pretreatment levels and a reduction in PVR predominates. All thiazides are equally effective in lowering BP.
    - ⊙ Hydrochlorothiazide, either alone or in combination with potassium-sparing diuretics, remains the most commonly prescribed thiazide because it has been proven to be the most cost effective and efficacious agent.
    - ⊙ With the exception of metolazone, thiazides lose their hypertensive activity as renal function declines below a creatinine clearance of 30 mL/min.
  - ▸ In general, loop diuretics are used less often than thiazides in treating HTN. Their use is reserved primarily for those individuals who have a creatinine clearance less than 30 mL/min or who have concomitant edema.
  - ▸ Of the potassium-sparing diuretics (triamterene, amiloride, and spironolactone), only spironolactone is effective in lowering BP. In addition, spironolactone appears to have cardioprotective characteristics in patients suffering from CHF irrespective of its antihypertensive benefit.

- ▸ The concomitant use of potassium-sparing agents minimizes (essentially neutralizes) the hypokalemia from thiazides.
- The most common side effects patients complain of are dizziness and frequent urination. Dehydration and hypotension may also occur. Because thiazide diuretics and loop diuretics result in potassium excretion, muscle weakness may be a warning sign that potassium is low. To prevent this, a potassium supplement is frequently prescribed with these diuretics.
- Of note, the use of diuretics is associated with an increased incidence of new diabetes mellitus and adverse changes in plasma lipids.
- Nonetheless, clinical studies continue to demonstrate the efficacy of the thiazide diuretics in reducing CV risk.[1a]

Calcium Channel Blockers

Calcium channel blockers (CCBs) are also considered a first-line treatment for HTN, and have proven to be more effective in lowering BP in blacks and the elderly, including those with isolated systolic HTN, than ACEIs, ARBs, and β-blockers.[28,33,46] Some agents are also used to treat angina, CHF, and arrhythmias, as shown in Table 5-7. These drugs can be divided into three distinct pharmacologic groups including dihydropyridines (e.g., amlodipine, felodipine, and nifedipine), phenylalkylamines (e.g., verapamil), and benzothiazepines (e.g., diltiazem); the latter two groups are often combined and referred to as nondihydropyridine CCBs.

The major properties of the CCBs include vasodilation of the coronary and peripheral arteries, reduced myocardial contractility, and slowed cardiac conduction.[108b]

- CCBs block voltage-sensitive calcium channels and decrease the movement of extracellular calcium into vascular smooth

TABLE 5-7: Calcium Channel–Blocking Agents: Indications and Adverse Reactions

Drug	Brand Name	Indications					Adverse Reactions*
		Angina	CHF	HTN	Arrhythmias	Other	
Dihydropyridine CCBs							Dizziness, headache, hypotension, facial flushing, palpitations, lower extremity edema, exacerbation of CHF, tachy- or bradyarrhythmias, AV conduction disturbances, constipation, gingival overgrowth
Amlodipine	Norvasc	✓		✓			
Benidipine	Coniel	✓		✓		1	
Felodipine	Plendil			✓			
Isradipine	DynaCirc			✓			
Manidipine	Manyper			✓			
Nicardipine	Cardene	✓	✓	✓			
Nifedipine	Procardia, Adalat	✓	✓	✓			
Nilvadipine	Nivadil	✓		✓			
Nimodipine	Nimotop			✓		1	
Nisoldipine	Sular			✓			
Lacidipine	Motens			✓		1	
Lercanidipine	Zanidip			✓			
Nondihydropyridine CCBs							
Verapamil	Calan, Isoptin, Verelan	✓		✓	✓		
Diltiazem	Cardizem, Dilacor	✓		✓	✓		
Bepridil	Vascor	✓					

✓, Indicated; 1, cerebrovascular disease; AV, atrioventricular; CCB, calcium channel blocker; CHF, congestive heart failure; HTN, hypertension.
*Can occur with any of these drugs.

muscle cells, resulting in vasodilation. In addition, the decrease in cardiac contractility reduces cardiac output. Thus, BP is lowered through reductions in both cardiac output and PVR.

- Vasodilation is greatest with the dihydropyridine agents, whereas alterations in cardiac conduction predominate with the nondihydropyridine agents. The potent vasodilator effects of nifedipine are similar for the coronary and peripheral arteries, diltiazem has less effect on the peripheral arteries, and verapamil has intermediary peripheral vascular effects.
- HR is decreased and cardiac conduction is lowered by verapamil and, to a lesser extent, by diltiazem.
- The dihydropyridine CCBs decrease the risk of CV events, particularly stroke, without having adverse effects on glucose metabolism.[28]
- Adverse effects are usually a simple extension of their basic pharmacologic properties, with hypotension, dizziness, headache, and constipation being common complaints. Other possible side effects include flushing, peripheral edema, palpitations, exacerbations of CHF, and tachy- or bradyarrhythmias.

Angiotensin-converting Enzyme Inhibitors

The renin–angiotensin system (RAS) is a major determinant of BP and intravascular volume, and medications directed at modifying its components are often used to control HTN.

The angiotensin-converting enzyme inhibitors (ACEIs) have been shown to reduce morbidity and to prolong life in patients with HTN. As shown in Table 5-8, they are also used to treat CHF, and some reduce the risk of cardiac events after acute myocardial infarction (MI) and revascularization procedures and prevent or delay the progression of nephropathy in patients with DM, so they are the drugs of choice in these patients with HTN.

- ACEIs inhibit the activity of plasma angiotensin-converting enzyme, thereby blocking the conversion of angiotensin I (Ang I) to angiotensin II (Ang II), which is a potent vasoconstrictor and stimulus for the release of aldosterone. ACEIs produce vasodilation and reduction of PVR as well as an increase in venous capacitance.
- They also prevent the breakdown of bradykinin and may stimulate the synthesis of local vasodilators including prostaglandins.
- Although all these actions may contribute to the hypotensive effects of ACEIs, local tissue angiotensin systems may also modulate much of the vascular response to these drugs.[89]
- ACEIs have been associated with significant hypotension in sodium- or volume-depleted individuals, but cough and sometimes dermatologic reactions are the more common adverse reactions associated with these agents. Infrequent but important adverse reactions include renal impairment, particularly

TABLE 5-8: Angiotensin-converting Enzyme Inhibitors: Indications and Adverse Reactions

Drug	Brand Name	Indications HTN	Indications CHF	Adverse Reactions*
Benazepril	Lotensin	✓		Hypotension, cough, hyperkalemia, headache, dizziness, fatigue, and nausea; rash and taste disturbances (particularly with captopril)
Captopril	Capoten	✓	✓	
Enalapril	Vasotec	✓	✓	Occasional renal impairment or angioedema
Fosinopril	Monopril	✓		
Lisinopril	Prinivil, Zestril	✓	✓	
Perindopril[†]	Aceon	✓	✓	
Quinapril	Accupril	✓	✓	
Ramipril[†]	Altace	✓	✓	
Trandolapril	Mavik	✓	✓	
Zofenopril[†]	Zofenil	✓	✓	

✓, Indicated; CHF, congestive heart failure; HTN, hypertension.
*Can occur with any of these drugs.
[†]Also used for stable coronary disease because of reduced risk of cardiac event following myocardial infarction or revascularization procedures.

in patients with renal artery stenosis and those taking a nonsteroidal antiinflammatory drug (NSAID) and a diuretic; hyperkalemia; and angioedema, which is induced by increased bradykinin levels.

Angiotensin II Receptor Blockers

Angiotensin II receptor blockers (ARBs) are the newest class of antihypertensive agents. At present, they are prescribed primarily for patients who do not tolerate ACEIs, but this is expected to change as outcome trials prove their value. They have shown efficacy in the treatment of a wide spectrum of hypertensive patients, including those with mild-to-moderate/severe HTN and isolated systolic HTN, as well as those who are black or Asian.[88a,91] Some are also valuable for the treatment of left ventricular dysfunction and CHF and for preventing or delaying the progression of diabetic nephropathy (Table 5-9).
- ARBs work by displacing Ang II from its specific Ang I receptor, which results in antagonism of all its known effects, leading to

vasodilation and inhibition of vasopressin secretion and reduced production and secretion of aldosterone. Thus, there is a dose-dependent reduction in PVR and increased salt and water excretion (and therefore reduced plasma volume) with little change in HR or cardiac output.
- In addition, the ARBs reduce vascular medial hypertrophy.
- Side effects are usually mild and similar to those of other antihypertensives: dizziness, headache, and/or hyperkalemia. More rare adverse reactions include first-dose orthostatic hypotension, rash, diarrhea, dyspepsia, myalgia, back pain, insomnia, and abnormal liver function. Similar to ACEIs, but more rare, is an increased risk of renal dysfunction and angioedema.

β-Adrenergic Receptor Antagonists

Previously prescribed as the first-line drug therapy for HTN, β-adrenergic blocking agents have dropped in favor because of studies showing that they do not reduce other CV outcomes as much

TABLE 5-9: Angiotensin 2 Receptor Blockers: Indications and Adverse Reactions

Drug	Brand Name	Indications HTN	Indications Other	Adverse Reactions*
Candesartan	Atacand	✓		Generally minimal: similar to those of ACE inhibitors although less frequent or pronounced, including cough; angioedema is rare
Eprosartan	Teveten	✓		
Irbesartan	Avapro	✓	Nephropathy in type 2 DM	Occasional fetal toxicity
Losartan	Cozaar	✓	Nephropathy in type 2 DM	
Olmesartan	Benicar	✓		
Telmisartan	Micardis	✓		
Valsartan	Diovan	✓	CHF	

✓, Indicated; ACE, angiotensin-converting enzyme; CHF, congestive heart failure; DM, diabetes mellitus; HTN, hypertension.
*Can occur with any of these drugs.

as other classes of antihypertensive medications. However, they may be considered for younger patients, especially those with intolerance or contraindications to ACEIs and ARBs, women of child-bearing potential, and patients with evidence of increased sympathetic nervous system (SNS) drive.[46,76a] They are also used to treat myocardial ischemia and infarction, CHF, and arrhythmias, as shown in Table 5-10.

- Although the major property of all β-blockers involves the blockade of β_1-receptors so that epinephrine and norepinephrine cannot bind to them, the exact mechanisms by which they reduce BP remain unknown. It is known that antagonism of cardiac β_1-receptors results in decreases in HR and cardiac output (by approximately 15% to 20%), and that blockade of β-receptors in the kidney inhibits the release of renin (by about 60%).[57] Specific agents may have slightly different or additional effects.

- Second-generation cardioselective β-blockers exhibit a higher binding affinity for the cardiac β_1-receptors, with fewer effects on β_2-receptors (located primarily in the bronchioles and the peripheral blood vessels), and thus are referred to as cardioselective β-blockers. They may be better tolerated by patients with reactive airway disease (e.g., asthma and COPD), in whom the use of nonselective agents can provoke bronchospasm, and by those with peripheral vascular disease. However, cardioselectivity is a relative property and is predictable only at lower doses; as the dosage of any cardioselective drug is increased, β_2-receptors will be inhibited as well.

- Some β-blockers exhibit intrinsic sympathomimetic activity (ISA), exerting low-level β-receptor stimulation, and thus cause smaller declines in HR, cardiac output, and renin levels than those without ISA.

- The third-generation nonselective vasodilating β-blockers have concomitant β_1-blocking activity. Because stimulation of β_1-receptors causes vasoconstriction and reduces lipoprotein lipase activity, a β-blocker with β_1-blocking activity offer benefits for individuals who have concomitant peripheral vascular disease or dyslipidemia. In addition, some of these agents have antioxidant properties and antiproliferative effects (e.g., carvedilol and labetalol).

- Nebivolol is a third-generation β_1-selective blocker, which has an added pharmaceutical property of inducing peripheral vasodilation by increasing NO release, which may also improve endothelial function and therefore provide further benefits compared with other agents. In addition, it does not adversely affect glucose metabolism.

- The most common side effect of the β-blockers is fatigue, which likely results from reductions in cardiac output and peripheral and cerebral blood flow. Other adverse effects include headache, dizziness, diarrhea, and sexual dysfunction (see Table 5-10).

- In addition, β-blockers, particularly nonselective agents, induce perturbations of carbohydrate and lipid metabolism, causing an increase in the incidence of type 2 diabetes and reducing high-density lipoproteins (HDLs) and raising low-density lipoproteins (LDLs) and triglycerides. In addition, they may mask the symptoms of hypoglycemia and delay recovery from insulin-induced hypoglycemia, so they should be used with great caution in

diabetics. However, the benefits of β-receptor antagonists in type 1 DM with MI may outweigh the risk in selected patients (see page 105). Of note, the third-generation agents appear to increase insulin sensitivity in patients with insulin resistance, and therefore they may become the drugs of choice in patients with type 2 DM.[11]

- Another problem with β-blockers is their tendency to provoke angina pectoris, acute MI, and occasionally sudden death when abruptly discontinued. Thus, it is important to wean patients from these drugs.

Other Antihypertensive Agents

Other classes of drugs can also be used to treat HTN, but are generally reserved for use when other drugs are ineffective, poorly tolerated, or considered unsafe. They are not recommended as monotherapy and are used primarily in combined therapy with diuretics, β-blockers, and other antihypertensive agents. These drugs include α_1-receptor antagonists, central and peripheral adrenergic inhibitors, and direct vasodilators (see Table 5-4).

α_1-Receptor Antagonists

Drugs that selectively block α_1-adrenergic receptors without affecting α_2-adrenergic receptors inhibit catecholamine-induced vasoconstriction and produce arterial vasodilation and reduced PVR, leading to a decrease in BP. Drugs that fall into this class include doxazosin (Cardura), prazosin (Minipress), and terazosin (Hytrin).

- An increase in venous capacitance frequently provokes orthostatic hypotension. Patients should be cautioned to change posture slowly from supine or sitting to the standing position. This orthostatic hypotensive phenomenon is especially prevalent in the initial dosing of these drugs. The "first-dose" response is characterized by severe hypotension, dizziness, or even syncopal episodes that occur within two two hours of the first dose or after subsequent increases in dose. Patients must be warned about the potential for this side effect and usually are instructed to take the first dose at bedtime.

- Other side effects include headache, dizziness, and asthenia; less frequent complaints include nausea, dyspnea, and drowsiness.

Because the α_1-receptor antagonists also induce relaxation of the smooth muscles in the neck of the urinary bladder and prostate, they are most often used for treating benign prostatic hypertrophy. Furthermore, doxazosin and terazosin induce apoptosis in prostatic smooth muscle, resulting in inhibition of cell proliferation, which is independent of α_1-receptor antagonism.

Central Adrenergic Inhibitors

Central adrenergic inhibitors, also referred to as central-acting agents or central α-agonists, act on the vasomotor center in the brain to inhibit SNS output and thus reduce HR and cardiac output. Methyldopa acts through an active metabolite to stimulate central inhibitory α-adrenergic receptors. These drugs are also used to manage panic attacks, hot flashes, and alcohol or other substance withdrawal symptoms.

- With the occasional exception of clonidine (Catapres), which is available as a transdermal patch, these agents are rarely used anymore.

TABLE 5-10: β-Adrenergic Blocking Agents

Drug	Brand Name	Mode of Action			Indications					Adverse Reaction*
		Adrenergic Receptor(s)	Membrane Stabilizing	ISA	HTN	Arrhythmia	Angina	MI	CHF	
First Generation, Nonselective Agents										
Nadolol	Corgard	β_1, β_2	0	0	✓	✓	✓			
Penbutolol	Levatol	β_1, β_2	0	+	✓	✓				
Pindolol	Visken	β_1, β_2	+	+++	✓	✓				
Propranolol	Inderal	β_1, β_2	++	0	✓	✓	✓	✓		
Sotalol	Betapace	β_1, β_2	0	0	✓	✓	✓			
Timolol	Blocadren	β_1, β_2	0	0	✓	✓	✓	✓		
Second Generation, β_1-selective Agents										
Acebutolol	Sectral	β_1†	+	+	✓	✓	✓			
Atenolol	Tenormin	β_1†	0	0	✓	✓	✓	✓		
Bisoprolol	Zebeta	β_1†	0	0	✓	✓	✓			
Esmolol	Brevibloc	β_1†	0	0		✓	✓			
Metoprolol	Lopressor, Toprol	β_1†	0	0	✓	✓	✓	✓	✓	
Third Generation, Nonselective Vasodilators‡										
Carteolol	Cartrol	β_1, β_2, α_1	0	++	✓		✓			
Carvedilol	Coreg, Dilatrend, Eucardic	β_1, β_2, α	++	0	✓			✓	✓	
Labetalol	Normodyne, Trandate	β_1, β_2, α_1	+	+	✓					
Third Generation, β_1-selective Vasodilators‡										
Betaxolol	Kerlone	β_1†	+	0	✓		✓			
Celiprolol	Selector	β_1†, ↑α_1	0	+	✓		✓			
Nebivolol	Bystolic, Nebilet	β_1†	0	0	✓		✓		✓	

Adverse Reaction*

General: Most are mild and transient

Cardiovascular: Bradycardia, CHF, ↑AV block, hypotension, cold extremities, paresthesia of hands. *Note:* Abrupt cessation can ↑ angina and risk of sudden death

CNS: Lightheadedness, depression, insomnia, fatigue, weakness, visual disturbances, hallucinations

Gastrointestinal: Nausea, vomiting, abdominal cramping, diarrhea, constipation

Respiratory: Bronchospasm with nonselective agents

Endocrine: Hyperglycemia, unstable diabetes, hypoglycemia

Genitourinary: Sexual dysfunction

Musculoskeletal: Joint pain, arthralgia, muscle cramps, tremor, twitching

Allergic: Rash, pharyngitis, and agranulocytosis, respiratory distress

0, None; +, low; ++, moderate; +++, high; ✓, indicated; ↑, increased; AV, atrioventricular; CHF, congestive heart failure; HTN, hypertension; ISA, intrinsic sympathomimetic activity; MI, myocardial infarction.

*Can occur with any of these drugs.

†Inhibits β_2-receptors (bronchial and vascular) at higher doses.

‡The third-generation drugs produce peripheral vasodilation through a variety of mechanisms, including α_1-adrenergic receptor blockade, increased nitric oxide release, β_2 agonism, and calcium ion entry blockade.

- Other agents in this category include methyldopa (Aldomet), guanabenz (Wytensin), and guanfacine (Tenex). Methyldopa is used primarily during pregnancy, having demonstrated efficacy and safety for both mother and fetus.
- Adverse side effects include dry mouth (xerostomia), dizziness, constipation, weakness, erectile dysfunction, and nasal congestion. In addition, methyldopa may cause an autoimmune inflammatory disorder and abnormal liver function, and clonidine may be associated with rebound HTN on discontinuation if dosage is not tapered.

Peripheral Adrenergic Inhibitors

The peripheral adrenergic inhibitors act to suppress the release of norepinephrine from peripheral sympathetic nerve endings, inhibiting SNS-mediated vasoconstriction. In addition, guanethidine directly reduces myocardial depletion of catecholamines.

- These drugs include guanadrel (Hylorel), guanethidine (Ismelin), and reserpine (Serpasil, Serpalan).
- Common side effects include orthostatic hypotension, gastrointestinal (GI) disturbances (nausea, vomiting, and diarrhea), weakness, and sedation.

Direct Vasodilators

Direct vasodilators relax or reduce the tone of arteriolar smooth muscle, possibly by interfering with calcium movement. The drugs that fall into this class of drugs include hydralazine (Apresoline), diazoxide (Hyperstat), minoxidil (Loniten), and nitroprusside (Nipride, Nitropress).

- Hydralazine is the only one of these drugs that is used on rare occasions to treat HTN, mainly hypertensive emergencies in pregnant women. However, it may be used in conjunction with nitrates for patients with CHF who cannot tolerate ACEIs or ARBs.
- Minoxidil has the undesirable side effect of promoting the growth and darkening of body hair; this has resulted in its reinvention as Rogaine for the treatment of balding.
- Nitroprusside and diazoxide are used primarily to treat hypertensive emergencies. Nitroprusside may be used in other situations in which short-term reduction of cardiac preload or afterload is needed.
- Side effects of the direct vasodilators are similar to those of other vasodilators, including reflex tachycardia, orthostatic hypotension, dizziness, weakness, nausea, headache, peripheral edema, and dyspepsia. In addition, hydralazine sometimes causes arthralgias and on rare occasions a lupus syndrome or polyneuropathy.[11] Minoxidil is sometimes associated with pericardial effusion, angina, edema, and CHF.

Combination Therapy

As mentioned previously, optimal antihypertensive therapy usually requires that patients take two or more (sometimes four) different agents. Concurrent use of drugs from different classes can take advantage of distinct complementary hemodynamic actions, resulting in additive effects on BP control at smaller doses, which produces fewer adverse side effects. Examples of these include diuretics and β-adrenergic inhibitors, diuretics and ACEIs, and β-blockers and vasodilators. However, not all combinations of drugs are equally efficacious because of their overlapping mechanisms of action (e.g., ACEIs and ARBs, β-blockers and ACEIs or ARBs).

Numerous fixed-dose combination medications are available, many of which are listed in Table 5-11. Their use increases adherence to treatment, especially in patients who are unwilling or unable to manage multiple medications.

- Potassium-sparing diuretics are used in conjunction with thiazide diuretics to offset hypokalemia.
- The concurrent use of a diuretic with an agent that negates the effects of the reactive rise in renin, such as an ACEI or ARB, is particularly beneficial in blacks and the elderly.
- The combination of a dihydropyridine CCB with an agent that interrupts the renin–angiotensin–aldosterone system (e.g., ACEI or ARB) is also an effective strategy and also offers the benefit of offsetting the pedal edema that can occur with the CCBs.
- β-Receptor antagonists enhance the efficacy of the $α_1$-blockers (hence the development of the third-generation nonselective β-blocker vasodilators).
- Cotreatment with diuretics minimizes the retention of salt and water that commonly occurs with vasodilators and some adrenergic antagonists.

ANTIANGINAL AGENTS

Angina pectoris is characterized by transient episodes of chest discomfort precipitated by myocardial ischemia, which usually occurs as the result of atherosclerotic narrowing of one or more coronary arteries, as described on page 103. Typically, angina develops when an atherosclerotic plaque obstructs at least 70% of the arterial lumen and is triggered by physical activity or emotional disturbance. In addition, the presence of atherosclerotic lesions can cause vasomotor dysfunction so that vasospasm is superimposed on the preexisting lesion, further restricting blood flow to the myocardium. Most patients have a least some episodes of asymptomatic myocardial ischemia (silent ischemia).

Medications for angina aim to provide symptomatic and prophylactic treatment by correcting and maintaining the balance between myocardial oxygen supply and demand (see Figure 4-14, page 104). These are listed in Table 5-12 and consist of organic nitrates, β-adrenergic receptor antagonists, calcium channel blockers, ACEIs, ranolazine, antiplatelet agents, and the statins, which may play a role in stabilizing vulnerable plaques.

- Drugs that reduce myocardial work, and thus the demand for oxygen, include the β-adrenergic receptor antagonists, CCBs, and nitrates, and those that increase oxygen delivery (i.e., coronary blood flow [CBF]) to the myocardium through vasodilation are the nitrates and CCBs.
- Combination therapy may be required for effective prophylaxis of angina and typically consists of a β-blocker and a dihydropyridine CCB, although a CCB and a long-acting nitrate may also be used.
- Standard treatment for chronic stable angina also includes medications that provide vascular protection through attenuation of the progression of atherosclerosis and potential stabilization of coronary plaques: aspirin, clopidogrel, ACEIs, HMG-CoA reductase inhibitors (statins), and dipyrimadole. The antiplatelet drugs and statins are presented in later sections.

TABLE 5-11: Combination Antihypertensive Agents

Combination Product	Brand Name(s)
Diuretic/Diuretic Combinations	
Triamterene/HCTZ	Dyazide, Maxzide
Spironolactone/HCTZ	Aldactone
Amiloride/HCTZ	Moduretic
β_1-Blocker/Diuretic Combinations	
Propranolol/HCTZ	Inderide
Metoprolol/HCTZ	Lopressor/HCT
Atenolol/chlorthalidone	Tenoretic
Nadolol/bendroflumethiazide	Corzide
Timolol/HCTZ	Timolide
Propranolol LA/HCTZ	Inderide LA
Bisoprolol/HCTZ	Ziac
Centrally Acting Drug/Diuretic Combinations	
Guanethidine/HCTZ	Esimil
Methyldopa/HCTZ	Aldoril
Methyldopa/CTZ	Aldoclor
Reserpine/CTX	Diupres
Reserpine/chlorthalidone	Demi-Regroton
Reserpine/HCTZ	Hydropres
Clonidine/chlorthalidone	Combipres
ACE Inhibitor/Diuretic Combinations	
Captopril/HCTZ	Capozide
Enalapril/HCTZ	Vaseretic
Lisinopril/HCTZ	Prinzide, Zestoretic
Fosinopril/HCTZ	Monopril/HCT
Quinapril/HCTZ	Accuretic
Benazepril/HCTZ	Lotensin/HCT
Moexipril/HCTZ	Uniretic
ARB/Diuretic Combinations	
Losartan/HCTZ	Hyzaar
Valsartan/HCTZ	Diovan/HCT
Irbesartan/HCTZ	Avalide
Candesartan/HCTZ	Atacand/HCT
Telmisartan/HCTZ	Micardis/HCT
Eprosartan/HCTZ	Teveten/HCT
Olmesartan/HCTZ	Benicar/HCT
Calcium Channel Blocker/ACE Inhibitor Combinations	
Amlodipine/Benazepril	Lotrel
Diltiazem/Enalapril	Teczem
Verapamil (ER)/Trandolapril	Tarka
Felodipine (ER)/Enalapril	Lexxel
Vasodilator/Diuretic Combinations	
Hydralazine/HCTZ	Apresazide
Prazosin/polythiazide	Minizide
Triple Combination	
Reserpine/hydralazine/HCTZ	Ser-Ap-Es

ACE, Angiotensin-converting enzyme; ARB, angiotensin II receptor blocker; CTZ, chlorothiazide; ER, extended release; HCTZ, hydrochlorothiazide; LA, long-acting.

- Research has revealed that myocardial ischemia alters the normal handling of sodium within the myocytes, leading to increased levels of intracellular sodium and calcium. The calcium overload causes increased actin–myosin filament interaction and impairs myocardial relaxation. This diastolic dysfunction reduces myocardial perfusion (as described on page 103) and increases oxygen demand.[6,106] Thus, a positive feedback loop is created, wherein ischemia perpetuates further ischemia. Newer antianginal agents (e.g., ranolazine) target these derangements in sodium and calcium.
- The hemodynamic effects of various antianginal medications at rest and during exercise are also described later in this chapter (see Table 5-22 on page 216).

β-Adrenergic Blocking Agents

β-Blockers reduce myocardial oxygen demand by inhibiting SNS stimulation of the heart through competitive blockade of the β-adrenergic receptors (see Table 5-12). β-Blockers are the most effective therapy for reducing myocardial ischemia both at rest and during exercise. However, there is a wide variety of activity and selectivity within the β-blocking drugs, as described on page 174 and shown in Table 5-10. Not all agents are effective in treating angina. Cardioselective β_1-blockers are frequently prescribed as they are often tolerated better.

- β-Blockers reduce myocardial ischemia by:
  - Reducing cardiac contractility, which lowers wall stress and thus myocardial oxygen demand
  - Slowing the HR, which reduces myocardial work and increases the diastolic period, which allows greater CBF
  - Reducing BP, which decreases afterload and eases myocardial effort both at rest and during exercise
- Thus, β-blockers curtail the number of angina attacks and improve exercise tolerance.
- In addition, patients who have stable angina along with certain comorbidities derive additional benefits from β-adrenergic blockade:
  - Patients with symptoms of congestive heart failure due to systolic left ventricular (LV) dysfunction show a reduction in HF-related mortality of about 35% with β-blocker therapy.[102]
  - Patients who take β-blockers post-MI experience significant reductions in subsequent myocardial ischemia, reinfarction, HF, and sudden death.[4,34]
- The side effects associated with these drugs are listed in Table 5-10.

Calcium Channel Blockers

CCBs are also valuable in the treatment of stable and unstable angina, as well as Prinzmetal's angina (i.e., coronary spasm). These drugs (see Table 5-7) act by dilating the coronary and peripheral arteries, thus increasing CBF and reducing PVR (see Table 5-12).

- The decrement in afterload that results from reduced PVR lowers myocardial oxygen demand.
- In addition, inhibition of the sinoatrial (SA) and atrioventricular (AV) nodes produced by the nondihydropyridine CCBs reduces HR, which further decreases the work of the heart.
- The various drugs differ in the type of effects they produce. Nicardipine and nifedipine produce the greatest systemic

TABLE 5-12: Antianginal Agents

Drug	Brand Name	Indications: Acute	Indications: Immediate Prophylaxis	Indications: Long-acting Prophylaxis	Indications: Other	Mechanisms of Action	Adverse Reactions
β-Blockers*				✓	HTN, CHF, tachyarrhythmias	↓ HR and ↑ diastolic period → ↑ CBF; ↓ contractility; ↓ BP at rest + during exercise (↓ afterload); ↓ myocardial O_2 demand	Per Table 5-10
Calcium channel blockers†				✓	HTN, CHF, arrhythmias	Coronary and collateral vessel vasodilation; Peripheral vasodilation; Verapamil, diltiazem: ↓ HR and myocardial contractility; Some drugs ↓ BP and thus afterload	Per Table 5-7
Ranolazine	Ranexa			✓		Selective inhibition of late sodium channels altered by myocardial ischemia so calcium excess is inhibited; Attenuation of electrical dysfunction due to excessive sodium	Dizziness, headache, constipation, nausea, asthenia, syncope, palpitations, tinnitus, vertigo, abdominal pain, dry mouth, peripheral edema, dyspnea
Organic Nitrates							
Nitroglycerin						All organic nitrates:	General: GI disturbances, headache, which may be severe and persistent, apprehension, vertigo, tachycardia, hypotension, arthralgia
Intravenous‡		✓			HTN, CHF	Vasodilation of CAs, collaterals, + stenotic sites to ↑ CBF	Adverse reactions are usually dose related and secondary to vasodilation
Sublingual	Nitrostat	✓	✓			Prevention of CA spasm	
Lingual spray	Nitrolingual	✓	✓			Venodilation → ↓ preload	
Buccal tablets§			✓			In large doses, systemic vasodilation → ↓ afterload	
Oral and ER/SR tabs	Nitroglyn, Nitro-Bid		✓	✓		↑ Exercise tolerance, ↓ ST segment depression	
Transdermal patch¶				✓			

Continued

TABLE 5-12: Antianginal Agents—Cont'd

Drug	Brand Name	Indications				Mechanisms of Action	Adverse Reactions
		Acute	Immediate Prophylaxis	Long-acting Prophylaxis	Other		
Topical ointment	Nitro-Bid, Nitrol		✓	✓			
Isosorbide dinitrate¶	Dilatrate, Isochron, Isordil, Sorbitrate		✓	✓	CHF, PAH, PortH		
Isosorbide mononitrate**	Imdur, Ismo, Monoket			✓	PortH		
Erythrityl tetranitrate††	Cardilate			✓			
Pentaerythritol tetranitrate‡‡	Peritrate SA, Duotrate			✓			
Amyl nitrate (inhalant)§§	Aspirols, Vaporole	✓					

BP, Blood pressure; CA, coronary artery; CBF, coronary blood flow; CHF, congestive heart failure; ER, extended-release; GI, gastrointestinal; HR, heart rate; HTN, hypertension; PAH, pulmonary hypertension; PortH, portal hypertension; SR, sustained release.

*See Table 5-10.
†See Table 5-7.
‡Intravenous nitroglycerin: Tridil, NitroBid.
§Buccal tablets (Nitrogard) are placed under the upper lip or between the teeth and gums and allowed to dissolve slowly.
¶Transdermal patch: Nitro-Dur, Transderm-Nitro, Nitrodisc, Minitran, Deponit.
¶Isosorbide dinitrate (Isordil, Sorbitrate, Dilatrate) comes in sublingual and chewable tablets and controlled-release capsules.
**Available in immediate release and extended release tablets.
††Available in sublingual and oral tablets.
‡‡Available in oral tablets and long-acting capsules and tablets.
§§Comes in a protective cloth-covered glass capsule, which is broken and inhale one to six times while seated.

vasodilation, whereas verapamil has the greatest negative inotropic effect. Nicardipine appears to produce the greatest increase in coronary blood flow.

- Refer to page 178 for a description of the CCBs and to Table 5-7 for a list of these agents and their indications, as well as their adverse effects.

Organic Nitrates

Organic nitrates produce potent vasodilation, including both the coronary and peripheral arteries as well as the venous system. They exert their effects by reducing myocardial oxygen demand due to reductions in preload and, at high does, afterload. They are often the first-line therapy for angina. Nitrates also produce vasodilation of stenotic segments of the coronary arteries and increase collateral blood flow, so perfusion of ischemic myocardium is enhanced.

- The effects of nitroglycerin (NTG) are almost immediate in terms of pain relief and favorable alterations in the electrocardiographic patterns, but are short in duration (less than 30 minutes). NTG can be used prophylactically in situations of increased demand, when chest discomfort is likely (e.g., before exercise or physical therapy).
  - ▸ Immediate-acting agents are available in intravenous, sublingual, spray, and buccal forms, as shown in Table 5-12.
  - ▸ Patients who have angina should have their short-acting emergency medication on their persons at all times. Therapists should be aware of the medication each patient uses and have access to it in case of emergency. The patient's medication can be easily administered by a third party in case of emergency.
- Various longer acting nitrates are also available to provide prophylaxis against angina.
  - ▸ The primary drug is isosorbide dinitrate, which is available in several forms, including sublingual, chewable, and oral capsules. The sublingual tablets are shorter acting than the chewable tablets, which are shorter acting than the controlled-release capsules.
  - ▸ Nitrates also come in the form of a topical ointment and as a more aesthetically pleasing patch.
- The main problem with nitrates is that tolerance often develops with continuous or intermittent around-the-clock use of these drugs, so they lose their effectiveness. Tolerance can be prevented by intermittent dosing, during which treatment is interrupted at night. However, this regimen leaves patients unprotected at night and early in the morning, when 7% to 10% of patients experience angina.
- The major adverse effects associated with NTG and other nitrates include headache, dizziness, weakness, palpitations, and severe hypotension and occasionally syncope. Hypotension and reflex tachycardia may aggravate angina.

Ranolazine

Ranolazine (Ranexa) is a novel antianginal agent that is used in the treatment of chronic stable angina that is refractory to more standard antianginal drugs (see Table 5-12).[6] By inhibiting the derangements in sodium and calcium that lead to intracellular calcium overload, ranolazine addresses the consequences of myocardial ischemia that act to perpetuate the ischemia.

- Ranolazine causes selective inhibition of the late sodium channels, which are altered by myocardial ischemia, and so prevents the resultant intracellular excesses of sodium and calcium.[6,106]
- Ranolazine improves diastolic ventricular relaxation, increasing peak filling rate and myocardial wall lengthening during isovolumic relaxation of ischemic regions of the LV.[6]
- It has demonstrated effectiveness in decreasing the frequency of angina attacks and increasing exercise tolerance in patients with CAD who are taking concomitant atenolol, amlodipine, or diltiazem.[106]
- Side effects of ranolazine include dizziness, headache, constipation, nausea, and asthenia. Less common are syncope, palpitations, tinnitus, vertigo, abdominal pain, dry mouth, peripheral edema, and dyspnea.
- Prolongation of the Q–T interval may occur but is not associated with increased arrhythmias; in fact, ranolazine appears to have an antiarrhythmic effect, resulting in significantly lower incidence of ventricular tachycardia, supraventricular tachycardia, and significant ventricular pauses.[100]

ACE Inhibitors

A number of studies have observed the value of ACEIs in reducing MIs and death in patients with heart failure. Subsequently, two major studies using ramipril and perindopril have confirmed the same findings in patients with chronic CAD with preserved LV function. Unfortunately, these findings are not universal; however, methodologic differences (ACEI agent used, dosage, and patient population) may account for the discrepancies.[106]

DRUGS USED TO TREAT CHRONIC HEART FAILURE

Chronic heart failure (CHF) develops through impairment of the left ventricle's ability to fill or empty properly (refer to Chapter 4 [Cardiopulmonary Pathology], page 108). As a consequence, cardiac output falls and left ventricular filling pressure rises, which is reflected back to the pulmonary vasculature. Inadequate cardiac output triggers compensatory neurohumoral responses involving the SNS and the renin–angiotensin–aldosterone system (RAAS), which work together to support cardiac output and mean arterial pressure (MAP) in order to maintain perfusion pressure to critical vascular beds, such as the CNS, myocardium, and kidneys.

- Under normal circumstances, cardiac output is maintained primarily by increasing LV end-diastolic (filling) volume (i.e., preload). If volume recruitment from the venous capacitance vessels is not effective in generating adequate preload to produce the needed cardiac output, the compensatory responses illustrated in Figure 5-3 are activated, according to the severity and duration of the hemodynamic stress.
- Activation of the SNS stimulates increases in HR and myocardial contractility and enhances myocardial relaxation, all of which serve to increase cardiac output. SNS output also increases systemic vascular resistance via peripheral vasoconstriction to maintain MAP.

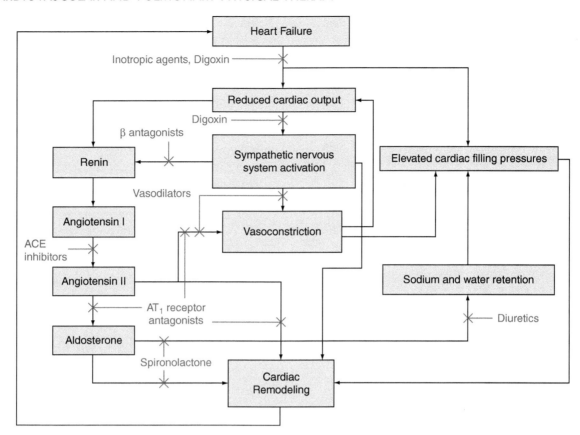

Figure 5-3: The pathophysiological mechanisms involved in congestive heart failure and the major sites of drug action. (From Brunton LL, Lazo JS, Parker KL. *Goodman and Gilman's The Pharmacologic Basis of Therapeutics.* 11th ed. New York: McGraw-Hill Professional; 2005.)

- Of importance, the existence of systolic contractile dysfunction complicates the situation, shifting the normal relationship between preload and stroke volume such that enhanced preload may not produce adequate stroke volume (see Figure 3-5 on page 43). SNS-mediated vasoconstriction aggravates the problem by increasing afterload and impeding LV ejection. Thus, a vicious cycle of inadequate cardiac output and neurohumoral activation is created.
- Additional compensatory responses that develop with chronic hemodynamic stress include myocardial hypertrophy provoked by pressure overload and chamber dilation induced by volume overload. If the abnormal loading conditions are not corrected, cardiomyocyte injury ensues and pump dysfunction develops.
- The RAAS responds by secreting more renin, which leads to augmented production of Ang I and II, ultimately effecting vasoconstriction to support MAP. Ang II also stimulates the generation of aldosterone, which increases sodium and fluid retention to expand intravascular volume and raise preload.
- Unfortunately, research has revealed that each of these compensatory responses also promotes disease progression by direct myocardial injury and stimulation of myocardial remodeling.

Traditional pharmacologic therapy for CHF has focused on the relief of symptoms and stabilization of hemodynamic abnormalities through inhibition of compensatory neurohumoral activation, as shown in Figure 5-3. More recent insights into the induction and propagation of CHF have redirected treatment to drugs that also slow disease progression, retard maladaptive ventricular remodeling, and reduce mortality. These benefits are accomplished by blocking the deleterious effects of vasoconstrictive hormones and stimulating production of vasodilator hormones, often with traditional medications as well as with some newer classes of drugs.

Guidelines for the treatment of chronic CHF advocate the use of ACEIs, β-blockers, aldosterone antagonists, and ARBs because of their remarkable success in reducing morbidity and mortality.[2,90,102] Other drugs may also be prescribed including other vasodilators, diuretics, digitalis and other inotropic agents, and phosphodiesterase inhibitors (Table 5-13), as well as antiplatelet and anticoagulant agents and statins. The last two types of these medications are presented later in the chapter.

The effects of various medications used to treat CHF on resting and exercise vital signs are presented at the end of this chapter (see Table 5-22 on page 216).

ACE Inhibitors

As already noted, activation of the RAAS plays a critical role in the pathogenesis of CHF. ACEIs are first-line treatment for all stages of CHF, including asymptomatic LV dysfunction, because of their

TABLE 5-13: Drugs Used to Treat Congestive Heart Failure

Drug	Mode of Action	Indications	Adverse Reactions
Afterload Reducers			
ACE inhibitors*	Blocks activation of RAAS → inhibition of vasoconstriction and vascular hypertrophy + reversal/prevention of ventricular remodeling and progressive dysfunction	All stages of SHF: ↓ HF disability, hospitalizations, + mortality, and to improve symptoms and functional capacity DHF: to improve relaxation	Per Table 5-8
β-Blockers†	↓ SNS stimulation of heart and blood vessels → reversal or prevention of ventricular remodeling and progressive dysfunction + ↓ peripheral vasoconstriction	Stages II + III SHF: ↓ HF disability, hospitalizations, + mortality, and to improve symptoms and functional capacity DHF: to ↓ HR and prolong filling in patients with ↑ HR	Per Table 5-10
ARBs‡	Prevention of vasoconstriction and vascular hypertrophy + reversal/ prevention of ventricular remodeling and progressive dysfunction	Stage II SHF: to ↓ disability + hospitalizations, and to improve symptoms and functional capacity	Per Table 5-9
Vasodilators§	↓ Peripheral vascular resistance → ↓ preload and afterload → ↓ stress on failing heart	CHF: can use concurrently with digitalis, diuretics	Reflex tachycardia, orthostatic hypotension, dizziness, weakness, nausea, headache, peripheral edema
Aldosterone Antagonists			
Spironolactone (Aldactone)	Inhibition of Na+ and fluid retention Inhibition of aldosterone-induced effects that contribute to ventricular remodeling	Symptomatic CHF	Per Table 5-6
Eplerenone (Inspra)		Post-MI patients with LV dysfunction	Hyperkalemia
Preload Reducers			
Diuretics¶	Promote excretion of excess fluid in vascular system → ↓ end-diastolic volume → ↓ workload on failing heart	Symptomatic CHF	Per Table 5-5
Positive Inotropic Agents: Cardiac Glycosides			
Digoxin (Lanoxin, others)	↑ Force and velocity of systolic contraction ↓ SNS activity	SHF with persistent symptoms despite all other medications; most effective in low-output failure Atrial fibrillation that is not controlled by β-blockers	Cardiac toxicity, GI effects (which mimic CHF) and CNS effects; headache, weakness, and visual disturbances
Positive Inotropic Agents: Phosphodiesterase Inhibitors			
Milrinone (Primacor); Amrinone (Inocor)	↑ Contractility + vasodilation of arteries, venous capacitance and pulmonary vascular beds	SHF with persistent symptoms despite all other medications	Arrhythmias, hypotension, headache, hypokalemia

↑, Increased; ↓, decreased; →, resulting in; ACE, angiotensin-converting enzyme; ARB, angiotensin II receptor blockers; CHF, chronic heart failure; DHF, diastolic heart failure; GI, gastrointestinal; HF, heart failure; HR, heart rate; LV, left ventricular; MI, myocardial infarction; RAAS, renin–angiotensin–aldosterone system; SHF, systolic heart failure; SNS, sympathetic nervous system.

*See Table 5-8.
†See Table 5-10.
‡See Table 5-9.
§Inorganic nitrates, mesiritide, hydralazine, calcium channel blockers.
¶Usually prescribed along with low sodium diet.
¶See Table 5-5.

proven ability to attenuate many of the key hemodynamic, mechanical, and functional disturbances that occur.

- By impeding the formation of Ang II, ACEIs suppress vasoconstriction and reduce PVR and therefore afterload. Consequently, stroke volume and cardiac output are enhanced.
- In addition, ACEIs inhibit aldosterone production, decrease SNS activity, and potentiate the effects of diuretics in CHF. However, it appears that there is a rebound effect in which aldosterone levels slowly return toward normal after the initiation of treatment.
- ACEIs also increase the levels of bradykinin, which stimulates production of NO, cyclic GMP, and other vasodilator substances. It is this effect that appears to be responsible for attenuation of ventricular remodeling and progression.
- Specifically, captopril, enalapril, lisinopril, and ramipril have proven to alleviate symptoms, improve clinical status, and reduce mortality in patients with HF, including those with diastolic LV dysfunction. They also delay diabetic nephropathy.[93]
- A list of these agents can be found in Table 5-8, which also presents their adverse effects (see pages 173 to 174).

β-Adrenergic Blockers

Because β-blockers inhibit the hyperactivation of the SNS that contributes to disease progression, they are recommended as standard therapy for CHF, including patients who appear clinically stable on ACEIs and diuretic therapy.

- β-Adrenergic stimulation is known to cause apoptosis of cardiac myocytes, which may be attenuated by β-blockade. β-Blockers modify the expression of genes that become altered by CHF, which may play a role in ventricular remodeling and turnover of extracellular matrix.[11]
- In addition, β-blockers improve cardiac metabolism by reestablishing carbohydrates as the primary source of energy (SNS activation in CHF causes a shift from carbohydrate to free fatty acid use), thus improving the efficiency of myocardial energetics so that more ATP is available for contraction.[42]
- Thus, long-term β-blocker therapy, especially with the β₁-selective agents, has been shown to reduce symptoms, improve myocardial function and LV remodeling, increase exercise tolerance, and reduce all-cause and CV mortality, sudden death, and hospitalizations.[2,42] Unfortunately, not all patients respond to β-blocker therapy.
- Yet, it is important to realize that symptomatic improvements may take weeks to months before they become apparent. In fact, most patients experience a deterioration in LV performance during the first weeks of treatment because of the withdrawal of β-adrenergic support.[90,93,111] LV function returns to pretreatment level by about the fourth week of treatment and then increases by approximately 10% over the next few months, during which LV diastolic and systolic volumes and mass steadily decrease.[36]
- Treatment using carvedilol in patients with CHF with normal LV ejection fraction has produced significant improvements in diastolic LV function, including improved relaxation and regression of ventricular remodeling.[88]
- The side effects of β-blocker therapy are listed in Table 5-10.

Angiotensin II Receptor Blockers

Most of the known physiological effects of Ang II, including its deleterious effects in CHF, are mediated by type 1 angiotensin (AT₁) receptors, whereas type 2 angiotensin (AT₂) receptors generally seem to counterbalance the biological effects of Ang II–mediated stimulation of the AT₁ pathway.

- Thus, antagonism of the RAAS at the level of the AT₁ receptor provides more complete inhibition of the effects of Ang II than do ACEIs, because it blocks all sources of Ang II.
- ARBs provide comparable mortality benefits compared with ACEIs and are recommended as the preferred alternative to ACEIs in patients who do not tolerate them.[91] ARBs also appear to be useful for the treatment of diastolic heart failure due to improvements in LV remodeling.[88]
- In addition, there is evidence that combined treatment with an ACEI and an ARB produces greater improvement in LV remodeling and reduces hospitalization, although it does not appear to reduce mortality.[2,91]
- The use of ARBs reduces, but does not eliminate, the occurrence of bradykinin-mediated side effect seen with ACEIs, mainly cough and angioedema. Other side effects occur less frequently and are less pronounced with the ARBs, as noted in Table 5-9 (see page 174).

Aldosterone Antagonists

Aldosterone is important in the pathophysiology of CHF, particularly structural remodeling, because of its effects on extracellular matrix, collagen deposition, myocardial fibrosis, and some other unique mechanisms.[2]

- Aldosterone blockers inhibit the effects of aldosterone, described previously, and check ventricular remodeling.
- Spironolactone results in significant reductions in morbidity and mortality in patients with NYHA class III–IV CHF from systolic LV dysfunction.[85,93] It has also been shown to retard ventricular remodeling after MI.[2]
- Eplerenone significantly reduces total mortality and sudden cardiac death in post-MI patients with systolic LV dysfunction.[85,93]
- Because both drugs improve ventricular remodeling with reductions in LV mass and hypertrophy, they improve diastolic function. In addition, these drugs counteract the rebound of aldosterone levels seen with ACEIs and ARBs, which is likely to increase their beneficial effects in patients with diastolic HF.[88]
- There is an increased incidence of hyperkalemia and renal dysfunction with aldosterone antagonists, so their use is avoided in patients with severe renal dysfunction or a history of severe hyperkalemia. Patients should be monitored carefully and should avoid the use of NSAIDs and other drugs that are associated with K^+ retention. Other side effects are listed in Table 5-6 (see page 172).

Vasodilators

The many drugs that produce vasodilation reduce afterload and often preload, which decreases myocardial work and enhances cardiac output and thus improves symptoms of CHF. However, only the combined use of isosorbide dinitrate and hydralazine (available commercially as BiDil) and the antiangiotensin drugs already presented have demonstrated mortality benefits.

- The organic nitrates (see Table 5-12, page 179) relax vascular smooth muscle, causing reductions in pulmonary and systemic vascular resistance, and therefore RV and LV afterload. They also reduce preload and LV filling pressure.
- Likewise, hydralazine decreases RV and LV afterload through its effects on vascular resistance; however, it has minimal effects on venous capacitance and therefore preload. Hydralazine augments contractility, reduces renovascular resistance, and increases renal blood flow. It is used for CHF patients with impaired renal function who do not tolerate ACEI therapy.
- The combination of isosorbide dinitrate and hydralazine produces regression of LV remodeling and increases survival. In addition, the antioxidant effect of hydralazine may decrease the nitrate tolerance that often limits its long-term effectiveness.
- Parenteral vasodilators, including nitroprusside and intravenous NTG, are used in intensive care settings when rapid reductions in ventricular filling pressures and systemic vascular resistance are indicated (e.g., severe HTN and decompensated HF). Nitroprusside is also effective in managing patients who develop mechanical complications, such as mitral regurgitation or ventricular septal defect, after acute MI.
- The major adverse effect of vasodilators is hypotension. Other side effects are described on page 177.

Diuretics

Although diuretics do not reduce mortality in CHF, they retain a central role in the management of the symptoms of pulmonary and systemic venous congestion.

- Diuretic therapy reduces extracellular fluid volume and therefore preload, which ameliorates the increases in end-diastolic filling pressure and ventricular wall stress that lead to LV hypertrophy and remodeling.
  - ▸ With the exception of ethacrynic acid, the loop diuretics, listed in Table 5-5 (see page 171), are widely used as chronic therapy to manage the congestive symptoms of both systolic and diastolic HF.
  - ▸ The thiazide diuretics, which require higher glomerular filtration rates than the loop diuretics, are used less frequently for CHF management, unless the two types are combined to provided additive benefits.
  - ▸ Because the potassium-sparing drugs are weak diuretics, they are not effective in reducing extracellular fluid. However, the aldosterone agonists spironolactone and eplerenone, previously discussed, offer benefits via mechanisms that are independent of their diuretic action.
- When rapid volume reduction is avoided, the reduction in LV filling volume produces little change in cardiac output, due to depression and flattening of the ventricular function curve (see Figure 3-5 on page 43).
- Many patients exhibit impaired responsiveness to diuretic therapy because of diminished renal function, poor absorption, or physiological adaptation to prolonged administration. Nonsteroidal antiinflammatory drugs can also contribute to diuretic resistance.

- The diuretics used for volume reduction do not alter the natural history of CHF. However, the improvements in ventricular geometry and wall stress may retard the progression of ventricular remodeling.
- The adverse effects of the various types of diuretics are provided in Table 5-6 (see page 172).

Positive Inotropic Agents

Myocardial contractility is depressed in systolic HF, and inotropic agents may be prescribed to enhance pump function. They are used to improve hemodynamics and to provide relief of symptoms in patients with advanced CHF who fail to respond to standard medications.

Digitalis

Digitalis (digoxin) is considered adjunct therapy for patients with persistent symptoms of CHF despite maximal therapy with the recommended drugs. It is also indicated for patients with atrial fibrillation that fails to achieve control with β-blockers.

- Digitalis is a cardiac glycoside that boosts myocardial contractility and cardiac output by increasing intracellular calcium concentration. It also attenuates SNS activity through inhibition of noncardiac Na^+,K^+-ATPase.
- In addition, digitalis prolongs the refractory period of the AV node (negative chronotropic effect) and is used to control the ventricular rate in atrial fibrillation.
- Although it does not reduce mortality, digitalis has been shown to improve CHF symptoms and exercise tolerance and to decrease hospitalizations.[93] However, there is some concern that it may increase mortality in women.
- The major danger of digitalis therapy is drug toxicity. The most serious manifestations of digitalis intoxication are cardiac arrhythmias, including conduction defects (AV block) and enhanced automaticity. The initial presenting symptoms are quite general and include GI symptoms (anorexia, nausea, and vomiting) as well as neurologic symptoms (headache, drowsiness, and confusion). Digoxin toxicity is also associated with visual green or yellow halos, which occur very late in an episode of toxicity.

Phosphodiesterase Inhibitors

Milrinone (Primocor) and inamrinone (formerly amrinone, Inocor) are parenteral phosphodiesterase (PDE) inhibitors that increase contractility, accelerate myocardial relaxation, and produce arterial and venous dilation, thus increasing cardiac output. Although they induce beneficial hemodynamic effects and improve symptoms, their use has been associated with increased mortality. Therefore, these agents are reserved mainly for the management of acute class IV CHF and symptomatic disease that persists despite maximal medical therapy. Milrinone is generally considered the drug of choice in these situations.

- These agents improve functional capacity and sense of well-being in patients with end-stage CHF. They are also used as a bridge to transplantation, increasing survival while awaiting a donor organ.
- The primary adverse reactions are cardiac arrhythmias (atrial fibrillation and flutter and ventricular tachycardia and fibrillation) and hypotension.

Dobutamine

Dobutamine is a positive inotropic agent that acts through direct stimulation of myocardial β_1-adrenergic receptors. It also reduces ventricular filling pressures without much change in HR. Dobutamine is used in intensive care settings to boost cardiac output, particularly when rapid deterioration of a patient's status requires immediate support, as in a large acute MI or increasing decompensation in severe CHF. It is the drug of choice in low-output states with hypotension or borderline BP.

Dopamine

Dopamine is a positive inotropic agent that has both α_1 and β_1 activity but also stimulates renovascular dopaminergic receptors, which produce dilation and increase renal blood flow. It is also administered by intravenous drip in critical care situations, usually in conjunction with more potent inotropic agents (e.g., dobutamine).

Antiplatelet Agents and Anticoagulants

The incidence of thromboembolic events (e.g., cerebrovascular accidents or venous thrombosis) is increased in patients with CHF. Contributory factors include intracardiac and peripheral blood flow deceleration, endothelial dysfunction, abnormalities of hemostasis, and platelet activation. Therefore, antiplatelet agents or anticoagulants are often prescribed for these patients.

- The evidence supporting the use of antiplatelet or anticoagulant therapies in heart failure is still limited. However, a number of clinical trials are currently underway that should provide some guidelines regarding their value.[32]
- At present, patients with HF due to ischemic heart disease are usually treated with antiplatelet agents, whereas patients with atrial fibrillation are placed on anticoagulation.
- Antiplatelet agents and anticoagulants are described in more detail on page 197.

Statins

Since the discovery of nonlipid (pleiotropic) effects of statins, their use for the treatment of patients with CHF has been under investigation. Accumulating evidence suggests that these agents can play an important role in preventing CHF or delay its progression.[101] Statins appear to be beneficial in both ischemic and nonischemic HF, including both systolic and diastolic dysfunction.[32]

- There is evidence that statins reduce the risk of all-cause mortality and hospitalization in patients with HF. They may also reduce the risk of nonfatal MI and stroke.
- Mechanisms that may induce these benefits include their effects on inflammatory responses (e.g., favorable modulation of signaling pathways involving NO, tissue-type plasminogen activator, endothelin-1, and plasminogen activator inhibitor-I), myocardial preservation (e.g., attenuation of ventricular remodeling, protection from myocardial apoptosis, and activation of endothelial cell NO production), and neurohumoral mediators and pathways (e.g., down-regulation of AT_1 receptors, reduction of SNS activity, and modification of vascular function of endothelin-1 receptors).[101]
- Statin therapy has been shown to prevent the development of HF after MI.
- The statins are presented in more detail in a later section of this chapter (see page 194).

Patients who survive acute coronary syndrome (ACS) have an increased risk of subsequent CV morbidity and mortality. Therefore, substantial research has been directed toward secondary prevention and myocardial protection. A number of lifestyle modifications and medications have demonstrated benefit in reducing risk of reinfarction, LV dysfunction, HF, and death.

- Among the many lifestyle modifications that have shown effectiveness in secondary prevention, cessation of smoking and control of HTN are probably the most crucial. Diet modification for lipid and weight control and regular exercise are also important.
- Daily laughter is a novel form of lifestyle modification that appears to reduce risk in patients with acute MI and those with DM through improvements in endothelial function.[108a]
- Some pharmacologic therapies aim to avoid further myocyte loss through apoptosis and inflammation, as described later. Strong evidence exists regarding the efficacy of β-blockers, ACEIs, ARBs, statins, and antiplatelet agents in patients who have suffered acute ST-elevation MI (STEMI).

Neurohumoral Blocking Agents

Depressed cardiac function after ST-segment elevation MI (STEMI) leads to a series of neurohumoral reflexes that activate the SNS and RAAS, increasing the levels of renin, angiotensin II, norepinephrine, endothelin, and aldosterone. Although these reflexes are initially helpful in maintaining MAP, prolonged activation eventually becomes maladaptive, leading to alterations in ventricular structure involving infarcted and noninfarcted areas of myocardium. The resultant contractile dysfunction, fibrosis, progressive dilation, hypertrophy, and distortion of the LV cavity (i.e., LV remodeling) are associated with inflated myocardial oxygen demand and recurrent ischemic events, ventricular dysfunction and HF, and increased risk of arrhythmias and sudden cardiac death.

- Pharmacologic inhibition of the neurohumoral pathways, using certain β-blockers (propranolol, timolol, and carvedilol) and ACEIs or ARBs, significantly reduces post-MI morbidity and mortality and is now included in clinical guideline recommendations as standards of care.[4,34] More comprehensive adrenergic blockade appears to offer superior benefits for post-MI patients with LV dysfunction and HF, as well as those with normal LV function, compared with β_1-blockade alone. Thus, the American College of Cardiology/American Heart Association (ACC/AHA) recommends that all patients with MI, irrespective of LV function, receive acute-phase and long-term management with β-blockers and ACEIs/ARBs as long as there are no contraindications.
- In addition, aldosterone antagonists are indicated for patients with LV dysfunction and HF in the absence of contraindications or intolerance.[10] In animal models, aldosterone blockade has been associated with reduced collagen deposition, norepinephrine levels, interstitial fibrosis, hypertrophy, LV dilation, and increased LV ejection fraction. Furthermore, spironolactone seems to improve endothelial dysfunction, reduces peripheral vasoconstriction and elevated vascular tone induced

by low levels of NO, and attenuates oxidative stress and resultant endothelial damage, inflammation, and fibrosis. Aldosterone receptor–blocking agents have been shown to substantially reduce morbidity and mortality in post-MI patients with LV dysfunction and HF when used in conjunction with β-blockers and ACEIs/ARBs, although these patients require close monitoring of renal function and serum potassium levels to avoid complications.

Statins

Because of the strong association of increased low-density lipoprotein (LDL) cholesterol level with CAD, a target level of LDL cholesterol of less than 100 mg/dL is recommended for all patients with clinically evident CAD. Post-ACS patients with higher levels should be discharged home on statin therapy with the goal of reducing the LDL level to less than 70 mg/dL.[4]

- Statins not only reduce LDL cholesterol levels but also raise high-density lipoprotein (HDL) cholesterol levels, low levels of which (<40 mg/dL) are often the primary lipid abnormality seen in post-ACS patients.
- In addition, statin therapy reduces levels of C-reactive protein, suggesting an antiinflammatory effect. Mounting evidence suggests other pleiotropic effects of statins that may also be important in reducing risk of CV morbidity and mortality, including maintenance of endothelial function, interruption of thrombogenesis, and stabilization of atherosclerotic plaques.[61]
- Statin therapy for patients with elevated LDL cholesterol produces significant reductions in CAD-related deaths and nonfatal MIs.[61]
- The statins are presented in more detail on pages 186 and 194.

Antiplatelet Agents and Anticoagulants

The benefits of aspirin in reducing vascular mortality and risk of ischemic events in patients with ST-elevation MI and other forms of ACS have been recognized since 1988 and reaffirmed by many studies.[19,27] More recent research has documented the advantage of clopidogrel in preventing reperfusion injury during fibrinolytic and primary percutaneous coronary interventions.[9,27]

- Low-dose aspirin therapy is recommended for all patients unless contraindications are present.
- Clopidogrel is indicated for patients who cannot take aspirin.

- Warfarin is used as an alternative in patients who can take neither aspirin nor clopidogrel. It is also prescribed for patients who require anticoagulation for abnormalities such as atrial fibrillation, LV thrombus, cerebral emboli, or extensive regional wall motion abnormality.[4] Warfarin may be combined with antiplatelet therapy in patients who are less than 75 years of age with low bleeding risk and are able to be monitored reliably.
- More information about antiplatelet agents and anticoagulants is offered on page 186.

ANTIARRHYTHMIC AGENTS

Myocardial cells have special properties (automaticity, excitability, and conductivity), which are responsible for the electrical activity of the heart that produces its pumping action.

- In the resting state, myocytes are polarized, being more negative on the inside of the cell and more positive on the outside, causing a resting membrane potential of −80 to −90 mV. This polarization is due to the higher concentrations of intracellular potassium ions (K^+) and proteins (negatively charged) and higher concentrations of extracellular sodium (Na^+) and chloride (Cl^-) ions.
- When a threshold potential occurs, pores or channels in the cell membrane are opened to allow shifts in ions, as shown in Figure 5-4. Thus, depolarization represents a reversal of the resting electrical charge, which then is followed by repolarization causing a return to the resting polarized state. The entire cycle of depolarization and repolarization constitutes an action potential, and it is the sum total of the action potentials from all areas of the heart that produces the waves of an electrocardiogram (ECG).
- Cardiac action potentials from different regions of the heart vary in shape because of differences in the ion channels, especially K^+ channels; action potentials of ventricular cells are composed of five phases:
  ▸ Phase 0 (the upstroke or spike): Depolarization, during which there is rapid influx of Na^+ through fast channels, which initiates the interaction of myosin and actin.
  ▸ Phase 1: Early repolarization, during which Na^+ influx ceases because of closure of the fast sodium channels, and potassium begins to reenter the cell and sodium begins to leave; it is part of the absolute refractory period.

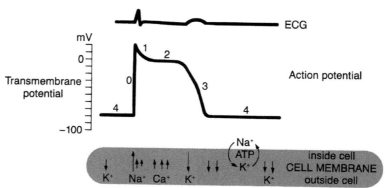

Figure 5-4: A myocardial action potential arising from the ventricles. The ion shifts that occur in each phase are depicted. (From American Heart Association: *Textbook of Advanced Cardiac Life Support.* Dallas, Texas: American Heart Association, 1990.)

▸ Phase 2: Plateau phase, when calcium continues to enter the cell through slow Ca^{2+} channels and repolarization continues relatively slowly; this phase is also part of the absolute refractory period.

▸ Phase 3: Late repolarization, during which the calcium channels close, potassium rapidly flows out of the cell, and then active transport via the sodium–potassium pump begins to restore potassium to the inside of the cell and sodium to the outside; this is the relative refractory period.

▸ Phase 4: Return to resting polarized state, corresponding to diastole, when sodium and calcium remain outside of the cell and potassium remains inside; the cell is ready to respond to the next stimulus.

• Perturbations of function of the Na^+, K^+, and Ca^{2+} ion channels can be produced by such things as acute ischemia, SNS stimulation, metabolic or electrolyte imbalances, drug toxicity, or myocardial scarring. In addition, heart disease can alter the concentration and distribution of cardiac ion channels.

• These perturbations provoke cardiac arrhythmias due to abnormalities of impulse generation (e.g., enhanced or abnormal automaticity), impulse conduction, or a combination of the two.

▸ Enhanced automaticity caused by abnormal phase 4 depolarization produces inappropriate sinus tachycardia and some idiopathic ventricular tachycardias.

▸ Abnormal automaticity induced by depression of the slope of diastolic depolarization so that the threshold voltage is shifted toward zero (hyperpolarizing the resting membrane potential), or by abnormal phase 4 depolarization, leads to atrial tachycardia and accelerated ideoventricular rhythms.

▸ Triggered arrhythmias, which occur as responses to the preceding cardiac impulse, can result from early after-depolarizations occurring during phase 2 or 3 when the action potential is prolonged due to bradycardia or certain drugs (e.g., torsades de pointes) or from delayed after-depolarizations occurring in phase 4 when excess calcium is released from the sarcoplasmic reticulum (e.g., digitalis-induced arrhythmias, and RV outflow tract ventricular tachycardia).[111]

▸ Reentry rhythms are produced by conduction abnormalities in which, given a requisite set of circumstances, an excitation wavefront fails to die out (per normal) but rather propagates continuously so that it continues to excite the heart by always encountering excitable tissue. For example, an anatomic accessory pathway of fast-response tissue can lead to atrial flutter, AV nodal reentrant tachycardia, Wolff-Parkinson-White syndrome tachycardia, and some forms of ventricular tachycardia (VT), depending on its location. Reentry can also occur as a result of functional circuit pathways formed by heterogeneities in conduction properties or refractoriness of neighboring cardiac tissues, or by a curved depolarization wavefront (e.g., atrial fibrillation [a-fib] or ventricular fibrillation [VF]).

▸ Rhythm disturbances can range from innocuous, asymptomatic events (that may or may not be detected or are found incidentally during a routine physical examination or ECG) to serious or life-threatening abnormalities.

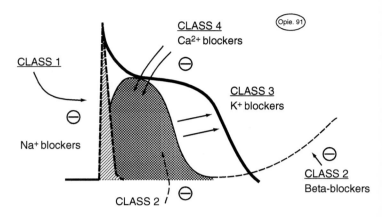

Figure 5-5: The action potential and its phases of activation of the excitable cell, with the sites of intervention of the four classic types of antiarrhythmic agents shown. Class I agents decrease phase 0 of the rapid depolarization of the action potential (rapid sodium channel). Class II agents, β-blocking drugs, have complex actions including inhibition of spontaneous depolarization (phase 4) and indirect closure of calcium channels, which are less likely to be in the "open" state when not phosphorylated by cyclic AMP. Class III agents block the outward potassium channels to prolong the action potential duration and hence refractoriness. Class IV agents, verapamil and diltiazem, and the indirect calcium antagonist adenosine, inhibit the inward calcium channel, which is most prominent in nodal tissue, particularly the atrioventricular node. Most antiarrhythmic drugs have more than one action. (From Opie LH, Gersh BJ. *Drugs for the Heart.* 6th ed. Philadelphia: Saunders; 2005.)

Antiarrhythmic drugs are classified according to their effects on the myocardial action potential and their mechanisms of action, which involve reduced conductance of the various ion channels (Figure 5-5, Box 5-3, and Table 5-14). The commonly used Vaughan Williams classification, which is based on the electrophysiological effects exerted by an arbitrary concentration of each drug, generally on normal cardiac tissue, is limited by its simplicity.

• Although drugs within the same group are similar, differences in pharmacologic effects occur among the various agents in each class, and these variations can lead to differences in clinical responses to specific drugs.

• In addition, many drugs exert multiple effects, so their pharmacology is more complex than that indicated by a simple drug classification scheme.

• Furthermore, the actions of many drugs differ in different cardiac tissue.

• The effects of various antiarrhythmic agents on resting and exercise vital signs are listed later in this chapter (see Table 5-22 on page 216).

An alternative classification system, called the Sicilian gambit, is based on the differential effects of antiarrhythmic drugs on ion channels, cardiac receptors, and transmembrane ion pumps, as detailed in Figure 5-6. Although it is based primarily on the predominant action of the drug, it also considers other ancillary

---

BOX 5-3: Currently Available Antiarrhythmic Agents, and Mechanism of Action: Generic and Trade Names

---

Class I: Local anesthetics or membrane-stabilizing agents that depress phase 0

    Subclass IA: Depress phase 0 and prolong action potential duration

        Disopyramide (Norpace)

        Procainamide (Pronestyl, Procan SR)

        Quinidine (Quinora, Quinidex Extentabs, Quinaglute Dura-Tabs, Cardioquin)

    Subclass IB: Depress phase 0 slightly and may shorten action potential duration

        Lidocaine (Xylocaine, Lidopen)

        Mexiletine (Mexitil)

        Phenytoin (Dilantin)

        Tocainide (Tonocard)

    Subclass IC: Marked depression of phase 0, slight effect on repolarization, and profound slowing of conduction

        Flecainide (Tambocor)

        Moricizine[†] (Ethmozine)

        Propafenone (Rythmol)

Class II: β-Blockers[‡] that depress phase 4 depolarization

    Acebutolol (Sectral)

    Esmolol (Brevibloc)

    Propranolol (Inderal, Inderal LA)

    Sotalol[§] (Betapace)

Class III: Prolongation of phase 3 (repolarization)

    Amiodarone[‖] (Cordarone)

    Bretylium (Bretylol)

    Sotalol[§] (Betapace)

    Dofetilide[*] (Tikosyn)

Class IV: Calcium channel blockers that depress phase 4 depolarization and lengthen phases 1 and 2 of repolarization

    Diltiazem (Cardizem, Cardizem CD, Dilacor SR)

    Verapamil (Calan, Isoptin, Verelan)

Digoxin: Prolongs effective refractory period of AV node and shortens refractory period in atrial muscle

Adenosine: Slows conduction through AV node and interrupts reentry pathways

---

*Was voluntarily withdrawn from the market but is available on a limited basis.

†Class I antiarrhythmic that shares characteristics of group IA, IB, and IC agents.

‡Antiarrhythmic effects occur in concentrations associated with β-blockade.

§Has both class II and III properties; class III properties occur at doses exceeding 160 mg.

‖Exhibits all properties of class III plus noncompetitive α- and β-adrenergic blockade.

---

actions that may be clinically germane, and it allows for the inclusion of other drugs, such as adenosine and digitalis, which were not considered in the Vaughan Williams classification.[64]

An important fact about antiarrhythmic agents is that, by their nature, they have the potential to cause or aggravate arrhythmias. Such proarrhythmic effects range from an increased frequency of premature ventricular contractions (PVCs) to the development of VT or VF, which may have fatal consequences. Most of the time, it is often not possible to distinguish a drug's proarrhythmic effect from the patient's underlying rhythm disorder.

Class I Agents

Class I drugs act predominantly to block the fast inward Na^+ channels, slowing the rate of rise of phase 0 and decreasing membrane excitability.[11,44,64] These agents are further classified into three subcategories, according to their electrophysiological effects (see Box 5-3 and Table 5-14). An additional agent, moricizine, shares some of the characteristics of class IA and IC.

Class IA Drugs

In the usual therapeutic concentrations, class IA agents (procainamide, quinidine, and disopyramide) lengthen the effective refractory period by two different mechanisms: first, they inhibit the fast sodium current and phase 0 upstroke of the action potential;

and second, they prolong the action potential by slowing repolarization (thus, lengthening the refractory period, as indicated by the Q–T interval).

- Common side effects include nausea, vomiting, and diarrhea. At higher doses, they can cause headache, vertigo, tinnitus, blurred vision, and disorientation.
- These drugs can cause proarrhythmic complications by prolonging the Q–T interval in predisposed individuals or by depressing conduction and promoting reentry.
- The use of class IA agents is steadily decreasing because of their generally unfavorable risk-to-benefit ratio and the availability of more effective and safer drugs.

Class IB Drugs

Class IB agents (lidocaine, mexiletine, and phenytoin) produce moderate inhibition of the fast Na^+ current and phase 0 depolarization (typical class I effect) while decreasing the action potential duration by shortening the refractory period. They also suppress conduction of triggering impulses.

- By shortening repolarization, these drugs protect against Q–T prolongation, which can provoke arrhythmias.
- Adverse reactions consist of dose-related manifestations of CNS toxicity, including drowsiness, dizziness, tremors, slurred speech, paresthesias, confusion, delirium, coma, and seizures.

TABLE 5-14: Electrophysiological Effects and Indications of Antiarrhythmic Agents

Group	Drug	Electrophysiological Effects			Indications								Adverse Reactions
		Automaticity	Conduction Velocity	Refractory Period	PACs	SVT	A-Flutter/Fib	PJCs, Junc Tach	PVCs	VT	Post-MI	Digitalis-induced Arrhythmias	
IA	Quinidine	↓	↓	↑↑	✓	✓	✓	✓	✓	✓			Proarrhythmic, GI upset is most common; CHF and hypotension are most serious; lupus erythematosus may develop
	Procainamide	↓	↓	↑↑		✓			✓				
	Disopyramide	↓	↓	↑↑		✓*				✓			
IB	Lidocaine	↓	↕	↔					✓				Primarily CNS reactions (drowsiness, dizziness, tremors, GI upset), increasing with higher doses)
	Mexiletine	↓	↕	←					✓	✓			
	Phenytoin	↓	↕	↔					✓			✓	
IC	Flecainide	↓	↓↓	↑↑		✓	✓	✓	✓	✓			Proarrhythmic, CNS reactions (dizziness, GI upset, fatigue, tremors, dry mouth), syncope, CHF
	Propafenone	↓	↓↓	←			✓	✓	✓	✓			
	Moricizine	↓	↓	↔↑					✓				
II†	Acebutolol	↓	↓	←					✓				
	Esmolol	↓	↓	←		✓		✓					
	Metoprolol	↓	↓	←					✓		✓		
	Propranolol	↓	↓	←		✓		✓	✓	✓	✓	✓	
	Timolol	↓	↓	←							✓		

Class	Drug						Side Effects
III	Amiodarone§	↓		↑		✓ ✓ ✓	GI upset, CNS symptoms (tremor, fatigue, ataxia)
	Bretylium	↑	↔↑	↓↑‡		✓ ✓	
	Sotalol	↓	↓	↑↑		✓ ✓	
IV	Verapamil	↓	↓	↑	✓	✓ ✓	Bradycardia, CHF, hypotension, edema, dizziness, GI upset, headache
	Diltiazem	↓	↔↑	↔↑	✓	✓	
Other	Digoxin	↓	↓	↑	✓	✓	See text, page 185
	Adenosine	↓	↓		✓		Not important due to very short half-life¶

↓, Decreased; ↑, increased; ↔, no change; ✓, indicated; a-fib, atrial fibrillation; a-flutter, atrial flutter; CHF, congestive heart failure; IV, intravenous; junc tach, junctional tachycardia; MI, myocardial infarction; PACs, premature atrial contractions; PJCs, premature junctional contractions; PVCs, premature ventricular contractions; SVT, supraventricular tachycardia; v-tach, ventricular tachycardia.

*Unlabeled use includes paroxysmal atrial tachycardia.
†Unlabeled uses of various β-blockers include ventricular arrhythmias (atenolol, metoprolol, timolol, and pindolol) and supraventricular tachycardias (bisoprolol).
‡Because of a complex balance of direct and indirect autonomic effects.
§Unlabeled uses include paroxysmal atrial tachycardia, atrial flutter, and atrial fibrillation.
¶Adenosine has an extremely short half-life (6-12 sec).

Drug	Channels Na* Fast	Med	Slow	Ca	K_r	K_s	α	β	M_2	P	Pumps Na+, K+-ATPase	LV Function	Sinus Rate	Extracardiac
Quinidine		●A			⊙		○		○			–	↑	⊙
Procainamide		●A			⊙							↓	–	⊙
Disopyramide		●A			⊙				○			↓	–	●
Lidocaine	○											–	–↓	○
Mexiletine	○											–	–	○
Phenytoin	○											–	–	⊙
Flecainide		●A			○							↓	–	○
Propafenone		●A			○			⊙				↓	↓	○
Moricizine	●I											↓	–	○
Propranolol	○							●				↓	↓	○
Nadolol								●				↓	↓	○
Amiodarone	○			⊙	●	⊙	⊙	⊙				–	↓	●
Bretylium					●		▣	▣				–	↓	○
Sotalol					●			●				↓	↓	○
Ibutilide					○							–	↓	○
Dofetilide					●							–	–	○
Azimilide					⊙	⊙	○					–	–	○
Verapamil	○			●				⊙				↓	↓	○
Diltiazem				⊙								↓	↓	○
Adenosine										□		–	↓	⊙
Digoxin									○		●	↑	↓	⊙
Atropine									●			–	↑	⊙

Figure 5-6: Actions of antiarrhythmic drugs on membrane ion channels, receptors, and ionic pumps in the heart and their clinical effects. Relative potency of blockade or extracardiac sided effects: ○, low antagonist; ⊙, moderate antagonist; ●, high antagonist; □, agonist; ▣, agonist–antagonist; A, activated state blocker; I, inactivated state blocker; –, minimal effect; ↑, increase; ↓, decrease; K_r, rapid component of delayed rectifier K^+ current; K_s, slow component of delayed rectifier K^+ current; M_2, muscarinic receptor subtype 2; P, A_1 purinergic receptor. (Adapted from Schwartz PJ, Zaza A. Haemodynamic effects of a new multifactorial antihypertensive drug. *Eur Heart J.* 1992;13[Suppl. A]:26.)

- Other than the occasional treatment of VT, these drugs are rarely prescribed anymore.

Class IC Drugs

Class IC agents (flecainide and propafenone) are powerful inhibitors of the fast sodium channels, causing marked depression of the phase 0 upstroke of the cardiac action potential. They also have a marked inhibitory effect on His-Purkinje conduction with QRS widening with relatively little effect on repolarization and the refractory period.

- These drugs have been found to increase mortality and the occurrence of nonfatal cardiac arrest when used in patients with CAD and thus are contraindicated in this population.
- These drugs are used mainly to control ventricular tachyarrhythmias resistant to other drugs.

- Adverse side effects include dizziness, nausea, vomiting, chest pain, fatigue, tremors, dry mouth, unusual taste, and visual disturbances. Proarrhythmias may cause syncope.

Moricizine

Moricizine is a class I antiarrhythmic agent with potent local anesthetic activity and myocardial membrane-stabilizing effects resulting from class IA and IC actions. It reduces the fast Na^+ current and prolongs AV nodal and His-Purkinje conduction times and QRS duration. There is slight prolongation of the Q–T interval (due to QRS widening) and the ventricular refractory period.

- Moricizine is reserved mainly for patients with life-threatening ventricular arrhythmias when other antiarrhythmics are ineffective, not tolerated, or contraindicated.

- Adverse reactions are similar to those of other class IA and IC agents.

Class II Agents

Class II agents, the β-blockers, inhibit sympathetic activity by blocking catecholamine binding at the β-adrenergic receptor sites, thus slowing the HR, delaying AV node conduction (with resultant slowing of the ventricular rate), and reducing contractility. As shown in Table 5-14, β-blockers may be used to prevent and control supraventricular arrhythmias (e.g., supraventricular tachycardia [SVT], rate control of atrial fibrillation and atrial flutter) and ventricular dysrhythmias (PVCs).[11,44,64] They are also used to manage digitalis-induced arrhythmias and ventricular arrhythmias associated with prolonged Q–T interval syndrome.

- β-Blockers approved for antiarrhythmic therapy or to prevent sudden death following MI consist of acebutolol (PVCs), esmolol (SVT), metoprolol (post-MI), propranolol (SVT, VT, post-MI), and timolol (post-MI).
- The use of β-blockers has increased significantly because of their beneficial effects of reducing oxygen demand in CAD, decreasing mortality after MI, and inhibiting SNS-mediated ventricular remodeling post-MI and in CHF.
- In addition, another β-blocker, sotalol, exerts antiarrhythmic effects consistent with class III agents.
- Adverse side effects are listed in Table 5-10.

Class III Agents

Class III compounds (amiodarone, bretylium, sotalol, ibutilide, dofetilide, and azilimide) are considered the most effective antiarrhythmic agents. They act by inhibiting K^+ and Na^+ channels, which results in prolongation of repolarization and the refractory period, lengthening the action potential duration and thus the Q–T interval.[11,44,64] Many of these drugs share additional properties with the other antiarrhythmic classes.

- Amiodarone is a structural analog of thyroid hormone. In addition to its class III actions, it also produces Na^+ channel blockade, noncompetitive antisympathetic action, and negative chronotropic properties of class IV agents.
  - ▸ It is effective in treating sustained VT or VF via intravenous (IV) administration, and the oral drug can be used for all other tachyarrhythmias, including control of many SVTs, rate control of a-fib and flutter, and cardioversion of a-fib. It is safe to use in post-MI and CHF patients.
  - ▸ Amiodarone is also an effective antianginal agent due to vasodilation of coronary and peripheral arteries.
  - ▸ Unfortunately, amiodarone has a wide spectrum of toxic effects, which affect a large percentage of patients. The most common side effects are GI intolerance, weight loss, visual disturbances, and CNS symptoms (tremor, fatigue, insomnia, ataxia, and vivid dreams). It can also produce asymptomatic elevation of liver enzymes and alterations in thyroid-stimulating hormone (TSH) or thyroid hormone.
  - ▸ The most dangerous adverse effect is pulmonary toxicity, which occurs in 5% to 10% of patients, particularly at higher doses and in older patients, and may occur at any time after starting treatment. It is manifested as dyspnea, nonproductive cough, and fever, although it may present as acute respiratory failure.

- Sotalol has combined class II and class III effects, producing β-blockade and prolongation of action potential duration, so it is especially effective in treating ventricular arrhythmias, including sustained VT. It also reduces defibrillation thresholds, improving treatment success for VF. It is also beneficial in a wide variety of SVTs. Adverse effects are those typical of other β-blockers (see Table 5-10). In addition, prolongation of the Q–T interval increases the incidence of torsades de pointes, especially if hypokalemia is present and in females, patients with renal impairment, and those with structural cardiac defects.
- Bretylium, which is no longer available, exerts class III actions and also blocks adrenergic neurons and has antifibrillatory effects.
- Ibutilide enhances the slow inward Na^+ channels rather than blocking the outward K^+ channels to cause an increase in the refractoriness of atrial and ventricular tissue and prolongation of the action potential. Administered by IV, it is used for rapid cardioversion of a-fib and flutter. Its main adverse effect is the increased risk of torsades de pointes.
- Dofetilide is a pure class III drug that has no extracardiac effects. It is used to maintain sinus rhythm in patients with a-fib. Because it has a narrow therapeutic window and must be dose adjusted for renal insufficiency and Q–T intervals, it can be used only by physicians with special training. The only adverse effect of significance is torsades de pointes.

Class IV Agents

The calcium channel blockers verapamil and diltiazem inhibit slow Ca^{2+} channel influx, depress depolarization, prolong repolarization, and slow conduction through the AV node.[11,44,64] They also depress myocardial contractility.

- These agents can prevent AV node and AV reentry and are used to slow the ventricular response to a variety of SVTs, including a-fib and flutter.
- Adverse reactions include bradycardia, CHF, hypotension, edema, dizziness, nausea, vomiting, headache, constipation, and heart block.

Digoxin

Digitalis prolongs the effective refractory period of the AV node and shortens the refractory period in the atria; it has minimal effects on the His-Purkinje system and ventricular muscle except at toxic concentrations.[11,37,44] It also increases vagal tone and thus slows the sinus rate. Digoxin is used primarily to reduce the ventricular rate in a-fib and flutter.

- Digoxin has a narrow therapeutic window and episodes of acute and chronic toxicity occur often and can cause serious arrhythmias, including sinus bradycardia and arrest, AV node block, and any type of tachycardia. The risk of toxicity is increased in patients with renal dysfunction, hypokalemia, advanced age, chronic lung disease, hypothyroidism, and amyloidosis.

- Medication interactions also occur with a number of drugs, including oral aminoglycosides, amiodarone, anticholinergics, benzodiazepines, CCBs, erythromycin, indomethacin, omeprazole, quinidine, and tetracycline.
- Side effects are presented on page 185.

Adenosine

Adenosine is a naturally occurring purine nucleoside that modulates many physiological responses. In the heart, it attaches to receptors in the AV node, slowing conduction through it and interrupting reentry pathways.[44,111] Administered as a rapid IV bolus, it is ultrashort-acting, with a half-life of 1 to 6 seconds.

- It is used to for the acute termination of reentrant paroxysmal SVTs and wide-complex tachycardia of unknown etiology.
- Adverse effects consist of flushing, dyspnea, and hypotension, but are short-lived. Transient asystole lasting up to 5 seconds is common, which can be disconcerting to a conscious patient and is usually accompanied by chest pressure and dyspnea. On rare occasions, it has triggered bronchospasm.

DYSLIPIDEMIC MEDICATIONS

Cholesterol and triglycerides are important serum lipids that are related to cardiovascular health. Cholesterol is an essential component of mammalian cell membranes and furnishes the substrate for bile acids and steroid hormones, including estrogen, testosterone, and cortisol. Triglycerides (TGs), which are composed of three free fatty acid (FFA) chains bound to glycerol, are oxidized as major sources of energy for metabolic processes, especially in the heart, liver, kidneys, and exercising muscles. Excess TGs are stored in fat cells (adipocytes).

Cholesterol and triglycerides are transported in the blood within lipoproteins, which are classified according to their density.[11,111] The protein components of lipoproteins, called apolipoproteins or apoproteins, provide structural stability and may assist the particles in lipoprotein–receptor interactions or enzymatic processes that regulate lipoprotein metabolism. Of note, the size and density of lipoprotein particles vary with their constituent parts (the amounts of cholesterol, TGs, phospholipids, and apoproteins).

- *Chylomicrons* transport dietary TGs and cholesterol from the intestines to the liver, cardiac, muscle, and adipose tissue, binding to lipoprotein lipase (LPL) in the capillaries, which hydrolyzes the FFAs for the production of energy in cardiac and muscle cells or for storage as TGs in the liver and adipocytes.
- *Very low density lipoproteins (VLDLs)* transport 85% of endogenously synthesized TGs in the plasma from the liver to peripheral tissues for storage in adipose tissue or for use in skeletal muscle (again, through the action of LPL). After most TGs are removed from VLDLs, they become intermediate-density lipoproteins (IDLs), which return to the liver where they are either cleared from the plasma or undergo delipidation to become LDL particles. High levels of VLDLs (>1000 mg/dL) can cause pancreatitis.
- *Low-density lipoproteins (LDLs)* are the major transporter of cholesterol in the blood, carrying it from the liver to tissues throughout the body, where it is hydrolyzed for use in a variety of cellular processes, including new cell membrane synthesis, steroid hormone production (in adrenal, ovarian, and testicular cells), and bile acid synthesis (in hepatocytes). The remaining LDLs are cleared by the liver, which has a large complement of LDL receptors. LDLs become atherogenic when they are modified by oxidation so they can be taken up by scavenger receptors on macrophages, leading to foam cell formation in arterial lesions.
- *Lipoprotein(a) [Lp(a)]* is an LDL particle with an apoprotein(a) [apo(a)], which appears to be an independent risk factor for CVD. It is thought to interfere with fibrinolysis of thrombi on the surface of atheromatous plaques.[11]
- *High-density lipoproteins (HDLs)* promote reverse cholesterol transport, the process by which excess cholesterol is acquired from cells and transferred to the liver for excretion. HDLs may also protect against atherogenesis by other mechanisms, including putative antiinflammatory, antioxidant, platelet antiregulatory, anticoagulant, and profibrinolytic activities.[11]

Disorders of lipid metabolism can lead to dyslipidemias, including elevated levels of LDL cholesterol (LDL-C) and triglycerides and low levels of HDL cholesterol (HDL-C), all of which are risk factors for atherosclerotic CVD. Clinical studies have led to the establishment of more stringent target levels for LDL-C and total cholesterol to HDL-C ratio and lower treatment thresholds, especially in high-risk and very high-risk patients, as shown in Table 5-15.

- Lifestyle modifications (diet and exercise) are the cornerstones to successful reduction of cholesterol levels; however, in most cases, pharmaceutical intervention is also necessary.
- There are five major categories of lipid-modifying agents. The most commonly used drugs are the statins (hydroxymethylglutamyl-coenzyme A [HMG-CoA] reductase inhibitors). Other agents are bile sequestrants, nicotinic acids (niacin), cholesterol absorption inhibitors, and fibric acid derivatives (Table 5-16).
- The pharmacologic effects of these agents on lipid and lipoprotein values appear in Table 5-17.

HMG-CoA Reductase Inhibitors (Statins)

The HMG-CoA reductase inhibitors, or statins, are the most effective and best tolerated antidyslipidemic agents. Statins suppress the conversion of HMG-CoA to mevalonate and thus inhibit the early and rate-limiting step in hepatic cholesterol synthesis.[11,31] Ultimately, this action leads to increased numbers and activity of LDL receptors in the liver, which pull LDL from the blood. There is some evidence that the statins may also reduce the production of VLDLs and enhance the removal of LDL precursors (VLDL, IDL, apoB-100, and apoE).

- Statins reduce LDL-C by 20% to 55% according to the dose. They also reduce VLDLs and TGs and increase HDL-C.
- A number of other cardioprotective properties have been attributed to statins:
  ‣ Improved endothelial function due to increased production of nitric oxide
  ‣ Increased stability of atheromatous plaques so they are less vulnerable to rupture

TABLE 5-15: Target LDL-C and TC:HDL-C Levels for Adults and Indications for Treatment According to Risk

			Treatment Indications	
Risk Category	**LDL-C Goal**	**TC: HDL-C**	**Lifestyle Modifications**	**Drug Therapy**

Very high risk:
• ASHD plus one of the following:
  ▸ Multiple risk factors
  ▸ Diabetes mellitus
  ▸ A poorly controlled single factor
  ▸ Acute coronary syndrome
  ▸ Metabolic syndrome
	<70 mg/dL*	<3.5	All individuals	All individuals

High risk: • ASHD or equivalent	<100 mg/dL*	<3.5	All individuals	All individuals
Moderately high risk: • 2+ risk factors • 10-yr risk of 10%-20%	<130 mg/dL (optional, <100 mg/dL)	<4.5	LDL-C ≥100 mg/dL or TC:HDL-C ≥4.5	≥130 mg/dL† or TC: HDL-C ≥6.0
Moderate risk: • 2+ risk factors • 10-yr risk <10%	<130 mg/dL	<4.5	≥130 mg/dL or TC:HDL-C ≥4.5	>160 mg/dL or TC: HDL-C ≥6.0
Low risk: • 0 or 1 risk factor	<160 mg/dL	<5.5	≥160 mg/dL or TC:HDL-C ≥5.5	≥190 mg/dL (optional, 160 to 189 mg/dL) or TC:HDL-C ≥7.0

From Brunton LL, Lazo JS, Parker KL. *Goodman and Gilman's The Pharmacologic Basis of Therapeutics.* 11th ed. New York: McGraw-Hill Professional; 2005.
ASHD, Atherosclerotic heart disease; HDL-C, high-density lipoprotein cholesterol; LDL-C, low-density lipoprotein cholesterol; TC = total cholesterol.
*If pretreatment LDL-C is near or below the goal value, a statin dose sufficient to lower LDL-C by 30% to 40% is recommended.
†A lower level (100 to 129 mg/dL) is recommended for patients if they also have one of the following: age greater than 60 years, three or more risk factors, a severe risk factor, triglycerides exceeding 200 mg/dL and HDL-C less than 40 mg/dL, metabolic syndrome, highly sensitive C-reactive protein exceeding 3 mg/L, or coronary calcium score (age/gender adjusted) greater than the 75th percentile.

▸ Inhibition of vascular smooth muscle proliferation and inhibition of apoptosis
▸ Attenuation of inflammatory processes contributing to atherogenesis
▸ Suppression of lipoprotein oxidation
▸ Inhibition of platelet aggregation and sometimes fibrinogen levels
• The most common side effects are gastrointestinal, which occur in 5% or less of patients. The most clinically significant adverse effect is myopathy, which occurs in about 0.01% of patients, usually those taking higher doses and concomitant drugs that diminish statin catabolism (e.g., fibrates, cyclosporine, digoxin, warfarin, and macrolide antibiotics); in rare cases, rhabdomyolysis develops. Severe muscle weakness or discomfort not associated with exercise in patients taking statins requires immediate evaluation to rule out rhabdomyalgias and discontinuation of the drug.
• Statins should be taken in the evening for maximal reduction of LDL because the activity of HMG-CoA reductase is greatest in the late evening and early morning.
• Combination treatment with bile acid sequestrants produces further reductions in LDL-C and TGs. The addition of niacin to statins is particularly beneficial in patients with elevated TGs and high HDL-C, but the risk of myopathy is increased when the statin dose exceeds 25% of maximum.

Bile Acid Sequestrants

Bile acid sequestrants (cholestyramine, colesevelam, and colestipol) block the absorption of bile from the gut so that it cannot be returned to the liver. This results in a compensatory increase in hepatic bile acid synthesis from cholesterol that leads to its further elimination, upregulation of LDL receptors, and a reduction in LDL-C.
• Because bile acid sequestrants are not absorbed from the GI tract, they do not produce systemic side effects. However, GI side effects consisting of constipation versus extreme diarrhea and flatulence make these agents less than desirable for patients.
• Bile acid sequestrants have the potential to interfere with absorption of medications from the GI tract. To minimize this possibility, patients should take other medications at least 1 to 2 hours before or 4 hours after the bile acid sequestrants.

Nicotinic Acid

Nicotinic acid (niacin, vitamin B_3) lowers cholesterol and TGs by inhibiting their lipolysis in adipose tissue, which reduces FFA transport to the liver and hepatic TG synthesis. This results in reduced VLDL production and lower LDL levels. Niacin also enhances LPL activity, resulting in increased clearance of chylomicrons and VLDL triglycerides, and raises the HDL-C level by decreasing its clearance in the liver.[11,31] Niacin is the only lipid-lowering drug that significantly decreases Lp(a) levels (by about 40%).[11]

TABLE 5-16: Medications Used to Treat Dyslipidemias

Type of Drug	Drug (Trade) Name	Mechanisms of Action	Adverse Reactions
HMG-CoA reductase inhibitors (statins)	Atorvastatin (Lipitor) Fluvastatin (Lescol) Lovastatin (Altocor, Mevacor) Pravastatin (Pravachol) Rosuvastatin (Crestor) Simvastatin (Zocor)	Block the synthesis of cholesterol, especially LDL and VLDL ↑ LDL clearance from plasma Also, ↓ inflammatory component of atherosclerotic plaques	Occur rarely, including reversible ↑ transaminases, myositis; some other drugs interact with statins to ↑ their plasma levels (e.g., antibiotics, antifungals, certain antivirals, grapefruit juice, cyclosporine, amiodarone, and others)
Bile acid–binding resins	Cholestyramine (Questran, Cholybar, Cuemid) Colesevelam (WelChol) Colestipol (Colestid)	Sequester cholesterol-laden bile salts in the bowel → ↑ excretion + ↓ reabsorption Used as adjuvant Rx in patients with severely ↑ TC due to ↑ LDL	Frequent GI symptoms (nausea, bloating, abdominal pain, constipation); ↑ TG levels, ↓ absorption of other medications (e.g., Coumadin, digitalis)
Cholesterol absorption inhibitors	Ezetimibe (Zetia)	Selectively inhibits intestinal sterol absorption Used to treat ↑ LDL not responsive to maximal statin dose	Upper respiratory infection, myalgia, extremity pain
Fibric acid derivatives	Clofibrate (Atromid, Clofibral, etc.)* Fenofibrate (Lipidil, Tricor) Gemfibrozil (Lopid, Tripid)	Interaction with factor that regulates transcription of some lipoproteins Used to treat ↑ TGs	Cutaneous manifestations, GI (abdominal discomfort, gallstones), erectile dysfunction, ↑ transaminases; interaction with anticoagulants, ↑ plasma homocysteine
Nicotinic acid (niacin)	Niacin, vitamin B (Niacor + many others)	Decreases hepatic secretion of VLDL and FFA mobilization Increases HDLs and TGs	Facial flushing, pruritus, gastritis, abnormal liver function, glucose intolerance, hyperuricemia
Combination drugs	Ezetimibe + simvastatin (Vytorin) Niacin + lovastatin (Advicor)		

↑, Increased; ↓, decreased; →, leads to or results in; FFA, free fatty acid; GI, gastrointestinal; HDL, high-density lipoprotein cholesterol; HMG-CoA, hydroxymethylglutaryl-coenzyme A; LDL, low-density lipoprotein cholesterol; Rx, treatment; TC, total cholesterol; TG, triglyceride; VLDL, very low density lipoprotein.
*Not used much anymore.

- Niacin is associated with two side effects that limit its usefulness: a flushing reaction that may be accompanied by itching and tingling and GI upset. The most serious adverse effect is hepatotoxicity, which is manifested as flulike symptoms of fatigue and weakness.
- Niacin should be used cautiously by diabetic persons because of increased insulin resistance leading to severe hyperglycemia.
- Niacin can precipitate gout attacks by interfering with renal excretion of uric acid.

Fibric Acid Derivatives

Fibric acid derivatives, or fibrates, stimulate peroxisome proliferator–activated receptors (PPAR) that are involved in lipid metabolism. They inhibit the production of VLDL in the liver and accelerate the removal of TGs from the blood, produce phenotypic change in LDL particles resulting in decreased synthesis of small dense atherogenic particles, and increase HDL-C levels.[31,90a]

- The fibric acid derivatives are the drug of choice for patients with severe hypertriglyceridemia who are at risk for pancreatitis. They are often used in conjunction with statins for more comprehensive dyslipidemic therapy.
- The effect of fibrates on lipoprotein levels varies widely, depending on the initial lipoprotein profile, the presence or absence of genetic hyperlipidemias, the associated environmental influences, and the specific drug used.
- Side effects include GI upset, increased risk of gallstones, cutaneous manifestations (rash, urticaria, and hair loss), myalgias, fatigue, headache, sexual dysfunction, and anemia. In addition, they may potentiate the effects of oral anticoagulants.

TABLE 5-17: Pharmacologic Effects of Antidyslipidemic Agents

Drug	Pharmacologic Effects					
	Lipids		Lipoproteins			
	Cholesterol	Triglycerides	VLDL	LDL	HDL	
HMG-CoA reductase inhibitors (statins)	↓	↓ 20%–37%	↓	↓ 20%–55%*	↑ 5%–15%	
Bile acid sequestrants	↓	↔↑	↔↑	↓ 15%–30%	↑ 3%–5%	
Cholesterol absorption inhibitors	↓	↓ 8%		↓ 18%	↑ 1%	
Nicotinic acid	↓	↓ 20%–50%	↓	↓ 5%–25%	↑ 15%–35%	
Fibric acid derivatives	↓	↓ 20%–50%	↓	↔[†]	↑ 10%–20%	

↑, Increased; ↓, decreased; ↔, no change; HDL, high-density lipoprotein cholesterol; HMG-CoA, hydroxymethylglutaryl coenzyme A; LDL, low-density lipoprotein cholesterol; VLDL, very low density lipoprotein.
[†]Minimal effect on LDL values, but beneficial effect on LDL particle size,changing from small atherogenic particles to larger, less atherogenic particles; also may ↓ total LDL particle numbers.

Cholesterol Absorption Inhibitors

Ezetimibe is a novel antidyslipidemic agent that inhibits cholesterol absorption in the small intestine (by about 70%). In addition, there is an upregulation of LDL receptor expression, which increases hepatic clearance of LDL-C from the plasma.

- Ezetimibe is usually prescribed as dual therapy with statins, with which it has complementary actions. Vytorin is a combination tablet containing ezetimibe and various doses of simvastatin, which produces a reduction of LDL-C up to 60%.
- The most common side effects are diarrhea, abdominal pain, back pain, joint pain, and sinusitis, which occur at similar rates as with a placebo. There are also rare allergic reactions.

ANTIPLATELET AGENTS AND ANTICOAGULANTS

Normal intact vascular endothelium is protected from thrombosis by a number of endothelium-controlled processes, which repel platelets from the vessel wall and maintain the fluid state of the blood. Nitric oxide (NO) and prostacyclin (prostaglandin-I_2, PGI_2) are among the potent, locally active platelet inhibitors (and vasodilators) that are produced by normal endothelial cells. The actions of these two substances, as well as of tissue-type plasminogen activator (t-PA), are induced by thrombin, which can either promote or prevent blood clotting, depending on the circumstances.

At the site of vascular damage, these antiplatelet substances are lost and platelets adhere to tissue factor exposed by the damaged endothelium. Binding of platelets to the injured vessel wall is facilitated by other proteins, such as von Willebrand factor. Rapid platelet activation and aggregation creates a platelet plug, which may be sufficient to seal small injuries.

Simultaneously, the interaction of tissue factor with factor VII activates the coagulation cascade (Figure 5-7), producing thrombin through stepwise activation of a series of circulating proteolytic enzymes. The final reaction is the activation of factor X to factor Xa, which can be catalyzed directly by the tissue factor–VIIa complex or indirectly by converting factor IX to IXa; factor Xa then stimulates the conversion of prothrombin to thrombin.

The prothrombotic activities of thrombin now predominate, and it plays a central role in the clotting process. Thrombin converts fibrinogen to fibrin, activates factors V, VIII, and XI, which generates more thrombin, and stimulates platelets. The activation of factor VII can also be induced by thrombin and factor Xa. Furthermore, through activation of factor XIII, thrombin promotes the formation of cross-linked bonds among the fibrin molecules, leading to clot stabilization.

Antiplatelet agents and anticoagulants, listed in Table 5-18, act at various steps in the coagulation cascade to inhibit platelet aggregation and thrombus formation and expansion. Antiplatelet drugs are the treatment of choice for the prevention and treatment of arterial thrombosis, although anticoagulants are also effective, and combination therapy offers added benefits. Anticoagulants are the primary agents used for prevention and treatment of venous thromboembolism and for prevention of cardioembolic events in patients with atrial fibrillation, prosthetic heart valves, and mural thrombus.

Antiplatelet Drugs

Intact vascular endothelium is protected from thrombosis by potent platelet inhibitors, prostacyclin, NO, carbon monoxide, and ADPase. However, vascular intimal injury disrupts the antiplatelet properties of the endothelium.

Atherothrombosis is a generalized and progressive process with an inflammatory component, which leads to platelet adhesion, activation, and aggregation, so that the presence of atheromatous plaques increases the risk of thrombus formation. Most acute coronary events are caused by acute thrombosis superimposed on an atheromatous plaque that has fissured or ruptured.

Antiplatelet therapy is used to inhibit the formation of platelet-rich thrombi for primary and secondary prevention of vascular events in patients with CAD, stroke or transient ischemic attack (TIA), and peripheral arterial disease (PAD).

Aspirin

Aspirin (acetylsalicylic acid) binds to and irreversibly inactivates cyclooxygenase (COX), the first step in the biosynthesis of

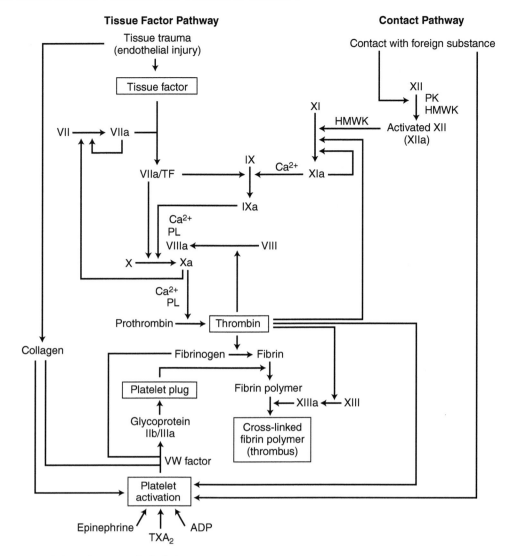

Figure 5-7: Hemostasis and thrombosis. Endothelial injury resulting from tissue trauma or a vascular event (e.g., atherosclerotic plaque rupture or fissure) triggers the release of collagen, which induces platelet activation and aggregation, and tissue factor, which activates the coagulation cascade, ultimately leading to thrombus formation. Small injuries may be sealed through rapid platelet aggregation and platelet plug formation, but larger injuries require the formation of fibrin leading to a cross-linked thrombus. As shown, both systems are mutually reinforcing. ADP, adenosine diphosphate; HMWK, high-molecular-weight kininogen; PK, prekallikrein; PL, platelet phospholipids (which are located on the surface of activated platelets); TXA_2, thromboxane A_2; VW, von Willebrand factor.

thromboxane A_2 (TXA_2, a potent agonist of platelet activation), resulting in inhibition of platelet activation and aggregation for 8 to 10 days.

- Aspirin prophylaxis prevents thrombus formation and reduces the incidence of MI, death, or both by 15% to 25% in patients with unstable angina, acute MI, or cerebrovascular disease, and in those undergoing angioplasty or coronary artery bypass graft (CABG) surgery.[21,43,77a]
- In addition, aspirin therapy has been shown to significantly reduce the risk of first MI and other CV events in both men and women, and combination therapy using clopidogrel with aspirin may be even more effective.[27]
- Aspirin use is associated with dose-related upper GI symptoms (nausea, heartburn, and epigastric pain), especially at doses exceeding 500 mg. Enteric-coated aspirin may cause less

gastric irritation than regular aspirin. The risk of bleeding, particularly GI bleeding, is also increased and does not appear to differ according to dose or formulation.

Thienopyridines

Clopidogrel and ticlopidine inhibit platelet activation through metabolites that block fibrinogen binding, leading to inhibition of platelet aggregation and clot formation.

- Clopidogrel and ticlopidine are used as an adjunct to aspirin therapy to prevent arterial thromboembolism during and for 1 year after acute MI, percutaneous translumenal coronary angioplasty (PTCA), or stroke. It is also an appropriate alternative for patients with contraindications or intolerance to aspirin, those who have a recurrent vascular event while taking aspirin, or those at high risk of recurrent vascular events (>20%/yr).

TABLE 5-18: Antiplatelet and Anticoagulant Drugs

Drug Type and Agents	Brand Name	Indications	Mechanism of Action	Adverse Effects
Antiplatelet Drugs				
COX inhibitors Aspirin		MI and post-MI, unstable angina, atrial fibrillation, PTCA, prosthetic heart valve, TIA, stroke	Irreversibly binds to COX → inhibits platelet activation and formation of thromboxane A_2 → ↓ platelet aggregation + ↓ clot formation	Gastric upset, gastritis, ↑ risk of bleeding, especially GI

Thienopyridines
  Clopidogrel
  Ticlopidine
	
	Plavix
	Ticlid
		Post-MI, PTCA, stroke	Blocks fibrinogen binding → ↓ platelet aggregation + ↓ clot formation	↑ Risk of bleeding; rare skin reactions, thrombotic thrombocytopenia purpura

GPIIb/IIIa receptor antagonists
  Abciximab
  Eptifibatide
  Tirofiban
	
	ReoPro
	Integrilin
	Aggrastat
		ACS, PTCA	Inhibits binding of fibrinogen and von Willebrand factor to GPIIb/IIIa receptors on platelet surface	↑ Risk of bleeding at arterial access site; thrombocytopenia

PDE inhibitors Dipyridamole	 Persantine	Prosthetic cardiac valve	Inhibits platelet uptake of adenosine → ↓ platelet aggregation	Dizziness, abdominal distress, headache, rash
Anticoagulants				

Heparin (unfractionated)
LMW heparin
  Enoxaparin
  Dalteparin
  Tinzaparin
	
	Lovenox
	Fragmin
	Innohep
		PTCA, CP bypass
		
		Prevention of VTE, PTCA
			Binds with antithrombin III and thrombin → inactivation of thrombin and factor Xa → ↓ clot formation and extension; platelet inhibition	↑ Risk of bleeding and hemorrhage; heparin-induced thrombocytopenia; skin reactions, general hypersensitivity reactions; heparin-induced osteoporosis

Heparinoids Danaparoid*	 Orgaran	Prevention of VTE	As for heparin	↑ Risk of bleeding, anemia, thrombocytopenia, hypersensitivity reactions
Factor Xa inhibitors Fondaparinux	 Arixtra		Blocks clotting factor Xa → interruption of coagulation cascade	Small ↑ risk of bleeding, anemia, fever, GI symptoms, edema, rash, insomnia

Direct thrombin inhibitors
  Argatroban
  Desirudin
  Lepirudin
  Bivalirudin
	
	Argatroban
	Iprivask
	Refludan
	Angiomax
		Heparin-induced thrombocytopenia, VTE prophylaxis, ACS, PTCA	Direct binding to free and clot-bound thrombin → ↓ clot formation, as well as clot lysis; platelet inhibition	↑ Risk of bleeding, anemia, thrombocytopenia, anaphylaxis, hypotension, chest pain, back pain, GI symptoms, headache

Vitamin K antagonists Warfarin	 Coumadin	Long-term anticoagulation: prosthetic cardiac valves, atrial fibrillation, mural thrombus	Inhibition of vitamin K–dependent clotting factors (II, VII, IX, X) → anticoagulation	↑ Risk of bleeding, dermatitis, allergic manifestations, skin necrosis

↓, Decreased; ↑, increased; →, leads to or results in; ACS, acute coronary syndrome; COX, cyclooxygenase; CP, cardiopulmonary; GI, gastrointestinal; GP, glycoprotein; LMW, low molecular weight; PDE, phosphodiesterase; PTCA, percutaneous translumenal coronary angioplasty and related interventions.
*No longer available in the United States.

- Adverse side effects include significantly increased risk of bleeding. In addition, ticlopidine may cause rare skin reactions and thrombotic thrombocytopenia purpura, and therefore it is not used as often as clopidogrel, especially in patients with ACS.

Glycoprotein IIb/IIIa Receptor Antagonists

Glycoprotein IIb/IIIa (GPIIb/IIIa) receptor antagonists, which are administered intravenously, prevent platelet aggregation by inhibiting the binding of fibrinogen and von Willebrand factor to GPIIb/IIIa receptors on the platelet surface.[43]

- These drugs are used in emergency and acute care situations in combination with aspirin or clopidogrel and heparin for the prevention of ischemic complications in patients with ACS undergoing percutaneous coronary interventions or sometimes those being managed with medical therapies.
  - Abciximab (ReoPro) is a humanized mouse antibody fragment with high binding affinity for the GPIIb/IIIa receptor on both activated and nonactivated platelets.
  - Eptifibatide (Integrilin) is a heptapeptide inhibitor of platelet GPIIb/IIIa receptors on activated platelets.
  - Tirofiban (Aggrastat) is a nonpeptide inhibitor of platelet GPIIb/IIIa receptors on activated platelets.
- The most common complication associated with these agents is bleeding at the arterial access site (e.g., groin hematoma), particularly with abciximab. They can also cause thrombocytopenia, which can occur up to 5 days after administration. More rare is acute severe thrombocytopenia, which occurs most often with abciximab, especially on reexposure.

Dipyridamole

Dipyridamole (Persantine) inhibits platelet uptake of adenosine and blocks ADP-induced platelet aggregation. Most often it is prescribed as Aggrenox, which is an extended-release formulation of dipyridamole combined with aspirin.

- It is typically used in combination with warfarin for the prevention of thromboembolism in patients with prosthetic cardiac valves.
- Dipyridamole can cause nausea, vomiting, severe headache, dizziness, and diarrhea, which often disappear with continued use. Because it sometimes causes angina, it should be used with caution in patients with severe CAD or recent MI. It also increases the risk of bleeding, especially when used in combination with other agents.

Anticoagulants

Anticoagulants work by interrupting the coagulation cascade, inhibiting thrombin formation and thrombus development, and are used to prevent or control venous and arterial thrombosis. Their effectiveness has been established for the primary and secondary prevention of venous thromboembolism (VTE: deep vein thrombosis and pulmonary embolism) in patients undergoing high-risk surgeries (e.g., total hip or knee replacement), for prophylaxis against systemic embolism in patients with prosthetic heart valves or atrial fibrillation, for primary prevention of acute MI in high-risk men, and for the prevention of stroke, recurrent MI, or death in patients with acute MI.[47,56,109]

Many anticoagulants require clinical monitoring of activated partial thromboplastin time (aPTT), prothrombin time (PT), and/or international normalized ratio (INR) in order to avoid hemorrhagic complications.

- Symptoms of minor bleeding include blood in urine, epistaxis (nosebleeds), gingival bleeding, petechiae, unusual bleeding or bruising, oozing from cuts or wounds, and uterine bleeding.
- Symptoms of major bleeding or hemorrhage consist of pain from involved organ(s) (e.g., GI tract, joints, CNS, ovary, pericardium, and retroperitoneum), dizziness, syncope, hypotension, weakness, signs of GI bleeding (e.g., black tarry stools, blood in stool or vomit, and "coffee ground" emesis), headache.

Heparin

Heparins act by binding simultaneously with plasma antithrombin III and thrombin to form a heparin–thrombin–antithrombin complex that inactivates thrombin and clotting factor Xa.[11,36,111] It also increases vessel wall permeability and inhibits platelet function. Heparin can also bind to fibrin, forming a fibrin–heparin–thrombin complex, but because both thrombin exosites are occupied in this state, the enzymatic activity of thrombin is relatively protected from inactivation by the heparin–antithrombin complex. Thus, heparins are effective mainly in preventing blood clot formation and extension, but not in dissolving them.

Heparins are often used to initiate chronic anticoagulant therapy until warfarin reaches the desired therapeutic level. Heparin therapy can be administered in two forms: unfractionated or low molecular weight.

- *Unfractionated heparin (UFH)* exhibits high nonspecific binding (it binds to macrophages, endothelial cells, and plasma proteins), resulting in an unpredictable anticoagulant response, the need for a loading dose, and the necessity for close laboratory monitoring with dose adjustments according to results.[26,47] In addition, nonspecific binding to plasma proteins is the most common cause of heparin resistance, in which extremely high doses of the drug (>35,000 IU over 24 h) are required to achieve adequate anticoagulation.
  - UHF is administered by intravenous (IV) or subcutaneous (SC) injection. The bioavailability is reduced when heparin is given subcutaneously.
  - The variability of the anticoagulant response mandates close anticoagulant monitoring, via the aPTT, which should be maintained at the target level (varies with drug lot number), or INR >1.5.
  - The advantages of UFH include rapid and complete neutralization via the administration of protamine (and thus it remains the anticoagulant of choice during cardiopulmonary bypass[47]), increased safety in patients with renal insufficiency (because it is not cleared by the kidneys), and direct inhibition of the contact activation pathway (thereby preventing thrombosis formation on catheter tips, stents, and filters).
  - The most serious adverse effect is heparin-induced thrombocytopenia (HIT), which is described following the LMWHs.
- *Low molecular weight heparins (LMWHs)* are produced by cleaving UFH into shorter chains, which leads to less nonspecific binding to cell surfaces and plasma proteins and greater bioavailability, as well as more predictable anticoagulant response.[11,47] They inhibit factor Xa more than they inhibit thrombin. They

have longer half-lives than UFH, so require only once or twice per day SC dosing.

▸ Three LMWHs are currently in use in the United States: enoxaparin (Lovenox), dalteparin (Fragmin), and tinzaparin (Innohep). Of these, enoxaparin has been associated with better outcomes, mainly because of a lower incidence of nonfatal MI, and is at least as safe as UFH in patients undergoing percutaneous coronary interventions.

▸ LMWH therapy is dosed according to weight and does not require routine monitoring of aPPT, PT, or INR.

▸ LMWHs offer equal to superior anticoagulation and benefits compared with UFH and are now the preferred initial anticoagulant therapy for VTE, because they tend to produce fewer hemorrhagic complications and do not require laboratory monitoring.[56,109] However, bleeding complications are not readily reversible as with UFH.

- The most frequent side effect of the heparins is increased risk of bleeding and hemorrhage, as described previously.

- In addition, hypersensitivity to UFH and LMWHs is increasingly common and results in a number of immune-mediated side effects. The most serious of these is heparin-induced thrombocytopenia (HIT), which is produced by an immunologic reaction against platelets. Although platelet counts are low, HIT is associated with increased risk of thrombosis generated by the destruction of platelets and leads to arterial thrombosis in up to 30% of affected patients (1% to 3% of patients treated with UFH).[20,26] It typically develops 5 to 14 days after beginning heparin therapy and is manifested as VTE and skin changes (bruising or necrosis at the injection site and in the fingers, toes, and nipples). HIT is not as common with low-dose SC heparin and LMWHs. Other immune-mediated side effects include cutaneous reactions (urticarial lesions, erythematous papules/plaques, and skin necrosis) and generalized hypersensitivity reactions.

- Heparin also binds to osteoblasts, which stimulates osteoclast activation and induces osteopenia, causing heparin-induced osteoporosis.[26] This occurs mainly in patients receiving moderately high doses of heparin for more than 1 to 3 months.

Heparinoids

Heparinoids are heparin derivatives, of which the only agent is danaparoid (Orgaran). Danaparoid is used to prevent VTE in high-risk surgical patients. Because it is essentially heparin free, it has minimal cross-reactivity with heparin and is therefore used to treat HIT. Its adverse side effects include hemorrhage, anemia, thrombocytopenia, and generalized hypersensitivity reactions. Its long half-life and lack of responsiveness to neutralization with protamine are troublesome disadvantages in the event of bleeding complications or overdose. Danaparoid is no longer available in the United States, although it continues to be used elsewhere.

Factor Xa Inhibitors

Factor Xa inhibitors block factor Xa either directly, by binding to its active site, or indirectly, via antithrombin-mediated inhibition of factor Xa, as occurs with fondaparinux (Arixtra). Inhibition of factor Xa interrupts the blood coagulation cascade, inhibiting thrombin formation and thrombus development (see Figure 5-7). Other indirect and direct factor Xa inhibitors are currently under

investigation, including rivaroxaban and apixaban. These drugs do not require routine laboratory monitoring.

- Fondaparinux is administered once daily via SC injection and has been shown to be at least as effective as LMWHs for the prevention and treatment of VTE, and shows promise in the management of ACS and in thrombolysis for acute STEMI.[23,47,56]

▸ It has a low risk for major bleeding, and minor bleeding occurs in only 3% of patients. In the event of bleeding or overdose or need for acute surgery, the anticoagulant effect may be partially reversed with recombinant factor VIIa.[47]

▸ Fondaparinux is generally well tolerated. The most common adverse side effects consist of anemia, fever, nausea, vomiting, edema, constipation, rash, and insomnia. Less common are hypokalemia, dizziness, hypotension, purpura, and confusion.

▸ Because fondaparinux does not bind to platelets, it has a low incidence of HIT.

▸ One limitation of fondaparinux is that it accumulates in patients with renal insufficiency, so it must be used with caution in the elderly and is contraindicated in severe renal dysfunction.

- Rivaroxaban (Xarelto) and apixaban are oral agents that are being evaluated for the prevention and treatment of VTE, for the prevention of stroke or systemic embolism in a-fib, and for the management of ACS. The promising results for rivaroxaban make it a likely replacement for warfarin for patients who require chronic anticoagulation.

Direct Thrombin Inhibitors

Direct thrombin inhibitors (DTIs) block the action of thrombin by binding directly to both free and clot-bound thrombin so it cannot interact with its substrates. They also have an antiplatelet effect due to their inhibition of thrombin-mediated platelet activation. All DTIs are administered parentally and, in the absence of increased risk of bleeding complications or renal dysfunction, they do not require laboratory monitoring.

There are two types of DTIs: bivalent agents, which bind to thrombin at both its active catalytic site and its docking site for other substrates such as fibrin (exosite 1), and univalent agents, which bind only to the active site.[20,25,111] Of note, thrombin also has a third site (exosite 2), which binds to heparin.

Bivalent DTIs

Bivalent DTIs bind not only to free (circulating) thrombin but also to clot-bound thrombin and thus can prevent and dissolve blood clots. Hirudin and the recombinant hirudins form irreversible bonds with these thrombin sites, eliminating its prothrombotic activities; the synthetic hirudin bivalirudin also binds at both thrombin sites, but binding at the active site is not maintained, and therefore only transient inhibition is produced.

- Hirudin, a naturally occurring peptide found in the salivary glands of medicinal leeches, is the most potent natural inhibitor of thrombin. Lepirudin (Refludan) is a recombinant hirudin. It is approved to treat patients with arterial or venous thrombotic complications of HIT.

- Desirudin (Iprivask, Revasc) is synthetic recombinant form of hirudin that is approved as prophylaxis against VTE in hip replacement surgery. It is also being studied in acute MI, unstable angina, and hemodialysis.

- Bivalirudin (Angiomax, Angiox) is a synthetic form or hirudin. Because it binds only transiently to thrombin and has a half-life of 25 minutes, bivalirudin is a good alternative to heparin during percutaneous coronary interventions. It has a lower incidence of severe bleeding (2.4%), allergic reactions, and thrombocytopenia than heparin.

Univalent DTIs

Because univalent DTIs bind only to the active catalytic site, they inactivate only fibrin-bound thrombin. Like bivalirudin, argatroban and melagatran dissociate from thrombin, leaving a small amount of free, enzymatically active thrombin available for blood-clotting interactions.

- Argatroban is equally effective in inhibiting platelet aggregation and thromboxane B_2 release in the presence of both free and clot-bound thrombin.[110] It used in patients with HIT and during ACS and percutaneous coronary interventions in patients who have or are at high risk of HIT.
- Other univalent DTIs are under investigation.
- Adverse side effects of DTIs occur less frequently than with heparin.
- As with all anticoagulants, the most frequent adverse event is bleeding, particularly from puncture sites and wounds. Anemia and hematoma also occur and occasionally severe bleeding. Thrombocytopenia is encountered only infrequently.
- Allergic reactions have also been reported, including skin and generalized hypersensitivity reactions. Rare instances of serious anaphylactic reactions that have resulted in shock or death have been reported during initial administration or on second or subsequent reexposure.
- Other possible side effects include hypotension, chest pain, back pain, nausea, vomiting, diarrhea, and headache.
- Most DTIs (hirudin, melagatran, and dabigatran) are cleared mainly through the kidneys, so they are likely to accumulate in patients with impaired renal function. Although bivalirudin is only partially excreted by the kidneys, its half-life is prolonged with severe renal impairment. Only argatroban is cleared predominantly by hepatic metabolism and thus requires dose adjustment in patients with hepatic dysfunction.

Warfarin

Warfarin (Coumadin) is a coumarin and vitamin K antagonist (VKA) and is the most frequently prescribed oral anticoagulant in the United States. Other VKAs include dicoumarol (Dicumarol), phenprocoumon (Marcoumar), and acenocoumarol, which are used in Europe. Vitamin K is a necessary element in the synthesis of clotting factors II (prothrombin), VII, IX, and X. VKAs slow the rate at which these factors are produced, thereby creating a state of anticoagulation.[3,49]

- The goal of anticoagulant therapy is to prevent clot formation or expansion at the lowest possible dose so that hemorrhagic complications are avoided.
- In general, the therapeutic goal is to achieve an INR of 2 to 3, although target values of 2.5 to 3.5 are often allowed for mechanical prosthetic valves.
- The use of VKAs is complicated by a narrow therapeutic index and an unpredictable dose–response relationship, giving rise to

frequent bleeding complications or insufficient anticoagulation. The dosing of warfarin is affected by a variety of drug interactions and other factors.

- ▸ Some drugs reduce its effect by interfering with absorption (e.g., cholestyramine) or increasing its clearance (e.g., barbiturates, rifampin, and carbamazepine), whereas other drugs potentiate its effect by inhibiting its clearance (e.g., amiodarone, phenylbutazone, sulfinpyrazone, metronidazole, and trimethoprim–sulfamethoxazole).
- ▸ Other drugs inhibit the synthesis or increase the clearance of vitamin K–dependent coagulation factors or interfere with other pathways of hemostasis.
- ▸ Additional factors that alter the pharmacokinetics of warfarin include genetic predisposition, diet (high vitamin K–content foods or enteral formulas, large amounts of avocado), and various disease states (e.g., hepatic dysfunction, hypermetabolic states produced by fever or hyperthyroidism, and CHF).
- The major adverse effect of warfarin is increased risk of bleeding, which occurs in 6% to 39% of patients and is strongly related to the intensity of anticoagulation.[49] Risk is heightened by advanced age (>65 to 75 yr); drugs such as aspirin, NSAIDs, penicillins in high dose, and moxalactam; and comorbid disease states (e.g., HTN, cerebrovascular disease, serious heart disease, and renal insufficiency).
- Other, less common side effects include dermatitis and allergic manifestations (skin rash, hives, and itching). A rare but serious adverse effect is skin necrosis that occurs on the third to eighth day of therapy.

▣ 5.3 VASOPRESSORS USED IN SHOCK

Circulatory shock is a state of inadequate tissue perfusion. It can be caused by (or cause) a decreased supply or an increased demand for oxygen and nutrients. The imbalance between oxygen supply and demand interferes with normal cellular function, which if widespread can result in multisystem organ failure and death. Shock usually results from inadequate cardiac output although sometimes low systemic vascular resistance (SVR) due to arterial vasodilation is responsible.

- Low cardiac output can occur as a result of impaired LV systolic function (cardiogenic shock due to CHF) or inadequate venous return leading to reduced cardiac preload (hypovolemic shock due to dehydration or hemorrhage or extracardiac obstructive shock, such as that produced by pericardial tamponade, which reduces right heart filling volume, or tension pneumothorax or pulmonary emboli, which impair RV cardiac output).
- On occasion, shock develops despite normal or elevated cardiac output. This situation typically results from abnormal redistribution of blood flow due to peripheral vasodilation (distributive shock due to sepsis, drug overdose, anaphylaxis, or neurogenic disorders, such as spinal cord injury), so that inadequate blood volume is available to perfuse the vital organs. It is characterized by warm rather than cold extremities, as SVR is reduced.
- In most types of shock, hypotension is present due to low cardiac output; however, this is not always the case, as

compensatory reflexes designed to maintain perfusion pressure will raise SVR and offset the drop in BP induced by low cardiac output.

- Although the causes of shock are varied, advanced shock tends to follow a common clinical course due to deterioration of body tissues from inadequate perfusion, including the CV system, so that a vicious cycle of progressively increasing shock develops. Yet, identifying the underlying cause may assist in the selection of general supportive therapy and is essential for instituting the most appropriate therapy.
  - ▶ Agents that enhance cardiac contractility (inotropes) are used to increase cardiac output and MAP and thus organ perfusion.
  - ▶ Drugs that augment BP by inducing arterial vasoconstriction (vasopressors) are used to increase SVR and thus venous return.
  - ▶ Relative or absolute volume depletion occurs in most shock states, especially in the early phase in which vasodilation is prominent. Adequate volume repletion is necessary to maintain cardiac output, urine flow, and the integrity of the microcirculation. Attempts to support the circulation with vasopressors or inotropes will be unsuccessful if the intravascular volume is depleted.

SYMPATHOMIMETIC AGENTS

Sympathomimetic agents induce stimulation of the α_1-adrenergic receptors to produce vasoconstriction and an increase in SVR and BP (at the expense of increasing afterload); β_1-adrenergic receptors to increase myocardial contractility, HR, and AV node conduction and thus cardiac output; and β_2-adrenergic receptors to effect vasodilation in the coronary arteries and skeletal muscle (which is usually overpowered by β-adrenergically stimulated vasoconstriction). Thus these drugs have variable hemodynamic effects, depending on their sites of action, as shown in Table 5-19. They are used in shock to treat hypoperfusion in normovolemic patients and in those unresponsive to fluid resuscitation.

Vasopressors and Inotropes

Vasopressors and inotropic agents are usually administered for resuscitation of seriously ill patients and for treatment of hypotension during anesthesia. All these drugs act directly or indirectly on the SNS, but the effects vary according to the adrenergic receptor(s) each drug stimulates.[18,51]

- Epinephrine (Adrenalin) stimulates α_1-, β_1-, and β_2-receptors and is used mainly in anaphylactic and septic shock. At low doses the β effects dominate so that HR and contractility are increased, producing an increase in systolic blood pressure (SBP), but diastolic blood pressure (DBP) may fall because of vasodilation of the skeletal muscle bed. At higher doses vasoconstriction induced by α-adrenergic stimulation becomes apparent. Side effects include ventricular arrhythmias and hypertension.
- Ephedrine acts directly on β_1- and β_2-receptors and indirectly on α-receptors by causing release of norepinephrine. It is often used to treat hypotension induced by spinal or epidural anesthesia and drug overdoses, as well as in pregnancy, as it does not reduce placental blood flow.
- Methoxamine, metaraminol, and phenylephrine act only on α_1-receptors to produce vasoconstriction and an increase in BP.

- ▶ Methoxamine and phenylephrine may also produce reflex bradycardia. Therefore, they are particularly beneficial for treating hypotension with tachycardia (e.g., SVT). Methoxamine is also useful during spinal anesthesia.
- ▶ Metaraminol also produces release of norepinephrine and epinephrine, and therefore increases BP and cardiac output with less risk of reflex bradycardia.

Centrally Infused Inotropes

Centrally infused inotropic agents, administered by intravenous infusion or occasionally bolus injection through a central line, are used to increase cardiac output and support MAP. They are generally short-acting, with their effects lasting from a few seconds to 1 to 2 minutes. They require close clinical monitoring, particularly the ECG and BP. The most common side effects are tachycardia, arrhythmias, and hypertension or hypotension. Some of these drugs also have vasopressor activity.

- Norepinephrine (Levophed) is a potent α_1-adrenergic agonist with minimal β-adrenergic agonist effects, which increases BP through vasoconstriction. It is used for the treatment of patients with septic shock who remain hypotensive after fluid resuscitation.
- Dopamine, a precursor of norepinephrine and epinephrine, is used to optimize MAP in patients with cardiogenic shock with severe hypotension and in those with hypovolemic or septic shock who remain hypotensive after volume resuscitation. It has variable effects, depending on the dosage.
  - ▶ At low dosages (0.5 to 2 µg/kg/min) dopamine produces dopaminergic receptor activation, causing vasodilation of the renal, mesenteric, cerebral, and coronary beds.
  - ▶ At dosages of 5 to 10 µg/kg/min, β_1-adrenergic effects dominate, inducing increases in HR and cardiac contractility. BP increases primarily as a result of the inotropic effect and, thus, it is useful in patients who have concomitant cardiac dysfunction.
  - ▶ At doses of about 10 µg/kg/min, α_1-adrenergic effects become apparent, leading to arterial vasoconstriction and elevation in BP.
- Dobutamine acts mainly on β_1 and β_2 receptors to increase cardiac output and reduce afterload. It is the first-line treatment for cardiogenic shock.

In cardiogenic shock or advanced shock from other causes associated with low cardiac output, sympathomimetic agents may be combined with vasodilators (e.g., nitroprusside or nitroglycerin) to improve myocardial performance and maintain BP.

PHOSPHODIESTERASE INHIBITORS

The PDE inhibitors milrinone and amrinone increase contractility and produce arterial and venous vasodilation in order to increase cardiac output independent of β-adrenergic receptor stimulation, as described on page 185.

VASOPRESSIN

Vasopressin, also known as antidiuretic hormone (ADH), increases water absorption in the kidneys and induces peripheral vasoconstriction by binding to V_1 receptors on vascular smooth muscle,

TABLE 5-19: Vasopressors Used in Shock

Drug	Trade Name	Sites of Action				Hemodynamic Response				Adverse Reactions
		α₁ Vasoconstriction	β₁ Contractility	β₁ Heart Rate	β₂ Vasodilation	Renal Perfusion	Cardiac Output	Systemic Vascular Resistance	Blood Pressure	
Dobutamine	Dobutrex	0-+	+++	0-+	+	0	↑	→	↑	Tachycardia, HTN, nausea, angina, headache
Dopamine*	Intropin, Dopastat	+-+++	+++	+-+++	0-+	↑	↑	↑↓	0-↑	Tachycardia, arrhythmias, angina, palpitations, dyspnea, nausea, headache, hypotension
Epinephrine	Adrenalin	+++	+++	+++	++	→	↑	→	↑↓	Hemiplegia, anxiety, headache, palpitations, arrhythmias
Norepinephrine	Levophed	+++	++	++	0	→	0-→	↑	↑	Bradycardia, headache, sulfite sensitivity and other allergic reactions
Ephedrine		+	++	++	0-+	→	↑	↑↓	↑	Palpitations, tachycardia, headache, vertigo, respiratory difficulty, confusion
Methoxamine	Vasoxyl	+++	0	0	0	→	0-→	↑	↑	Hypertension, severe headache, sweating, gastrointestinal upset
Phenylephrine	Neo-Synephrine	+++	0	0	0	→	→	↑	↑	Bradycardia, excitability, restlessness, headache, arrhythmias
Inamirinone	Inocor	0	+++	0-+	++	0	↑	→	→	Thrombocytopenia, arrhythmias, hypotension, rare hepatotoxicity
Milrinone	Primacor	0	+++	+-+++	++	0	↑	→	→	Ventricular arrhythmias, hypotension, headache
Vasopressin	Pitressin	(+++)†	0	0	0	↑	?	↑	↑	

+++, Pronounced effect; ++, moderate effect; +, slight effect; 0, no effect; ↑, increase; ↓, decrease; ↑↓, either increase or decrease; HTN, hypertension.

*The actions of dopamine vary with dose (see text).

†Vasopressin acts by stimulating V_1 receptors on vascular smooth muscle rather than through adrenergic actions.

diverting blood flow from noncritical vascular beds to vital organs.[48] It also modulates NO production and potentiates adrenergic and other vasoconstrictor agents. BP is increased not only through restoration of impaired vasoconstrictor mechanisms (induced by vasopressin deficiency occurring in shock) but also through inhibition of pathological vasodilator responses that occur with vasodilatory shock.

- Vasopressin is used in hypovolemic or septic shock not responsive to high doses of norepinephrine or dopamine
- Because it increases MAP without provoking other adverse hemodynamic effects, such as increased pulmonary capillary wedge pressure or cardiac index, it may offer benefits for the treatment of cardiogenic shock (under investigation).
- Adverse side effects are not common but can be serious, including severe cutaneous and limb ischemia and necrosis, hepatic necrosis, and neurotoxicity.
- Terlipressin (Glypressin) is a synthetic vasopressin analog that increases BP via vasoconstriction but at the expense of increased cardiac index and myocardial oxygen consumption.

NITROPRUSSIDE

Nitroprusside is used when rapid, short-term reduction of cardiac preload or afterload is needed, as with acutely decompensated CHF. It produces arterial and venous vasodilation, resulting in a reduction in systemic and pulmonary vascular resistance and an increase in aortic wall compliance. Thus it increases both RV and LV output. However, intramyocardial afterload–reducing effects may lead to "coronary steal" in which blood flow is diverted from epicardial coronary segments with high-grade atherosclerotic lesions.

- Because nitroprusside is metabolized to thiocyanide, cyanide toxicity can develop, which causes neurotoxicity with tinnitus, contraction of the pupils, and hyperreflexia. Hypothyroidism can develop because of interference with iodine uptake.
- Excessively rapid reduction of BP can cause abdominal pain, apprehension, diaphoresis, dizziness, headache, muscle twitching, nausea, palpitations, restlessness, retching, and chest discomfort.
- Other side effects include bradycardia, tachycardia, skin rash, ileus, decreased platelet aggregation, increased intracranial pressure, venous streaking, and skin irritation.

5.4 DRUGS USED WITH ORGAN TRANSPLANTATION

The success of organ transplantation, including heart and lung transplants, depends in large part on effective immunosuppressive regimens. A number of immunosuppressant drugs are available to prevent and treat organ rejection. In addition, they may be used to inhibit immune-mediated responses occurring in other diseases, such as systemic lupus erythematosus, rheumatoid arthritis, and other autoimmune diseases.

Immunosuppressive therapy for transplantation is achieved with combined regimens, typically consisting of three drugs: a calcineurin inhibitor (usually tacrolimus), an antiproliferative agent (most commonly mycophenolate mofetil), and a corticosteroid. The highest levels of immunosuppression are required immediately after transplantation, and then the doses are decreased over time until the lowest maintenance levels of suppression necessary to prevent rejection are identified for each patient.[1,62,74,77,104] Episodes of acute rejection, which occur in more than one third of patients, require augmentation of immunosuppression, usually with increased dosage of corticosteroids.

Most immunosuppressive agents provide nonspecific suppression of the immune system by inhibiting T cell lymphocyte activation, clonal expansion, or differentiation into effector cells, and therefore leave patients susceptible to infectious complications. Pulmonary infections are a major cause of morbidity and mortality in transplant recipients. Other long-term complications that limit the success of transplantation include adverse effects of maintenance immunosuppressive drugs (e.g., nephrotoxicity, HTN, hyperlipidemia, accelerated atherosclerotic CVD, bone disease, diabetes, and infections), chronic allograft rejection (cardiac allograft vasculopathy, affecting 32% of heart transplant patients within the first 5 yr and 43% within the first 8 yr; bronchiolitis obliterans syndrome [BOS], affecting more than 50% of lung transplant patients who survive the acute transplant period), and malignancies.

Research is seeking to come up with new immunosuppressive drugs that specifically target allograft T cells, and regimens that provide similar short-term results but with minimal long-term deterioration and secondary abnormalities, such as nephrotoxicity, HTN, hyperlipidemia, and CVD, so that long-term graft and patient survival are increased. There is also research investigating methods of inducing sustained tolerance to the transplanted organ by exploiting central and peripheral mechanisms that normally maintain immune homeostasis and tolerance to self-antigens.[38] Many centers now use steroid avoidance, minimization, and withdrawal protocols.

INDUCTION THERAPY

One of the most controversial components of transplantation immunosuppression is induction therapy. In both heart and lung transplantation in 2006, 57% of patients received antibody induction therapy, usually with Thymoglobulin or monoclonal antibody (MAb) therapy directed against the interleukin (IL)-2 receptor, in addition to standard immunosuppression, with the aim of creating a state of immune hyporesponsiveness against the allograft.[77] The goal is to reduce the incidence of acute rejection, especially during the first 4 to 6 weeks after surgery, protect against nephrotoxicity by delaying the introduction of the calcineurin inhibitors, and decrease the occurrence of chronic rejection effects. However, many clinicians remain concerned about the increased risk of infection and posttransplant complications, such as lymphoproliferative disorders, with some agents.

Polyclonal Antibodies

The polyclonal antibodies anti–thymocyte globulin (ATG) and anti–lymphocyte globulin (ALG) are immunoglobulins created by immunizing rabbits (or sometimes horses) with human lymphoid cells. They induce a rapid and profound lymphopenia by interacting with a variety of T cell–specific surface molecules, triggering complement- and antibody-dependent cytolysis. ATG also seems to contain antibodies against a variety of lymphocyte costimulatory molecules, which may induce anergy or immune tolerance.[74] ATG and ALG are used less often now in transplantation than are monoclonal antibodies (see later), but are used in the treatment of T cell–mediated autoimmune diseases, such as aplastic anemia.

Monoclonal Interleukin-2 Receptor Antibodies

Monoclonal IL-2 receptor antibodies, daclizumab and basiliximab, are thought to work by binding of the anti-CD25 MAbs to the IL-2 receptor on the surface of activated, but not resting, T cells.[11] Significant T cell depletion does not appear to be an important mechanism of their action.

- Daclizumab (Zenapax) is a humanized murine (mouse) complementarity-determining region (CDR)–human IgG$_1$ chimeric MAb (90% human, 10% murine). It is usually administered in five doses starting immediately preoperatively and then at biweekly intervals.
- Basiliximab (Simulect) is a chimeric human–mouse MAb directed against the α chain of the IL-2 receptor, CD25. It is usually administered preoperatively and on days 0 and 4 after transplantation.

Muromonab CD3

Muromonab CD3 (OKT3) is the first MAb to be approved for use in humans. It is a murine monoclonal immunoglobulin antibody, which specifically reacts with the T cell receptor–CD3 complex on the surface of circulating T cells, blocking antigen recognition and subsequent T cell proliferation and differentiation, so that almost all T cells are transiently removed from the circulation. T cells that reappear during treatment are CD3-negative and are not capable of T cell activation.

- Common side effects of polyclonal and MAbs include fever, chills, and hives (due to cytokine release induced by T cell activation), especially with the initial dose(s), and mild pulmonary and GI symptoms. In addition, they can produce various cardiopulmonary, hematologic, renal, and psychoneurological side effects, which are usually self-limiting but occasionally can be life-threatening. There have been some cases of lymphoproliferative diseases. OKT3 is associated with increased incidences of infection with cytomegalovirus (manifesting as hepatitis, pneumonia, or enteritis) and herpes simplex virus (usually as herpes stomatitis) during the first 2 to 3 weeks after administration.

Monoclonal Anti-CD52 Antibodies

Alemtuzumab (Compath-1H) is a humanized MAb that targets CD52, a glycoprotein expressed on lymphocytes, monocytes, macrophages, and natural killer cells, and causes profound long-term depletion of lymphocytes and transient depletion of B cells and monocytes. It is approved for use in the treatment of chronic lymphocytic leukemia and is being used off label in solid organ transplantation, both for induction therapy and as part of a maintenance immunosuppressive regimen. There is evidence that its use facilitates reduction of maintenance immunosuppression and is effective in treating refractory acute rejection and stabilizing or improving BOS in lung allografts.[104] Compared with daclizumab induction followed by a traditional triple-drug regimen, Compath-1H showed a significant reduction in the incidence of acute rejection, while maintaining comparable rates of survival and lung allograft survival.

CALCINEURIN-INHIBITING THERAPY

The calcineurin inhibitors (CNIs) cyclosporine and tacrolimus are the mainstays of posttransplant immunosuppression. They bind to immunophilin proteins within lymphocytes, resulting in inhibition of calcineurin, a calcium-dependent phosphatase that activates inflammatory interleukins, tumor necrosis factor, and the nuclear factor of activated T cells (NFAT).[74] The end result is selective T cell immunosuppression through inhibition of cell maturation and proliferation. Thus, they have a lower risk of myelosuppression or bacterial and fungal infection in comparison with azathioprine.[62,74]

Cyclosporine

Cyclosporine (Sandimmune, Neoral, Gengraf) is the immunosuppressive agent that ushered in the modern era of organ transplantation by increasing the rates of early engraftment, extending kidney graft survival, and allowing the development of cardiac and liver transplantation. However, it also causes serious side effects that contribute to high CV morbidity and mortality and long-term use leads to accelerated loss of kidney graft function. The use of inhaled cyclosporine is being investigated in lung transplant patients, and there is evidence that it produces significant improvements in survival and chronic rejection-free survival without increased rates of acute rejection. Side effects consist of local irritation with transient cough, sore throat, or dyspnea.

Tacrolimus

Tacrolimus (Prograf, FK506) is a macrolide antibiotic that binds with an immunophilin to block calcineurin. Although it produces similar survival rates at 1 and 2 years as cyclosporine, tacrolimus shows a trend toward decreased acute rejection and it may produce a significant reduction in the incidence of BOS in lung transplant patients.[74] It exhibits similar long-term outcomes for survival, allograft rejection, and cardiac allograft vasculopathy as cyclosporine in a standard immunosuppressive protocol but is associated with a significant decrease in renal impairment at 5 years.[62] It is commonly used in triple-drug immunosuppressive regimens and otherwise is sometimes used as a rescue agent in the treatment of either acute or chronic rejection, decreasing the incidence of acute rejection episodes and slowing the progression of BOS.

- The use of CNIs is associated with a number of adverse effects, including nephrotoxicity (acute or chronic renal dysfunction, which can range from mild to severe), HTN, neurotoxicity (involuntary tremor, paresthesias, headache, delirium, rare seizures, especially in the elderly), hyperlipidemia, hepatic toxicity, gingival hyperplasia, hirsutism, and increased risk of lymphoma. Tacrolimus is less likely to produce HTN and hyperlipidemia, but has a higher incidence of posttransplant diabetes.
- Both agents, particularly cyclosporine, have variable absorption, and therefore monitoring of blood levels is recommended. A microemulsion formula of cyclosporine has greater bioavailability and more predictable pharmacokinetics than the original oil-based preparations; it is better tolerated and is associated with lower rates of rejection that required treatment.[62]

ANTIPROLIFERATIVE AGENTS

Antiproliferative agents, or proliferation inhibitors, are antimetabolites that inhibit the proliferation of activated immune cells by interfering with different aspects of either DNA or RNA synthesis. These include mycophenolate mofetil (MMF), mycophenolate sodium (MFS), and azathioprine, which are used in maintenance immunosuppression.

Mycophenolate Mofetil and Mycophenolate Sodium

MMF (Cellcept) and enteric-coated MFS (Myfortic) metabolize to mycophenolic acid (MPA), an enzyme that prevents proliferation of activated T cells and B cells. Side effects include GI disturbances (esophagitis, gastritis, and diarrhea), bone marrow suppression, and increased infections, especially viral. MMF has comparable survival rates, possibly lower acute rejection rates, but higher opportunistic infections, mostly due to cytomegalovirus (CMV), than azathioprine. The incidence of GI problems appears unchanged with enteric-coated MFS compared with MMP.[96] MMF is now preferred over azathioprine.

Azathioprine

Azathioprine (Imuran, Azasan) releases a metabolite that blocks de novo and salvage pathways of purine synthesis and inhibits DNA replication, suppressing the proliferation of lymphocytes and monocytes.[74,96] It is used mainly in patients who don not tolerate MMF or MFS and those with low immunological risk who are not receiving treatment with allopurinol for bone marrow suppression. Adverse effects consist of bone marrow suppression, lymphomas, and skin cancers.

PROLIFERATION SIGNAL INHIBITORS

Proliferation signal inhibitors (PSIs), sirolimus and everolimus are macrolide immunosuppressants that bind to the same immunophilin as tacrolimus, but with PSIs, the resultant complexes inhibit mammalian target of rapamycin (so they are also referred to as inhibitors of mammalian target of rapamycin [mTOR]). This results in inhibition of lymphocyte proliferation and cell cycle arrest during the gap 1 (G_1, cell growth) phase.[62,74] PSIs also have antiproliferative effects on smooth muscle cells, blocking their cell cycle, so they offer an important advantage of reducing cardiac allograft vasculopathy.

Sirolimus

Sirolimus (Rapamune) produces significant reductions in rates of acute rejection compared with azathioprine and less renal dysfunction and HTN but a higher incidence of hyperlipidemia and bone marrow suppression than cyclosporine. When used in regimens with minimal or no CNI therapy (the combination of which significantly reduces allograft survival), sirolimus was associated with improved long-term allograft function and survival and low risk of rejection.

Everolimus

Everolimus (Certican) is associated with significantly lower rates of cytomegalovirus infection than azathioprine, but higher bacterial infection rates and serum creatinine levels.[62]

- The action of the PSIs is complementary to that of the CNIs.
- Adverse side effects include bone marrow suppression leading to pancytopenia, renal dysfunction with proteinuria, hemolytic–uremic syndrome, hyperlipidemia, GI distress, delayed wound healing (including airway anastomosis dehiscence in lung transplant patients), pulmonary toxicity (less with everolimus), and anemia. They have also been implicated in reduced testosterone production, mouth ulcers, and skin malignancies.

CORTICOSTEROIDS

Corticosteroids produce potent immunosuppression, which is used for prevention of organ rejection and in severe autoimmune diseases. They suppress cellular immunity and promote humoral immunity.[96] They also have strong antiinflammatory effects, as described for asthma (see page 161). The vast majority of transplant patients receive a corticosteroid as part of their maintenance immunosuppressive regimen for at least 6 to 12 months posttransplantation, and then many patients are weaned off steroids in order to avoid the serious adverse reactions that occurs with long-term therapy. Of note, there may be an increased risk of acute rejection when low-dose therapy is further reduced or discontinued.[96]

- Corticosteroids suppress cell-mediated immunity by inhibiting genes that control growth factors, a number of cytokines, most importantly IL-2, and adhesion molecules, which leads to a reduction in T lymphocyte proliferation.
- They also suppress humoral immunity, ultimately resulting in diminished B cell clone expansion and antibody synthesis.
- The side effects of long-term corticosteroid use are listed on page 162, which include diabetes, HTN, peptic ulcer disease, osteoporosis, accelerated atherosclerotic CVD, and poor wound healing.

OTHER MEDICATIONS

Organ transplant recipients also require a number of other medications:

- Antimicrobial therapy is frequently required for infectious complications.
- More than half of patients receiving cyclosporine will require treatment for HTN within 1 year of transplantation, which is managed by standard antihypertensive therapy, such as ACE inhibitors and CCBs.
- Most transplant patients show elevated lipid levels due to cyclosporine and corticosteroid therapy, and most patients, regardless of their lipid levels, are now being treated with statins because of their effects of reducing the incidence of atherosclerosis. In addition, pleiotropic effects, including immunomodulation, may be of benefit in preventing graft rejection. There is evidence that statins reduce the incidence of both acute and chronic rejection in lung transplant patients and reduce the progression of cardiac allograft vasculopathy.[74,97]
- Antihyperglycemic agents are used to treat patients who develop new-onset diabetes.
- Various other medications may be used to manage other symptoms associated with immunosuppressive agents, such as allergic reactions, GI upset, edema, and anemia.

5.5 DRUGS USED TO TREAT DIABETES MELLITUS

Diabetes mellitus (DM) is a condition of excessive glucose in the blood, which results in damage to the blood vessels, heart, kidneys, eyes, and peripheral nerves, as well as increased susceptibility to infections, particularly of the skin and gums, as described in Chapter 4 (see page 130). CVD complications account for approximately 80% of deaths among patients with DM.[72]

Therefore, aggressive risk factor reduction is extremely important in these patients, particularly reduction of BP to less than 130/80 mm Hg, smoking cessation, and optimization of lipid levels. Statins are recommended for all patients with DM (see page 132).

It is now known that postprandial hyperglycemia, even with well-controlled fasting blood glucose levels, is associated with increased CVD risk. Furthermore, treatments that specifically target postprandial glycemic excursions, the amplitude of which is an important predictor of oxidative stress (more so than even chronic hyperglycemia), reduce CVD events and atherosclerotic surrogates.[24,69,108] Tight control of blood glucose levels through intensive treatment delays the onset and slows the progression of microvascular and macrovascular complications of both types of DM.[24,107] Intensive insulin therapy also reduces mortality in patients with diabetes who suffer acute MI.[81]

The American Association of Clinical Endocrinologists recommend a hemoglobin A_{1c} (HbA$_{1c}$, which indicates the percentage of glycosylated hemoglobin) target of less than 6.5%, and the American Diabetes Association accepts a goal of less than 7%. It is estimated that a 1% increase in HbA$_{1c}$ portends a 17% increase in the risk of fatal MI.[71]

The treatment of type 1 DM, which is caused by autoimmune destruction of pancreatic beta cells, requires insulin replacement therapy. In addition, pramlintide is a new drug that is approved for use in conjunction with meal-time insulin in patients with type 1 (and type 2) DM.

The management of type 2 DM, which is characterized by abnormalities in hepatic glucose production, insulin resistance, and a progressive decline in beta cell function over time, centers on diet modification and exercise, as well as weight loss for overweight patients. Pharmacologic therapy is initiated if these interventions are not successful in achieving target HbA$_{1c}$ levels within 3 to 6 months. The treatment of type 2 DM consists of a variety of oral agents and some injectable drugs, often used in combination, that stimulate insulin secretion, improve insulin action, or delay digestion and absorption of carbohydrates. Insulin is also used in combination therapy for type 2 DM.

Major factors that lead to the slowly progressive hyperglycemia that characterizes type 2 DM include the progressive loss of beta cell function; nonadherence to dietary, exercise, and medication prescriptions; and weight gain. Studies indicate that up to 40% of patients do not adhere to their glucose-lowering medication, and the rate is much higher for certain agents, regimens, and populations.[55] Physical therapists can play an important role in the management of DM by reinforcing the importance of treatment compliance and including appropriate exercise prescriptions as part of all PT treatment plans.

INSULIN

The cornerstone of therapy for all individuals with type 1 DM and many patients with advanced type 2 DM is insulin, which acts to lower blood glucose levels by inhibiting hepatic glucose production (gluconeogenesis) and by promoting glucose uptake and metabolism in skeletal muscle and adipocytes. Although insulin can be administered intravenously or intramuscularly when necessary, long-term treatment is usually achieved via subcutaneous injection. Insulin preparations are available in a variety of forms, which vary according to their duration of action and by their species of origin (human or porcine).

Human insulin (which does not actually come from humans but is synthetic insulin almost identical to that produced by the human pancreas, that is manufactured by DNA technology) is currently used almost exclusively in the United States. Animal (mainly porcine) insulin is expected to be eliminated by pharmaceutical companies, despite the lack of scientific proof regarding the advantages and safety of "human" insulin.

- By far the most common form of therapy is daily injection of insulin preparations, listed in Table 5-20.[81,84] By using some combination of short-, intermediate-, and long-acting insulin, an attempt is made to mimic the normal endogenous physiological insulin profile, with sharp peaks at meal times and basal levels in between and overnight, as shown in Figure 5-8.
  - ▶ Because it is absorbed slowly after SC injection, rapid-acting regular insulins are injected 30 to 45 minutes before an anticipated meal. At standard doses, their activity peaks after 2 to 3 hours and they have a duration of action of 6 to 8 hours, well beyond the late postprandial period (see solid lines, profiles C and D). There is a great deal of intraindividual variation in these time frames, and they are dose dependent. As the insulin is cleared and the action of the counterregulatory hormones (glucagon, epinephrine, norepinephrine, cortisol, and growth hormone) takes over, blood sugar returns toward normal, usually in about 3 to 5 hours.
    - ⊙ In addition, the maximal effect is only about two thirds the normal postprandial insulin levels, so there is a relative insulin deficiency and postprandial hyperglycemia may occur, especially if the meal is larger or contains more carbohydrates than anticipated. The same problem occurs when the insulin is injected closer to the mealtime, without an adequate injection–meal interval to be effective.
    - ⊙ Rapid-acting insulin is usually injected along with an intermediate- or long-acting insulin in order to maintain basal metabolic requirements and prevent hyperglycemia between meals and at night, as shown in profiles C and D, respectively.
    - ⊙ Rapid-acting insulin analogs, described later, can be used instead of regular insulin and more closely approximate the normal physiological insulin profile.
    - ⊙ Rapid-acting insulins and insulin analogs are also used in subcutaneous insulin infusion pumps (see profile E).
  - ▶ Intermediate-acting insulins dissolve more slowly after SC injection and therefore are injected only once or twice per day (see dot/dash line, profile C). They include neutral protamine Hagedorn (NPH) and lente insulins.

TABLE 5-20: Common Insulin Preparations and Their Properties

Type and Agent	Trade Name	Action (h)*		
		Onset	Peak Effect	Duration
Rapid-acting Insulin				
Regular soluble (crystalline)	Humalin R, Novolin R	0.5–1.0	2–3	6–8
Rapid-acting Insulin Analogs				
Lispro	Humalog	0.2–0.5	0.5–2	3–4
Aspart	NovoLog	0.2–0.5	0.5–2	3–5
Glulisine	Apidra	0.2–0.5	0.5–2	3–4
Intermediate-acting Insulin				
NPH (isophane)	Humulin N, Novolin N	1.5	4–10	16–24
Lente	Humulin L, Novolin L	1.5–3	7–15	16–24
Long-acting Insulins				
Protamine zinc		3–4	14–20	24–36
Ultralente		3–4	9–15	22–28
Long-acting Insulin Analogs				
Glargine (Lantus)		3–4	No peak	20–30
Detemir (Levemir)		3–4	No peak at lower doses	12–24
Mixtures†				
70/30		0.5–1.0	3–12	16–24
50/50		0.5–1.0	2–12	16–24
Insulin Analogs†				
75/25		0.2–0.5	0.5–2	16–24
70/30		0.2–0.5	0.5–2	16–24

NPH, Neutral protamine Hagedorn.
*These are approximate figures for human insulins and insulin analogs. There is considerable variation from patient to patient and from time to time in a given patient.
†These are premixed combinations of nPH (the first number) and regular (the second number) insulin or insulin analogs.

⊙ Their onset of action ranges from 2 to 4 hours, and their activity usually peaks at about 6 to 7 hours and can last up to 20 hours.[11,81]

⊙ Human intermediate-acting insulins have a more rapid onset and shorter duration than porcine agents.

▸ Long-acting insulins, ultralente and protamine zinc suspensions, have a slower onset and a prolonged peak of action. They are used to provide a low basal concentration of insulin throughout the day in order to meet basal metabolic requirements and to avoid periods of insulin deficiency and hyperglycemia (see dashed line, profile D).

⊙ The long-acting insulins have a wide variability in onset (6 to 10 h), peak action (10 to 16 h), and duration of activity (18 to 24 h), so they are often considered less predictable for use as basal insulin.[11,81]

⊙ Long-acting insulin analogs are also available (see later).

▸ Thus, profiles C through E in Figure 5-8 illustrate that besides lower peak insulin levels after injections, there are often periods of insulin excess between doses, during which hepatic glucose production and mobilization of other substrates are inhibited and hypoglycemia can occur.

• Rapid-acting insulin analogs (lispro, aspart, and glulisine) have been designed to address these deficiencies. They are absorbed much more rapidly than human insulin (onset of action within 15 to 30 minutes and peaking within 1 to 2 hours), resulting in a more rapid rise in plasma insulin concentrations and an earlier hypoglycemic response.[45,81] They also achieve higher maximal effects and have a shorter duration of action (3 to 5 h), simulating more closely the normal physiological responses. In addition, they show significantly less variability in absorption at the injection site.

▸ These agents are much more convenient than standard insulin in that they can be injected immediately before or even after a meal, when it is clear how much food is actually consumed (this is particularly valuable in patients with gastroparesis or loss of appetite, who often eat less than anticipated and might otherwise experience postprandial hypoglycemia).[8,11] Optimal dosing is dependent on carbohydrate counting.

▸ The advantages of insulin analogs are even more evident when a high-carbohydrate meal is consumed (e.g., a "fast food" meal of pizza, cola, and carbohydrate-rich dessert,

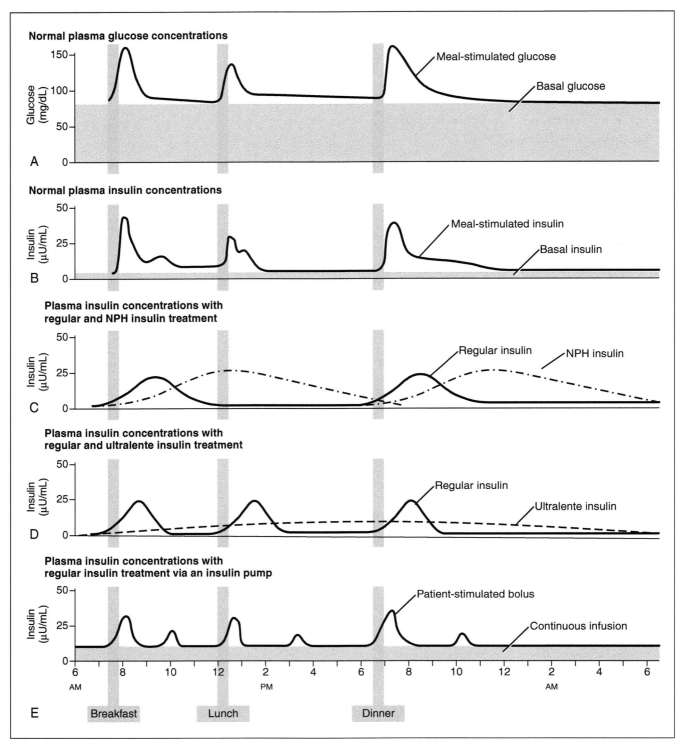

Figure 5-8: Normal plasma glucose concentrations, endogenous insulin secretion, and exogenous insulin levels produced by various treatment regimens as a function of time and food intake. **A**, Normal plasma glucose concentrations consist of the basal level and meal-stimulated increases. **B**, In healthy individuals, insulin is secreted as the postprandial glucose concentration rises, which acts to increase glucose utilization and return the blood glucose concentration to its basal level. **C–E**, In patients with diabetes mellitus, insulin treatment seeks to mimic the natural secretion of insulin as closely as possible, with different treatment regimens producing different curves, as shown. **C**, Insulin levels resulting from two daily injections of regular insulin and neutral protamine Hagedorn (NPH) insulin, which are given before breakfast and the evening meal. **D**, Insulin levels produced by treatment based on three daily injections of regular insulin, administered before each meal, and one injection of ultralente insulin given at bedtime. **E**, Insulin levels resulting from treatment via an insulin pump, which delivers a constant infusion to fulfill basal insulin requirement as well as patient-activated small bolus injections before meals, snacks, and bedtime. (From Brenner GM. *Pharmacology.* 2nd ed. Philadelphia: Saunders; 2006.)

typical of that consumed by most teenagers), producing a greater reduction in total blood sugar excursion and lower peak glucose concentrations.[11,45]

- ▸ Lispro (Humalog), aspart (NovoLog), and glulisine (Apidra) produce similar insulin profiles and have similar effects on glucose control and frequency of hypoglycemia, with a lower rates of nocturnal hypoglycemia.[11] These agents can be used in insulin pumps and insulin pens (e.g., FlexPen, NovoPen, OptiClick Pen). A potential disadvantage of using these agents in insulin pumps is that pump malfunction and interruption of insulin delivery in patients with type 1 DM will result in ketoacidosis faster than when regular insulin is used.

- ▸ Patient populations especially likely to benefit from the improved pharmacodynamics of the insulin analogs include those with renal impairment (who tend to have prolonged insulin action due to reduced clearance), pregnant women (in whom more normal glycemic levels are important for avoiding adverse maternal and fetal outcomes), and the elderly (who often have unpredictable eating habits).

- ▸ However, a number of systematic reviews have shown only minor benefits over human insulin in the majority of diabetic patients.[12,13,52,103] In addition, there are some concerns about potential carcinogenic and proliferative effects, as well as inhibition of thrombocyte function.[81]

- *Long-acting insulin analogs* are also available to meet basal insulin requirements. Glargine (Lantus) and detemir (Levemir) have been engineered to provide a more normal basal insulin concentration with no peak when absorbed from a SC depot, so their use is associated with lower incidences of nocturnal hypoglycemia.[8,12] However, they have not been shown to improve glycemic control.[50,99]

- *Intensive insulin therapy,* which allows for adjustment of insulin doses throughout the day on the basis of the results of frequent blood glucose monitoring (at least three times daily) and other factors, achieves the most normal physiological levels of insulin but requires maximal patient participation and cooperation. This treatment involves multiple daily injections (MDIs) comprising basal and prandial insulin doses or the use of continuous subcutaneous insulin infusion (CSII) that delivers a continuous basal level of insulin as well as boluses at mealtimes, both of which can be adjusted according to different circumstances.

- ▸ Insulin doses are adjusted according to the results of frequent monitoring of blood glucose levels, taking into account the pattern of need, size and composition of the impending meal, and anticipated activity level.

- ▸ Implantable pumps offer a great deal of flexibility: They can be programmed to cover a prebreakfast rise in blood sugar, the basal insulin output can be reduced during exercise to prevent hypoglycemia, and the insulin dose can be easily adjusted to cover a high-fat or high-protein meal.

- ▸ Either regular insulin or an insulin analog can be used to provide rapid-acting insulin for MDI therapy and for CSII pumps.

- ▸ A large majority of patients prefer CSII over MDI therapy, finding it more convenient, more flexible in terms of food intake and exercise, less painful, and with fewer social limitations.[8] Patients can disconnect insulin pumps for up to 1 hour for such activities as showering, swimming, and sexual activity. Of importance, patients must still monitor their blood glucose levels at least four times daily (before each meal and at bedtime), and the pump setup and injection site should be changed every 2 or 3 days for proper effect.[54]

- ▸ A disadvantage of intensive insulin therapy is a much higher risk of severe hypoglycemia (blood glucose <50 mg/dL) than regular rapid-acting insulin.

- ▸ Insulin mixtures that combine intermediate-acting and rapid-acting regular insulin or insulin analogs are commercially available and serve to reduce mixing errors and improve dosing accuracy. They are prescribed primarily to patients with type 2 DM using twice-daily dosing regimens.

- Alternative routes of administration are being investigated.
  - ▸ An oral insulin spray, Oralin, is available; however, its bioavailability is low and its absorption is unreliable.[81]
  - ▸ Inhaled insulin systems involve the use of a variety of liquid and powder preparations, several unique delivery devices, and different technical methodologies. A number of different products are currently in phase III clinical trials, and Exubera has been approved for patients over 18 years of age and who do not have lung disease. However, Pfizer stopped marketing Exubera in January 2008, saying it did not meet customers' needs (they did not like the clumsy inhalation device) or financial expectations. In addition, there was growing concern about its tendency to slightly impair lung function. Since then, two other companies have halted their development of inhaled insulin. Side effects include coughing, dyspnea, shortness of breath, and dry mouth. Exercise increases transport and the risk of hypoglycemia. A major problem with Exubera was the inability to deliver precise doses.
  - ▸ Other routes of insulin administration are under investigation, including oral, transdermal, sublingual, intranasal, and rectal routes, but so far they have not been successful.

- The most common side effect of insulin therapy is hypoglycemia, which is usually mild but can be severe and life-threatening.
  - ▸ Hypoglycemia typically occurs in the late postprandial period or overnight when there is a relative insulin excess compared with normal basal levels. It can also develop when less food is eaten than expected, an inappropriately large dose of insulin is injected, food is not consumed before the onset of insulin activity (especially with insulin analogs), or there is increased glucose uptake (e.g., exercise performed during peak insulin levels, which normally requires a decrease in insulin dose, fever, hyperthyroidism).
  - ▸ The risk of hypoglycemia is increased with intensive insulin therapy and autonomic neuropathy.
  - ▸ A number of medications can increase the hypoglycemic effect of insulin, including oral antidiabetic agents, ACE inhibitors, disopyramide, fibrates, fluoxetine, monoamine oxidase (MAO) inhibitors, propoxyphene, salicylates (aspirin and NSAIDs), somatostatin analogs (e.g., octreotide), and sulfonamide antibiotics.
  - ▸ β-Blockers, clonidine, lithium salts, and alcohol may either potentiate or weaken the hypoglycemic effectiveness of insulin.

▸ Of importance, sympatholytic drugs, such as β-blockers, clonidine, guanethidine, and reserpine, may mask the symptoms of hypoglycemia and delay recovery from insulin-induced hypoglycemia.

▸ Refer to page 134 for the clinical manifestations of hypoglycemia.

- Hyperglycemia can also develop, particularly if insufficient insulin is administered or carbohydrate intake is higher or more frequent than expected.

  ▸ In addition, some medications can reduce insulin's hypoglycemic effect, causing hyperglycemia: corticosteroids, danazol, diuretics, sympathomimetic agents (epinephrine, albuterol, and terbutaline), isoniazid, phenothiazine derivatives, somatropin, thyroid hormones, estrogens and progestogens (oral contraceptives and hormone replacement therapy), HIV-1 protease inhibitors, and nicotine.

  ▸ Hyperglycemia can also occur if a patient's insulin pump becomes disconnected from the injection site.

- Other adverse effects include insulin allergy and resistance, injection site reactions (redness, swelling, and itching), skin thickening or dimpling or changes in the amount of body fat at the sites of injection, and edema.

OTHER ANTIDIABETIC AGENTS

Oral medications and injectables are used for type 2 DM. During the early stages of type 2 DM (see Chapter 4, page 130), therapies to improve beta cell function, using an oral antihyperglycemic agent along with diet and exercise interventions, are usually effective in controlling blood glucose levels. However, as the disease progresses, combinations of agents and, ultimately, insulin replacement therapy are often required. Because glycemic function changes continuously throughout the course of type 2 DM, constant monitoring and adjustments of the therapy are crucial to maintain glycemic control, which typically worsens within 5 years of initiating antihyperglycemic therapy.

Insulin Sensitizers

The insulin sensitizers enhance insulin action through inhibition of gluconeogenesis (formation of glucose or glycogen from fats and proteins) and glycogenolysis (conversion of glycogen to glucose) or facilitation of glucose uptake in skeletal muscle and adipocytes.

Biguanides

Metformin (Glucophage) is the only biguanide available in the United States and is typically used as the initial therapy for hyperglycemia, along with lifestyle modification. Although its mechanism of action is not known, it decreases hepatic gluconeogenesis and, to a lesser extent, glycogenolysis. It improves insulin sensitivity in skeletal muscle, which may be related to a reduction in circulating free fatty acid (FFA) levels.[15] It is given three times daily before meals or, in the extended release formulation, once daily.

- Advantages of metformin include modest weight loss due to appetite suppression (however, this appears to dissipate over time), a reduction in hyperinsulinemia related to insulin resistance, or both. It also exerts favorable influences on lipids.

- The ability of metformin to increase insulin action may be responsible for reduced CV events and all-cause mortality rates in obese subjects.

- The most common side effect is GI intolerance (nausea, metallic taste, abdominal discomfort, and diarrhea), which occurs in varying degrees in approximately 20% to 30% of patients and is dose dependent.[15] Less frequent side effects include interference with vitamin B_{12} absorption and anemia. On rare occasions it causes lactic acidosis, which is fatal in 30% to 50% of patients.

Thiazolidinediones

Thiazolidinediones (TZDs), also referred to as glitazones, act by binding to peroxisome proliferator–activated receptor-γ (PPARγ) nuclear receptors, which regulate the transcription of insulin-responsive genes involved in the control of glucose production, transportation, and use. The resultant reduction in circulating FFAs is thought to enhance insulin receptor signaling in skeletal muscle and adipocytes, increasing general insulin sensitivity, and to improve beta cell function. In animal models and human cell lines, TZDs inhibit vascular smooth muscle and endothelial cell migration and proliferation and reduce atherosclerosis.[72]

Two TZDs are currently available: rosiglitazone (Avandia) and pioglitazone (Actos).[15] The prototype agent in this class, troglitazone (Rezulin), was removed from the market because of rare, idiosyncratic hepatotoxicity.

- TZDs are often used as initial monotherapy, which produces lower failure rates than metformin and glyburide.

- The two agents have different effects on lipids. Rosiglitazone increases HDL-C and LDL-C while having no effect on TGs. Pioglitazone has a neutral effect on LDL-C, decreases TGs, and increases HDL-C more so than rosiglitazone. Both agents may reduce the level of small, dense LDL particles, which are thought to be the most atherogenic lipoprotein component in DM.

- In addition, they appear to improve many surrogate markers for CVD, including plasminogen activator inhibitor, C-reactive protein, endothelial function, smooth muscle proliferation, and carotid intimal–medial thickness.[72] Whether these findings will translate into clinically significant reductions in CVD events is under investigation.

- One side effect of TZDs is weight gain (about 2 kg). However, the specific, unique increase in adiposity associated with TZDs is characterized by differentiation to insulin-sensitive smaller adipocytes and redistribution of fat from the viscera to subcutaneous deposits, which is associated with lower CVD risk and improved adipocytokine profiles.[72]

- A major adverse effect is new or worsening edema (occurring in 2.5% to 5% of patients when used as monotherapy and in up to 16.2% of patients with combined insulin therapy) and, much less commonly, CHF.[72,84] Thus, they are contraindicated in patients with class III or IV CHF. Less frequent problems include induction of ovulation in women with polycystic ovary syndrome, elevation of liver enzymes, and rare instances of new or worsening macular edema.

Insulin Secretagogues

Agents that increase insulin secretion address primarily the progressive decline in pancreatic beta cell function that is characteristic of type 2 DM. The insulin secretagogues stimulate insulin production, which lowers blood glucose and improves glucose uptake by skeletal muscles.[11,15,65] They are usually used as an adjunct to optimized insulin sensitizer therapy with metformin or a TZD.

Sulfonylureas

Sulfonylureas bind to sulfonylurea receptor-1 on pancreatic beta cells, stimulating them to produce more insulin, with all agents except glyburide exerting a glucose-dependent effect. First-generation drugs consist of acetohexamide (Dymelor), chlorpropamide (Diabinese), tolazamide (Tolinase), and tolbutamide (Orinase). The second-generation agents include glyburide (DiaBeta, Micronas, Glynase), glipizide (Glucotrol), and glimepiride (Amaryl).

- These drugs are effective in lowering blood glucose and microvascular events but do not reduce mortality or macrovascular complications They do not have a significant effect on lipids.
- A major disadvantage of these drugs is weight gain, although glipizide and glimepiride cause less of a problem.
- Hypoglycemia may occur with these drugs, especially glyburide, if meals are skipped.

Nonsulfonylurea Secretagogues

Nonsulfonylurea secretagogues (also referred to as glinides) include repaglinide (Prandin) and nateglinide (Starlix). They are taken just before meals or large snacks with a high carbohydrate content and stimulate rapid insulin production by binding to beta cell receptors. Having short half-lives, they produce less hypoglycemia, limit exposure to hyperinsulinemia, and cause less weight gain than the sulfonylureas.

- These drugs are useful for patients with high postprandial glucose levels, erratic eating schedules, and concern about gaining weight. They are often prescribed in combination with metformin or a TZD.
- Repaglinide and nateglinide are usually well tolerated with minimal side effects (asthenia, headache, fatigue, upper respiratory infection, and diarrhea). Liver enzymes occasionally rise, and there have been rare hypersensitivity reactions. There may be a slight increased risk of myocardial ischemia with repaglinide, and uric acid levels may be increased with nateglinide.

To lower the risk of hypoglycemia, the dose of insulin secretagogues may need to be reduced before exercise, particularly in patients who are near or at goal HbA$_{1c}$. A common strategy is to take half the usual dose on days that will include exercise. Patients most at risk for hypoglycemia with these agents are the elderly and those with renal or hepatic impairment.

Inhibitors of Glucose Absorption

Inhibitors of glucose absorption reduce the need for insulin by inhibiting glucose absorption from the GI tract.

α-Glucosidase Inhibitors

α-Glucosidase inhibitors inhibit an enzyme in the small intestine, delaying the absorption of carbohydrate and so reducing the bioavailability of glucose. The two agents in this category are acarbose (Precose, Glucobay) and miglitol (Glyset).

- One study suggests that acarbose is associated with a significant reduction in the risk of HTN and CVD.[15]
- Although they do not cause hypoglycemia or weight gain, they have significant GI side effects (flatulence, abdominal discomfort, and diarrhea) that limit their clinical appeal. Other side effects are rare.

Incretin Potentiators

Incretins are GI-secreted insulinotropic hormones that are important in glucose homeostasis, stimulating insulin secretion by pancreatic beta cells and suppressing glucagon secretion by the alpha cells. Glucagon-like peptide-1 (GLP-1) is one of two gut hormones that are mainly responsible for augmenting insulin release when glucose is ingested. Exogenous GLP-1 has been shown to increase insulin release and to normalize fasting blood glucose levels, even in patients with long-standing type 2 DM. It also inhibits glucagon secretion, delays gastric emptying, and blunts postprandial glucose excursions.[15,53] In addition, GLP-1 induces weight loss through appetite suppression.[46a] It may also reduce beta cell apoptosis and promote beta cell proliferation. A major limitation to the use of GLP-1 is its rapid degradation by dipeptidyl-peptidase IV (DPP-4).

Incretin therapy uses two approaches to enhance GLP-1 effects while preventing rapid breakdown by DPP-4: GLP-1 receptor agonists that are resistant to DPP-4 inhibition and inhibition of endogenous DPP-4 activity, thus prolonging the effects of native GLP-1.

GLP-1 Receptor Agonists

Exenatide (Byetta) is a full agonist for the GLP-1 receptor that is resistant to DPP-4, and it is injected twice daily and approved solely for use in combination therapy. It appears to delay gastric emptying and, combined with the glucagon suppression effects, is very effective in blunting postprandial glycemic excursions. It has also shown effectiveness in reducing HbA$_{1c}$ levels when used in combination with metformin, sulfonylureas, or TZDs. Liraglutide is currently in phase III clinical trials, and other agents are also being developed.

- Exenatide is as effective as adding basal insulin (glargine) to combination oral therapy and is particularly beneficial for patients with morbid obesity and poorly controlled type 2 DM due to induction of weight loss. It does not appear to increase the risk of hypoglycemia, unless used in combination with a sulfonylurea, or to blunt the glucagon response to hypoglycemia, either at rest or during exercise.
- An advantage of exenatide is weight loss, which is more pronounced in patients with greater body mass index, and continues over 2 years of treatment (up to 5 kg).
- The main side effect is nausea, which usually improves over time, although rare instances of unremitting nausea with or without vomiting have been reported, most often in patients with underlying gastroparesis.

Dipeptidyl-Peptidase IV Inhibitors

DPP-4 inhibitors are oral agents that block the degradation of GLP-1 and gradually increase both fasting and postprandial endogenous GLP-1 levels. They reduce blood glucose levels, possibly more than do the GLP-1 agonists, by enhancing beta cell insulin production and suppressing alpha cell glucagon secretion. In addition, they have been shown in animal models to stimulate beta cell proliferation and differentiation, which may help preserve beta cell mass and function.[79]

Sitagliptin (Januvia) is a once-daily oral drug that produces modest reductions in fasting glucose and HbA$_{1c}$ levels, with greater effectiveness when used in combination with insulin sensitizers (e.g., metformin and pioglitazone).[15,53] Vildagliptin (Galvus) is currently in phase III testing, and a number of other agents are under investigation.

- An advantage of sitagliptin is appetite suppression leading to weight loss (mean, 1.5 kg).
- It is generally well tolerated with a similar incidence of hypoglycemia as placebo. The most common side effects are stuffy or runny nose and sore throat, headache, diarrhea, upper respiratory tract infection, joint pain, and urinary tract infection.

Amylin Agonists

Amylin is a peptide neurohormone that is cosecreted with insulin from pancreatic beta cells in response to dietary intake, costored with insulin, and shares the same processing enzymes. Amylin circulates in both nonglycosylated and glycosylated forms, the latter of which is the biologically active compound. It lowers blood glucose by slowing gastric emptying, inhibiting glucagon secretion, and suppressing appetite by providing a feeling of satiety.[53,98] Normal fasting amylin levels fall between 4 and 25 pmol/L. It is eliminated mainly through the kidneys.

Pramlintide (Symlin) is a human amylin analog that was specifically engineered to overcome the tendency of amylin to self-aggregate. It is injected along with meal-time insulin (but cannot be combined in the same syringe) in both type 1 and type 2 DM and usually allows patients to use less insulin.

- A major advantage of amylin agonists is weight loss due to its effect on satiety. Reductions in body weight greater than 5% often occur, especially in morbidly obese individuals and in those receiving combined therapy with metformin.[15]
- A serious disadvantage is the requirement for a separate injection of each dose.
- The main side effect is nausea, which improves over time. It is also associated with increased risk of hypoglycemia, particularly during the first month of treatment.

Combination Therapy

When monotherapy is no longer effective in controlling hyperglycemia (HbA$_{1c}$ $\geq$6.5% to 7%), combination therapy is initiated. Most of the drug classes can be combined to take advantage of their different mechanisms of action in managing both fasting and postprandial blood glucose levels. Several combinations are commercially available in single tablet form, as shown in Table 5-21.

Until recently, insulin was not added until combination oral therapy failed to adequately control blood glucose; however, intensive insulin therapy is now recommend earlier in the disease process, especially in women, at the time combination therapy is initiated, because it is most likely to be successful in attaining glycemic control.[67,108] The prevention of postprandial glycemic

excursions, known to occur even in patients with well-controlled fasting blood glucose levels, is crucial for inhibiting the development of macrovascular complications.[24,69,108] Furthermore, insulin exerts a protective effect on beta cell survival and function.

5.6 MEDICATIONS AND EXERCISE RESPONSES

Many medications, particularly those used to treat cardiovascular disease, affect resting vital signs and the hemodynamic and ECG responses to exercise, as shown in Table 5-22.[1b]

- Many medications used to treat pulmonary disease have minimal effects on resting and exercise HR and BP. However, the anticholinergic agents and β-adrenergic agonists (i.e., sympathomimetic agents) may increase resting and exercise HR, and the β-adrenergic agonists may affect BP, producing higher or lower values at rest or during exercise. In addition, the xanthine derivatives may provoke PVCs.
- Antihistamines do not affect hemodynamics, but cold medications with sympathomimetic agents (e.g., pseudoephedrine and phenylephrine) may increase HR and BP.
- By their nature, antihypertensive agents reduce resting and exercise BP. Some agents, like the β-blockers and nondihypdropyridine CCBs, also lower resting and exercise HRs; whereas others, like the dihydropyridine CCBs and some vasodilators, may increase resting and exercise HRs. Other drugs, like diuretics, ACE inhibitors, and α–adrenergic blockers, usually have no effect on HR. Exercise tolerance is rarely affected, except for some patients taking β-blockers, who may experience a reduction in exercise tolerance.
- Medications used to treat angina that reduce myocardial oxygen demand by reducing afterload and thus BP are also antihypertensive agents. Thus, HR is affected as described previously. The exception is the nitrates, which may increase resting and sometimes exercise HR. In patients with angina, all of these drugs reduce ECG evidence of myocardial ischemia and increase exercise tolerance.
- The drugs used to treat CHF include many of the antihypertensive agents, discussed above, and positive inotropic agents. Digitalis reduces HR in patients with a-fib and possibly CHF and may cause non-specific ST-T wave changes at rest and ST-T depression during exercise. Exercise tolerance may be improved with all of these drugs.
- Most antiarrhythmic agents have little effect on HR and BP, although a few, like propafenone and amiodarone, reduce resting and exercise HRs, and quinidine may increase resting and exercise HRs and reduce BP. In addition, some of these drugs may cause prolongation of the QRS and QT intervals (e.g., disopyramide, procainamide, and moricizine).
- In general, dyslipidemic agents do not affect HR, BP, or ECG; however, clofibrate may provoke arrhythmias and angina in patients with prior MI, and nicotinic acid may lower BP.
- Likewise, antiplatelet agents and anticoagulants and anti-hyperglycemic agents, including insulin and oral agents, have no effect on hemodynamics.

TABLE 5-21: Antihyperglycemic Medications for Type 2 Diabetes Mellitus

Type and Drugs	Trade Name	Actions	Adverse Effects
Insulin Sensitizers			
Biguanides		↓ Hepatic glucose output (i.e., ↓ gluconeogenesis + some ↓ glycogenolysis); ↓ fatty acid oxidation; ↑ insulin sensitivity in skeletal muscle	GI symptoms, especially during initiation of treatment; rare lactic acidosis, especially if renal insufficiency exists; hypoglycemia only with combination therapy
Metformin	Glucophage		
Thiazolidinediones		Alter regulation of genes involved in control of glucose production, transportation, and use; ↑ fatty acid uptake; ↑ insulin sensitivity; may improve beta cell function	Generally well tolerated; new or worsening peripheral edema, possible ↑ HF; occasional hepatotoxicity; possible hypoglycemia several weeks after adding a TZD to a sulfonylurea
Rosiglitazone	Avandia		
Pioglitazone	Actos		
Insulin Secretagogues			
Sulfonylureas		Act on beta cells to ↑ insulin production	Hypoglycemia, usually subclinical or minor but occasionally life-threatening with ↑ risk in patients with irregular eating habits and excessive alcohol intake; uncommon sensitivity reactions; weight gain (≈1 to 4 kg)
Acetohexamide	Dymelor		
Chlorpropamide	Diabinese		
Tolazamide	Tolinase		
Tolbutamide	Orinase		
Glyburide	Micronase, DiaBeta	Second generation, more potent sulfonylureas, which act as above	
Glipizide	Glucotrol		
Glimepiride	Amaryl		
Nonsulfonylureas (Glinides)		Fast-acting, short-duration ↑ insulin production	Hypoglycemia (lower incidence than sulfonylureas); sensitivity reactions (usually transient); possible small weight gain
Repaglinide	Prandin		
Nateglinide	Starlix		
Glucose Absorption Inhibitors			
α-Glucosidase inhibitors		Delay absorption of carbohydrates in small intestine → ↓ rise in postprandial glucose levels	GI symptoms (flatulence, abdominal discomfort, sometimes diarrhea), which subside over time; hypoglycemia only if therapy combined with sulfonylurea or insulin
Acarbose	Precose, Glucobay		
Miglitol	Glyset		
Incretin potentiators		↑ Insulin release with glucose ingestion, ↓ postprandial glucagon release, delay gastric emptying	Nausea, which usually improves over time, but rare instances of unremitting nausea, mainly in patients with gastroparesis
GLP-1 receptor agonists			
Exenatide	Byetta		
DPP-4 inhibitors		↑ Insulin release + ↓ glucagon release in glucose-dependent manner	Generally well tolerated; stuffy or runny nose, sore throat, URI, headache, diarrhea, joint pain, UTI
Sitagliptin	Januvia		
Amylin agonists		Slows gastric emptying, inhibits glucagon secretion, suppresses appetite	Nausea, which usually improves over time; hypoglycemia, especially during first month of treatment
Pramlintide	Symlin		
Combination Drugs			
Glyburide/metformin	Glucovance	Per individual drugs	See individual drugs
Glipizide/metformin	Metaglip		
Metformin/rosiglitazone	Avandamet		
Rosiglitazone/glimepiride	Avandaryl		
Pioglitazone/metformin	Actoplus Met		

↑, Increased; ↓, decreased; →, leads to or results in; DPP-4, dipeptidyl-peptidase IV; GI, gastrointestinal; GLP-1, glucagon-like peptide-1; HF, heart failure; TZDs, thiazolidinediones; URI, upper respiratory infection; UTI, urinary tract infection.

TABLE 5–22: Effects of Medications on Heart Rate, Blood Pressure, the Electrocardiogram (ECG), and Exercise Capacity

Medications	Heart Rate	Blood Pressure	ECG	Exercise Capacity
Bronchodilators	↔ (R and E)	↔ (R and E)	↔ (R and E)	Bronchodilators ↑ exercise capacity in patients limited by bronchospasm
Sympathomimetic agents*	↑ or ↔ (R and E)	↑, ↔, or ↓ (R and E)	↑ or ↔ HR (R and E)	↔
Anticholinergic agents	↑ or ↔ (R and E)	↔ (R and E)	↑ or ↔ HR	
Xanthine derivatives			May produce PVCs (R and E)	
Steroidal anti-inflammatory agents	↔ (R and E)	↔ (R and E)	↔ (R and E)	↔
Cromolyn sodium	↔ (R and E)	↔ (R and E)	↔ (R and E)	↔
Antihistamines	↔ (R and E)	↔ (R and E)	↔ (R and E)	↔
Cold medications with sympathomimetic agents	Effects similar to those described in sympathomimetic bronchodilators (above), although magnitude of effects is usually smaller.			
β-blockers (including carvedilol and labetalol)	↓† (R and E)	↓ (R and E)	↓HR† (R), ↓Ischemia† (E)	↑ in patients with angina; ↓ or ↔ in patients without angina
Nitrates	↑ (R), ↑ or ↔ (E)	↓ (R); ↑ or ↔ (E)	↑ HR (R) ↑ or ↔ HR (E) ↓ ischemia† (E)	↑ in patients with angina; ↔ in patients without angina; ↑ or ↔ in patients with CHF
Calcium channel blockers				
Dihydropyridine CCBs	↑ or ↔ (R and E)	↓ (R and E)	↑ or ↔ HR (R and E) ↓ ischemia‡ (E)	↑ in patients with angina; ↔ in patients without angina
Nondihydropyridine CCBs	↓ (R and E)	↓ (R and E)	↓ HR (R and E) ↓ ischemia‡ (E)	↑ in patients with angina, ↔ in patients without angina
Digitalis	↓ in patients with a-fib and possibly CHF Not significantly altered in patients with sinus rhythm	↔ (R and E)	May produce nonspecific ST-T wave changes (R) May produce ST segment depression (E)	Improved only in patients with atrial fibrillation or in patients with CHF
Diuretics	↔ (R and E)	↔ or ↓ (R and E)	↔ or PVCs (R) May cause PVCs and "false-positive" test results if hypokalemia occurs May cause PVCs if hypomagnesemia occurs (E)	↔, except possible ↑ in patients with CHF

Vasodilators, nonadrenergic	↑ or ↔ (R and E)	↓ (R and E)	↑ or ↔ HR (R and E)	↔, except ↑ or ↔ in patients with CHF
ACE inhibitors and Angiotensin II receptor blockers	↔ (R and E)	↓ (R and E)	↔ (R and E)	↔, except ↑ or ↔ in patients with CHF
α-Adrenergic blockers	↔ (R and E)	↓ (R and E)	↔ (R and E)	↕
Antiadrenergic agents without selective blockade of peripheral receptors	↓ or ↔ (R and E)	↓ (R and E)	↓ or ↔ HR (R and E)	↕
Antiarrhythmic agents	All antiarrhythmic agents may cause new or worsened arrhythmias (proarrhythmic effect)			
Class I				
IA	↑ or ↔ (R and E)	↑ or ↔ (R) ↔ (E)	↑ or ↔ HR (R); May prolong QRS and QT intervals (R); Quinidine may result in "false negative" test results (E); Procainamide may result in "false positive" test results (E)	↕
IB	↔ (R and E)	↔ (R and E)	↔ (R and E)	↕
IC	↓ or ↔ (R and E)	↔ (R and E)	Moricizine may prolong QRS and QT intervals (R), ↔ (E); Propafenone and flecainide: ↓ HR (R) and ↓ or ↔ HR (E)	↕
Class II	See β-Blockers (previous page)			
Class III	↓ (R and E)	↔ (R and E)	↓ HR (R)	↕
Class IV	See calcium channel blockers (previous page)		↔ (E)	↕
Antilipidemic agents	Clofibrate may provoke arrhythmias, angina in patients with prior myocardial infarction. Nicotinic acid may ↓ BP. All other hyperlipidemic agents have no effect on HR, BP, and ECG.			
Psychotropic medication				
Minor tranquilizers	May ↓ HR and BP by controlling anxiety; no other effects			
Antidepressants	↑ or ↔ (R and E)	↓ or ↔ (R and E)	Variable (R); May cause "false positive" test results (E)	
Major tranquilizers	↑ or ↔ (R and E)	↓ or ↔ (R and E)	Variable (R); May cause "false positive" or "false negative" test results (E)	

Continued

TABLE 5–22: Effects of Medications on Heart Rate, Blood Pressure, the Electrocardiogram (ECG), and Exercise Capacity—Cont'd

Medications	Heart Rate	Blood Pressure	ECG	Exercise Capacity
Lithium	↔ (R and E)	↔ (R and E)	May result in T wave changes and arrhythmias (R and E)	
Nicotine	↑ or ↔ (R and E)	↑ (R and E)	↑ or ↔ HR; May provoke ischemia, arrhythmias (R and E)	↔, except ↓ or ↔ in patients with angina
Thyroid medications	↑ (R and E)	↑ (R and E)	↑ HR; May provoke arrhythmias	↔, unless angina worsened
Only levothyroxine			↑ ischemia (R and E)	
Alcohol	↔ (R and E)	Chronic use may have role in ↑ BP (R and E)	May provoke arrhythmias (R and E)	↔
Anti-hyperglycemia agents **Insulin and oral agents**	↔ (R and E)	↔ (R and E)	↔ (R and E)	↔
Antiplatelet agents and Anticoagulants	↔ (R and E)	↔ (R and E)	↔ (R and E)	↔
Pentoxifylline	↔ (R and E)	↔ (R and E)	↔ (R and E)	↑ or ↔ in patients limited by intermittent claudication
Antigout medications	↔ (R and E)	↔ (R and E)	↔ (R and E)	↔
Caffeine	Variable effects depending on previous usage		May provoke arrhythmias	Variable
Anorexiants/diet pills	↑ or ↔ (R and E)	↑ or ↔ (R and E)	↑ or ↔ (R and E)	

Modified from American College of Sports Medicine. ACSM's *Guidelines for Exercise Testing and Prescription.* *7th* ed. Baltimore, Md: Lippincott Williams & Wilkins; pp. 261–66, 2006.

↑ = increase, ↔ = no effect, ↓ = decrease, BP = blood pressure, CHF = congestive heart failure, E, during exercise; R, at rest. HR = heart rate, PVC = premature ventricular contraction.
*Inhaled short-acting β-adrenergic agonists have little effect; higher doses or oral or intravenous administration are likely to induce tachycardia and arrhythmias.
†Beta-blockers with ISA lower resting HR only slightly
‡May prevent or delay myocardial ischemia (see text)

REFERENCES

1. Aliabadi AZ, Zuckermann AO, Grimm M. Immunosuppresive therapy in older cardiac transplant patients. *Drugs Aging.* 2007;24:913-932.

1a. ALLHAT Officers and Coordinators for the ALLHAT Collaborative Research Group. Major outcomes in high-risk hypertensive patients randomized to angiotensin-converting enzyme inhibitor or calcium channel blocker vs. diuretic: the Antihypertensive and Lipid-lowering Treatment to Prevent Heart Attack Trial. *JAMA.* 2002;288:2981-2997.

1b. American College of Sports Medicine. *ACSM's Guidelines for Exercise Testing and Prescription.* 7th ed. Baltimore, MD: Lippincott Williams & Wilkins; 2006.

2. Anand IS, Florea VG. Traditional and novel approaches to management of heart failure: successes and failures. *Cardiol Clin.* 2008;26:59-72.

3. Ansell J, Hirsh J, Poller L, et al. The pharmacology and management of the vitamin K antagonists. The Seventh ACCP Conference on Antithrombotic and Thrombolytic Therapy. *Chest.* 2004;126: 204S-233S.

4. Antman EM, Anbe DT, Armstrong PW, et al. ACC/AHA guidelines for the management of patients with ST-elevation myocardial infarction—executive summary: a report of the American College of Cardiology/American Heart Association Task Force on Practice Guidelines (Writing Committee to Revise the 1999 Guidelines for the Management of Patients with Acute Myocardial Infarction). *Circulation.* 2004;110:588-636.

5. Anzueto A, Rubin BK. Mucokinetic agents and surfactant. In: Rubin BK, van der Schans CP, eds. *Therapy for Mucus-clearance Disorders.* London: Informa Health Care; 2004.

6. Belardinelli L, Shryock JC, Fraser H. The mechanism of ranolazine action to reduce ischemia-induced diastolic dysfunction. *Eur Heart J.* 2006;8 (suppl A):A10-A13.

6a. Bell SC, Senini SL, McCormack JG. Macrolides in cystic fibrosis. *Chron Respir Dis.* 2005;2:85-98.

7. Benedict N, Seybert A, Mathier MA. Evidence-based pharmacologic management of pulmonary arterial hypertension. *Clin Ther.* 2007;29:2134-2153.

8. Bode BW. Use of rapid-acting insulin analogues in the treatment of patients with type 1 and type 2 diabetes mellitus: insulin pump therapy versus multiple daily injections. *Clin Ther.* 2007;29(suppl D):S135-S144.

9. Boden WE, Hoekstra J, Miller CD. ST-elevation myocardial infarction: the role of adjunctive antiplatelet therapy. *Am J Emerg Med.* 2008;26:212-220.

10. Brandimarte F, Blair JEA, Manuchehry A, et al. Aldosterone receptor blockade in patients with left ventricular systolic dysfunction following acute myocardial infarction. *Cardiol Clin.* 2008;26:91-105.

11. Brunton LL, Lazo JS, Parker KL. *Goodman and Gilman's The Pharmacologic Basis of Therapeutics.* 11th ed. New York: McGraw-Hill Professional; 2005.

12. Canadian Agency for Drugs and Technologies in Health. Long-acting insulin analogues for the treatment of diabetes mellitus: meta-analyses of clinical outcomes—update of CADTH technology report no. 92. *COMPUS Rep.* 2008;2(1).

13. Canadian Agency for Drugs and Technologies in Health. Rapid-acting insulin analogues for the treatment of diabetes mellitus: meta-analyses of clinical outcomes. Update of CADTH technology report no. 97. *COMPUS Rep.* 2008;2(2).

14. Carroll W, Lenney W. Drug therapy in the management of acute asthma. *Arch Dis Child Educ Pract Ed.* 2007;92:82-96.

15. Cefalu WT. Pharmacotherapy for the treatment of patients with type 2 diabetes mellitus: rationale and specific agents. *Clin Pharm Ther.* 2007;81:636-649.

16. Chin KM, Rubin LJ. Pulmonary arterial hypertension. *J Am Coll Cardiol.* 2008;51:1527-1538.

17. Chobanian AV, Bakris GL, Black HR, et al. The seventh report of the Joint National Committee on Prevention, Detection, Evaluation, and Treatment of High Blood Pressure. *Hypertension.* 2003;42:1206-1252.

18. Cooper BE. Review and update on inotropes and vasopressors. *AACN Adv Crit Care.* 2008;19:5-15.

19. Coull BM, Williams LS, Goldstein LB, et al. Anticoagulants and antiplatelet agents in acute ischemic stroke. Report of the Joint Stroke Guideline Development Committee of the American Academy of Neurology and the American Stroke Association (a division of the American Heart Association). *Stroke.* 2002;33:1934-1942.

20. Crawford MH, DiMarco JP, Paulus WJ. eds. *Cardiology.* 2nd ed. St. Louis: Mosby; 2004.

21. De Meyer SF, Vanhoorelbeke K, Broos K, et al. Antiplatelet drugs. *Br J Haematol.* 2008;142(4):515-528, Epub May 30.

22. Denlinger LC, Sorkness CA, Chinchilli VM, et al. Guideline-defining asthma clinical trials of the National Heart, Lung, and Blood Institute's Asthma Clinical Research Network and Childhood Asthma Research and Education Network. *J Allergy Clin Immunol.* 2007;119:3-11.

23. Dhillon S, Plosker GL. Fondaparinux—use in thromboprophylaxis in acute medical patients. *Drugs Aging.* 2008;25:81-88.

24. Diabetes Control and Complications Trial/Epidemiology of Diabetes Interventions and Complications Study (DCCT/EDIC) Research Group. Intensive diabetes treatment and cardiovascular disease in type 1 diabetes in the DCCT/EDIC Study. *N Engl J Med.* 2005;353:2643-2653.

25. Di Nisio M, Middeldorp S, Büller HR. Direct thrombin inhibitors. *N Engl J Med.* 2005;353:1028-1040.

26. Eikelboom JW, Hankey GJ. Low molecular weight heparins and heparinoids. *Med J Aust.* 2002;177:379-383.

27. Ellahham S. Role of antiplatelet agents in the primary and secondary prevention of atherothrombotic events in high-risk patients. *South Med J.* 2008;101:273-283.

28. Epstein M. Dihydropyridine calcium channel antagonists in the management of hypertension. *Drugs.* 2007;67:1309-1327.

29. Epstein M, Campese VM. Evolving role of calcium antagonists in the management of hypertension. *Med Clin North Am.* 2004;88:149-165.

30. Etter J-F. Cytisine for smoking cessation. *Arch Intern Med.* 2006;166:1553-1559.

31. Evans M, Roberts A, Rees A. Pharmacological management of hyperlipidemias. *Br J Diabetes Vasc Dis.* 2003;3:204-210.

32. Farmakis D, Filippatos G, Lainscak M, et al. Anticoagulants, antiplatelets, and statins in heart failure. *Cardiol Clin.* 2008;26:49-58.

33. Ferdinand KC, Armani AM. The management of hypertension in African Americans. *Crit Pathw Cardiol.* 2007;6:67-71.

34. Fonarow GC. Comprehensive adrenergic blockade post myocardial infarction left ventricular dysfunction. *Cardiol Clin.* 2008;26:79-89.

35. Frishman WH. Smoking cessation pharmacotherapy—nicotine and non-nicotine preparations. *Prev Cardiol.* 2007;10:(2 suppl 1):10-22.

36. Fuster V, Alexander RW, O'Rourke RA, eds. *Hurst's The Heart.* 11th ed. New York: McGraw-Hill; 2004.

37. Gheorghiade M, van Veldhuisen DJ, Colucci WS. Contemporary use of digoxin in the management of cardiovascular disorders. *Circulation.* 2006;113:2556-2564.

38. Golshayan D, Buhler L, Lechler RI, et al. From current immunosuppressive strategies to clinical tolerance of allografts. *Transplant Int.* 2007; 20:12-24.

39. Gomberg-Maitland M, Olschewski H. Prostacyclin therapies for the treatment of pulmonary arterial hypertension. *Eur Respir J.* 2008;31:891-901.

40. Gotfried MH. Macrolides for the treatment of chronic sinusitis, asthma, and COPD. *Chest.* 2004;125:52S-61S.

41. Grimes GC, Manning JL, Patel P, et al. Medications for COPD: a review of effectiveness. *Am Fam Physician.* 2007;76:1141-1148.

42. Hamad E, Mather PJ, Srinivasan S, et al. Pharmacologic therapy of chronic heart failure. *Am J Cardiovasc Drugs.* 2007;7:235-248.

43. Hankey GJ, Eikelboom JW. Antiplatelet drugs. *Med J Aust.* 2003;178:568-574.

44. Haugh KH. Antiarrhythmic agents at the turn of the twenty-first century. *Crit Care Nurs Clin North Am.* 2002;14:53-69.

45. Heise T. Getting closer to physiologic insulin secretion. *Clin Ther.* 2007;29 (suppl D):S161-S165.

46. Higgins B, Williams B. Pharmacologic management of hypertension. *Clin Med.* 2007;7:612-616.

46a. Hinnen D, Nielsen LL, Waninger A, et al. Incretin mimetics and DPP-IV inhibitors: new paradigms for the treatment of type 2 diabetes. *J Am Board Fam Med.* 2006;19:612-620.

47. Hisch J, O'Donnell M, Eikelboom JW. Beyond unfractionated heparin and warfarin: current and future advances. *Circulation.* 2007;116: 552-560.

48. Holmes CL, Landry DW, Granton JT. Science review: vasopressin and the cardiovascular system. 2. Clinical physiology. *Crit Care.* 2004;8:15-23.

49. Horton JD, Bushwick BM. Warfarin therapy: evolving strategies in anticoagulation. *Am Fam Physician.* 1999;59:635-648.

50. Horvath K, Jeither K, Berghold A, et al. Long-acting insulin analogues versus NPH insulin (human isophane insulin) for type 2 diabetes: a Cochrane review. *Cochrane Database Syst Rev.* 2007;2:CD005613.

51. Iakobishvili Z, Hasdai D. Cardiogenic shock: treatment. *Med Clin North Am.* 2007;91:713-727.

52. Institute for Quality and Efficiency in Health Care (IQWiG). Rapid-acting insulin analogues in diabetes mellitus type 1—superiority not proven. www.iqwig.de/index.449.en.html.

53. Inzucchi SE, McGuire DK. New drugs for the treatment of diabetes mellitus. II. Incretin-based therapy and beyond. *Circulation.* 2008;117:574-584.

54. Jones R, Mustafa N. A fresh look at continuous subcutaneous insulin infusion. *JAAPA.* 2008;21(3):36-42.

55. Joy SV. Clinical pearls and strategies to optimize patient outcomes. *J Am Acad Nurs Pract.* 2007;19(11 suppl 1):15-20.

56. Kanaan AO, Silva MA, Donovan JL, et al. Meta-analysis of venous thromboembolism prophylaxis in medically-ill patients. *Clin Ther.* 2007;29:2395-2405.

57. Kaplan NM. Systemic hypertension: therapy. In: Zipes DP, Libby P, Bonow PO, Braunwald E, eds. *Braunwald's Heart Disease* 7th ed. Philadelphia: Saunders; 2005.

58. Kass DA, Champion HC, Beavo JA. Phosphodiesterase type 5: expanding roles in cardiovascular regulation. *Circ Res.* 2007;101:1084-1095.

59. Kearney CE, Wallis CE. Deoxyribonuclease for cystic fibrosis. *Cochrane Database Syst Rev.* 2000;2:CD001127.

60. Kelly HW. Rationale for the major changes in the pharmacotherapy section of the National Asthma Education and Prevention Program guidelines. *J Allergy Clin Immunol.* 2007;120:989-994.

61. Kerst LL, Mauro VF. Coronary event secondary prevention with statins irrespective of LDL-cholesterol. *Ann Pharmacother.* 2004;38:1060-1064.

62. Kobashigawa JA, Patel JK. Immunosuppression for heart transplantation: where are we now? *Nat Clin Pract Cardiovasc Med.* 2006;3:203-212.

63. Köhnlein T. Welte T: α-1 Antitrypsin deficiency: pathogenesis, clinical presentation, diagnosis, and treatment. *Am J Med.* 2008;12:3-9.

64. Kowey PR, Marinchak RA, Rials SJ, et al. Classification and pharmacology of antiarrhythmic drugs. *Am Heart J.* 2000;140:12-20.

65. Krentz AJ, Bailey CJ. Oral antidiabetic agents: current role in type 2 diabetes mellitus. *Drugs.* 2005;65:385-411.

66. Lancaster T, Stead L, Cahill K. An update on therapeutics for tobacco dependence. *Expert Opin Pharmacother.* 2008;9:15-22.

67. Levine JP. Type 2 diabetes among women: clinical considerations for pharmacological management to achieve glycemic control and reduce cardiovascular risk. *J Womens Health.* 2008;17: 249-260.

68. Lincoln TM. Cyclic GMP and phosphodiesterase 5 inhibitor therapies: what's on the horizon? *Mol Pharmacol.* 2004;66:11-13.

69. Massi-Benedetti M, Orsini-Federici M. Treatment of type 2 diabetes with combination therapy: what are the pros and cons? *Diabetes Care.* 2008;31(suppl 2):S131-S135.

70. Matthay MA. β-Adrenergic agonist therapy as a potential treatment for acute lung injury. *Am J Respir Crit Care Med.* 2006;173:254-255.

71. McDonnell ME. Combination therapy with new targets in type 2 diabetes: a review of available agents with a focus on pre-exercise adjustment. *J Cardiopulm Rehabil Prevent.* 2007;27:193-201.

72. McGuire DK, Inzucchi SE. New drugs for the treatment of diabetes mellitus. I. Thiazolidinediones and their evolving cardiovascular implications. *Circulation.* 2008;117:440-449.

73. McLaughlin VV, Oudiz RJ, Fronst A, et al. Randomized study of adding inhaled iloprost to existing bosentan in pulmonary arterial hypertension. *Am J Respir Crit Care Med.* 2006;174:1257-1263.

74. Meyer NJ, Bhorade SM. Evolving immunosuppressive regimens for lung transplantation. *Semin Respir Crit Care Med.* 2006;27: 470-479.

75. Moore WC. Update in asthma 2007. *Am J Respir Crit Care Med.* 2008;177:1068-1073.

76. Moore WC, Peters SP. Update in asthma 2006. *Am J Respir Crit Care Med.* 2007;175:649-654.

76a. Moser M, Setaro J. Continued importance of diuretics and β-adrenergic blockers in the management of hypertension. *Med Clin North Am.* 2004;88:167-187.

77. Mulligan MS, Shearon TH, Weill D, et al. Heart and lung transplantation in the United States, 1997–2006. *Am J Transplant.* 2008;8:977-987.

77a. Nagarankanti R, Sodhi S, Lee R, et al. Chronic antithrombotic therapy in post-myocardial patients. *Cardiol Clin.* 2008;26: 277-288.

78. National Asthma Education and Prevention Program. *Expert Panel Report 3. Guidelines of the diagnosis and management of asthma.* Bethesda, MD: National Institutes of Health: National Heart, Lung, and Blood Institute. Publication No 07-4051. Available from: www.nhlbi.nih.gov/guidelines/asthma/asthgdln.htm; 2007.

79. Ng VWS, Kong APS. Dipeptidyl peptidase (DPP)-IV inhibitor: a novel class of oral anti-hyperglycemic agents. *Drug Rev.* 2007;12(5):33-34.

80. O'Bryne PM. Acute asthma intervention: insights from the STAY Study. *J Allergy Clin Immunol.* 2007;119:1332-1336.

81. Oiknine R, Bernbaum M, Mooradian AD. A critical appraisal of the role of insulin analogues in the management of diabetes mellitus. *Drugs.* 2005;65:325-340.

82. Oncken C, Gonzles D, Nides M, et al. Efficacy and safety of the novel selective nicotinic acetylcholine receptor partial agonist, varenicline, for smoking cessation. *Arch Intern Med.* 2006;166: 1571-1577.

83. Perkins GD, McAuley DF, Thickett DR, et al. The β-agonist lung injury trial (BALTI): a randomized placebo-controlled clinical trial. *Am J Respir Crit Care Med.* 2006;173:281-287.

84. *Physician's Desk Reference 2008.* 62nd ed. Montvale, NJ: Thomson PDR; 2008.

85. Pitt B. Aldosterone blockade in patients with chronic heart failure. *Cardiol Clin.* 2008;26:15-21.

86. Poole PJ, Black PN. Oral mucolytic drugs for exacerbations of chronic obstructive pulmonary disease: systematic review. *BMJ.* 2001;322:1-6.

87. Qaseem A, Snow V, Shekelle P, et al. Diagnosis and management of stable chronic obstructive pulmonary disease: a clinical practice guideline from the American College of Physicians. *Ann Intern Med.* 2007;147:633-638.

88. Rapp JA, Gheorghiade M. Role of neurohumoral modulators in heart failure with relatively preserved systolic function. *Cardiol Clin.* 2008;26:23-40.

88a. Ramasubbu K, Mann DL, Deswal A. Anti-angiotensin therapy: new perspectives. *Cardiol Clin.* 2007;25:573-580.

89. Re RN. Tissue renin angiotensin systems. *Med Clin North Am.* 2004;88:19-38.

90. Remme WJ. Beta blockers or angiotensin-converting inhibitor/angiotensin receptor blocker: what should be first? *Cardiol Clin.* 2007;25:581-594.

90a. Remick J, Weintraub H, Setton R, et al. Fibrate therapy. An update. *Cardiol Rev.* 2008;16:129-141.

91. Ribeiro AB. Angiotensin II antagonists—therapeutic benefits spanning the cardiovascular disease continuum from hypertension to heart failure and diabetic neuropathy. *Curr Med Res Opin.* 2006;22:1-16.

92. Rogers DF. Mucoactive agents for airway mucus hypersecretory disease. *Respir Care.* 2007;52:1176-1197.

93. Rosen D, Decaro MV, Graham MG. Evidence-based treatment of chronic heart failure. *Compr Ther.* 2007;33:2-11.

94. Rosenkranz S. Pulmonary hypertension: current diagnosis and treatment. *Clin Res Cardiol.* 2007;96:527-541.

95. Rubin BK. The pharmacologic approach to airway clearance: mucoactive agents. *Respir Care.* 2002;47:808-817.

96. Samaniego M, Becker BN, Djamali A. Drug insight: maintenance immunosuppression in kidney transplant recipients. *Nat Clin Pract Nephrol.* 2006;2:688-699.

97. Schmauss D, Weis M. Cardiac allograft vasculopathy: recent developments. *Circulation.* 2008;117:2131-2141.

98. Schmitz O, Brock B, Rungby J. Amylin agonists: a novel approach in the treatment of diabetes. *Diabetes.* 2004;53(suppl 3):S233-S238.

99. Schooff MD, Gupta L. Are long-acting insulin analogues better than isophane insulin? *Am Fam Physician.* 2008;77:447-449.

100. Scirica BM, Morrow DA, Hod H, et al. Effect of ranolazine, an antianginal agent with novel electrophysiological properties, on the incidence of arrhythmias in patients with non-ST-segment-elevation acute coronary syndrome. Results from the Metabolic Efficiency with Ranolazine for Less Ischemia in Non-ST-Elevation Acute Coronary Syndrome-Thrombolysis in Myocardial Infarction 36 (MERLIN-TIMI 36) randomized control trial. *Circulation.* 2007;116:1647-1652.

101. Shanes JG, Minadeo KN, Moret A, et al. Statin therapy in heart failure: prognostic effects and potential mechanisms. *Am Heart J.* 2007;154:617-623.

102. Shavelle DM. Long term medical treatment of stable coronary disease. *Heart.* 2007;93:1473-1477.

103. Siebenhofer A, Plank J, Berghold A, et al. Short acting insulin analogues versus regular human insulin in patients with diabetes mellitus. *Cochrane Database Syst Rev.* 2004;4:CD003287.

104. Snell GI, Westall GP. Immunosuppression for lung transplantation: evidence to date. *Drugs.* 2007;67:1531-1539.

105. Stevens TP, Sinkin RA. Surfactant replacement therapy. *Chest.* 2007;131:1577-1582.

105a. Taut FJH, Rippin G, Schnenk K, et al. A search for subgroups of patients with ARDS who may benefit from surfactant replacement therapy. A pooled analysis of five studies with recombinant surfactant protein-C surfactant (Venticute). *Chest.* 2008;134:724-732.

106. Trujillo TC, Dobesh PP. Traditional management of chronic stable angina. *Pharmacotherapy.* 2007;27:1677-1692.

107. UK Prospective Diabetes Study Group. Intensive blood-glucose control with sulphonylureas or insulin compared with conventional treatment and risk of complications in patients with type 2 diabetes (UKPDS 33). *Lancet.* 1998;352:837-853.

108. Uwaifo GI, Ratner RE. Differential effects of oral hypoglycemic agents on glucose control and cardiovascular risk. *Am J Cardiol.* 2007;99 (suppl):51B-67B.

108a. Vilachopoulos C, Xaplanteris P, Alexopoulos N, et al. Divergent effects of laughter and mental stress on arterial stiffness and central hemodynamics. *Psychosom Med.* 2009;71:446-453.

108b. Weber MA. Calcium channel antagonists in the treatment of hypertension. *Am J Cardiovasc Drugs.* 2002;2:415-431.

109. Wein L, Wein S, Haas SJ, et al. Pharmacological venous thromboembolism prophylaxis in hospitalized medical patients. *Arch Intern Med.* 2007;167:1476-1486.

110. Yeh RW, Jang I-K. Argatoroban: update. *Am Heart J.* 2005;151:1131-1138.

111. Zipes DP, Libby P, Bonow PO, Braunwald E, eds. *Braunwald's Heart Disease.* 7th ed. Philadelphia: Saunders; 2005.

ADDITIONAL READINGS

Ciccone C. *Pharmacology in Rehabilitation.* 3rd ed. Philadelphia: F.A. Davis; 2002.

Gibson GJ, Geddes DM, Costabel U, et al., eds. *Respiratory Medicine.* 3rd ed. Philadelphia: W.B. Saunders; 2003.

Gladson B. *Pharmacology for Physical Therapists.* St. Louis: MO, Saunders; 2006.

Guyton AC, Hall JE. *Textbook of Medical Physiology.* 10th ed. Philadelphia: Saunders; 2000.

McPhee SJ, Papdakis MA, Tierney Jr LM, eds. *Current Medical Diagnosis and Treatment 2008.* 48th ed. McGraw-Hill; 2008.

Murray JF, Nadal JA, eds-in-chief. *Textbook of Respiratory Medicine.* 3rd ed. Philadelphia: Saunders; 2000.

CHAPTER 6

Cardiopulmonary Assessment

Because cardiopulmonary disease is so prevalent in our society, it is likely that a significant portion of the patients referred for physical therapy have some form of disease or dysfunction related to these systems, although many may not have been diagnosed yet. For example, only 25% to 48% of patients with cerebrovascular disease have a history of coronary artery disease, but 75% have been documented to have notable disease by angiography.[19,40] Therefore, assessment of the cardiopulmonary system is important to include in the physical therapy evaluations of all patients more than 40 years of age and younger patients with coronary risk factors, possible cardiopulmonary symptomatology, or disease or disorders that can affect the cardiopulmonary system, as presented in Chapter 4 (Cardiopulmonary Pathology).

This chapter includes descriptions of the relevant elements of a cardiopulmonary assessment for physical therapists (PTs): the medical chart review; patient/family interview; physical assessment, including an activity and endurance evaluation; as well as important "red flags" (i.e., precautions and contraindications) that may indicate increased risk for adverse events during exercise. Not all assessment techniques are indicated for every patient, and some require equipment that may not be available in all practice settings. When one element of a cardiopulmonary assessment is not feasible, the remaining elements become more important. For example, the therapist working in the outpatient or home care setting usually does not have access to the patient's medical record and may be given minimal information regarding the patient's medical history other than the diagnosis for which treatment is requested; thus, the patient/family interview and physical assessments take on greater significance.

6.1 MEDICAL CHART REVIEW

When the patient is in the hospital, a careful review of the physician and nursing admission and progress notes, as well as physician orders and results of various diagnostic tests, can provide the therapist with valuable knowledge about the patient's medical status and possible treatment needs even before the therapist meets him or her. Important findings that may influence the therapist are presented in the following sections, according to their location in the medical chart.

ADMISSION NOTES

The physician and nursing admission notes usually offer the most complete summary of the patient's medical history and physical examination.
- Specific medical information that is of particular value includes the admitting diagnosis, the date of admission, the patient's symptoms or medical complaints, the patient's past medical and surgical history, and medications being taken at the time of admission. Important considerations for each of these are presented in Table 6-1.
- The level of disability of cardiac patients is often described in terms of the New York Heart Association (NYHA) functional classifications, which are found in Table 6-2.
- Also commonly found in the admission notes are the patient's coronary risk factors and social history, and sometimes, occupation, home environment, and family situation. Some of the questions that should be considered are as follows:
  - Does the patient smoke? If so, what (cigarettes, cigars, pipe)? Has the patient ever smoked? How many pack-years (number of packs per day times the number of years)?
  - Does the patient have any other risk factors for cardiovascular (CV) disease (e.g., hypertension [HTN], family history, elevated cholesterol, obesity, diabetes mellitus [DM]; see Table 4-7 on page 103) or pulmonary disease (e.g., occupational exposure to known irritants or allergens; residential exposure to high levels of air pollution; heart failure; musculoskeletal or integumentary disorders affecting the chest; recurrent pulmonary infections; premature birth; immunosuppression)?
  - Does the patient have other chronic medical problems that are associated with cardiopulmonary dysfunction (e.g., obesity, neuromuscular disorders, connective tissue disease, or previous cancer treatment with chemotherapy or radiation therapy to the chest; see pages 127 to 149)?
  - What is the patient's history of alcohol use? (High intake is associated with an increased incidence of HTN, cardiomyopathy, and aspiration pneumonia.)
  - Does the patient use any illicit drugs? (Marijuana use can result in chronic obstructive pulmonary disease [COPD]; cocaine use is associated with coronary spasm and arrhythmias, which can lead to acute myocardial infarction [MI] and sudden death.)
  - Is the patient's lifestyle active or predominantly sedentary? (Physical inactivity is a risk factor for CV disease.)
  - What social support systems does the patient have? Are there people who can provide help if needed? Will the patient require home health services?
  - Will the lifestyle habits of those close to the patient support or interfere with recommended changes for the patient?
  - What is the patient's occupation? What are the physical requirements of the job? Will the patient be able to return to that job or will a change need to be made?
  - Where does the patient live? With whom? Are there physical barriers that may be a problem?
  - Who is the patient's medical insurance provider? Will the insurance provider cover continued therapy after discharge? How many treatments?
- The relevant data from the patient's physical examination (often listed as *systems review*, or *review of systems*, ROS)

TABLE 6-1: Important Medical Information Found in a Patient's Medical Chart

Information	Important Considerations
Admitting diagnosis	Is the diagnosis related to cardiovascular or pulmonary disease?
	Does the diagnosis have any cardiovascular or pulmonary complications associated with it? (See pages 127-149)
Admission date	How long has the patient been in the hospital? (The longer the hospitalization, the greater the likelihood of major medical problems or complications)
Patient symptoms or complaints	What were the patient's complaints prompting admission?
	Does the patient have any symptoms that can be attributed to cardiac disease (e.g., chest discomfort, shortness of breath, palpitations, lightheadedness, as on page 46) or lung disease (e.g., dyspnea, wheezing, cough, sputum production, as on page 10)?
	Specific descriptors offered by the patient are particularly helpful, because they provide medical personnel with vocabulary that is meaningful to the patient (e.g., "chest tightness" might not be considered to be "chest pain" by the patient)
Past medical and surgical history	Does the patient have any past history of cardiovascular or pulmonary problems, or other diseases with possible cardiopulmonary complications, whether or not related to the admission diagnosis (e.g., HTN, metabolic syndrome, or DM)?
	Will other medical problems limit the patient's ability to exercise (e.g., arthritis, neurologic or neuromuscular disease)?
	Does the patient have any known risk factors for cardiovascular or pulmonary disease?
Medications	Was the patient taking any medications on a regular basis before admission?
	Do any of the previously prescribed medications indicate possible cardiovascular or pulmonary disease (e.g., HTN, angina, heart failure, bronchospasm, DM, or infection)?
	What medications is the patient currently taking?
	Will any of the currently prescribed medications affect the patient's physiological responses to physical therapy interventions, such as exercise or Hubbard tank? (See pages 156-221)
	Is the patient receiving oxygen therapy? What amount and by what method (e.g., 3 L/min by nasal cannula, 60% by face mask)?

DM, Diabetes mellitus; HTN, hypertension.

TABLE 6-2: NYHA Functional Classification of Heart Disease, With Relationship to Exercise Tolerance

Functional Classification	Description	Approximate Exercise Tolerance
I	Patient with cardiac disease but without any resulting limitations of physical activity; ordinary physical activity does not cause undue fatigue, palpitations, dyspnea, or anginal pain	6–10 METs
II	Slight limitations of physical activity; comfortable at rest, but ordinary physical activity results in fatigue, palpitations, dyspnea, or anginal pain	4–6 METs
III	Marked limitation of physical activity; comfortable at rest, but less than ordinary physical activity causes symptoms, as above	2–3 METs
IV	Unable to carry out any physical activity without discomfort; symptoms of cardiac insufficiency or of angina may be present even at rest; if exertion is undertaken, discomfort increases	<2 METs

MET, Metabolic equivalent of energy expenditure (1 MET = approximately 3.5 mL O_2/kg/min).

include the general observations, chest, cardiovascular system, abdomen, extremities, and others, which are described in Table 6-3.

- Blood serum data that may indicate cardiopulmonary dysfunction include arterial blood gases, myocardial enzymes, white blood cell count, and renal function tests.

▸ Patterns of abnormalities seen in cardiac or pulmonary disease include the following:
  ⊙ Increased myocardial enzymes (e.g., troponins I and T [cTnI and cTnT] and creatine phosphokinase [CPK]; see page 407), white blood cell count and sedimentation rate in acute MI

TABLE 6-3: **Important Information Obtained From a Review of the Patient's Physical Examination**

Important Considerations

Are there any findings that might suggest cardiovascular or pulmonary disease or result in increased workload on these systems?

General appearance	Obesity, cachexia, barrel-shaped chest, signs of breathing difficulty (e.g., tachypnea, use of accessory muscles of respiration, intercostal retractions)
Vital signs	↓ Or ↑ heart rate, blood pressure, or respiratory rate; presence of fever
Skin	Cold and clammy in low-cardiac output states; pale, blue, and cold if peripheral vasoconstriction; cyanosis if marked arterial hypoxemia; or xanthomas in familial hypercholesterolemia
Head, eyes, ears, nose, and throat (HEENT)	Abnormal funduscopic eye examination (e.g., retinal arteriolar changes in HTN and DM)
	Abnormal neck examination (e.g., jugular venous distension in right or biventricular heart failure, exaggerated venous pulse waves in pulmonary HTN or right-sided valvular disease, or prominent carotid pulsations in aortic incompetence)
	Signs of upper respiratory infection (which might be seeding lower respiratory tract)
Chest, lungs	Abnormal chest examination (e.g., ↓ chest or diaphragmatic excursions in chronic obstructive pulmonary disease, prominent pulsations in cardiac hypertrophy, thrills in valve disease)
	Abnormal breath sounds (e.g., decreased, bronchial, or adventitious breath sounds; see page 247)
Cardiovascular	Abnormal heart sounds (e.g., murmurs in valvular disease, third and/or fourth heart sounds if diastolic dysfunction or reduced ventricular compliance, friction rubs in pericarditis; see page 249)
	Abnormal peripheral pulses (e.g., decreased if atherosclerotic disease or aortic stenosis, bounding in aortic incompetence)
Abdomen	Enlarged liver and spleen, ascites in right heart failure
Extremities	Abnormal extremity examination (e.g., peripheral edema, digital clubbing)

↓, Decreased; ↑, increased; HTN, hypertension; DM, diabetes mellitus.

⊙ Possible hypoxemia, hypercapnia, respiratory acidosis, increased white blood cell count, and bacteremia in acute pulmonary disease

⊙ Increased sedimentation rate, white blood cell count, and streptolysin O titers in acute rheumatic fever

⊙ Increased blood urea nitrogen, proteinuria, and granular casts in cardiac failure

⊙ Possible hypoxemia, hypercapnia, compensated respiratory acidosis, and polycythemia in chronic pulmonary disease

⊙ Elevated levels of total and low-density lipoprotein (LDL) cholesterol and reduced level of high-density lipoprotein (HDL) cholesterol, as well as possible glucose intolerance and increased levels of high-sensitivity C-reactive protein (CRP), triglycerides, homocysteine, and fibrinogen, in cardiovascular disease, including coronary artery disease (CAD), stroke, and peripheral arterial disease (PAD)

⊙ Increased serum creatinine and blood urea nitrogen, decreased creatinine clearance, and proteinuria in renal insufficiency, plus anemia in renal failure

▶ A number of other serum abnormalities may be associated with cardiopulmonary dysfunction or impaired exercise tolerance.

⊙ Increased K^+ (especially if decreased Ca^{2+}), decreased K^+, decreased Mg^{2+}, and toxic digitalis levels (which may be potentiated by decreased K^+ or Mg^{2+}) may cause arrhythmias.

⊙ Anemia (reduced hematocrit and hemoglobin) can result in fatigue and dyspnea.

⊙ Very low levels of phosphorus may depress myocardial function.

⊙ Metabolic acidosis (e.g., diabetic ketoacidosis) elicits hyperventilation, whereas metabolic alkalosis (e.g., excess sodium bicarbonate during cardiopulmonary resuscitation) can lead to hypoventilation.

⊙ Abnormally low platelet counts (e.g., patients receiving chemotherapy for cancer) can increase the risk of bleeding induced by exercise.

⊙ Abnormal coagulation studies may indicate an elevated risk of blood clotting versus bleeding, depending on the direction of the abnormality.

• Finally, the results of any diagnostic tests and procedures performed before or at the time of admission are often described in the admission note. Important considerations related to various cardiovascular and pulmonary studies are listed in Table 6-4 (refer to Chapter 2 [Pulmonology] and Chapter 3 [Cardiovascular Medicine] for descriptions of specific diagnostic tests). Also refer to pages 227 to 233 for information related to the interpretation of arterial blood gases, pulmonary function tests, and 12-lead electrocardiograms.

PROGRESS NOTES

Within the physician and nursing progress notes are the details of the patient's hospital course, ongoing clinical laboratory data,

TABLE 6-4: Important Considerations Related to Cardiopulmonary Diagnostic Tests and Procedures

Diagnostic Test/Procedure	Important Cardiopulmonary Considerations
Arterial blood gases (ABGs)	Is oxygenation normal (Pao_2 >80 with O_2 saturation [SaO_2] >97%) or adequate (Pao_2 >60 with SaO_2 >90%)? If SaO_2 <85%, exercise is usually contraindicated.
	Are $Paco_2$ and pH within normal limits (35–45 mm Hg and 7.35–7.45, respectively)?
	Are alterations acute or chronic (see pages 228–229)?
	Was the patient receiving supplemental oxygen when the ABGs were drawn?
	Does the patient need oxygen during treatment? Is the dose of oxygen sufficient to prevent desaturation during activity?
Bronchoscopy	Are there endobronchial abnormalities (mucus, tumor, aspirated foreign body, other lesions)? If there is mucous plugging, more aggressive bronchial hygiene is indicated.
	Were other diagnostic tests performed (bronchial brushings, needle aspiration, or biopsy)? What were the results?
	Were any therapeutic procedures performed?
Cardiac catheterization	Are the chamber and vessel pressures normal?
	Are there any gradients across the valves?
Ventriculography	Is ventricular performance normal (EF >40%–50%, normal wall motion)?
	Is there evidence of valvular regurgitation?
Angiography	Are there any obstructions in the coronary arteries? If so, how many, in which vessels, and to what degree?
	Are coronary artery bypass grafts patent?
Chest radiography (CXR)	Are there any abnormalities?
	• Infiltrates, atelectasis, consolidation, air bronchogram, interstitial markings and nodules, pleural effusion, or masses may be visualized in acute pulmonary disease
	• Flattened diaphragms and hyperinflated chest are seen in COPD, along with possible blebs and bullae in emphysema; possible peribronchial thickening in asthma, chronic bronchitis, bronchiectasis
	• Pulmonary fibrosis (e.g., reticular markings, honeycomb shadowing) or pleural thickening may be seen in RLD with ↓ lung compliance
	• ↑ Chamber or heart size, ↑ pulmonary vascular markings, infiltrates, and/or pleural effusions are commonly observed in cardiac disease, particularly if LV failure is present
Computed tomography (CT)	Are there any structural abnormalities (parenchymal, pleural, mediastinal, hilar, lung carcinomas or metastatic lesions, emphysematous bullae)?
Echocardiography: M-mode, two- and three-dimensional, Doppler, transesophageal	Are chamber sizes and wall thicknesses normal (see page 51)? Chamber dilation and ventricular hypertrophy are compensatory adaptations that occur as a result of volume or pressure overload
	Are all cardiac valves functioning normally? Are there any structural abnormalities?
	What is the EF? (normal is at least 40%–50%)
	Are there areas of abnormal wall motion (e.g., hypokinesis, akinesis, or dyskinesis)?
Contrast	Are there any intracardiac shunts or other flow abnormalities?
Intracardiac	Are there any coronary lesions? What is their composition (lipid, calcium, or medial hypertrophy)?
Stress	Do abnormalities (wall motion, EF, valvular flow) develop or increase after exercise?
Duplex ultrasound	Are there abnormalities of vascular structure and flow (e.g., DVT, atherosclerotic lesions)?
Electrocardiography (ECG)	Is there evidence of acute, evolving, or old MI?
	Are there any signs of chamber enlargement or hypertrophy?
	Are there any arrhythmias or conduction disturbances? Do they improve over time or with therapeutic interventions?
	Are there any other abnormalities (e.g., myocardial ischemia, axis deviation, or prominant U-wave)
	Are there any lesions in the coronary arteries or bypass grafts?

Continued

TABLE 6-4: Important Considerations Related to Cardiopulmonary Diagnostic Tests and Procedures—Cont'd

Diagnostic Test/Procedure	Important Cardiopulmonary Considerations
Electron beam CT (EBCT), multidetector or multislice spiral CT (MDCT, MSCT)	Are there any structural abnormalities (chamber size, ventricular mass, congenital lesions)?
	Is ventricular performance normal (EF >40%–50%, normal wall motion)?
Exercise testing	How well did the patient perform (e.g., how many minutes on what protocol)?
	Why did the patient stop (i.e., what limited performance)?
	Were the patient's responses to exercise normal (see pages 261-282)?
	Were there any abnormalities (ECG, metabolic [O_2 consumption, CO_2 production], O_2 pulse, etc.)?
	What was the maximal MET level achieved?
Gallium and other radionuclide (^{111}In WBC, ^{99m}Tc DTPA, ^{201}Tl) scans	Is pulmonary inflammation/infection (as seen in AIDS, interstitial lung disease, sarcoidosis, etc.)?
Infarct-avid imaging (pyrophosphate, antimyosin antibody scans)	Are there areas of myocardial necrosis (indicating acute MI within past 7–10 d)?
Magnetic resonance imaging (MRI)	Are there structural abnormalities (mediastinal great vessels, venae cavae, central pulmonary arteries, soft tissues of chest wall)?
Cardiac magnetic resonance (CMR)	Are there any structural abnormalities (chamber volume, wall thickness, valves, pericardial + intracardiac masses)?
	Is ventricular performance normal (EF, wall motion)?
Cine MRI	Are there any vascular lesions (carotid, coronary, intracerebral, great and peripheral vessels)?
Positron emission tomography (PET)	What is the metabolic activity of lung masses (pulmonary nodules, non–small cell lung cancer)?
	Are there areas of myocardial perfusion and substrate use abnormalities (indicating ischemic or hibernating myocardium)?
	Are there signs of autonomic neuropathy?
Pulmonary arteriography	Are there any structural abnormalities within the pulmonary arteries (pulmonary embolus, arteriovenous malformation, pulmonary varices)?
	What is the patient's pulmonary vascular anatomy? (may need to define before lung surgery).
Pulmonary function tests (PFTs)	Are there abnormalities that indicate obstructive or restrictive dysfunction? (See pages 11-17)
	In COPD: ↑ Vital capacity and total lung capacity, mostly due to ↑ residual volume and functional residual capacity, and ↓ expiratory flow rates
	In RLD: ↓ Lung volumes and capacities and ↓ diffusing capacity, usually with normal or ↑ FEV_1/FVC
	Mixed defects show a combination of obstructive and restrictive abnormalities
	How do the current results compare with previous PFTs, if available?
Radionuclide angiography (RNA) or ventriculography (RNV), multiunit gated analysis (MUGA) scan	What is the ejection fraction? (normal is at least 40%–50%).
	Does it increase during exercise?
	Are there areas of abnormal wall motion?
Single-photon emission computer tomography (SPECT)	Are there defects in pulmonary perfusion or ventilation?
	Are there any defects of myocardial perfusion? Are they reversible? (reversible defects indicate ischemic but viable myocardium)
	If there is evidence of MI (i.e., irreversible defect), how large is it?
Thallium scan	Are there any perfusion defects after exercise? Are they reversible? (See preceding entry for SPECT)

Continued

TABLE 6-4: Important Considerations Related to Cardiopulmonary Diagnostic Tests and Procedures—Cont'd

Diagnostic Test/Procedure	Important Cardiopulmonary Considerations
Thoracentesis/pleural biopsy	What are the characteristics of the pleural fluid (exudate or transudate, evidence of blood, infectious agents, immunological components)?
	Are there abnormal cells or organisms in the pleural membrane (e.g., infectious, malignant)?
Ultrasonography	Is there a pleural effusion or pleural thickening?
Ventilation–perfusion $\dot{V}/\dot{Q}$ scan	Are there any defects in either ventilation or perfusion?
	What was the diagnostic conclusion?

↓, Decreased; ↑, increased; ABG, arterial blood gas; AIDS, acquired immunodeficiency syndrome; COPD, chronic obstructive pulmonary disease; DTPA, diethylenetriaminepentaacetic acid; DVT, deep venous thrombosis; ECG, electrocardiogram; EF, ejection fraction; FEV_1, forced expiratory volume in 1 second; FVC, forced vital capacity; LV, left ventricular; MET, metabolic equivalent of energy expenditure; MI, myocardial infarction; MRI, magnetic resonance imaging; $Paco_2$, partial pressure of arterial carbon dioxide; PFT, pulmonary function testing; Pao_2, pressure of arterial oxygen; RLD, restrictive lung dysfunction; T1, thallium; WBC, white blood cell.

the results of diagnostic tests and procedures, and therapeutic interventions (e.g., surgical procedures, changes in medications, electrolyte replacement, and nutritional support). In addition, the patient's actual diagnosis may not be determined until a few days of hospitalization have passed.

Also of importance, any complications that develop or secondary diagnoses that are identified are documented in these pages. These may have notable implications for physical therapy interventions. Some common examples are as follows:

- Fever is a common postoperative occurrence for all types of surgery and is often due to acute pulmonary complications; all therapists should encourage their patients to breathe deeply, cough, move around in bed, and get in and out of bed as much as possible and also request them to cough (while providing splinting of the incision if necessary) after any change of position or rehabilitation activity.
- Large discrepancies between fluid intake and output, resulting in either fluid overload (a common postoperative finding) or dehydration, will impair the patient's tolerance for activity.
- Patients with major complications after acute myocardial infarction (e.g., significant arrhythmias, systolic hypotension, pulmonary edema, cardiogenic shock, or postinfarction angina or extension of MI) have a higher risk of serious morbidity and mortality and therefore require close monitoring and slower progression during PT activities.
- Some monitoring or therapeutic interventions can affect PT treatment interventions and therefore will require modifications of the treatment plan to accommodate appropriate precautions. Examples include arterial or central venous lines, endotracheal intubation and ventilatory support, pacemaker insertion, ventricular assist device support, or bed rest limitations.

PHYSICIAN ORDERS

A running chronicle of the prescribed and discontinued medications and their doses, as well as of any ordered tests and procedures and prescribed activity level, can be found in the physician orders. When the specific decisions regarding patient management are not clearly defined in the physician progress notes, the order sheets will usually disclose them. In addition, a list of the patient's prescribed medications can be found on the nurses' medication cart.

OTHER REPORTS

The remaining sections of the patient's medical chart typically contain the records of vital signs and intake and output (if ordered), reports of diagnostic tests and procedures, surgical reports, physician consultation reports, and the evaluation and treatment notes of allied health professionals, such as physical, occupational, speech, and respiratory therapists.

Some diagnostic test results are particularly valuable for PTs to understand and the ability to interpret their significance can be crucial to providing appropriate treatment interventions and modifications and anticipating a patient's physiological responses to exercise. These include arterial blood gases, pulmonary function tests, and 12-lead electrocardiograms, and basic information related to their interpretation is presented.

Arterial Blood Gases

Patients with pulmonary disease may have arterial blood gas (ABG) values in their charts, which provide data related to a patient's oxygenation and ventilatory and acid–base status (see next page). The values are obtained by analysis of an arterial blood sample or by direct-reading electrodes from arterial cannulation to give an indication of the patient's baseline levels, to monitor the patient's status when acutely ill, and to document the efficacy of therapeutic interventions, as in critical care units, or to provide information about the patient's oxygenation status during exertion, as in exercise testing with ABG sampling.

- Normal values for ABGs are found on page 17.
- Four simple steps can be used to analyze ABGs, which are described in Table 6-5 and illustrated in Figure 6-1.
- The following are a few specific abnormalities documented by ABGs:
  - ▸ *Hypoxemia* is defined as a partial pressure of arterial oxygen (Pao_2) less than 80; common causes include hypoventilation (e.g., muscle weakness or paralysis, CNS disorders, and

TABLE 6-5: **Four Simple Steps for Analyzing Arterial Blood Gases**

Steps for Analyzing ABGs	Interpretation
Look at pH to assess acid–base status	pH <7.40 indicates acidosis pH >7.40 indicates alkalosis (although the normal range is 7.35 to 7.45, for this purpose only 7.40 is considered normal)
Examine the $Paco_2$: First, as an indicator of ventilatory status	$Paco_2$ = 35 to 45 mm Hg indicates adequate ventilation; no primary respiratory problem and no respiratory compensation for a metabolic problem
	$Paco_2$ <30 mm Hg indicates alveolar hyperventilation
	$Paco_2$ >50 mm Hg indicates alveolar hypoventilation, ventilatory failure
Next, interpret the levels in relation to pH to determine the cause of abnormal values	$Paco_2$ >45 mm Hg and pH <7.40 indicate respiratory acidosis
	$Paco_2$ >45 mm Hg and pH >7.40 indicate respiratory retention of CO_2 to compensate for metabolic alkalosis
	$Paco_2$ <35 mm Hg and pH >7.40 indicate respiratory alkalosis
	$Paco_2$ <35 mm Hg and pH <7.40 indicate respiratory elimination of CO_2 to compensate for metabolic acidosis
Check the HCO_3^- level	Normal HCO_3^- values (22 to 26 mEq/L) indicate no primary metabolic problem and no metabolic compensation for a respiratory problem
	Abnormal HCO_3^- values are interpreted in relation to pH:
	HCO_3^- <22 mEq/L and pH <7.40 indicate metabolic acidosis
	HCO_3^- <22 mEq/L and pH >7.40 indicate renal compensation for respiratory alkalosis
	HCO_3^- >26 mEq/L and pH >7.40 indicate metabolic alkalosis
	HCO_3^- >26 mEq/L and pH <7.40 indicate renal compensation for respiratory acidosis
Assess Pao_2 and Sao_2	Normal: 80 to 100 mm Hg at sea level with Sao_2 >95%
	Pao_2 = 60 to 80 mm Hg indicates mild hypoxemia, Sao_2 will be 90% to 95% (if no shift in the HbO_2 curve)
	Pao_2 = 40 to 60 mm Hg indicates moderate hypoxemia, Sao_2 will be 60% to 90% (if no shift in the HbO_2 curve)
	Pao_2 <40 mm Hg indicates severe hypoxemia, Sao_2 will be ≤60% (if no shift in the HbO_2 curve)

ABGs, Arterial blood gases; HbO_2, oxyhemoglobin; HCO_3^-, bicarbonate; $Paco_2$, partial pressure of arterial carbon dioxide; Pao_2, partial pressure of arterial oxygen; Sao_2, arterial oxygen saturation.

chest wall abnormalities), pulmonary disease with ventilation–perfusion mismatching or impaired diffusion, decreased atmospheric O_2 (altitudes >6500 feet above sea level) and right-to-left shunting (e.g., cyanotic congenital heart disease).
- ⊙ Pao_2 of 60 to 79 is considered mild hypoxemia.
- ⊙ Pao_2 of 40 to 59 is considered moderate hypoxemia.
- ⊙ Pao_2 less than 40 is considered severe hypoxemia.
▸ *Alveolar hypoventilation* is indicated by a partial pressure of arterial carbon dioxide ($Paco_2$) greater than 45 (i.e., hypercapnia); causes of persistent hypercapnia include COPD, diseases restricting chest wall expansion (e.g., kyphoscoliosis, ankylosing spondylitis, spinal cord injury, and neuromuscular disorders), CNS abnormalities, metabolic alkalosis, myxedema, and primary alveolar hypoventilation (see Respiratory Failure, page 95). Acute hypercapnia has a number of physiological consequences, including impaired diaphragmatic function, pulmonary vasoconstriction, systemic and cerebral vasodilation, increased intracranial pressure, depressed consciousness, and stimulation of the sympathetic nervous system.[7]

▸ *Alveolar hyperventilation* is indicated by a $Paco_2$ less than 35; it is caused by an increase in respiratory drive, which can be induced by hypoxemia, pulmonary disease (e.g., asthma, pneumonia, interstitial pneumonitis or fibrosis, and pulmonary embolism), cardiovascular disorders (e.g., CHF and hypotension), metabolic abnormalities (e.g., acidosis and hepatic failure), neurologic and psychogenic disorders, various drugs (e.g., salicylates, methylxanthine bronchodilators, and β-adrenergic agonists), pain, fever, sepsis, and pregnancy.
▸ *Ventilatory, or hypercapnic respiratory, failure* is diagnosed if $Paco_2$ exceeds 50 and can be precipitated by increased work of breathing (e.g., acute or chronic pulmonary disease causing significant ventilation–perfusion mismatching), reduced energy supply (e.g., low cardiac output and CHF), and impaired muscular efficiency (e.g., hyperinflation of chest, respiratory muscle weakness or fatigue, and flaccidity of abdominal muscles). Refer to page 95.
▸ *Acidemia* refers to a pH less than 7.35, whereas *alkalemia* refers to a pH greater than 7.45, which can be either respiratory

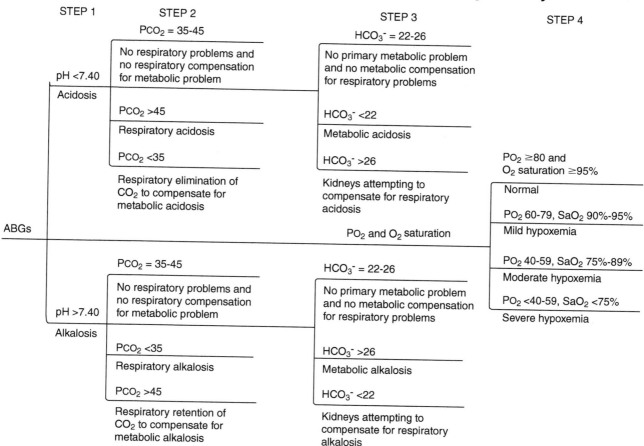

Figure 6-1: Steps involved in analyzing arterial blood gases (ABGs): (1) look at pH, (2) examine partial pressure of carbon dioxide (Pco_2) (mm Hg), (3) check bicarbonate (HCO_3^-) (mEq/L), and (4) assess partial pressure of oxygen (Po_2) (mm Hg) and arterial oxygen saturation (Sao_2) (%).

TABLE 6-6: **Summary of Acid–Base Changes in the Blood**

	pH	$Paco_2$	[HCO_3^-]
Acidosis			
Acute respiratory	↓	↑	WNL
Compensated respiratory	WNL*	↑	↑
Acute metabolic	↓	WNL	↓
Compensated metabolic	WNL*	↓	↓
Alkalosis			
Acute respiratory	↑	↓	WNL
Compensated respiratory	WNL†	↓	↓
Acute metabolic	↑	WNL	↑
Chronic metabolic	↑	↑	↑

↓, Decreased; ↑, increased; HCO_3^-, bicarbonate; $Paco_2$, partial pressure of arterial carbon dioxide; WNL, within normal limits.
*and pH <7.40.
†and pH >7.40.

or metabolic in origin. A summary of acid–base changes that are seen with various disorders is shown in Table 6-6.

⊙ Respiratory acidosis is present when the pH is less than 7.40 and $Paco_2$ is more than 45, which results from hypoventilation due to a number of causes (see page 311).

⊙ Metabolic acidosis exists when the pH is less than 7.40 and bicarbonate ion (HCO_3^-) is less than 22. It can result from increased acid production due to ketoacidosis (e.g., diabetes, alcohol abuse, and starvation), lactic acidosis (e.g., circulatory or respiratory failure, shock, drugs and toxins, and enzyme defects); or that associated with other disorders (e.g., severe anemia, pulmonary disease, and neoplasms) or renal failure. It can also be induced by retention of chloride (normal anion gap) due to renal tubular dysfunction (e.g., renal tubular acidosis, hypoaldosteronism, and potassium-sparing diuretics), loss of alkali (e.g., diarrhea, ureterosigmoidoscopy, enteric fistula, ileostomy, ileal loop bladder, and carbonic anhydrase inhibitors), or excess intake (e.g., ammonium chloride and cationic amino acids).

⊙ Respiratory alkalosis occurs when the pH is greater than 7.40 and $Paco_2$ is less than 35, which is induced by alveolar hyperventilation.

⊙ Metabolic alkalosis is present when the pH is greater than 7.40 and bicarbonate ion (HCO_3^-) is greater than 26. The metabolic abnormalities that can cause excessively high pH include those associated with volume (and chloride) depletion (e.g., vomiting, nasogastric suction, diuretic therapy, and abrupt decrease in $Paco_2$ during treatment of chronic respiratory acidosis) or hyperadrenocorticism leading to renal acid excretion (e.g., Cushing's syndrome and hyperaldosteronism), severe potassium depletion, and excessive alkali intake (e.g., bicarbonate or precursors, alkalizing salts, and milk-alkali syndrome).

- Patients with oxygen saturations less than 86% to 90% at rest (chronic vs. acute disease, respectively) usually require supplemental O_2 or an increase in O_2 dosage during exertion to avoid further desaturation. In addition, there is evidence that the use of supplemental O_2 during exercise by nonhypoxemic patients with moderate to severe COPD allows patients to perform high-intensity exercise training and thus achieve greater improvements in exercise capacity and breathing pattern.[29]
- It is important for PTs to be able to distinguish normal versus abnormal values for ABGs and to appreciate how abnormalities can affect an individual's ability to perform exercise and rehabilitation activities.

Pulmonary Function Tests

Pulmonary function tests (PFTs) are described on pages 11 to 17. The information provided by PFTs is helpful to PTs in establishing realistic treatment goals and an appropriate treatment plan according to the patient's current pulmonary problems and degree of impairment.

- A simplified method of examining PFT data is shown in Table 6-7.
- Patterns of pulmonary function abnormalities for obstructive, restrictive, and combined defects are depicted in Table 6-8.
  ▸ Obstructive lung disease is typically characterized by decreased expiratory flow rates, FEV_1/FVC (forced expiratory volume in 1 s/forced vital capacity) less than 70%, and increased RV (residual volume) and often RV/TLC (residual volume/total lung capacity).
  ▸ Restrictive lung disease is usually distinguished by reduced lung volumes, especially inspiratory reserve volume (IRV), inspiratory capacity (IC), and TLC, with normal or increased FEV_1/FVC.
  ▸ Combined abnormalities are generally marked by reduced expiratory flow rates and FEV_1/FVC along with normal or decreased TLC and increased RV/TLC.

TABLE 6-7: **Sequence for Examining Pulmonary Function Test Data**

Sequence of Analysis	Implications
1. Is VC normal?	VC may be ↓ in either RLD or OLD
2. Is ventilatory flow normal?	80% of predicted is taken as the lower limit of normal for FEV_1 and FVC, with the FVC being within 5% of the VC. An FEV_1/FVC ratio <65% is diagnostic of OLD
	The lower limit of normal for $FEF_{25-75\%}$ is 60%–65% of predicted
	The FVC recording should be examined for any flattening as well as prolongation of time required to expire the FVC, and the MEFV curve should be examined for concavity; both indicate possible OLD. Uneven, slurred, or notched curves and poor reproducibility indicate poor cooperation, effort, or both
	Some reversibility of airway obstruction is indicated by an ↑ in FEV_1 of >12%–15% after administration of a bronchodilator in individuals with near-normal spirometry or ≥200 mL in those with more severe disease
	FVC and FEV_1 are also ↓ in RLD, but the FEV_1/FVC ratio is usually normal or ↑
	FEF is often ↓ in OLD and sometimes in moderate to severe RLD when there is ↓ cross-sectional area of the small airways
3. Are the lung volumes normal?	RV and FRC are often ↑ in OLD, pulmonary vascular congestion, and expiratory muscle weakness; RV is ↓ in RLD resulting in ↓ TLC
	Proportional ↓ in most lung volumes indicates RLD. ↑ TLC >120% predicted or above the 95% confidence limit as a result of ↑ RV indicates hyperinflation, especially if the RV/TLC ratio is ↑. An ↑ RV/TLC ratio with normal TLC indicates that air trapping is present
	↑ RV with normal FEV_1 may occur in asthma in remission
4. Is gas distribution normal?	Check the results of the single-breath nitrogen test or nitrogen washout test, as well as the closing volume. Both RLD and OLD can result in uneven distribution of ventilation
5. Is gas transfer normal?	A normal diffusing capacity excludes significant $\dot{V}/\dot{Q}$ abnormality or interstitial lung disease
	Assess the arterial blood gases
6. Are other tests indicated?	An exercise test may be helpful in clarifying complaints of dyspnea
	Studies of lung mechanics and measurement of VC with the patient sitting and supine can determine whether there is paralysis of the diaphragm
	Bronchoprovocation testing for reactive airway disease may be indicated in patients with bouts of coughing and dyspnea, especially on exertion, who have normal spirometry when asymptomatic

↑, Increased; ↓, decreased; FEF, forced expiratory flow; $FEF_{25\%-75\%}$, forced expiratory flow from 25% to 75% of vital capacity; FEV_1, forced expiratory volume in 1 second; FRC, functional residual capacity; FVC, forced vital capacity; MEFV, maximal expiratory flow volume; OLD, obstructive lung dysfunction; RLD, restrictive lung dysfunction; RV, residual volume; TLC, total lung capacity; VC, vital capacity.

TABLE 6-8: Patterns of Pulmonary Function Abnormalities

Function	Normal	Obstruction	Restriction	Combined
FVC	≥75%–80% pred	nl–↓	↓	↓
FEV_1	≥75%–80% pred	↓	↓	↓
FEV_1/FVC	≥75%	↓	nl–↑	↑
$FEF_{25\%–75\%}$	≥60%–65% pred	↓	nl–↓	↓
TLC	80%–120% pred	nl–↑	↓	nl–↓
RV	80%–120% pred	↑	nl–↓	nl, ↓, or ↑
RV/TLC	25%–40%	↑	nl	↑

↓, Lower than normal; ↑, higher than normal; FEV_1, forced expiratory volume in 1 second; $FEF_{25\%–75\%}$, forced expiratory flow between 25% and 75% of the forced vital capacity; FVC, forced vital capacity; nl, normal; pred, predicted normal value; TLC, total lung capacity; RV, residual volume.

- The changes typical of obstructive and restrictive lung disease are illustrated in Figures 2–8, 2–9, and 2–10 (see pages 13 and 16)

Twelve-lead Electrocardiogram

Usually copies of any electrocardiograms (ECGs) obtained since admission are found in the patient's chart. Even when the therapist is not formally trained in the interpretation of 12-lead ECGs, repeated review of the recordings along with the interpretation, especially if obtained serially, and asking questions of friendly nurses and physicians often results in increasing recognition of a number of abnormalities and an appreciation of changes that occur over time.

- Some specific abnormalities that can be identified with a 12-lead ECG include the following:
  ▸ Left ventricular hypertrophy (LVH)
    ⊙ LVH is characterized by tall R waves in leads V_5 and V_6 and deep S waves in lead V_1 (Figure 6-2); sometimes there are ST–T wave changes in the opposite direction of the QRS (strain pattern). Many different ECG criteria have been developed to diagnose LVH, most of which have high specificity (not many false positives) but low to moderate sensitivity (and therefore many false negatives); a simple criterion with high accuracy (60%) is the Cornell voltage criterion, which recognizes LVH when the sum of the voltages of the R wave in lead aVL and the S wave in lead V_3 is greater than 2.0 mV for females or 2.8 mV for males.[17]
    ⊙ LVH is caused by excessive pressure or volume load on the left ventricle (LV) (e.g., hypertension, aortic stenosis, and severe aortic incompetence) or hypertrophic cardiomyopathy.
    ⊙ ECG changes occur late in the progression of LVH, so there is likely to be significant diastolic and probably systolic dysfunction by the time of their appearance; patients with ECG criteria for LVH have significantly increased risk for cardiovascular morbidity and mortality.
    ⊙ The presence of strain pattern at rest (abnormal ST–T wave changes in the direction opposite to the QRS complex) interferes with the detection of ischemic ST–T changes.
  ▸ Right ventricular hypertrophy (RVH)
    ⊙ Severe RVH is characterized by right axis deviation, prominent R waves in leads aVR, V_1 and V_2, and abnormally small R and deep S waves in leads I, aV_L, V_5 and V_6

(Figure 6-2); ST–T wave changes in the direction opposite of the QRS complex are often seen when RVH is severe (strain pattern).
    ⊙ RVH results from pressure or volume load on the right ventricle (RV) (e.g., pulmonary hypertension, severe lung disease, pulmonary or mitral stenosis, severe mitral regurgitation, and LV failure) or hypertrophic cardiomyopathy.
  ▸ Left atrial abnormality
    ⊙ Left atrial (LA) abnormality is characterized by a prolonged P wave (>0.12 s) in lead II; prominent notching of the P wave in leads I and II (lead II is the most obvious and is called *P mitrale*), and in leads V_4 to V_6; and a deep, broad terminal trough of the P wave in lead V_1 (duration ≥0.04 s; depth ≥1 mm), as shown in Figure 6-3.
    ⊙ These changes are actually due to conduction abnormalities within the atria rather than to hypertrophy or dilation and are caused by pressure or volume overload.
  ▸ Right atrial abnormality
    ⊙ Right atrial (RA) abnormality is characterized by tall peaked P waves in leads II (>0.25 mV, called *P pulmonale*), aVF (>0.20 mV), and V_1 (>0.10 mV), as shown in Figure 6-3.
    ⊙ It may be found in severe lung disease, pulmonary embolus, pulmonary hypertension, and severe tricuspid or pulmonary valve disease.
  ▸ Left bundle branch block (LBBB)
    ⊙ When disease interferes with conduction of the electrical impulse down the left bundle branch, electrical activation occurs first in the RV and then travels to the LV (opposite of normal), resulting in a markedly wide and distorted QRS complex. Thus, LBBB is characterized by QRS exceeding 0.12 seconds, a broad notched R in V_5 and V_6 plus a wide, slurred S in V_1, and abnormal T waves, often in the opposite direction of the predominant QRS voltage, as illustrated in Figure 6-2.
    ⊙ LBBB occurs in coronary disease, any cause of LVH, and congenital heart disease, or it may be idiopathic. It can be transient (e.g., acute myocardial infarction, congestive heart failure, myocarditis, or drug toxicity) or rate related (i.e., it develops at faster heart rates [HRs] only).
    ⊙ Because of the abnormal ST–T waves, LBBB may mask ischemic ST changes.

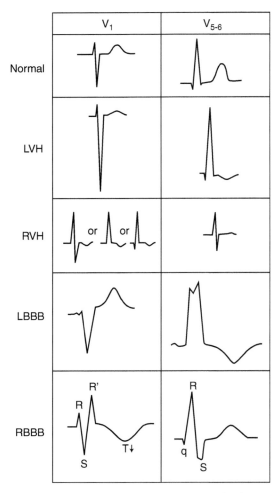

Figure 6-2: ECG changes seen in leads V_1 and leads V_5 and V_6 with ventricular hypertrophy and bundle branch blocks. Left ventricular hypertrophy (LVH) increases the amplitude of electrical forces directed to the left and posteriorly, producing tall R waves in V_5 and V_6 and deep S waves in V_1, whereas right ventricular hypertrophy (RVH) often shifts the QRS vector to the right, producing an R, RS, or qR complex in V_1 and an S in V_5 and V_6; T wave inversion may be present in leads with a prominent R wave. In left bundle branch block (LBBB), electrical activation occurs first in the right ventricle and then travels in a delayed manner to the left ventricle, resulting in a markedly wide and distorted QRS with T wave in the opposite direction in both leads; and in right bundle branch block (RBBB), delayed activation of the right ventricle causes widening of the QRS with an rSR′ and inverted T in V_1 and wide, slurred S in V_5 and V_6.

▸ Right bundle branch block (RBBB)
  ⊙ Disease affecting the right bundle branch leads to delayed activation of the RV, so the initial activation of the LV proceeds normally, but that of the RV occurs later than usual. Thus, RBBB is characterized by QRS greater than 0.12 seconds, rSR′ or notched R in V_1 and V_2 along with wide, slurred S waves in V_5 and V_6 (see Figure 6-2).
  ⊙ RBBB may be seen in coronary disease, hypertensive heart disease, any cause of RVH, and congenital heart

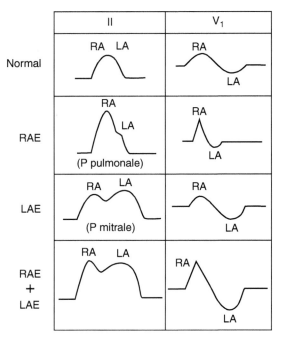

Figure 6-3: Changes in P-wave morphology typical of atrial enlargement (or, more accurately, atrial overload) as they appear in leads II and V_1. RAE, Right atrial enlargement; LAE, left atrial enlargement; RAE + LAE, biatrial enlargement.

disease; or it may be idiopathic (found in up to 10% of normal individuals). It may be transient (e.g., pulmonary embolism and exacerbation of COPD) or rate elated (as described previously for LBBB).
▸ Myocardial ischemia
  ⊙ Subendocardial myocardial ischemia is characterized by at least 1.0 mm (1 mV) of horizontal or downsloping ST-segment depression 0.08 second after the J point, and/or T wave inversion (see Figure 6-4 as well as Figure 3-13 on page 49).[2]
  ⊙ ST depression usually develops during or immediately after activity or mental or emotional stress and resolves within minutes of rest or taking nitroglycerin.
  ⊙ The amount of myocardium that experiences ischemia can be identified on a 12-lead ECG, as is typically monitored during exercise stress testing. The more leads with ischemic ST changes, the more severe the disease.[2]
  ⊙ ST-segment depression does not reliably predict the specific location of angiographic CAD.[2,62]
  ⊙ The value of ECG changes during exercise testing in asymptomatic individuals with fewer than two risk factors is questionable; positive tests have a poor predictive value (about 23%) for having significant CAD, but negative tests have an excellent predictive value (about 99%) for not having CAD.[2] The sensitivity of exercise-induced ST-segment changes is improved when patients are exercised to maximal exertion, multiple leads are monitored, and test data other than ECG changes (e.g., exercise capacity, HR and blood pressure [BP] responses, and symptomatology) are included as diagnostic criteria.

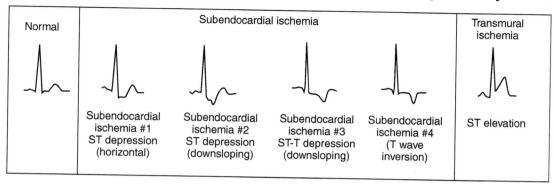

Figure 6-4: Changes in the ST segment and T wave during myocardial ischemia. Subendocardial ischemia causes ST-segment depression (which may be slowly upsloping, horizontal, or downsloping) and/or T wave flattening or inversion. Severe transient transmural ischemia can produce ST elevation (similar to the early changes in acute myocardial infarction), which returns to normal with resolution of the ischemia.

⊙ Significant transmural ischemia (involving the full thickness of the myocardial wall) may produce a transient injury current with exercise-induced ST-segment elevation (see Figure 6-4) that localizes to a specific area of myocardium and resolves after rest or administration of nitroglycerin.[2,62]

⊙ In persons with baseline ST abnormalities (e.g., LVH, LBBB, nonspecific interventricular conduction delay, and digitalis therapy), further ST changes are not necessarily indicative of myocardial ischemia and therefore are difficult to interpret.

▸ Myocardial infarction (MI)

⊙ Acute transmural MI is characterized by abnormal Q waves (≥ 0.03 s in duration and ≥ 2 mm in depth) with ST elevation (≥ 1 mm at 0.02 s after the J point) in two contiguous leads in the area of infarct and reciprocal ST depression in the area opposite to the infarct (Figure 6-5).[34]

⊙ Acute subendocardial MI (involving only the innermost layer of the myocardium) is characterized by ST depression and inverted T waves in the area of infarct ("non–Q-wave" infarct). Because these changes are similar to those seen in myocardial ischemia, although they persist despite rest or nitroglycerin, and are accompanied by similar symptoms, the term *acute coronary syndrome* is now preferred.

⊙ The ECG pattern of acute MI evolves over days to months (see Figure 4-17 on page 107).

⊙ In addition, localization of acute MI is possible using 12-lead ECG, as described in Table 6-9. By appreciating the location and extent of infarcted tissue, the therapist is better able to understand what impact the loss of myocardium will have on cardiac function.

6.2 PATIENT/FAMILY INTERVIEW

After review of the medical chart, the therapist will have some impressions of the patient's medical status and major problems and is ready to meet the patient and family. The purpose of the interview with the patient and family is to clarify the information obtained from the medical chart and fill in any missing information so an appropriate assessment techniques and treatment interventions can begin to be identified.

Of particular concern are any signs or symptoms the patient might reveal and their possible causes, many of which are presented in Table 6-10.[22b,37,40a] Of note, on occasion the patient/family interview provides a completely different picture of the patient's status than the impression created by the medical chart review. Other important benefits of the interview include

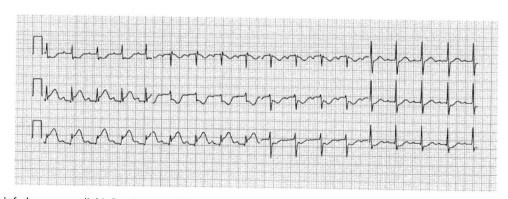

Figure 6-5: Acute inferior myocardial infarction with ST-segment elevation and peaked T waves in leads II, III, and aVF and reciprocal ST-segment depression in leads I, aVL, and V_1 and V_2. (From Jaffe AS, Davidenko J, Clements I. Diagnosis of acute coronary syndromes including acute myocardial infarctions. In Crawford MH, DiMarco JP, Paulus WJ, editors. *Cardiology.* 2nd ed. Edinburgh: Mosby; 2004.)

TABLE 6-9: Localization of Myocardial Infarction by ECG

Area of Infarction	Diagnostic ECG changes	Likely Coronary Artery
Anterior/anteroseptal	ST elevation in V_{1-3}	LAD
Anterolateral	ST elevation in I, aVL, and V_{4-6}	LAD
Lateral	ST elevation in I, aVL, and V_{5-6}	LAD
Extensive anterolateral	ST elevation in I, aVL, and V_{1-6}	LMCA
Inferior	ST elevation in II, III, and aVF	LAD or PDA
Inferolateral	ST elevation in II, III, aVF, and V_{4-6}	LAD
Posterior	ST depression in V_{1-3}	Circ
Posterolateral	ST depression in V_{1-3} and ST elevation in V_{4-6}	Circ
Right ventricular	ST elevation in V_1 and V_4R; usually occurs in association with inferior MI	RCA

Circ, left circumflex; ECG, electrocardiogram; LAD, left anterior descending; LMCA, left main coronary artery; PDA, posterior descending artery; RCA, right coronary artery.

TABLE 6-10: Common Patient Complaints and Possible Causes and Differentiating Features

Complaint	Possible Causes and Differentiating Features
Chest pain/discomfort	**Cardiac disease**

Myocardial ischemia: Pressure, tightness, heaviness in the chest that comes on with exertion, emotional distress, or eating, usually at same rate–pressure product, and is relieved within minutes by rest or NTG; may radiate to shoulder, arm, neck, back, jaw, teeth; often associated with dyspnea, fatigue, ST-segment depression

- Myocardial infarction: Severe, crushing pain that persists despite three administrations of NTG and is often accompanied by nausea ± vomiting, diaphoresis, hypotension, dyspnea, ST-segment elevation, or sometimes depression

Pericarditis: Chest pain that typically extends to left shoulder and sometimes down left arm; worsens on lying down, swallowing food, coughing, or with deep breathing; improves with sitting, leaning forward, or lying on right side; is not affected by exertion; is accompanied by fever

- Mitral valve prolapse: Pain, often of brief duration, that is stabbing or needle-like below the left breast and is unrelated to body position or activity

Myocarditis or endocarditis: chest tightness with dyspnea, low-grade fever, malaise, and possible arthralgias

LV outflow obstruction: myocardial ischemia (above) with LVH on echo or ECG

Pulmonary disease

Pleurisy: Sharp pain arising near the rib cage that increases with deep inspiration, often accompanied by fever, chills, malaise, cough

Pulmonary embolism or infarction: Sudden severe pain, usually accompanied by sudden dyspnea, hemoptysis, tachycardia, cyanosis, hypotension, anxiety

- Pneumothorax: Sudden severe pain that may radiate to shoulder, neck, or abdomen, usually accompanied by dyspnea and dry hacking cough, although small or slowly developing pneumothorax may produce minimal symptoms

- Pulmonary hypertension: Chest pain that may mimic angina, occurring with exertion and not at rest, accompanied by dyspnea, but is not relieved with NTG

- Lung cancer or pulmonary metastases: Pleural pain (see previous entry for pleurisy) with dyspnea and persistent cough

Other causes

Chest wall pain: More superficial, well-localized pain that can be evoked by chest palpation or deep breaths and may worsen with trunk motions; typically occurs after exertion and lasts for hours and is not relieved by rest or NTG

Dissecting aortic aneurysm: Sudden excruciating, deep pain, usually in the back or lower part of the abdomen (abdominal aortic aneurysms), which may radiate into the groin, buttocks, or legs; thoracic aortic aneurysms produce severe pain that penetrates to the back of the neck or between the scapulae

Continued

TABLE 6-10: Common Patient Complaints and Possible Causes and Differentiating Features—Cont'd

Complaint	Possible Causes and Differentiating Features
	Referred pain from the esophagus: Squeezing, aching substernal pain ("heart burn") that is precipitated by eating certain foods, swallowing hot or cold liquids, emotional stress; may radiate to one or both arms or to the back; may be relieved by antacids, NTG (due to relaxation of smooth muscle), and change of position from supine to upright; may be accompanied by pain on swallowing, dysphagia, and reflux of stomach acids
	Epigastric pain: Substernal, lower thoracic or upper abdominal discomfort that may radiate to the back; not associated with activity; often relieved by antacids or food
	Herpes zoster infections: Pain, itching, and hyperesthesia followed by skin eruptions that occur along a unilateral dermatome
Cough	**Pulmonary disease**
	Acute or chronic pulmonary infections: May be dry-sounding and nonproductive (e.g., pneumonia) or full-sounding and productive of purulent sputum (e.g., exacerbation of chronic bronchitis or CF)
	Pulmonary parenchymal inflammatory processes (e.g., asthma with tight-sounding productive cough that is often provoked by exercise or exposure to cold air or allergens, usually accompanied by wheezes; chronic bronchitis with full-sounding productive cough that is usually worse in the early mornings; interstitial lung disease with dry, irritating cough)
	Other (e.g., tumors, foreign body aspiration, pulmonary infarction): Nonproductive, although hemoptysis may be present
	Cardiovascular disease
	Left ventricular failure: Persistent, spasmodic cough, especially when recumbent; often productive of white or pink frothy sputum
	Thoracic aortic aneurysm: Dry, nonproductive cough due to compression of the trachea or bronchi
	Postnasal drip: Productive cough that is most prominent in early morning, sensation of secretions coming from nasopharynx that provoke throat clearing or coughing
	Gastroesophageal problems: Nonproductive cough occurring mostly at night or after meals (due to microaspiration or irritation of cough receptors in lower esophagus)
	Medications (e.g., ACE inhibitors, β-blockers, chemotherapeutic agents causing interstitial lung disease): Usually dry, nonproductive cough
Dyspnea, shortness of breath	**Cardiac dysfunction**
	LV systolic dysfunction (e.g., CAD, CHF, hypertensive heart disease, dilated cardiomyopathy, valvular dysfunction, myocarditis): Dyspnea occurs on exertion initially (i.e., DOE) but may develop at rest during uncontrolled CHF; often accompanied by lightheadedness or dizziness, fatigue/weakness, hypotension, possible wheezing; worse on lying flat (i.e., orthopnea)
	Impaired LV filling (i.e., diastolic dysfunction, as in HTN, LV hypertrophy, restrictive cardiomyopathy, pericardial tamponade, constrictive pericarditis): Dyspnea same as for systolic dysfunction (see previous entry)
	Pulmonary disease
	Chronic obstructive pulmonary disease: Discomfort of not being able to get enough air, often accompanied by uncomfortable sensation that another breath is urgently needed before exhalation is completed; develops with exertion initially but may occur at rest once cor pulmonale is present
	Restrictive lung dysfunction: Feeling of inability to get enough air in accompanied by tachypnea, especially on exertion
	Mixed obstructive–restrictive defects (e.g., pulmonary edema, occupational lung disease): Specific symptoms (see previous two entries) vary with the specific pathology and dominant features
	Other causes
	Anemia: Rapid, deep breathing to compensate for ↓ oxygen-carrying capacity of blood
	↑ Demand for oxygen (e.g., exercise, sepsis): deeper breaths with increased RR
	Peripheral arterial disease: ↑ Breathing induced by lactic acidosis, which is provoked by anaerobic metabolism when insufficient O_2 is delivered to exercising muscles
	Metabolic acidosis: Rapid, deep breathing to blow off excessive CO_2 resulting from buffering of acidosis
	Deconditioning: ↑ Ventilation due to inefficiency of oxygen transport system at all levels

Continued

TABLE 6-10: Common Patient Complaints and Possible Causes and Differentiating Features—Cont'd

Complaint	Possible Causes and Differentiating Features
	Psychogenic: Hyperventilation with precisely regular RR except for possible breath-holding episodes if anxiety reaction and very irregular breathing with periods of hyperventilation and hypoventilation if malingering
Edema, swelling (weight gain >3 lb in 1 d is earliest indicator of fluid retention)	RV or biventricular failure (e.g., CAD, CHF, valvular disease, cardiomyopathy, pulmonary HTN, cor pulmonale): Edema develops in feet, ankles, and legs when upright or after DOE, increasing as the day progresses, and often diminishing during the night; associated with DOE, fatigue/weakness, and lightheadedness or dizziness; digits are often cool and cyanotic (due to low cardiac output and venous congestion); hepatomegaly, abdominal edema (i.e., ascites), and JVD may also be present
	Fluid overload (e.g., kidney disease, postoperative state): Edema occurs in dependent tissues; associated with multiple other systemic manifestations in renal failure (see page 135)
	Venous disease (venous valve incompetence, venous obstruction, thrombophlebitis): Edema may be unilateral or bilateral; increases when limb is dependent and decreases with periods of elevation; there may be pain during ambulation
	Lymphatic incompetence: Edema may be unilateral or bilateral, depending on location of obstruction, which can be caused by trauma, infection, neoplasm, radiation, or surgery; exacerbated by limb dependency and improved by elevation and use of compression garment
	Other (e.g., medications, cirrhosis, inflammation, trauma, malnutrition, hypoproteinemia, anemia)
Fatigue, weakness	Poor LV function (e.g., CAD, CHF, hypertensive heart disease, valvular dysfunction, cardiomyopathy, myocarditis): Tends to be related to exertion (due to inadequate cardiac output)
	Arrhythmias (e.g., paroxysmal supraventricular tachycardia, frequent ventricular ectopy) that reduce cardiac output
	Cor pulmonale and RV dysfunction limiting RV, and therefore LV, output
	Multiple other causes
	Depression, anxiety, emotional stress: Fatigue tends to be constant
	Illness/disease causing reduced delivery of oxygen and/or nutrients to muscles or impaired use of nutrients for energy production, etc. (e.g., anemia, dehydration [diarrhea, vomiting], fever; hypothyroidism, hypoxemia, hyperglycemia, hypocalcemia)
	• Sleep deprivation (e.g., sleep disorders, fibromyalgia): Fatigue is usually mental and physical
	Inadequate nutrition (and thus impaired energy production): increases on exertion
	Medications (e.g., β-blockers, other antihypertensives causing orthostatic hypotension)
	Treatment interventions (e.g., chemotherapy or radiation therapy): often improves with regular exercise
	• Chronic fatigue syndrome: Severe, incapacitating fatigue that persists for >6 mo that is not relieved by rest and is aggravated by physical or mental activity; frequently accompanied by cognitive dysfunction, joint and muscle pain, sore throat, tender lymph nodes, headaches
	• Mitral valve prolapse: Profound fatigue not associated with exercise or stress that occurs in some patients because of abnormal autonomic nervous system function
	Deconditioning (impaired delivery and utilization of oxygen and nutrients for energy production)
Hemoptysis	Pulmonary infections (e.g., bronchiectasis, TB, fungus), bronchogenic carcinoma, rupture of lung abscess, pulmonary infarction
	Mitral stenosis, Eisenmenger's syndrome, aortic aneurysm
Leg pain on exertion	Peripheral arterial disease: Intermittent claudication (pain, ache, sense of fatigue or other discomfort that occurs in the affected muscle group with exercise and resolves within several minutes of rest); may be rest pain with severe disease (pain or paresthesias, usually in the foot or toes, that occurs with critical limb ischemia; worsens on leg elevation and improves with leg dependency).
	Arthritis of the knees or hips: Pain usually localizes to the affected joint(s) and can be elicited by palpation and range-of-motion maneuvers
	Musculoskeletal injuries (e.g., muscle fiber microtears, stress fracture): Usually characterized by localized tenderness

Continued

TABLE 6-10: Common Patient Complaints and Possible Causes and Differentiating Features—Cont'd

Complaint	Possible Causes and Differentiating Features
	Lumbosacral radiculopathy (e.g., sciatica due to degenerative joint disease, herniated disc, spinal stenosis): Pain in the buttock, hip, thigh, calf, and/or foot with walking, often after very short distances, or even with standing; sometimes referred to as *neurogenic pseudoclaudication*
	Venous insufficiency: Venous claudication that results from impaired blood flow provoked by venous HTN and congestion; often associated with LE edema and venous stasis pigmentation
	Extravascular compression (e.g., anterior compartment syndrome)
	Peripheral neuropathy (e.g., diabetes mellitus)
Lightheadedness, dizziness	Hypotension (causing reduced perfusion and therefore oxygen delivery to the brain)
	Decreased cardiac output (e.g., LV dysfunction or outflow obstruction, RV failure, orthostasis, Valsalva maneuver)
	Excessive peripheral vasodilation, which reduces venous return and therefore cardiac output
	Cerebral ischemia (cerebral or vertebral artery insufficiency, thrombosis, embolism, or hemorrhage)
	Hyperventilation (causing hypocapnia and alkalemia)
	Hypoglycemia (insufficient glucose supply for adequate brain function)
Orthopnea or PND	CHF (increased venous return and preload challenging severely impaired LV)
	COPD (increased venous return and preload challenging severely impaired RV)
Pallor or cyanosis	Inadequate cardiac output (e.g., LV dysfunction or outflow obstruction, RV failure): Causes generalized pallor or peripheral cyanosis (bluish tint in fingertips, toes, nose, nail beds)
	Reduced peripheral perfusion (e.g., PAD, venous congestion): Causes pallor or cyanosis in affected limb
	Hypoxemia: Causes central cyanosis seen in mucous membranes, such as tongue and lips
	Pulmonary disease (insufficient gas exchange producing O_2 saturation <85%)
	Congenital heart disease with right-to-left shunting
	Anemia (reduced O_2 delivery to peripheral tissues)
Palpitations	Premature atrial contractions/complexes
	Premature ventricular contractions/complexes
	Paroxysmal atrial/supraventricular tachycardia
	Atrial fibrillation or flutter
	Ventricular tachycardia
Syncope, near syncope	Severely reduced cardiac output causing hypoperfusion of the brain
	Arrhythmias (e.g., profound bradycardia, second- or third-degree AV block, rapid tachycardia of any origin, asystole, ventricular fibrillation)
	• LV failure or outflow obstruction (e.g., aortic stenosis, hypertrophic obstructive cardiomyopathy, coarctation of the aorta)
	• Other CV disease (cardiac tamponade, aortic dissection)
	• Orthostatic hypotension, vasovagal reaction, Valsalva maneuver
	• RV outflow obstruction or failure (pulmonary stenosis, acute pulmonary embolus, pulmonary HTN)
	Cerebrovascular accident, transient ischemic attack, seizure
	Hyperventilation (see previous entries for lightheadedness/dizziness)
	Hypoglycemia (see previous entries for lightheadedness/dizziness)
	Unknown etiology

ACE, Angiotensin-converting enzyme; AV, atrioventricular; CAD, coronary artery disease; CF, cystic fibrosis; CHF, congestive/chronic heart failure; COPD, chronic obstructive pulmonary disease; CV, cardiovascular; DOE, dyspnea on exertion; ECG, electrocardiogram; echo, echocardiography; HTN, hypertension; JVD, jugular venous distension; LE, lower extremity; LV, left ventricular; NTG, nitroglycerin; PAD, peripheral arterial disease; PND, paroxysmal nocturnal dyspnea; RR, respiratory rate; RV, right ventricular; TB, tuberculosis.

Data from Goodman CC, Snyder TEK. *Differential Diagnosis for Physical Therapists: Screening for Referral.* St. Louis: Saunders; 2007; and Hillegass E. Assessment procedures. In Hillegass EA, Sadowsky HS, editors. *Essentials of Cardiopulmonary Physical Therapy.* 2nd ed. Philadelphia: Saunders; 2001.

establishing rapport with the patient and family, discerning their level of understanding of the medical problem(s), and ascertaining their goals and expectations for rehabilitation.

Many clinicians working in outpatient facilities use questionnaires to expedite data gathering. These allow patients to describe in advance all symptoms, medical conditions, surgeries, occupational and leisure activity habits, medications, and many other factors that may affect the selection of appropriate PT interventions in a manner that permits the patient sufficient time to recall details. The therapist can then go over relevant information during the patient/family interview, further increasing its accuracy.

Typically, interview questions should be open ended and straightforward. For example:

- What prompted you to come to the hospital/seek physical therapy?
- Do you ever have problems with shortness of breath, chest pain or discomfort, lightheadedness or dizziness, getting tired easily, palpitations, etc.?
- Do you experience any type of discomfort or pain with exertion? If it occurs during ambulation, at what distance, speed, or incline? What about stairs?
- Can you describe your symptoms for me?
- What brings on your symptoms? What kinds of things are you doing immediately before or at the time of the onset of your symptoms?
- Are your symptoms aggravated by certain positions, such as lying flat or on one side or the other?
- How long have you had these symptoms?
- Do the symptoms interfere with things you would like to do? Such as?
- Have you discovered any ways to relieve the symptoms?
- What has your doctor told you about your problem?
- Have you ever received physical therapy for this problem or any other problem?
- Have you ever smoked? How much and for how long?
- What would you say your major difficulty is right now?
- What would you like us to work on before you go home?
- What are your goals for your recovery?

 6.3 RED FLAGS

On the basis of the information obtained from the medical chart review, the patient/family interview, or both, the therapist might identify potential problems related to patient evaluation and treatment planning. Diagnoses and situations that present relative contraindications to exercise or require caution are listed in Table 6-11. Depending on the circumstances and the therapist's experience and comfort level, the therapist may decide to proceed slowly with careful monitoring of the patient's responses to positional changes and minimal activities. If these results are normal or nearly normal, the therapist may decide to proceed with the activity evaluation. If there is any question about the patient's status, consultation with the referring physician is recommended. However, certain circumstances present absolute contraindications to exertion of any kind, as listed in Table 6-12, and require physician clearance before proceeding with PT evaluation and treatment.

Beyond the primary diagnosis and information related it, one of the most important details to ascertain from a patient's medical history is the presence of problems that might limit her/his ability to perform rehabilitation activities and therefore necessitate modifications in the treatment plan. Of prime importance is the identification of a history of cardiopulmonary dysfunction or any cardiovascular risk factors (see Table 4-7 on page 103) that might increase the risk of adverse exercise responses or cardiovascular events.

RISK STRATIFICATION FOR CARDIAC EVENTS DURING EXERCISE PARTICIPATION

The American College of Sports Medicine (ACSM) recommends stratifying individuals without known cardiovascular disease into one of three risk categories,[2] which will indicate the level of monitoring that the therapist should perform during the evaluation. Those who fall into the high-risk category will require closer clinical monitoring than those with low risk, although all should receive assessment of vital signs, both at rest and during activity.

- *Low risk:* Men less than 45 years of age and women less than 55 years of age who are asymptomatic and have no more than one cardiovascular risk factor listed in Table 4-7 (see page 103)
- *Moderate risk:* Men age 45 years or older and women age 55 years or older, or those who have two or more risk factors from Table 4-7
- *High risk:* Individuals with one or more major signs or symptoms suggestive of cardiovascular disease (cardiac, peripheral vascular, or cerebrovascular disease), pulmonary disease (COPD, asthma, interstitial lung disease, or cystic fibrosis), or metabolic disorders (diabetes mellitus, thyroid disorders, or renal or liver disease).

Cardiac patients can also be stratified according to risk for exercise-induced complications.[63] The higher the risk category, the more closely they should be monitored during exercise and physical therapy interventions.

- Low-risk level
  ‣ Individuals with a history of a cardiac abnormality and
  ‣ No significant left ventricular (LV) dysfunction (resting ejection fraction [EF] ≥50%)
  ‣ Presence of normal physiological responses and functional status of at least 7 METs (metabolic equivalents for energy expenditure) on exercise testing
  ‣ No history of myocardial ischemia or other significant symptoms of exercise intolerance (unusual shortness of breath, lightheadedness, or dizziness) during exercise testing and recovery
  ‣ No history of resting or exercise-induced complex arrhythmias
  ‣ No history of congestive heart failure
  ‣ Status/post uncomplicated MI or revascularization procedure
  ‣ Absence of clinical depression
- Intermediate-risk level
  ‣ Mildly to moderately depressed LV function (resting EF 40% to 49%)
  ‣ Presence of angina or other significant symptoms of exercise intolerance only at high levels of exertion (≥7 METs)

TABLE 6-11: Patient Diagnoses or Situations That Present Relative Contraindications to Exercise or That Require Caution

Diagnosis	Important Considerations
Acute MI within past 2–3 mo	Area of infarction is still undergoing remodeling with scar formation, so vigorous activities should be avoided
Alcoholic hangover	The patient is clearly not functioning normally and may be dehydrated. The patient's physiological responses to activity may be exaggerated
h/o angina, especially if recent	There is potential for myocardial ischemia, particularly on exertion; therefore, monitoring of vital signs and symptoms is important
Angina (recurrent) after an MI	Additional myocardium is at risk for infarction, so extreme caution is warranted
Arrhythmias	The patient's BP should be taken to determine whether an arrhythmia is hemodynamically significant (see page 113)
Cardiac valve disease	Most defects are tolerated well for decades, but some (e.g., severe aortic stenosis or mitral regurgitation) can cause major problems if the patient overexerts. Lack of symptoms along with normal BP responses during exertion indicate safety to proceed
Cerebral dysfunction: Dizziness, vertigo	The patient runs an increased risk of falling. Cause could be related to cardiovascular dysfunction*
Drug intake	Decongestants, bronchodilators, and diet pills increase the work of the heart, usually through ↑ HR, and may ↑ the HR response to activity
Edema, weight gain of sudden onset	Increasing edema and weight gain >3 lbs in 24 hr could indicate onset of RV or biventricular heart failure
Emotional turmoil	The patient is already under the influence of increased sympathetic nervous system stimulation with elevated demands on the cardiovascular and respiratory systems
Environmental extremes: Weather, air pollution	Workload on the heart is increased even at rest; exercise responses may be exaggerated
Evidence of end-organ damage in HTN: Retinopathy, renal impairment, LV hypertrophy	BP must be controlled at rest and during exercise to avoid further end-organ damage
Mural thrombus	RV thrombus creates potential for pulmonary emboli; LV thrombus may result in cerebral or peripheral emboli
Overindulgence: heavy meal within 2 h, caffeine	Workload on the heart is increased even at rest; exercise responses may be exaggerated
Positive exercise test after acute MI	Additional myocardium is at risk for infarction, so extreme caution is warranted
h/o pulmonary edema, CHF	Careful monitoring of vital signs and symptoms is indicated to prevent overexertion
Recent pericarditis or myocarditis	During recovery from cardiac inflammation, activity should be low level and physiological monitoring of exercise responses should be performed in order to determine how much activity the patient can perform safely
Severe sunburn	Fluid shifts to the peripheral tissues (i.e., edema) and pain increase the workload of the heart at rest

↑, Increased; BP, blood pressure; CHF, congestive heart failure; h/o, history of; HR, heart rate; HTN, hypertension; LV, left ventricular; MI, myocardial infarction; RV, right ventricular.
*See Table 6-10.

▸ Mild to moderate level of silent ischemia during exercise testing or recovery (<2-mm ST-segment depression from baseline)
▸ Functional capacity less than 5 or 6 METs on graded exercise test 3 or more weeks after MI
▸ Failure to comply with exercise intensity prescription
• High-risk level
   ▸ Severely depressed LV function (EF <40%)
   ▸ Presence of angina or other significant symptoms at low levels of exertion (<5 METs) or during recovery
   ▸ Presence of abnormal physiological responses with exercise testing (e.g., chronotropic incompetence or flat or decreasing

systolic BP with increasing workloads) or during recovery (e.g., severe postexercise hypotension or persistent tachycardia)
▸ High level of silent myocardial ischemia (≥2-mm ST-segment depression from baseline) during exercise testing or recovery
▸ History of complex ventricular arrhythmias at rest or appearing or increasing with exercise
▸ History of cardiac arrest or sudden cardiac death
▸ Complicated or high-risk MI or revascularization procedure (e.g., anterior infarction, large infarct size, infarct extension, congestive heart failure [CHF], cardiogenic shock, and/or complex ventricular arrhythmias)
▸ Presence of congestive heart failure

TABLE 6-12: Absolute Contraindications to Exercise

Absolute Contraindications	Important Considerations
Unstable or rest angina	Myocardial oxygen demand exceeds supply during minimal exertion or even at rest; therefore, patient will not tolerate much physical therapy
A recent significant change in the resting ECG suggesting significant ischemia, recent MI (within 2 d), or other acute cardiac event	There is a high risk for complications during exertion until status is determined and stabilized
Dangerous arrhythmias causing symptoms of hemodynamic compromise (e.g., sustained supraventricular tachycardia, ventricular tachycardia, second- or third-degree heart block)	Exercise demands ↑ cardiac output that cannot be produced when the heart is not pumping effectively, as in hemodynamically significant arrhythmias
Symptomatic CHF/pulmonary edema	The heart is unable to pump adequate cardiac output to meet metabolic demands at rest or during minimal activity, let alone those of physical therapy
Suspected or known dissecting aneurysm	Increasing BP, as with exertion, places additional stress on an already weakened arterial wall, which could provoke rupture
Severe aortic stenosis or obstructive hypertrophic cardiomyopathy	There is an ↑ risk of exercise-induced syncope and sudden death
Acute pulmonary embolus or pulmonary infarction	There is an ↑ risk of arrhythmias and sudden death
Uncontrolled diabetes mellitus	When blood sugar is >250–300 mg/dL, an insulin deficiency impairs glucose uptake by exercising muscles so that ↑ hepatic glucose production exceeds peripheral utilization, so exertion will provoke even more marked hyperglycemia
Uncontrolled HTN: Resting SBP >200 mm Hg and/or resting DBP >110 mm Hg	LV and arterial wall tensions are already extremely high at rest and will increase further during exertion. In addition, if any end-organ damage exists, there is risk of ↑ morbidity
Persistent hypotension after MI (SBP <90 mm Hg)	This is an indication of very poor LV function at rest and poor ability to tolerate the demands of exertion
Acute systemic infection, accompanied by fever, body aches, or swollen lymph glands	With acute illness, the cardiovascular and immune systems are subjected to increased demands, so exercise is not recommended
Acute pericarditis or myocarditis	Increasing the demands on an inflamed heart is not advised

↑, Increased; BP, blood pressure; CHF, congestive heart failure; DBP, diastolic blood pressure; ECG, electrocardiogram; HTN, hypertension; LV, left ventricular; MI, myocardial infarction; SBP, systolic blood pressure.

▸ Presence of signs or symptoms of postevent/postprocedure ischemia
▸ Presence of clinical depression

6.4 PHYSICAL THERAPY EXAMINATION

The physical therapy examination of cardiopulmonary function includes a wide variety of tests and measures, as delineated in the *Guide to Physical Therapist Practice*, including those assessing ventilation and respiration/gas exchange, circulation, muscle performance, range of motion, posture, self-care and home management, and aerobic capacity/endurance.[4] PTs perform many of the same cardiopulmonary measures conducted by physicians and nurses: inspection, palpation, percussion, and auscultation. However, PTs go beyond these measures to assess the functional impact of any cardiopulmonary abnormalities, as well as those of other systems, on patient performance. Furthermore, each time the therapist sees the patient, the patient's status is reassessed before, during, and after the treatment session so that appropriate modifications can be incorporated as the need arises.

INSPECTION

Although objective observations of a patient's appearance are an essential component of all physical therapy evaluations, they are especially important in patients with possible cardiopulmonary dysfunction, because subtle changes often represent important variations in clinical status. During the assessment process, inspection serves to detect problems that require further evaluation using more specific PT tests and measures.

• Important components of cardiopulmonary inspection and specific observations include the following:
  ▸ General appearance
    ⊙ Level of consciousness (e.g., alert, automatic, confused, delirious, stuporous, semicomatose, comatose)
    ⊙ Body type (e.g., obese, normal, cachectic)
    ⊙ Level of distress (e.g., cardiac: chest discomfort, dyspnea, lightheadedness, or dizziness; pulmonary: use of accessory muscles, pursed-lip breathing, speech interrupted to take breaths, decreased breath control, signs of respiratory distress [listed in Box 6-1])

BOX 6-1: Clinical Manifestations of Respiratory Distress

- Dyspnea, shortness of breath
- Tachypnea
- Use of accessory muscles of respiration
- Retractions (suprasternal, subcostal, substernal, intercostal)
- Nasal flaring
- Cyanosis
- Stridor
- Change in mental status (agitation, confusion, diminished level of arousal, orientation, or ability to follow commands)

TABLE 6-13: Clinical Manifestations of Hypoxemia

Pao$_2$ (mm Hg)	Signs and Symptoms
80–100	Normal
60–80	Moderate tachycardia
	Dyspnea
50–60	Malaise, nausea
	Possible onset of respiratory distress
	Central cyanosis with or without peripheral cyanosis
	Lightheadedness, vertigo
	Restlessness
	Poor judgment, motor incoordination, slower reaction times
	Fatigue, somnolence, apathy
35–50	Respiratory distress
	Arrhythmias
	Marked confusion, agitation
25–35	Marked respiratory distress
	Peripheral vasoconstriction, ↓ renal blood flow + urine output
	Poor oxygenation, lactic acidosis
	Lethargy, loss of consciousness
<25	Hypoventilation, apnea (due to depression of respiratory centers)
	Bradycardia, myocardial depression, shock
	Cardiac arrest

↓, Decreased; Pao$_2$, partial pressure of arterial oxygen.

⊙ Any monitoring or support equipment in use (e.g., supplemental oxygen, cardiac monitor, oxygen saturation monitor, arterial line, pulmonary arterial or central lines, mechanical ventilation, intraaortic balloon pump, ventricular assist device)

⊙ Presence of incisions, wounds, dressings, casts, etc.

⊙ Other (e.g., pallor, cyanosis, sweating/diaphoresis, flushing, tremors)

▸ Head and neck

⊙ Facial expressions indicating distress or fatigue

⊙ Central cyanosis (lips, tongue) indicating hypoxemia (Table 6-13)

⊙ Use of accessory muscles of respiration, muscular hypertrophy

⊙ Jugular venous distension (distended above the level of the clavicles when sitting or in semi-Fowler position ≥45°)

▸ Chest

⊙ Position of trachea (e.g., midline vs. deviated to one side)

⊙ Configuration (e.g., normal vs. congenital abnormalities [pectus excavatum or carinatum] or barrel-shaped chest with anteroposterior [AP] diameter at least twice that of the transverse diameter and widening of the rib angles) (Figure 6-6)

⊙ Symmetry at rest and with respiration (e.g., asymmetry due to chest trauma, thoracic surgery, scoliosis, or underlying lung pathology)

⊙ Respiratory-related movements (e.g., suprasternal, subcostal, substernal, or intercostal retractions)

⊙ Nonrespiratory movements (e.g., visible pulsations)

▸ Breathing pattern

⊙ Respiratory rate (normal for adults: 12–20 breaths/min; late childhood: 15–25; early childhood: 20–40; newborns: 30–60; rates >25 breaths/min in adults may indicate primary pulmonary dysfunction, metabolic acidosis, or systemic stress [e.g., sepsis or shock] whereas rates <10 breaths/min may denote CNS abnormality or metabolic alkalosis)

⊙ Inspiratory muscles employed (e.g., normal relaxed breathing with abdominal rise followed by symmetric expansion

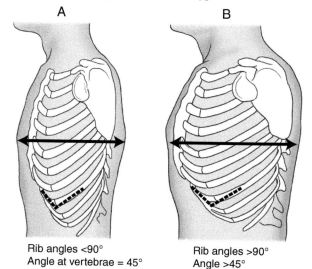

Rib angles <90°
Angle at vertebrae = 45°

Rib angles >90°
Angle >45°

Figure 6-6: A, A normal chest configuration with normal anteroposterior (AP) diameter, rib angles less than 90°, and attaching at the vertebrae at an approximately 45° angle (so the diaphragm has a normal domed shape). **B,** A chronically hyperinflated chest with increased AP diameter, rib angles greater than 90°, and vertebral attachment angles greater than 45° (causing the diaphragm to be flattened).

TABLE 6-14: Common Breathing Patterns

Breathing Pattern	Characteristic Features
Eupnea	Normal rate, depth, and rhythm of breathing
Apnea	Cessation of breathing after an expiration, interrupted by eventual inspiration or becomes fatal
Tachypnea	Increased breathing rate, usually shallow with regular rhythm (as in restrictive lung dysfunction)
Bradypnea	Slow rate, shallow or normal depth, regular rhythm (as in drug overdose)
Hyperpnea	Increased breathing due to increased depth, but usually not increased rate
Cheyne-Stokes (periodic) respiration	Cyclic waxing and waning of depth of breathing with periods of apnea interspersed between cycles (seen in severe CNS lesions)
Apneustic breathing	Cessation of breathing after an inspiration, interrupted by periodic expiration (seen in brainstem disorders)
Biot's breathing	Irregular breathing with slow, shallow breaths and periods of apnea (seen in meningitis)
Cluster breathing	Clusters of normal breaths separated by irregular pauses (seen in high medullary or low pontine lesions)
Hyperventilation	Fast, deep breathing so that ventilation exceeds metabolic needs (e.g., anxiety attack)
Kussmaul breathing	Marked continuous hyperventilation with increased rate and depth of breathing in order to eliminate excess carbon dioxide (e.g., diabetic ketoacidosis)
Doorstop respirations	Normal breathing rate and rhythm but with abrupt cessation of inspiration, usually due to pain (seen in pleurisy)
Prolonged expiration	Breathing marked by fast inspiration and slow, prolonged expiration so that normal rate, depth, and rhythm is maintained (seen in COPD)
Pursed-lip breathing	Use of almost-closed (pursed) lips during expiration to maintain positive pressure within the bronchioles and thus prevent premature collapse of the weakened airways; seen in patients with emphysema
Paradoxical breathing	Two types: Inward motion of the abdomen with expansion of the rib cage on inspiration (seen in diaphragmatic fatigue or isolated paralysis with intact accessory muscles) Strong contraction of the diaphragm so that abdomen rises with collapse of upper chest on inspiration (seen with strong diaphragm but absence of intercostal spaces; e.g., C_5 or lower quadriplegia)
Respiratory alternans	Cyclic alternation between a series of diaphragmatic breaths (i.e., solely abdominal rise) and a series of predominantly accessory muscle breaths (i.e., mostly rib cage movements); seen in respiratory muscle fatigue

COPD, Chronic obstructive pulmonary disease.

of the lateral ribs without recruitment of any accessory muscles vs. obvious use of accessory muscles [which may be hypertrophied] indicating increased work of breathing)

⊙ Characteristics of expiration (e.g., normal passive expiration vs. active contraction of abdominals, prolonged expiration)

⊙ Inspiratory-to-expiratory (I/E) ratio (normal, 1:2; with obstructive disease expiration becomes prolonged so I/E ratio increases to 1:3 or 1:4; with tachypnea expiration is shortened so I/E ratio decreases to 1:1, leading to increased air trapping in COPD). The I/E ratio also decreases with respiratory distress as the patient struggles to breathe in and the expiratory phase shortens, which creates a vicious cycle.

⊙ Presence of abnormal breathing patterns (Table 6-14 and Figure 6-7). The clinical manifestations of respiratory muscle fatigue are listed in Box 6-2.

▸ Cough
⊙ Characteristics (e.g., strength/force, depth, length, dry vs. full-sounding)
⊙ Production of secretions (e.g., dry versus productive, with quantity, color, smell, consistency of sputum)

▸ Extremities
⊙ Peripheral pulses
⊙ Nicotine stains on fingers
⊙ Digital clubbing (Figure 6-8)
⊙ Edema
⊙ Cyanosis indicating poor peripheral perfusion (e.g., low cardiac output, peripheral vascular disease, congenital heart defects, Raynaud's phenomenon)
⊙ Trophic changes (muscle atrophy, hair loss, dry skin, skin color changes with limb elevation [blanching] vs. dependence [rubor] due to peripheral arterial disease)
⊙ Painful swollen joints (e.g., pseudohypertrophic pulmonary osteodystophy)

▸ Posture
⊙ Presence of any structural abnormalities (e.g., scoliosis or kyphosis)
⊙ Position of choice (e.g., leaning forward with arms supported; seen in patients with COPD)

▸ Range of motion

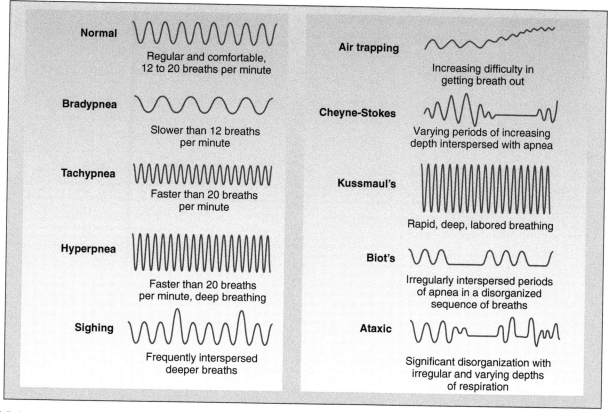

Figure 6-7: Various breathing patterns observed in patients. (Modified from Seidel HM, Ball JW, Dains JE, et al. *Mosby's Guide to Physical Examination.* 4th ed. St. Louis: Mosby; 1999.)

BOX 6-2: Clinical Manifestations of Respiratory Muscle Fatigue

- Rapid, shallow breathing
- Out-of-phase or incoordinated chest wall movements (paradoxical breathing, respiratory alternans
- Increased accessory muscle activity
- Dyspnea
- Signs and symptoms of hypoxemia (see Table 6-13)
- Signs and symptoms of carbon dioxide narcosis (hypercapnia):
  - ▸ Flushed/red skin coloring
  - ▸ Tachycardia
  - ▸ Hypertension or hypotension
  - ▸ Diaphoresis
  - ▸ Decreased mental status, confusion, drowsiness, coma
  - ▸ Headache
  - ▸ Muscular twitching, coarse myoclonic jerking, asterixis
  - ▸ Papilledema if chronic

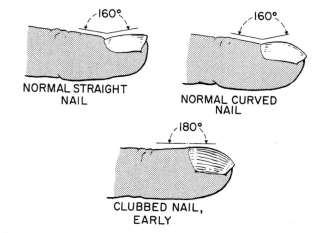

Figure 6-8: Digital clubbing compared with a normal finger with a straight nail or a curved nail. Note the base angle of at least 180°. Clubbing becomes more pronounced as lung disease progresses. (From Cherniack RM, Cherniack L. *Respiration in Health and Disease.* 3rd ed. Philadelphia: Saunders; 1983.)

⊙ Presence of any gross limitations of spine, shoulders, and neck
▸ Strength
⊙ Functional level as opposed to specific manual muscle testing

⊙ Presence of respiratory muscle weakness or dyscoordination especially in patients with neurologic or neuromuscular impairment (e.g., via gross assessment of inspiratory muscle strength and cough force)
▸ Mobility
⊙ Functional mobility (e.g., in bed, transfers, gait): Level of independence, use of any assistive devices

AUSCULTATION

Auscultation entails listening to the patient's chest with a stethoscope. To accurately identify a patient's lung or heart sounds, the therapist should have a stethoscope with properly fitting earpieces, adequate but not excessive tubing without cracks, and both a diaphragm and a bell. In addition, the room should be quiet and the patient should be positioned properly.

Lung Sounds

Auscultation of lung sounds can be accomplished with a basic stethoscope, which serves mainly as a filter to eliminate extraneous noises. With a little practice and some tutoring by a friendly nurse or physician, all PTs can become proficient at assessing lung sounds.

- The topographic relationships between the chest wall and the pulmonary segments are depicted in Figure 6-9.
- The proper technique consists of the following steps:
  ‣ Ideally, the patient should be in a quiet room in a sitting position with bare skin exposed and should breathe deeply but slowly through an open mouth.
  ‣ Using the diaphragm of the stethoscope, systematically listen to the entire lung space (anterior and then posterior and lateral, or vice versa) with at least one breath per

bronchopulmonary segment (as shown in Figure 6-10), alternating between similar locations on the right and left sides and comparing intensity, pitch, and quality, while moving from the upper to lower chest.
  ‣ If breath sounds are difficult to auscultate, the patient should be reminded to take deeper breaths through an open mouth (while avoiding hyperventilation).
  ‣ Specific precaution should be taken, as indicated:
    ⊙ Patients who are weak or have poor balance or orthostatic intolerance should be offered additional support in the sitting position to prevent falling.
    ⊙ The therapist should move slowly from one pulmonary segment to the next in order to avoid patient dizziness as a result of hyperventilation from deep breaths being performed too rapidly.
    ⊙ Appropriate draping should be maintained during auscultation so females are not embarrassed by having the chest bared.
- Common errors in auscultating lung sounds include the following:
  ‣ Listening to breath sounds through the patient's gown (the stethoscope should be placed directly against the patient's chest wall)

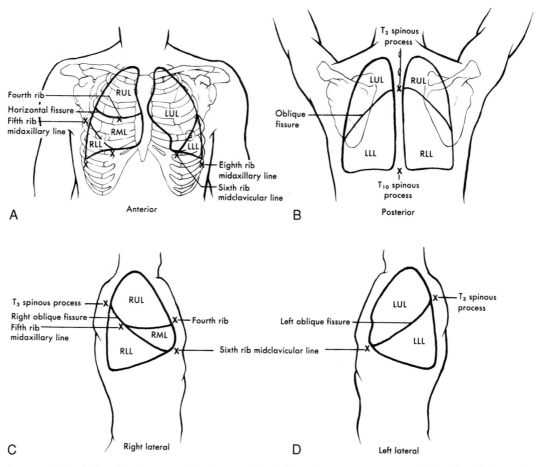

Figure 6-9: The topographic relationships between the chest wall and the pulmonary segments. **A,** Anterior. **B,** Posterior. **C** and **D,** Right and left lateral, respectively. (From Andreoli KG, Fowkes VK, Zipes DP, et al. *Comprehensive Cardiac Care: A Textbook for Nurses, Physicians, and Other Health Practitioners.* 6th ed. St. Louis: Mosby; 1987.)

- Lung sounds are divided into breath sounds and added, or adventitious, sounds:
  ▸ Over most lung areas, breath sounds are soft and rustling and are termed normal or vesicular (Figure 6-11). However, breath sounds over the area of the mainstem and segmental bronchi (upper intrascapular area) are somewhat more intense and higher in frequency and are called *bronchovesicular*.
  ▸ Abnormal conditions of the lungs can result in decreased, absent, or bronchial breath sounds, as described in Table 6-15.
  ▸ In addition, there may be adventitious sounds, such as crackles and wheezes, superimposed on normal or abnormal breath sounds.
  ▸ Vocal sounds are poorly transmitted through normal lungs (they are muffled, distant, and indistinct) but are transmitted more distinctly when there is consolidated lung tissue due to exudate (i.e., pneumonia) or mass (e.g., tumor):
    ⊙ Bronchophony (clearer transmission when the patient says "99")
    ⊙ Egophony (transmission of an "A" sound when the patient says "E")
    ⊙ Whispered pectoriloquy (greater transmission of whispered vocalizations)
- The lung sounds that occur with various pathologies can be found at the end of this chapter (see Table 6-34).
- Lung sounds should be evaluated both before and after treatment.
  ▸ With appropriate treatment, the pathological process may improve or resolve, and thus the posttreatment auscultative findings may differ from those noted before treatment.
  ▸ On the other hand, it is possible, on rare occasions, that the treatment procedures can result in a new acute pulmonary complication (e.g., bronchospasm or pneumothorax), which would be revealed during the reassessment.
  ▸ Overexertion in a patient with cardiac dysfunction may be manifested as the development of crackles at the lung bases after activity. The cause is poor left ventricular (LV) function with increasing filling pressures during activity resulting in increased pulmonary vascular pressures and exudation of fluid from the pulmonary capillaries into the interstitial space and possibly the alveoli.

Heart Sounds

Auscultation of the heart can provide valuable information regarding a patient's cardiac anatomy and function. Even if a PT is not skilled in auscultating heart sounds, s/he should be able to interpret the physician's observations in a patient's medical chart. The examiner listens to the individual heart sounds, noting their intensity, quality, and timing in the cardiac cycle as well as any additional sounds that are present.

- The technique for listening to heart sounds consists of the following steps:
  ▸ The patient should be lying in the supine position, with bare chest exposed, in a quiet, comfortable room and should breathe quietly through the nose.
  ▸ The entire chest is auscultated, using the diaphragm of the stethoscope and paying particular attention to the high-

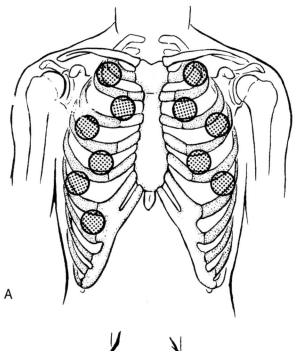

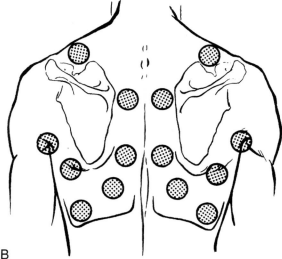

Figure 6-10: Areas to auscultate for breath sounds. **A,** Anterior chest. **B,** Posterior thorax. At least one breath should be taken per bronchopulmonary segment, comparing right and left sides while moving from upper to lower chest. (From Buckingham EB. *A Primer of Clinical Diagnosis.* 2nd ed. New York: Harper & Row; 1979.)

  ▸ Allowing stethoscope tubing to rub against bed rails or patient's gown (tubing should be kept free from contact with any objects during auscultation)
  ▸ Attempting to auscultate in a noisy room (television or radio should be turned off, other people in the room should be asked to maintain quiet or to leave the room)
  ▸ Interpreting chest hair sounds as adventitious lung sounds (chest hair can be wetted before auscultation if thick)
  ▸ Auscultating only the "convenient" areas (alert patients should sit up; comatose patients should be rolled onto their sides to auscultate posterior lobes)

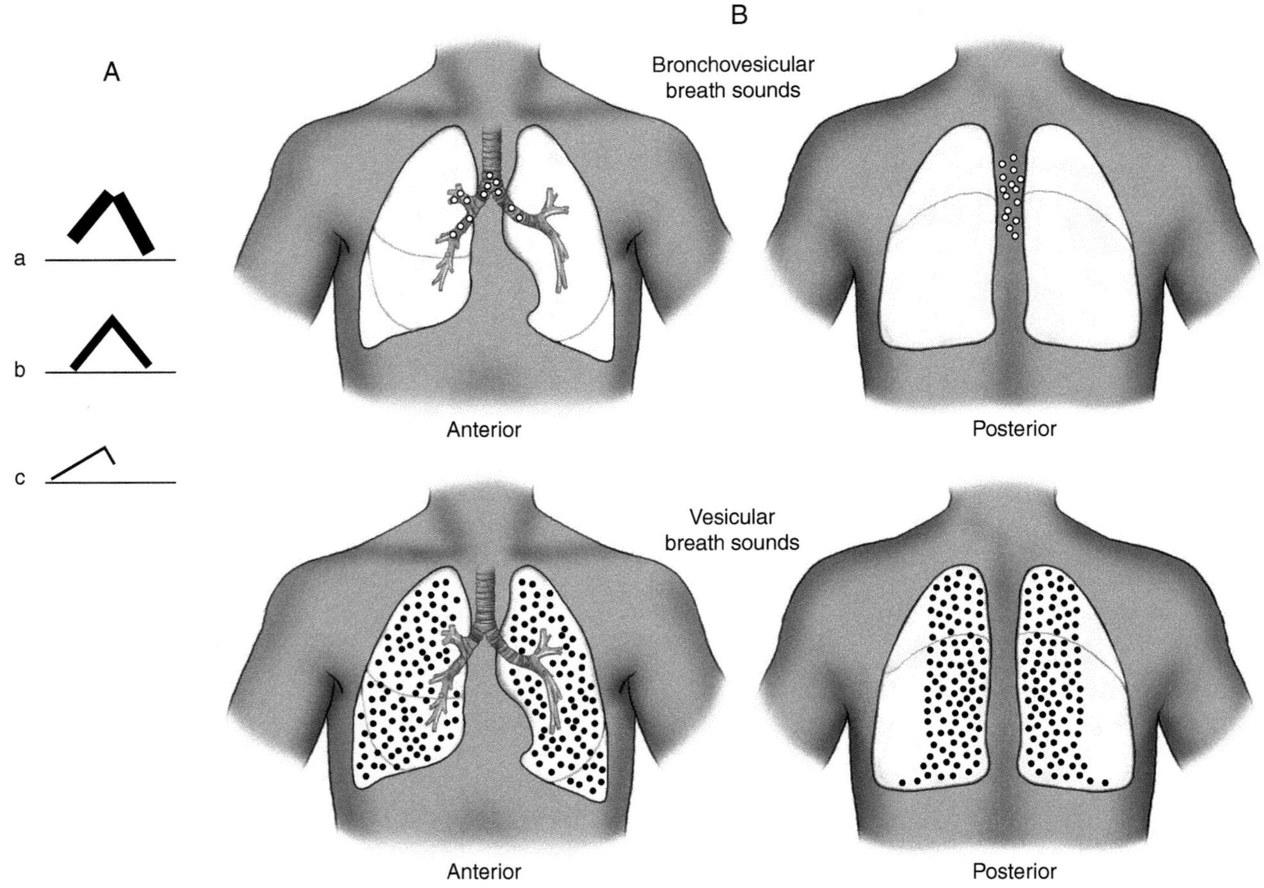

Figure 6-11: Normal breath sounds. **A,** Breath sound diagrams: Normal tracheobronchial *(a)*, bronchovesicular *(b)*, and vesicular *(c)* breath sounds. The upstroke represents inspiration and the downstroke expiration; the thickness of the line indicates the intensity of the sound. **B,** The positions on the anterior and posterior chest walls at which normal bronchovesicular and vesicular breath sounds are identified. (Redrawn from Wilkins RL, Hodgkin JE, Lopez B. *Lung Sounds: A Practical Guide.* St. Louis: Mosby; 1988.)

pitched sounds; the bell of the stethoscope is then used to accentuate lower frequency sounds.

▸ The clinician listens to five main topographic areas (Figure 6-12):
  ⊙ The *aortic area* is located near the second intercostal space just to the right of the sternum.
  ⊙ The *pulmonic area* is found at the second intercostal space to the left of the sternum.
  ⊙ The *third left intercostal space* can reveal murmurs of either aortic or pulmonary origin.
  ⊙ The *tricuspid area* is located at the lower left sternal border around the fourth or fifth intercostal space.
  ⊙ The *mitral area* is found at the apex of the heart, usually in the fifth left intercostal space, medial to the midclavicular line.

▸ Auscultation should be performed systematically so that each area is included, and attention is directed to both the intensity and timing, as well as any splitting, of the first and second heart sounds, and to any extra sounds and murmurs that may be present.

• The various heart sounds are described in Table 6-16, along with the most common causes of abnormalities.

• Although many cardiac sounds can change with the increased demands of physical activity, they are not typically auscultated during activity. However, it is important to reassess the cardiac sounds after exercise.

▸ The most significant change is the onset of a third heart sound (S_3) as a result of activity. This extra heart sound occurs during the rapid filling phase of the ventricles after the atrioventricular valves open and may indicate the development of diastolic dysfunction with reduced ventricular compliance because of delayed or impaired myocardial relaxation (e.g., myocardial ischemia, hypertension, valvular stenosis, cardiomyopathy) or difficulty filling a ventricle with increasing end-systolic volume (e.g., CHF, cardiomyopathy, valvular disease, congenital heart disease).[34] Thus, pulmonary pressures become elevated and new crackles may also be auscultated following exertion, as described previously (see page 245).

▸ Another significant finding is the onset of a new murmur following exertion (e.g., mitral regurgitation due to ischemia affecting the papillary muscles).

TABLE 6-15: Lung Sounds and Their Descriptions

Type of Sound	Description
Breath Sounds	
Normal or vesicular	Soft, low-pitched sounds heard throughout inspiration and the first third of expiration over most lung areas
Bronchovesicular	Medium-intensity and medium-pitched sounds with equal inspiratory and expiratory components without an intervening pause, which are heard over the carina and largest bronchi
Decreased	Lower intensity than normal, vesicular sounds; heard in hyperinflation (e.g., COPD) or hypoinflation (e.g., atelectasis, pneumothorax, and pleural effusion)
Absent	Lack of breath sounds; due to interference with transmission (e.g., large pleural effusion, pneumothorax, severe hyperinflation, obesity)
Bronchial	Loud, somewhat harsh, high-pitched, "tubular" sounds with equal inspiratory and expiratory components and an intervening pause; heard over areas of consolidation
Added Sounds	
Crackles	Discontinuous, nonmusical, crackling sounds (similar to the sound caused by rubbing several hairs together) heard most often on inspiration, which may result from the sudden opening of closed airways (e.g., atelectasis, fibrosis, pulmonary edema, or compression by pleural effusion) or the movement of secretions in the airways during inspiration and expiration; also called *rales*
Wheezes	Continuous, musical sounds of variable pitch and duration, which can be monophonic or polyphonic and heard on either inspiration, expiration (most common), or both; polyphonic wheezes occur when there is diffuse airway narrowing (as by bronchospasm or secretions), whereas monophonic wheezes are heard when there is localized stenosis; low-pitched wheezes are sometimes called *rhonchi*
Pleural rub	Inspiratory and expiratory grating, creaking sounds, like two pieces of sandpaper or leather being rubbed together, which are heard over the lower lateral lung areas and indicate pleural inflammation or reaction
Stridor	A continuous, monophonic, high-pitched crowing sound heard predominantly during inspiration, which is usually caused by inflammation and edema of the larynx and trachea (e.g. croup, epiglottitis, or after extubation) or other causes of upper airway obstruction
Vocal Sounds	
Normal	Soft, muffled, and indistinct sounds
Decreased	Weaker or softer than normal sounds; heard over pleural effusion, pneumothorax, and atelectasis, as well as fibrosis and airway obstruction
Absent	Lack of transmission of any vocal sounds; occurs over pleural effusion, pneumothorax, atelectasis, and obstructed airway
Increased	Louder, distinct voice transmission; heard over areas of consolidated lung tissue and pulmonary fibrosis
Bronchophony	Occurs when a patient is asked to say "99" and the words are transmitted clearly
Egophony	Demonstrated when a patient is asked to say "E" and it is heard as "A" (sometimes called E-to-A changes)
Whispered pectoriloquy	Evident when a patient is asked to whisper, and the words are distinctly heard with a stethoscope

COPD, Chronic obstructive pulmonary disease.

Heart Murmurs

Heart murmurs are vibrations of longer duration than the heart sounds and often represent turbulent flow across abnormal valves caused by congenital or acquired cardiac defects.

- The principal heart murmurs are presented in Figure 6-13.
- Heart murmurs are graded according to their intensity:
  - ▸ Grade 1: Murmur is barely audible with special effort.
  - ▸ Grade 2: Murmur is faint but easily heard.
  - ▸ Grade 3: Murmur is moderately loud.
  - ▸ Grade 4: Murmur is very loud; there may be a thrill.
  - ▸ Grade 5: Murmur is extremely loud; but one edge of the stethoscope must be on the chest to hear.
  - ▸ Grade 6: Murmur is exceptionally loud and is audible with the stethoscope just above the chest.

PALPATION

Abnormalities identified through the medical chart review, inspection, and auscultation can be further assessed by palpation. Through palpation, the clinician can determine the position of

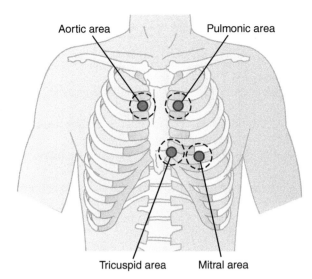

Figure 6-12: Areas to auscultate for sounds generated from the aortic, pulmonic, tricuspid, and mitral valves. In the normal heart, the mitral area is the apical pulse point and the point of maximal impulse (PMI). (From Guyton AC, Hall JE. *Textbook of Medical Physiology.* 11th ed. Philadelphia: Saunders; 2006.)

the trachea; the primary breathing pattern and active respiratory muscles; the extent and symmetry of chest expansion; the transmission of voice sounds as vibrations to the chest wall (i.e., vocal or tactile fremitus); the presence of chest wall pain, subcutaneous emphysema, or unstable rib fractures; the location of the cardiac apical impulse (i.e., the point of maximal impulse); and the status of the peripheral pulses.

Tracheal Deviation

- Tracheal position is evaluated to determine the presence of mediastinal shift, which occurs when there are differences in intrathoracic pressure or lung volumes between the two sides of the thorax.
- The techniques for palpation of tracheal position are as follows:
  ‣ The patient is seated upright with the neck slightly flexed (to relax the sternocleidomastoid muscles) and the chin in midline.
  ‣ The examiner inserts the tip of a fully extended index finger into the suprasternal notch, just medial to one sternoclavicular joint, and presses inward toward the cervical spine.
  ‣ The same technique is then repeated on the other side.
- The direction of tracheal deviation depends on the underlying pathology.
  ‣ Deviation occurs toward the side of the abnormality when there is loss of lung volume on one side (e.g., atelectasis, fibrosis, or surgical excision of lung tissue).
  ‣ Deviation is away from the side of the abnormality when there is an increase in volume on one side of the thorax (e.g., tension pneumothorax and pleural effusion).
  ‣ The mediastinum may be shifted to the right in older patients when no lung pathology exists as a result of elongation of an atherosclerotic aortic arch.

Breathing Pattern

- Palpation of upper and lower chest and abdominal movements reveals an individual's breathing pattern at rest and during deep breathing.
- By placing one hand on the midsternal area of the chest and the other in the abdominal area, the therapist notes the ratio of movement of the lower to upper chest.

TABLE 6-16: **Heart Sounds and Causes of Abnormalities**

Heart Sound	Comments
S_1 (first heart sound)	Associated with mitral and tricuspid closure and corresponds with the onset of ventricular systole
	MV sound (M_1) is best heard at apex whereas TV sound (T_1) is best heard at left lower sternal border
	↑: Mitral stenosis with mobile leaflets, LA myxoma, MV prolapse, short P–R interval, any condition causing tachycardia and vigorous ventricular contraction
	↓: Prolonged P–R interval, fibrotic or calcified MV, severe LV dysfunction, left bundle branch block, mitral regurgitation, ↓ sound conduction through chest wall
S_2 (second heart sound)	Associated with aortic and pulmonary valve closure and corresponds with the start of ventricular diastole
	Heard loudest in the aortic and pulmonic areas and is often split into two components, aortic (A_2) followed by pulmonic (P_2), with ↑ splitting on inspiration and ↓ splitting on expiration
	↑ A_2: Systemic HTN, congenital defects with the aorta arising anteriorly (e.g., transposition of the great arteries), aortic dilatation
	↑ P_2: Pulmonary HTN, thin-chested individuals
	↓ A_2: Aortic stenosis
	↓ P_2: Pulmonic stenosis

Continued

TABLE 6-16: Heart Sounds and Causes of Abnormalities—Cont'd

Heart Sound	Comments
S_2 (second heart sound)—Cont'd	
Fixed splitting	Delayed P_2 or early A_2:
	Acute pulmonary embolus, right bundle branch block, atrial septal defect, pulmonic stenosis
Wider splitting	Delayed PV closure:
	Proximal right bundle branch block, LV paced or ectopic beats, acute massive pulmonary embolus, RV failure, and some congenital heart defects
	Early AoV closure:
	Mitral regurgitation, ventricular septal defect
Parodoxical splitting	Delayed aortic closure:
	Left bundle branch block, RV paced or ectopic beats, LV outflow tract obstruction (e.g., aortic stenosis, obstructive hypertrophic cardiomyopathy), hypertensive heart disease, CAD, peripheral vasodilation, poststenotic dilation of the aorta, patent ductus arteriosus
S_3 (third heart sound): "ventricular gallop"	Associated with early rapid diastolic filling of the ventricles
	A low-pitched sound best heard with the patient lying on the left side so that the apex of the heart is closest to the chest wall
	May be heard in children and adults <40 yr of age, in which case it is termed *physiologic*
	Also commonly heard if:
	Impaired LV function of any cause with ↑ end-systolic volume (e.g., CAD, CHF, congenital heart disease, valvular disease, systemic or pulmonary HTN, cardiomyopathy)
	Constrictive pericarditis
	Hyperdynamic states (e.g., severe anemia, liver disease, thyrotoxicosis, systemic arteriovenous fistula, pregnancy)
S_4 (fourth heart sound): "atrial gallop"	Associated with ventricular filling due to atrial contraction
	A low-pitched sound heard late in diastole just before S_1
	Commonly heard if:
	LV or RV hypertrophy (e.g., outflow tract obstruction, systemic or pulmonary HTN, hypertrophic cardiomyopathy)
	Ischemic heart disease (e.g., acute myocardial ischemia or infarction, coronary artery bypass surgery)
	Hyperdynamic states (see previous entry for S_3)
	Acute valvular regurgitation (e.g., MV, AoV, TV)
	Arrhythmia (e.g., heart block, atrial flutter)
Summation gallop	Fusion of S_3 and S_4 and implies volume overload and need for more vigorous atrial contraction (e.g., dilated cardiomyopathy), especially with tachycardia
Ejection sounds	Associated with the opening of a stenotic semilunar valve or ejection of blood into a dilated aorta or pulmonary artery
Midsystolic clicks	Associated with maximal excursion of prolapsed valve leaflets and elongated chordae tendinae (e.g., MV prolapse)
Opening snaps	Diastolic sound associated with the opening of stenotic atrioventricular valves (e.g., mitral or tricuspid stenosis); occur before the S_3, if present

↑, Increased intensity; ↓, decreased intensity; AoV, aortic valve; CAD, coronary artery disease; CHF, congestive heart failure; HTN, hypertension; LA, left atrial; LV, left ventricular; MV, mitral valve; PV, pulmonary valve; RV, right ventricular; TV, tricuspid valve.

▸ Normally, quiet breathing is characterized by inspiratory abdominal distension (as the diaphragm descends and increased intraabdominal pressure forces the abdominal contents outward) followed by upward and outward movement of the lower ribs, which increases the transverse diameter of the chest. In many people there is minimal movement of the upper chest, whereas in others, particularly obese individuals and women with large breasts, upper chest movement may be more pronounced, producing increased anteroposterior expansion.

▸ In patients with COPD with lung hyperinflation, the barrel-shaped chest leads to flattening of the diaphragm, which reduces its mechanical advantage and force-generating

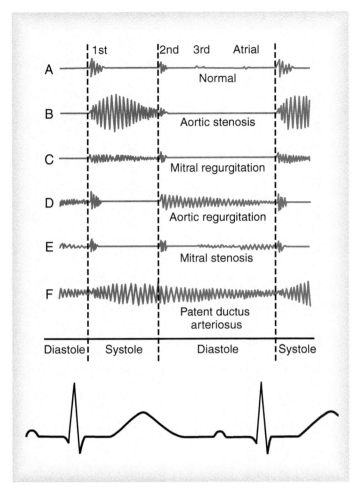

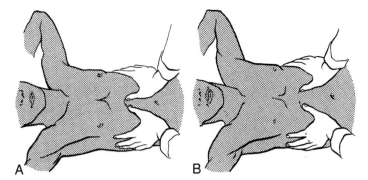

Figure 6-14: Palpation of diaphragmatic motion. **A,** At rest. **B,** At the end of a deep inspiration. (From Cherniack RM, Cherniack L. *Respiration in Health and Disease.* 3rd ed. Philadelphia: Saunders; 1983.)

Figure 6-13: Phonocardiograms from normal and abnormal heart sounds, shown in relation to the ECG. (Modified from Guyton AC, Hall JE. *Textbook of Medical Physiology.* 11th ed. Philadelphia: Saunders; 2006.)

ability and in severe hyperinflation causes its direction of force to become horizontal so that contraction produces an inward pull of the lower ribs. Therefore, these patients become more dependent on the upper rib cage contribution to chest expansion, rather than the lower chest or abdominal contribution.[25,27]

- Palpation of the lower, posterolateral chest motion can provide an overall sense of thoracic expansion and of the inspiratory-to-expiratory ratio (see page 242) and can be used therapeutically to offer sensory stimulation to facilitate lower lung expansion (see page 317).

Respiratory Muscle Activity

Palpation of respiratory muscle activity is used to assess diaphragmatic function and the presence of accessory muscle recruitment.

- Diaphragm (Figure 6-14)
  - With the patient lying supine and flat, the examiner places both hands lightly over the anterior chest with thumbs over costal margins so that their tips almost meet at the xiphoid. The patient is instructed to take a deep inspiration while the examiner's hands are allowed to move with chest expansion.

- Because of its dome shape, contraction of the diaphragm causes descent of the central tendon and elevation and outward rotation of the lower ribs. Therefore, normal diaphragmatic function results in equal upward motion of each costal margin, which produces an increase in the thoracic circumference of 2 to 3 in. Inward motion of the costal margins during inspiration occurs when the diaphragm is no longer dome-shaped, as in hyperinflation (e.g., COPD), or when there is fluid or air in the pleural space (i.e., pleural effusion or pneumothorax).
- Scalene muscles
  - With the patient sitting and facing away, the examiner places his or her hands on the upper trapezius muscles so that the fingers rest on the clavicles and the thumbs meet near the midline posteriorly. Activity of the scalene muscles is assessed as the patient takes at least two quiet breaths.
  - Normally, the scalene muscles are only minimally active during quiet breathing, mostly acting (in conjunction with the parasternal intercostals) to counteract the inward motion of the upper chest that would result from an unopposed drop in intrapleural pressure produced by diaphragmatic descent (as seen in individuals with high spinal cord lesions).[55] More pronounced scalene contraction signals the recruitment of the accessory muscles of inspiration, and therefore an increase in the work of breathing.

Chest Wall Excursion

- Movement of the chest wall, chest wall excursion (CWE), can be affected by a number of conditions. Unilateral restriction may occur when there is underlying lobar pneumonia, atelectasis, or fibrosis or with trauma or a surgical incision. Bilateral restriction occurs in patients with extensive pulmonary fibrosis, as well as in those with COPD and hyperinflated lungs.
- During palpation of CWE, the extent of movement, timing, and symmetry are assessed.
- Palpation of CWE is performed segmentally, comparing one side with the other during quiet and deep breathing, as illustrated in Figure 6-15.

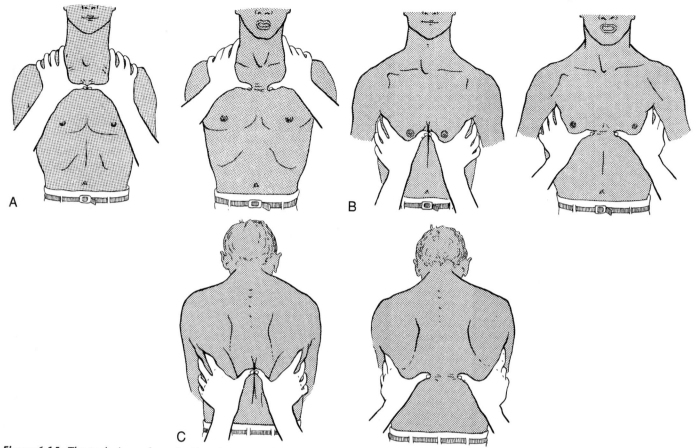

Figure 6-15: The techniques for palpating the expansion of the upper lobes **(A);** the right middle lobe and left lingula **(B);** and the lower lobes **(C).** (Modified from Cherniack RM, Cherniack L. *Respiration in Health and Disease.* 3rd ed. Philadelphia: Saunders; 1983.)

▸ Upper lobes
  ⊙ With the patient sitting or lying facing the examiner, the therapist places his/her palms anteriorly over the first four ribs with the fingertips extended over the trapezius muscles.
  ⊙ The skin is stretched downward until the palms are in the infraclavicular areas and then drawn medially until the tips of the extended thumbs meet in the midline.
  ⊙ With the elbows and shoulders maintained in a relaxed position, the therapist asks the patient to take a deep inspiration and allows his/her hands to reflect the movement of the underlying lung.
▸ Right middle lobe and lingular segment
  ⊙ The therapist places his/her widely outstretched fingers of both hands over the posterior axillary folds and his/her palms over the anterior chest wall.
  ⊙ The skin is then drawn medially until the tips of the extended thumbs meet in the midline.
  ⊙ Again, with the elbows and shoulders maintained in a relaxed position, the therapist asks the patient to take a deep inspiration and allows his/her hands to reflect the movement of the underlying lung.
▸ Lower lobes
  ⊙ With the patient sitting with his/her back to the therapist, the therapist places both hands high up in the axilla with outstretched fingers over the axillary folds.

  ⊙ The skin is then drawn medially until the extended thumbs meet in the midline.
  ⊙ Again, with the elbows and shoulders maintained in a relaxed position, the therapist asks the patient to take a deep inspiration and allows his/her hands to reflect the movement of the underlying lung.
▸ Normally, both lungs should expand equally, and thus the therapist's thumbs and hands will move with equal timing the same distance from each other during both quiet and deep breathing. Diminished or delayed movement of one side often provides the earliest evidence of a localized pathology that is reducing lung compliance.
▸ CWE can also be measured with a tape measure to quantify motion in different areas of the thorax. The tape measure is wrapped around the thorax in a level position and pulled just taut (but not restricting chest expansion) at three anatomic sites[14]:
  ⊙ The angle of Louis on the sternum, located at the second rib, for upper chest motion, which is produced by bucket handle motion
  ⊙ The xiphoid process for mid-chest expansion, which is due predominantly to bucket handle motion
  ⊙ The midpoint between the xiphoid process and the umbilicus for lower chest expansion, where most of the bucket handle motion occurs

▶ The individual is instructed to inspire normally to obtain a measure of chest motion during tidal breathing.

▶ The tape measure is allowed to move with chest expansion and the distance from end expiration to end inspiration is recorded; adding an inexpensive spring-loaded metal flange to the end of the tape can increase the accuracy of measurement.

▶ Chest wall motion is then obtained, as described previously, during maximal inspiration.

▶ If it is difficult to obtain measurements at all three anatomic sites, data from the upper and lower sites will provide information regarding pump handle and bucket handle motion.

Chest Wall Pain

• Patients sometimes report chest pain during the initial interview or as therapy gets underway. Chest pain can result from numerous cardiac, pulmonary, and other causes, as listed in Table 6-10, and sometimes patients experience more than one of these conditions at the same time. It is important for PTs to be able to differentiate between neuromusculoskeletal and systemic causes of chest pain, the latter of which may require referral to a physician.

• Information that may assist in differentiating neuromusculoskeletal and systemic problems include the individual's past medical history and presence of any cardiovascular or pulmonary risk factors, the clinical presentation, vital signs, chest pain pattern, and any associated signs and symptoms (e.g., fever, chills, upper respiratory or gastrointestinal complaints, dyspnea, and lightheadedness).

▶ Obtain a description of the patient's pain (e.g., type, extent, location, precipitating factors, and mechanisms of relief)

▶ Ask the patient to outline the borders of the painful area(s).

• Palpation is valuable in identifying chest wall pain. Starting well away from the affected area and moving toward it, the therapist palpates the ribs and intercostal spaces by pressing firmly downward. In addition, the effects of deep breathing, coughing, breath holding, and ipsilateral arm motion on the pain are noted.

▶ Chest wall pain due to musculoskeletal dysfunction is usually nonsegmental, localized to the anterior chest, and aggravated by deep inspiration but unrelated to exercise.

▶ A localized area of intense pain accompanied by a grating sensation with expiration is usually indicative of a rib fracture.

▶ Localized intercostal tenderness may represent fibrositis of an intercostal muscle.

▶ Pain due to subluxation of a costal cartilage can be reproduced by squeezing the ribs on either side of the dislocation.

▶ Chest pain due to nerve root irritation is more superficial and often radiates segmentally according to dermatomal distribution; it is aggravated by upper body exertion only, and sensory loss or hyperesthesia may occur over the affected dermatome.

▶ Other abnormalities are sometimes detected during palpation of CWE, vocal fremitus, or chest wall pain.

⊙ Subcutaneous air, or emphysema, is perceived as a crackling sensation that can be heard, as well as felt, and results from intrapulmonary rupture of air spaces (e.g., chest

trauma, acute asthma, and surgical incision). It is usually found above the sternum and clavicles or in the neck.

⊙ Unstable rib fractures can be detected by "popping" of the segment during inspiration and coughing.

Fremitus

Palpable vibrations resulting from the transmission of voice sounds to the chest wall are known as *vocal* or *tactile fremitus*.

• To identify fremitus, the examiner places either the palms or the hypothenar eminences of his/her hands lightly on symmetric areas of the chest wall. The patient is then instructed to say "99," and the intensity of the vibrations detected in each hand are compared as the examiner moves his or her hands over several areas of the chest (apical, anterior, lateral, and posterior).

• Under normal conditions, equal vibrations of moderate intensity are perceived during speech, but not during quiet breathing.

• Various pathologies will cause a change in intensity or quality of fremitus:

▶ Increased fremitus is noted when there is increased density of the underlying lung tissue (e.g., consolidation) caused by exudate or mass.

▶ Fremitus is decreased or absent when there is fluid or air in the pleural space or when there is atelectasis due to bronchial obstruction.

▶ When vibrations are detected during quiet breathing, it is termed *rhonchal fremitus*.

Cardiac Impulse

Palpation of the apical impulse of the heart is also included in the chest examination.

• Palpation of the apical impulse of the heart is performed with the patient sitting up and leaning forward or lying on the left side; the therapist uses the pads of his or her fingers to explore the third to sixth intercostal spaces from the left midaxillary line to the middle of the sternum.

▶ The most lateral point where a definite localized systolic pulsation is felt identifies the apex of the heart, or the point of maximal impulse (PMI).

▶ The intensity of the apical impulse can be assessed with the palm of the hand.

• The apical impulse is normally located in the fourth or fifth left intercostal space near the midclavicular line and consists of a brief, localized, early systolic outward thrust of moderate intensity; it may be exaggerated in thin, young individuals and when the individual is lying on the left side.

• Alterations in LV function will often be manifested by a shift in the PMI.

▶ Lateral displacement of the apical impulse without tracheal deviation most likely indicates LV hypertrophy.

▶ The apical impulse will be hyperkinetic when there is increased LV stroke volume (e.g., aortic or mitral regurgitation, severe anemia, anxiety, and exercise).

▶ The apical impulse will be sustained (i.e., lasting past the first half of systole) but normal in location when there is concentric hypertrophy and normal chamber size (e.g., hypertension and aortic stenosis). It will be laterally displaced and sustained with LV enlargement due to systolic LV dysfunction; a sustained outward movement or thrust of an extended area (>2 to 3 cm in diameter) is referred to as an *LV heave* or *lift*.

▸ The most common causes of a hypokinetic apical impulse are abnormal chest configuration and lung disease, although it is also seen in obesity, pericardial effusion or constriction, and shock.

▸ An LV aneurysm may produce an extended area of pulsation at the LV apex or a sustained systolic bulge several centimeters superior to the LV impulse (an ectopic impulse).

▸ Normally the RV is not palpable after the first few months of life. Right ventricular (RV) hypertrophy or enlargement is present when a sustained outward movement is palpated in the left parasternal area or in the subxiphoid region. Exaggerated motion of the entire parasternal area may occur with increased RV output (e.g., atrial septal defect or tricuspid regurgitation).[65]

• The apical impulse will shift according to tracheal deviation when there is mediastinal shift due to lung disease (see earlier).

Peripheral Pulses and Circulation

It is important to assess the adequacy of arterial blood flow in individuals with a history of cardiovascular disease and those with multiple cardiovascular risk factors. After visual inspection of the extremities for skin color and trophic changes, palpation of the peripheral pulses (e.g., femoral, popliteal, posterior tibial and dorsalis pedis for the lower extremities, and brachial and radial for the upper extremities) as well as the carotids should be performed. It is important to realize that the results are difficult to quantify, lack reliability between examiners, and have poor sensitivity. However, the measurement of segmental blood pressure gradient, ankle-to-arm blood pressure ratio (ankle/brachial index), and Doppler flowmetry augment their value, especially when pre- and postexercise data are compared.

• The arterial pulse is produced by the pulse pressure (the difference between the arterial systolic and diastolic pressures), which is usually 35 to 45 mm Hg. It is assessed by palpating over the artery with the index, and often middle, finger using various degrees of pressure until the maximal pulse is sensed. Both sides should be examined and compared for intensity and timing.

▸ Normal arterial pulses are strong and consistent.

▸ The peripheral pulses may be difficult to palpate if there is peripheral arterial disease (PAD) or low stroke volume (e.g., LV failure, hypovolemia, or valve stenosis). Weak inconsistent pulses occur with ventricular dysfunction.

▸ A higher intensity pulse occurs when the pulse pressure is increased because of increased stroke volume (e.g., exercise, anemia, fever, and aortic regurgitation), reduced arterial elasticity (e.g., hypertension and aging), or rapid runoff of blood from the arterial system (e.g., patent ductus arteriosis and arteriovenous fistulas).

▸ In coarctation of the aorta, the femoral pulses will be weaker and delayed compared with the radial pulses.

▸ The pulse will be irregular when arrhythmias are present (see page 262).

▸ On occasion, palpable turbulence (a thrill) is detected, which may indicate hyperdynamic circulation or cardiac valve dysfunction.

• *Doppler flowmetry* involves the use of a handheld continuous-wave Doppler ultrasound probe (rather than a stethoscope) to listen, during deflation of a BP cuff, for the onset of arterial flow, which is often not evident by a palpable pulse when there is significant arterial obstruction.

• The *ankle-brachial*, or *ankle-arm, index* (ABI or AAI, respectively) is obtained by measuring BP at the brachial artery in both upper extremities (UEs) and the posterior tibial and dorsalis pedis arteries in both lower extremities (LEs) and computing an average ankle-to-arm BP ratio. Doppler flowmetry is typically used to detect arterial blood flow and to improve accuracy. The systolic blood pressure (SBP) of the LE is divided by the higher of the two brachial SBP values. The ABI is often used to gauge the severity of PAD.

▸ Normally the ankle systolic pressure is at least as high as the brachial pressure, and therefore the ABI is 1.0 or more.

▸ An ABI less than 0.90 is diagnostic of PAD; values of 0.5 to 0.8 are typical in patients with claudication, and values less than 0.5 usually indicate critical limb ischemia.[23,65]

▸ An absolute SBP less than 50 mm Hg is also consistent with significant PAD.

▸ In addition, the lower the ABI, the greater the incidence of clinical cardiovascular disease.[52]

• The *segmental BP gradient* is determined by measuring BP at successive levels of the extremity, typically one or both LEs. After the patient rests in a supine position for 15 minutes, BPs are obtained via BP cuffs placed at the high-thigh, above-knee, below-knee, and ankle positions and palpating either the dorsalis pedis or posterior tibial pulse. Again, the addition of Doppler flowmetry improves accuracy when the pulses are difficult to detect.

▸ Dividing the pressure at each level by the highest systolic arm pressure provides an index for each level.

▸ Because the BP cuff width (even a thigh cuff) is often not the appropriately 120% of the diameter of the limb at the thigh level, the BP at this level is often 30 to 40 mm Hg higher than the brachial pressure. A high-thigh index less than 1.2 is considered abnormal and may reflect aortoiliac disease.

▸ In the LEs, a 20-mm Hg pressure gradient between successive levels on the same extremity is considered a significant pressure drop and correlates with flow-limiting PAD. In the UEs, a 10-mm Hg pressure gradient is significant.[65]

▸ Successive significant decrements are indicative of multilevel disease.

▸ In addition, a difference in pressure of more than 20 mm Hg between readings of both LEs at the same level is significant for unilateral PAD. However, adequate collateralization may obscure the pressure difference even when significant lesions are present.

▸ Segmental pressure measurements are useful in serial evaluations of patients over time and are reliable indicators of change resulting from various treatment interventions, including exercise. A change in index exceeding 0.15 at the same cuff level on repeat assessment to the next is considered significant.

- By evaluating segmental BP gradients, ABI, or both after arterial stress testing involving treadmill exercise (usually at 2 mph at a 10% to 12% grade for 5 min or until the patient is forced to stop), pharmacologic agents, or reactive hyperemia (the transient increase in blood flow that occurs after arterial occlusion), it is possible to detect subclinical disease and disease that is obscured by marked collateralization.
  - ▸ BP normally increases in both the arms and legs with exercise even though there is peripheral vasodilation.
  - ▸ When there is significant PAD, ABI usually decreases more than 20% from baseline and takes more than 2 to 3 minutes to recover, even though pulses may be palpable.
- In diabetics with medial sclerosis and patients with chronic renal insufficiency, arterial calcification often prevents compression during BP cuff inflation, and therefore the ABI and segmental BPs have limited usefulness. *Toe occlusive pressure* measurements and the *toe–brachial index (TBI)* may provide more reliable indications of foot perfusion in diabetics. However, this technique requires arterial waveform photoplethysmographic equipment, which is expensive and not available in many facilities.
- Inspection can also reveal changes that indicate arterial disease.
  - ▸ Impaired perfusion may produce peripheral cyanosis in the affected limb, which will feel cool to the touch below the level of the occlusion. The patient may complain of numbness or tingling in the affected area.
  - ▸ Chronic arterial insufficiency results in diminished nutritional supply to the skin, so that it becomes shiny, thin, pale, and hairless and the nails may become thickened, brittle, and ridged; thinning of the digits may be evident.
  - ▸ During acute arterial occlusion, the extremity will exhibit marked pallor regardless of limb position.
- Another technique that can be used to ascertain the adequacy of peripheral perfusion involves assessment of the changes in skin color that occur as a result of limb elevation and dependency.
  - ▸ Elevation of the extremity to approximately 45° allows the venous blood to drain and facilitates an accurate assessment of the degree of arterial flow: A normal extremity will remain pink or show slight blanching, whereas an extremity affected by significant PAD will quickly lose all color and appear dead grayish white.
  - ▸ Then, when placed in a dependent position, a normal extremity will quickly take on a pink flush, whereas an extremity with arterial disease will become very red (dependent rubor) although its appearance may take more than 30 seconds. The time it takes for blood to return to the extremity (normally <20 s) is directly related to the severity of PAD.
- Delayed capillary refilling time is also an indicator of impaired peripheral circulation.
  - ▸ To test capillary filling, press down on a nail bed and release.
  - ▸ Normally the nail bed will blanch (whiten) with pressure and normal color will return within 3 seconds of release of pressure.
- Patients may complain of pain during ambulation (i.e., intermittent claudication), especially at faster speeds, up inclines, or during stair climbing.

PERCUSSION

The final component of the chest examination is percussion, which allows the clinician to further evaluate any abnormal findings in terms of their relationship to changes in lung density. The pitch of the sound produced by percussion is determined by the ratio of air-containing tissue to solid tissue in the underlying area. Thus, areas of altered density can be identified, and the extent of the abnormality can be defined. In addition, percussion can be used to demonstrate the level of the diaphragm and its maximal excursion from end-expiratory to end-inspiratory positions.

- Percussion is most commonly performed indirectly by the mediate percussion technique, which is illustrated in Figure 6-16. However, it can also be performed by direct, or immediate, percussion, during which the middle finger taps directly on the chest wall.
- The proper technique for assessing lung density consists of the following:
  - ▸ Lightly position the pad of the middle finger of the nondominant hand along the intercostal space over the area in question while all other fingers are held away from the chest wall.
  - ▸ Position the other hand with the wrist in dorsiflexion; then using the wrist as the fulcrum, strike the middle finger of the nondominant hand repeatedly with the tip of the middle finger of the dominant hand, recoiling instantly after each tap.
  - ▸ Systematically percuss from side to side along each intercostal space from apex to base of the lungs, both anteriorly and posteriorly, comparing the pitch, intensity, and duration of the sound produced
- Well-aerated lung tissue produces a low-pitched, resonant sound that is similar to a muffled drum, whereas more dense organs such as the heart, liver, and subcostal abdominal viscera yield a duller sound, and less dense organs such as the stomach produce a more tympanic sound.

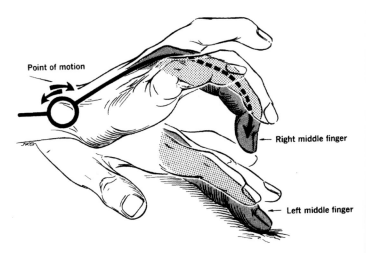

Figure 6-16: Hand position for performing mediate percussion. (From Buckingham EB. *A Primer of Clinical Diagnosis.* 2nd ed. New York: Harper & Row; 1979.)

- A higher pitched, dull-to-flat note (i.e., a "thud") denotes an area of increased density, as in atelectasis, consolidation, or pleural effusion.
- A loud, long, and hollow hyperresonant, or tympanic, note indicates decreased density (i.e., the presence of more air), as in pneumothorax or hyperinflated lungs.
- The steps involved in assessing diaphragmatic excursion include the following:
  - With the patient sitting, the examiner performs percussion down the chest until dullness is encountered.
  - The patient is then asked to exhale completely while the examiner defines the limit of diaphragmatic ascent.
  - After the patient takes a deep breath and holds it, the examiner tracks diaphragmatic motion and identifies the extent of descent.
- Diaphragmatic excursion is the distance between maximal expiration and maximal inspiration, which is normally 3 to 5 cm.
  - Diaphragmatic excursion is reduced bilaterally in COPD.
  - If there is unilateral diaphragmatic paralysis, the diaphragm may be fixed in an elevated position or move paradoxically, rising above its resting level when a deep inspiration is performed.
- The normal resonance pattern of the chest is depicted in Figure 6-17.
- The changes in resonance that occur with various pathologies can be found at the end of this chapter in Table 6-34.

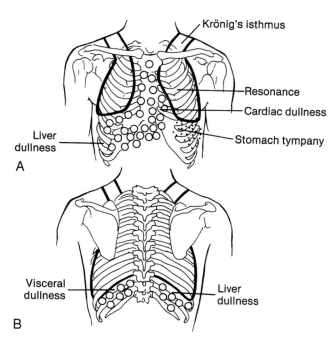

Figure 6-17: Normal resonance pattern of the chest. **A,** Anteriorly; **B,** posteriorly. *Circles,* areas of dullness; *small dots,* tympanic, or hyperresonant, areas. (From Irwin S, Tecklin JS. *Cardiopulmonary Physical Therapy: A Guide to Practice.* 4th ed. St. Louis: Mosby; 2004.)

6.5 EXERCISE ASSESSMENT

Because exercise is an essential component of nearly every physical therapy treatment plan and has the potential to provoke problems in individuals with cardiopulmonary dysfunction (many of whom are not diagnosed), it is important to assess the physiological responses to exercise, particularly in individuals over the age of 45 years and younger and in persons with coronary risk factors, possible cardiopulmonary symptomatology, and diseases or disorders that can affect the cardiopulmonary systems, as presented in Chapter 4. As depicted in Table 6-17, a number of disorders are associated with exercise intolerance.

There are several means of assessing exercise responses, including exercise stress testing and less formal activity and endurance evaluations. In addition, timed walk tests (e.g., the 6- or 12-minute walk test) are used to document functional status.

Regardless of the method used, it is important to monitor the physiological responses, including any abnormal signs or symptoms, before, during, and after exercise. It is not unusual for abnormalities to develop or become more marked during the first few minutes after exercise.

EXERCISE STRESS TESTING

In some centers, exercise stress testing, sometimes including the direct measurement of oxygen consumption ($\dot{V}O_2$), is administered by PTs with competency in the necessary cognitive and technical skills. However, equipment and monitoring requisites preclude the performance of exercise stress testing in most clinical settings. When they are performed by PTs, exercise tests are usually submaximal rather than maximal because of requirements for medical supervision and emergency equipment and the level of risk for the person being tested.

- Maximal stress tests require the individual to exercise to the point of maximal volitional fatigue and thus yield better estimates of maximal oxygen consumption ($\dot{V}O_{2\,max}$) and increased sensitivity in the diagnosis of coronary artery disease in asymptomatic individuals.
  - Physician supervision is recommended for individuals with moderate and high risk for untoward events during exercise participation (see page 238).[2,35a]
  - A number of protocols are used for exercise stress testing, depending on the fitness level of the individual and the preference of the clinician. Several protocols and the predicted oxygen cost of each stage of are presented in Figure 3-15 on page 50.
    ⊙ The standard Bruce protocol, which begins at 1.7 mph at a 10% grade, is the most common treadmill protocol used in the testing of apparently healthy individuals.
    ⊙ Individuals with limited exercise tolerance due to cardiopulmonary dysfunction or other chronic medical problems are often tested using the Naughton, McHenry, or modified Bruce protocol, which has two easier stages before stage 1 of the standard protocol (1.7 mph at 0% grade and 1.7 mph at 5% grade)
    ⊙ Many physicians and researchers prefer to perform exercise testing with a cycle ergometer, as there is less movement

TABLE 6-17: Disorders Limiting Exercise Tolerance, Pathophysiology, and Discriminating Measures

Disorders	Pathophysiology	Measures That Deviate From Normal
Pulmonary		
Obstructive lung disease	↓ Ventilatory capacity due to airflow limitation, increased ventilatory requirement due to $\dot{V}/\dot{Q}$ mismatching, hypoxic stimulation to breathing	↓ $\dot{V}O_{2\,max}$, ↑ V_D/V_T, ↑ $P(a–ET)co_2$, ↑ $P(A–a)o_2$, ↓ breathing reserve ($MVV − \dot{V}E_{2\,max}$), ↓ HR at maximal WR (↑ HR reserve), abnl (trapezoidal) expiratory flow pattern
Restrictive lung disease	↓ Lung volumes, especially IC and TLC; $\dot{V}/\dot{Q}$ mismatching, hypoxemia	↓ $\dot{V}O_{2\,max}$, ↑ V_T/IC, RR >50 at maximal WR, ↓ breathing reserve, ↑ V_D/V_T, ↑ $P(a–ET)co_2$, progressively ↓ Pao_2 and ↑ $P(A–a)o_2$ with ↑ WRs
Chest wall defects	Respiratory pump dysfunction due to muscle weakness or ↓ chest wall compliance	↓ $\dot{V}O_{2\,max}$, ↑ V_T/IC, ↑ RR at low WRs, nl $\Delta\dot{V}O_2/\Delta WR$, ↓ breathing reserve, ↓ HR at maximal WR, nl Pao_2
Diseases of pulmonary circulation	↓ Pulmonary perfusion leading to $\dot{V}/\dot{Q}$ mismatching	↑ $\dot{V}E$ at submaximal WRs, ↑ V_D/V_T, ↑ $P(a–ET)co_2$, progressively ↓ Pao_2 and ↑ $P(A–a)o_2$ with ↑ WRs, ↓ $\dot{V}O_{2\,max}$, ↓ AT, more shallow $\Delta\dot{V}O_2/\Delta WR$ as WR is ↑ toward maximum, ↓ O_2 pulse ($\dot{V}O_{2\,max}/HR$)
Cardiac		
Coronary insufficiency	Relative imbalance between myocardial oxygen supply and demand, causing myocardial ischemia	May have chest pain and ischemic ECG changes, ↓ $\dot{V}O_{2\,max}$, ↓ AT, ↓ O_2 pulse, more shallow $\Delta\dot{V}O_2/\Delta WR$ as WR is ↑ toward maximum, ↑ $HR/\dot{V}O_2$, ↑ breathing reserve, metabolic acidosis at low WRs → ↑ WRs → $\dot{V}E$, abnl BP responses
Valvular	Cardiac output limitation due to ↓ effective SV	↓ $\dot{V}O_{2\,max}$, ↓ AT, ↓ O_2 pulse, more shallow $\Delta\dot{V}O_{2\,max}/\Delta WR$ as WR is ↑ toward maximum, ↑ $HR/\dot{V}O_2$, ↑ breathing reserve, metabolic acidosis at low WRs → ↑ $\dot{V}E$, abnl BP responses
Myocardial	Cardiac output limitation due to ↓ EF and SV	
Other		
Obesity	↑ Energy cost to move body; if severe, restrictive lung dysfunction and pulmonary insufficiency	↑ $\dot{V}O_2$ per workload, nl O_2 pulse when predicted from ht, ↓ $\dot{V}O_{2\,max}/wt$ and AT/wt but nl $\dot{V}O_{2\,max}/ht$ and AT/ht (unless extremely obese), ↑ $P(A–a)o_2$ at rest which normalizes during exercise, nl V_D/V_T
Peripheral arterial disease	Impaired ability to ↑ blood flow to working muscles	Leg pain (claudication), ↓ $\Delta\dot{V}O_2/\Delta WR$, ↓ $\dot{V}O_{2\,max}$, ↓ AT, possible hypertensive BP response
Anemia	↓ Oxygen-carrying capacity	↓ Hemoglobin and hematocrit, ↓ $\dot{V}O_{2\,max}$, ↓ AT, ↓ O_2 pulse, nl V_D/V_T, $P(a - et)CO_2$, and $P(A-a)O_2$
Musculoskeletal disorders	Musculoskeletal coupling inefficiency; inflammation	↓ Mechanical efficiency ($\dot{V}O_2$ per workload), ↓ maximal WR; possible pain and abnl movement patterns
Chronic metabolic acidosis	Due to poorly controlled DM, CRF, CHF, or ingestion of certain drugs	↓ HCO_3^-, steep $\dot{V}E/\dot{V}CO_2$ relationship, nl $P(a–ET)co_2$ and $P(A–a)o_2$, nl V_D/Vt
Deconditioning	Inactivity or prolonged bed rest leading to loss of ability to effectively redistribute systemic blood flow	↓ $\dot{V}O_{2\,max}$, ↓ AT, ↓ O_2 pulse, ↑ breathing reserve, metabolic acidosis at lower WRs → ↑ $\dot{V}E$
Anxiety reaction	Hyperventilation and respiratory alkalosis with precisely regular RR, although possible breath-holding episodes	Abrupt tachypnea that sometimes starts at rest, ↓ $Paco_2$, respiratory alkalosis
Malingering, poor effort	Very irregular breathing with periods of hyperventilation and hypoventilation	AT not achieved or ↑ compared with $\dot{V}O_{2\,max}$, ↑ breathing and HR reserve; often irregular breathing pattern with periods of tachypnea and bradypnea producing wide swings in $Paco_2$ and $Petco_2$ unrelated to changes in WR

Data from American Thoracic Society/American College of Chest Physicians ATS/ACCP statement on cardiopulmonary exercise testing. *Am J Respir Crit Care Med.* 167:211–277, 2003; Wasserman K: Dyspnea on exertion. Is it the heart or the lungs? *JAMA* 248:2039–2043, 1982; Wasserman K, Hansen JE, Sue DY, et al.: *Principles of Exercise Testing and Interpretation.* Philadelphia, Lea & Febiger, 1987; and Weisman IM, Zeballos RJ: An integrative approach to the interpretation of cardiopulmonary exercise testing. *Prog. Respir. Res.* 32:300–322, 2002.

↓, Decreased; ↑, increased; →, leading to; Δ, change in; abnl, abnormal; AT, anaerobic threshold; BP, blood pressure; CHF, chronic heart failure; CRF, chronic renal failure; DM, diabetes mellitus; ECG, electrocardiogram; EF, ejection fraction; HR, heart rate; ht, height; IC, inspiratory capacity; MVV, maximal voluntary ventilation; nl, normal; $P(A–a)o_2$, alveolar–arterial oxygen difference; $Paco_2$, partial pressure of arterial carbon dioxide; $P(a–ET)co_2$, arterial–end-tidal carbon dioxide difference; Pao_2, partial pressure of arterial oxygen; $Petco_2$, partial pressure of end-tidal carbon dioxide; RR, respiratory rate; SV, stroke volume; TLC, total lung capacity; $\dot{V}co_2$, carbon dioxide production; V_D/V_T, ratio of dead space volume to tidal volume; $\dot{V}E$, minute ventilation; $V_{E\,max}$, maximal minute ventilation; $\dot{V}O_2$, oxygen consumption; $\dot{V}O_{2\,max}$, maximal oxygen consumption; $\dot{V}/\dot{Q}$, ventilation–perfusion; WR, work rate; wt, body weight.

of the patient's arms and thorax, making it easier to obtain better ECG recordings and BP measurements; in addition, balance problems are less of an issue. However, most patients are not as familiar with stationary cycling as they are with walking, and they may not be as willing to push themselves to perform as vigorous a test as on the treadmill or they may develop localized leg fatigue at a lower workload.

▶ The addition of gas analysis during exercise testing provides actual values for $\dot{V}O_{2\,max}$, as well as for anaerobic threshold and a variety of other parameters (see page 17).

- Submaximal exercise tests aim to document the clinical responses during at least two, preferably three, submaximal workloads and can be used to predict maximal workload and $\dot{V}O_{2\,max}$.

▶ Typically, the individual performs a standardized submaximal exercise test on a cycle ergometer or treadmill, stopping at 70% HR reserve (85% of age-predicted maximal HR), and then the values are predicted on the basis of the resultant data and an appropriate regression equation that is specific to the type of ergometer and testing protocol used.

⊙ A commonly used equation that is based on the standard Bruce protocol is as follows[32]:

$$\dot{V}O_{2\,max}\,(mL/kg/min) = 14.8 - 1.379(\text{time in min}) \\ + 0.451(\text{time}^2) - 0.012(\text{time}^3)$$

Standard error of estimate (SEE) = 3.35 mL/kg/min

⊙ For individuals who require handrail support during treadmill testing according to the Bruce protocol, the following equation has been validated[50]:

$$\dot{V}O_{2\,max}(mL/kg/min) = 2.282(\text{time in min}) + 8.545$$

$$SEE = 4.92\,mL/kg/min$$

▶ The results can also be used to document improvements in status (by comparing the submaximal exercise responses to specific workloads over time or the workload achieved at the selected submaximal HR) and to make adjustments to the individual's exercise prescription.

Refer to pages 18 and 49 for more information about exercise stress testing.

ACTIVITY AND ENDURANCE EVALUATION

Another method of assessing exercise responses that is readily performed by PTs is an activity or endurance evaluation, as detailed in Table 6-18, which involves clinical monitoring of the patient's physiological responses to progressively increasing submaximal intensities of activity or aerobic exercise.

- In patients with symptomatic heart or lung disease and those who are hospitalized or recently discharged, the assessment usually begins with an activity evaluation to determine the appropriateness of the patient's physiological responses to low-level exercise before proceeding to the endurance evaluation.

▶ The patient performs 10 or more repetitions of sitting knee extensions and/or knee lifts and the therapist measures the clinical responses toward the end of the exercise.

▶ The individual then performs 10 or more repetitions of uni- or bilateral UE exercise and again the therapist obtains clinical measurements toward the end of exercise (the person performs unilateral exercise with the opposite arm while the BP reading is obtained).

▶ If the patient can tolerate more activity, the therapist proceeds on to the endurance evaluation.

- In other individuals, including those who are sedentary and those with medical problems associated with mild to moderate limitation of activity tolerance, the exercise assessment can begin with the endurance evaluation.

- Vital signs (VSs), including HR, BP, respiratory rate (RR or f), oxygen saturation as determined by pulse oximetry (SpO_2), and possibly ECG, rating of perceived exertion (RPE), and symptomatology are monitored before, during, and after the exercise assessment.

▶ During exercise VSs should be obtained while the person continues to walk/exercise or marches in place.

▶ If it is not possible to obtain an accurate BP during activity, the other VSs should be obtained first and then the BP should be taken by inflating the BP cuff while the person is still exercising or marching and deflating the cuff slowly as soon as s/he stops the activity.

- To quantify the distance and/or speed of ambulation, the patient can be timed and the distances can be calculated. The author routinely maps out various "loops" used for hallway ambulation in the various treatment areas (e.g., physical therapy department and hospital units), notes their distances, and creates charts that can be used to determine walking pace and total distance covered, as depicted in Figure 6-18.

6-MINUTE WALK TEST

- Timed walk tests, such as the 6- and 12-minute walk tests (6 MWT and 12 MWT, respectively), are objective exercise field tests that are used to measure functional status, to document treatment outcomes, and to establish prognosis in patients with limited exercise tolerance, including those with heart and lung disease.

- Timed walk tests require minimal equipment: a stopwatch or countdown timer, a mechanical lap counter, two cones to mark the turnaround points, a chair that can be easily moved along the walking course, worksheets on a clipboard, a Borg Scale for RPE and other appropriate symptomatology scales (e.g., dyspnea, chest pain, and claudication), a stethoscope and sphygmomanometer, and safety equipment (telephone, oxygen, and automated electronic defibrillator).

- Clients are asked to walk along a path or corridor, back and forth and pivoting quickly around the cones, at a pace that allows them to cover as much distance as possible in the specified period of time, giving their best effort possible. They are allowed to slow down, stop, and rest as necessary, but the clock continues to run.

- The following are the American Thoracic Society guidelines for the 6 MWT[5]:

▶ Measure out a level walking path at least 100 ft in length that is free of obstruction, such as an infrequently used hallway or corridor.

TABLE 6-18: Activity and Endurance Evaluation

Procedure	Comments
Activity Evaluation	
Monitor the patient's HR and rhythm, BP, and any signs and symptoms while supine, then sitting, and finally standing	There are a number of methods of monitoring a patient's physiological responses to activity
Auscultate the patient's lungs and heart before and after activity	*Heart rate:*
Monitor the patient's physiological responses while the patient performs simple active exercises* or during some activity of daily living, such as dressing, combing or brushing hair, or brushing teeth	HR can be measured by palpation, usually of the radial pulse, by auscultation of the cardiac apex, via the digital display of an ECG or oxygen saturation monitor, or directly from an ECG rhythm strip
Sometimes, the patient's responses to a Valsalva maneuver or hyperventilation are also assessed	*Heart rhythm:* The most accurate means of monitoring cardiac rhythm is by watching an ECG monitor and printing out rhythm strips
Record and interpret all responses throughout the entire evaluation	Alternatively, if ECG equipment is not available, the pulse can be palpated or the heart can be auscultated for 30–60 s
Terminate the evaluation any time responses are identified that indicate continued activity would be inappropriate or unsafe	*Blood pressure:* BP is usually monitored with an arm cuff and a sphygmomanometer or with an automatic BP monitor
	In critical care units, patients often have an indwelling arterial line with a digital display of systolic, diastolic, and mean arterial pressure, which can be used to monitor BP responses
Endurance Evaluation	
If the patient's responses to the activity evaluation (see previous entry) are determined to be safe and appropriate, the evaluation may continue by having the patient perform progressive ambulation in the hallway or some other form of graded aerobic activity (e.g., stationary cycling, treadmill walking)	Inpatients are usually evaluated during ambulation initially, because this is convenient and permits assessment of the patient's balance and coordination, level of independence, and functional efficiency (i.e., speed and distance)
Starting at a comfortable, relaxed pace, have the patient ambulate for 2–3 min and then measure the patient's responses while the patient continues walking	Ideally, the endurance evaluation should be structured so that the patient can perform at least two different intensities of exercise before fatigue sets in
Include an RPE[†]	Be certain to take physiological measurements while the patient is still walking or at least marching in place because the values will drop rapidly when activity is terminated
Ask the patient to increase exercise intensity (i.e., walking pace or cycling resistance) and continue for another 2–3 min, at which time responses are again measured	
Repeat this procedure until the patient reaches an RPE of "somewhat hard" (13 on a scale of 6–20) or "somewhat strong" (4 on a scale of 1–10)	To quantify the distance and speed of ambulation for hallway ambulation, the distances of various "loops" can be measured and charts can be created to plot the number of loops or distance walked in so many minutes[‡]
Continue at this pace until the patient begins to feel fatigued. Note the total exercise time	The total walking time completed and the ending pace can be used to create an endurance exercise prescription for the patient

BP, Blood pressure; ECG, electrocardiography; HR, heart rate; RPE, rating of perceived exertion.
*See text.
[†]See Box 6-3.
[‡]See page 281.

▸ Mark a starting line as well as intervals of 10 ft along the path (to facilitate the determination of the final distance walked).
▸ Wearing comfortable clothes and appropriate shoes for walking, patients should use their normal assistive devices for ambulation. They should also use their current medications, including oxygen and preexercise bronchodilators, as directed, and eat only a light meal and avoid strenuous exercise within 2 hours of testing.
▸ Resting VSs measurements should be obtained after the patient has rested in a chair for 10 minutes, during which forms can be filled out, final preparations made, and instructions explained.

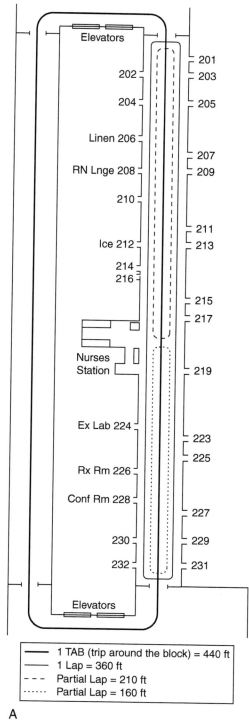

Elevators

202
204
Linen 206
RN Lnge 208
210
Ice 212
214
216

Nurses
Station

Ex Lab 224

Rx Rm 226

Conf Rm 228

230
232

Elevators

201
203
205

207
209

211
213

215
217

219

223
225

227

229
231

— 1 TAB (trip around the block) = 440 ft
— 1 Lap = 360 ft
- - - Partial Lap = 210 ft
······ Partial Lap = 160 ft

A

Figure 6-18: **A,** Example of a walking map posted on a hospital unit or in a rehabilitation department, which maps out various loops for ambulation and their distances.

Continued

▸ The timer is started as the patient leaves the starting line, and the examiner remains there throughout the test, paying full attention to the patient and not talking to anyone else.

▸ The lap counter is clicked or a mark is made on the worksheet with each lap completed.

▸ At the end of each minute of the test, the patient's progress is announced and standardized encouragement is offered in an even voice (e.g., "You are doing well. You have 5 minutes to go." or "Keep up the good work. You have only 2 minutes to go.").

▸ When the timer shows 15 seconds to completion of the test, the patient should be informed that the test is approaching completion and when told, he or she is to stop right at that spot.

# Laps	Distance (in feet)	Miles	Time (in min.) for specific diatance (will indicate speed)				
			1.0 mph	1.5 mph	2.0 mph	2.5 mph	3.0 mph
1	360	.07	4.1	2.7	2.0	1.6	1.4
2	720	.14	8.2	5.5	4.1	3.3	2.7
3	1080	.20 (⅕)	12.3	8.2	6.1	4.9	4.1
4	1440	.27 (~¼)	16.4	10.9	8.2	6.5	5.5
5	1800	.34 (⅓)	20.5	13.6	10.2	8.2	6.8
6	2160	.41	24.5	16.4	12.3	9.8	8.2
7	2520	.48 (~½)	28.6	19.1	14.3	11.5	9.5
8	2880	.55	32.7	21.8	16.4	13.1	10.9
9	3240	.61	36.8	24.5	18.4	14.7	12.3
10	3600	.68 (~⅔)	40.9	27.3	20.5	16.4	13.6
11	3960	.75 (¾)	45.0	30.0	22.5	18.0	15.0
12	4320	.82 (~⅘)	49.1	32.7	24.5	19.6	16.4
13	4680	.89	53.2	35.5	26.6	21.3	17.7
14	5040	.95	57.3	38.2	28.6	22.9	19.1

B

# TABs	Distance (in feet)	Miles	Time (in minutes) for specific distance (will indicate speed)				
			1.0 mph	1.5 mph	2.0 mph	2.5 mph	3.0 mph
1.0	440	.08 (1/12)	5.0	3.3	2.5	2.0	1.7
1.5	660	.13 (⅛)	7.5	5.0	3.8	3.0	2.5
2.0	880	.17 (⅙)	10.0	6.7	5.0	4.0	3.3
2.5	1080	.20 (⅕)	12.3	8.2	6.1	4.9	4.1
3.0	1320	.25 (¼)	15.0	10.0	7.5	6.0	5.0
4.0	1760	.33 (⅓)	20.0	13.3	10.0	8.0	6.7
6.0	2640	.50 (½)	30.0	20.0	15.0	12.0	10.0
8.0	3520	.67 (⅔)	40.0	26.7	20.0	16.0	13.3
9.0	3960	.75 (¾)	45.0	30.0	22.5	18.0	15.0
12.0	5280	1.00	60.0	40.0	30.0	24.0	20.0

C

Figure 6-18—cont'd **B,** A chart showing the distance walked along a hospital ward corridor according to the number of laps. Walking pace can also be determined by locating the time it took to complete the distance walked and looking up to the top of the column to find the corresponding speed. For example, if an individual walks two laps (720 ft) and it takes 6 minutes, the walking speed can be determined by looking to the right of two laps to find the time closest to 6 minutes, which is 5.5 minutes; because the walk actually took a little longer than 5.5 minutes, the individual was walking at a pace a little slower than 1.5 miles per hour (mph). **C,** A chart showing the distance walked around a hospital area according to the number of "trips around the block" (TABs). Walking pace is also determined according to the procedures described in **B.**

▶ When the timer signals, the patient is told to stop and the stopping point is marked. A chair is provided for the patient to sit on if s/he looks fatigued or uncomfortable.

▶ The immediate posttest HR, BP, SpO_2 if monitored, and Borg RPE, dyspnea, and fatigue levels are recorded. The total distance walked is calculated (no. of laps × the distance of each lap + the additional distance of the last partial lap). The number of rest stops taken and the use of supplemental oxygen or assistive devices should also be noted.

• The 6 MWT is the most extensively researched and established walk test and is better tolerated than the 12 MWT in patients with respiratory and CV disease. Distance walked is strongly correlated with $\dot{V}O_{2\,max}$ and correlates moderately to strongly with measures of function. However, correlations with spirometry and measures of dyspnea have produced conflicting results.

• Some studies have shown that the reliability of the 6 MWT (and other walk tests) may be improved by having the patient perform one or more practice walks before testing and by providing standardized encouragement (see earlier) every 30 to 60 seconds[39,42,58]; however, not all authors report benefits for practice walks.[5,46]

- When repeating the test to document outcome measures, the initial test conditions should be duplicated, including time of day, lap distance, use of pretest bronchodilators or supplemental oxygen and dose, type and frequency of encouragement, and so on.
- Two- and three-minute walk tests have been validated for use with the frail elderly and individuals with neurologic impairments.[12,42,46]

CLINICAL MONITORING

For the data obtained from exercise testing or the activity and endurance evaluation to be meaningful, accurate physiological monitoring must be performed before, during, and after exercise. The proper techniques for patient monitoring are presented for HR and rhythm, BP, and RR. In addition, ECG monitoring is described for therapists who have access to the equipment. (*Note:* Most hospitals have functional, but older ECG monitoring equipment hidden away in storage areas that can be resurrected for use during exercise. The first choice is usually a telemetry ECG unit; however, hardwiring is perfectly acceptable for monitoring activities using little space, such as treadmill walking and stationary cycling.) In addition, normal values, both at rest and in response to activity, are characterized.

Heart Rate

HR can be determined by palpation of the arterial pulse (usually at the radial artery), auscultation of the heart with a stethoscope, use of a HR monitor or pulse oximeter, or via ECG monitoring.

- The pulse is assessed by palpating with the index and middle fingers placed lightly over the artery; both sides should be examined. The pulse rate is usually palpated for 15 seconds and the result multiplied by 4 to produce a HR in beats per minute (bpm). Refer to page 253 for information regarding arterial pulse palpation and abnormal findings.
- For auscultation of the HR, the stethoscope is placed to the left of the sternum just above the level of the nipple. This method is most accurate when the heart sounds are clearly audible and there is minimal movement of the torso.
- Simple HR monitors rely on electrodes held in place with a chest strap and a HR watch to display the values. More complex models display peak and average HR, training zones, intensity and duration, caloric consumption, and more and are able to store data that can be downloaded to a personal computer. In addition, electronic exercise equipment, including treadmills, cycle ergometers, elliptical trainers, and stair steppers, often have HR monitors built into their handholds.
- For therapists working in cardiac or pulmonary rehabilitation or in a critical care unit, the availability of ECG monitoring allows for simple accurate determination, as well as arrhythmia recognition. Telemetry ECG monitoring is usually available in step-down units, but the monitors may not be within easy viewing during PT treatments; however, sometimes a nurse or aide is available to obtain ECG strips during treatment.

Some rehabilitation departments have their own portable ECG equipment, which can be carried to the patient's room or used in the department.

- Some patients in the acute care setting have bedside pulse oximetry for monitoring oxygen saturation, which usually displays a digital readout of HR, and this can be used to monitor HR responses to activity (see page 18).
- Some specific suggestions to increase the accuracy of HR monitoring include the following:
  ▶ If the pulse is difficult to palpate while the patient is walking, it can be counted while the patient marches in place, using auscultation of the heart, or, as a last resort, obtaining a count during the first 15 seconds of recovery. (*Note:* HR may begin to fall almost immediately on cessation of exercise so accuracy will be affected.)
  ▶ If the pulse rate becomes increasingly irregular, all of the impulses may not be peripherally palpable, and auscultation of the heart may afford a more accurate HR when compared with an ECG strip; however, the peripherally palpated rate may provide a better indication of the effective heart rate, because nonpalpable beats are usually associated with lower stroke volume than normal beats.
  ▶ If the digital display of an ECG or oxygen saturation monitor is being used to monitor HR responses, the therapist should be aware of the possibility of inaccuracies resulting from movement artifact or impaired perfusion during activity (see page 280).

HR Responses to Exercise

- Normal resting HR values and responses to activity are described in Table 6-19.
  ▶ In general, HR increases proportional to exercise intensity.
  ▶ Most activities included in the typical activity evaluation are low in intensity, requiring an increase in metabolic rate of less than three to four times the resting rate (i.e., <3 to 4 METs, as explained on page 361). Therefore, the rise in HR in response to these activities should be fairly minimal (<20 to 30 bpm).
- The hemodynamic responses to static versus dynamic exercise are illustrated in Figure 6-19. The maximal increase in HR during isometric exercise is typically about 50% of that noted during symptom-limited exercise testing.[57]
- Abnormal HR responses to activity occur as either excessive or inadequate increases in HR or delayed recovery of HR after exercise.
  ▶ Some individuals who are anxious about performing an exercise test may exhibit higher HR and BP at the onset of exercise (due to sympathetic nervous system stimulation), which then stabilize within the first minute.
  ▶ An exaggerated increase in HR at low exercise intensities may be seen in patients who are physically deconditioned, hypovolemic, or anemic, as well as in those who have impaired ventricular function or are in atrial fibrillation. The elevated HR may persist for several minutes after exercise.
  ▶ In some patients HR fails to increase appropriately with increasing exercise intensity. Chronotropic incompetence is

TABLE 6-19: **Heart Rate: Normal Values and Responses to Exercise**

Normal	Comments
Resting: 50–100 bpm	Varies with age, health status, fitness level, balance of sympathetic and parasympathetic nervous system activity, circulating catecholamine levels, level of hydration, effects of any medications being taken, and other factors
	More fit individuals tend to have lower resting HRs than sedentary individuals, probably due to ↓ sympathetic activity and ↑ ventricular filling resulting in ↑ cardiac efficiency
	↑ Resting HR means the heart is working harder (i.e., faster) in order to eject normal cardiac output
Dynamic exercise: HR increases in direct proportion to workload	The normal ↑ is 10 ± 2 bpm per MET ↑ in workload for untrained individuals
	HR response is often blunted in those who perform regular aerobic exercise, because of training effect increasing stroke volume
	A leveling off of HR rise with an ↑ in workload usually signals the approach of $\dot{V}O_{2\,max}$
	Abnormal HR responses: Tachycardic: HR rises more rapidly than expected; usually seen in the severely deconditioned and those who have cardiovascular disease with limited ability to ↑ stroke volume; therefore, must ↑ HR to ↑ cardiac output
	Bradycardic: A blunted HR response to increasing workload (<8 bpm/MET); seen most commonly in patients taking β-adrenergic blockers
	Chronotropic incompetence: A true bradycardic response with a peak exercise HR that is >20 bpm below the age-predicted HR_{max} in individuals who are limited by volitional fatigue and are not taking any β-blocker medications. It is considered very ominous for severe CAD
	Instances in which palpable HR seems to ↓ during exertion, but ECG monitoring usually reveals increasing arrhythmias, some of which are not perceived peripherally (due to peripheral resistance)
Static/isometric exercise: less pronounced ↑ in HR than with dynamic exercise	Caused by lower cardiac output requirements and associated with higher BP responses (due to ↑ peripheral resistance)

Data from American College of Sports Medicine: *ASCM's Guidelines for Exercise Testing and Prescription,* 7th Ed. Philadelphia, Lippincott Williams & Wilkins, 2006; and American College of Sports Medicine: *ASCM's Resource Manual for Guidelines for Exercise Testing and Prescription,* 4th Ed. Philadelphia, Lippincott Williams & Wilkins, 2001.
↓, Decreased; ↑, increased; BP, blood pressure; bpm, beats per minute; CAD, coronary artery disease; ECG, electrocardiographic; HR, heart rate; HR_{max}, maximal HR; MET, metabolic equivalent for oxygen consumption (1 MET, 3.5 mL O_2/kg/min); $\dot{V}O_{2\,max}$, maximal oxygen uptake.

defined as an inability to increase HR to at least 85% of age-predicted maximum (given high motivation by the individual) or an abnormally blunted HR response to increasing workload.[18] It is associated with an increased mortality risk in patients with cardiovascular disease.

▸ Abnormal HR recovery is manifested as a slow deceleration of HR after stopping exercise, which can be calculated by subtracting the HR at 1 minute of recovery from the peak HR ($HR_{recovery} = HR_{peak} - HR_{1\text{-}min\ recovery}$). Abnormal $HR_{recovery}$ values are related to increased risk of mortality and include the following[18]:
  ⊙ 12 or fewer bpm during upright cooldown activity
  ⊙ Less than 19 bpm when patient assumes a supine position immediately after exercise (as during stress echocardiography)
  ⊙ 22 bpm or less at 2 minutes of recovery
▸ Loss of sustained vigor of palpable pulse can occur when BP falls because of inadequate cardiac output (e.g., LV dysfunction, LV outflow obstruction, and arrhythmia).

Heart Rhythm

Using palpation, it is possible only to detect regularity versus irregularity of the rhythm and to state whether the irregularities occur in a regular (predictable) or irregular (unpredictable) pattern. Interpreting the irregularity in terms of the actual arrhythmia that is present is not possible without an ECG. Therefore, ECG monitoring is strongly advised, at least for screening, for any patient with a history of arrhythmias and for those who exhibit irregularities of pulse or any other abnormal signs or symptoms during activity.

• Heart rhythm is normally regular or with only occasional asymptomatic irregularities.
• During exertion, there should be little change in rhythm.
• Abnormal rhythm responses include the onset of arrhythmias (or more accurately called *dysrhythmia*) during or immediately after exertion or an increase in frequency or change in type of arrhythmia with an increase in activity or immediately after exercise.
• On occasion, a patient will have arrhythmias at rest that decrease or resolve with increasing heart rates, as with exertion.

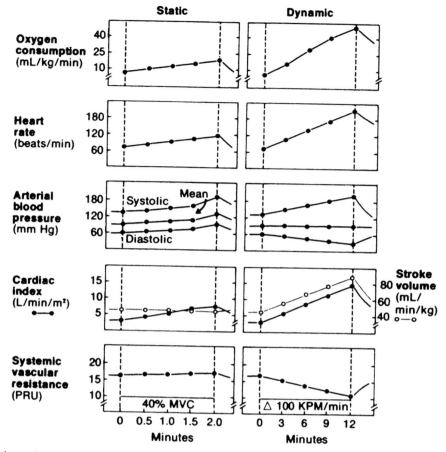

Figure 6-19: The hemodynamic responses to static exercise (isometric handgrip at 40% of maximal contraction) versus progressive dynamic exercise (stationary cycling with 100-kpm/min increase in workload). (From Longhurst LC, Mitchell JH. Does endurance training benefit the cardiovascular system? *J Cardiovasc Med.* 1983:8:227. Reprinted with permission from Physicians World Communication Group.)

ECG Monitoring

The availability of ECG monitoring markedly simplifies the task of performing a monitored patient evaluation, as it allows the therapist to concentrate on taking accurate BP measurements and noting signs and symptoms while the ECG recorder provides the HR and rhythm responses. The therapist merely needs to mark each ECG strip with the activity being monitored.

- Typically, a single lead is monitored and rhythm strips are printed out. The lead systems commonly used to monitor patients during activity are illustrated in Figure 6-20.
  - ▸ In lead I, the negative and positive electrodes are placed in the second intercostal space (ICS) on the right and left, respectively, at or lateral to the midclavicular line.
  - ▸ In lead II, the negative electrode is the same as lead I and the positive electrode is placed in the lowest ICS at the anterior axillary line.
  - ▸ In the modified chest lead V_1 (MCL$_1$) the negative electrode is placed in the second ICS on the left and the positive electrode is placed in the fourth ICS at the right sternal border.
  - ▸ In the modified chest lead V_6 (MCL$_6$) the negative electrode is placed in the second ICS on the left and the positive electrode is placed in the fifth ICS at the midaxillary line.

- ▸ When using hardwire ECG monitoring, the negative electrode is usually white and most often is placed on the right side of the chest ("white is right") and the positive electrode is red or black; if there is a ground electrode, it is usually green and it can be placed anywhere on the chest (often on the lower right chest).
- In general, any lead with a tall upright ventricular voltage (R wave) is acceptable for most patients; an exception is the patient with known myocardial ischemia (as noted on a stress test, etc.) in whom it is often advisable to monitor the area known to exhibit ischemic changes. This can be accomplished by using one of the standard leads or by creating a different lead in which the vector from the negative to the positive electrodes points to the area in question (the ground electrode, if present, can be placed anywhere).
- Caution is warranted when interpreting ST-segment changes obtained from ECG telemetry units. Most modern units contain special filters and amplifiers that dampen muscle artifact and provide a cleaner rhythm strip; however, these units do not accurately portray ST-segment changes. Only units without special filters (often called "diagnostic" telemetry units) and hardwire units can be used for valid ST-segment interpretation (if calibrated appropriately).

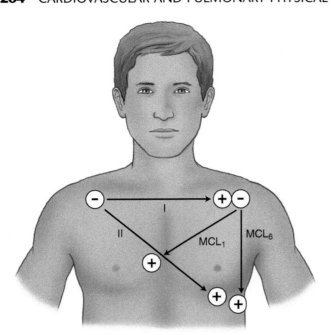

Figure 6-20: Bipolar lead systems commonly used for bedside or rehabilitation electrocardiogram (ECG) monitoring. See text for specific electrode placement sites.

- Sometimes single-lead ECG strips can be difficult to decipher because of artifact due to muscle tremors or patient movement (including shivering, hiccups, sneezing, and coughing), loose electrodes, or 60-cycle electrical interference.

▸ Artifact occurs as small to broad baseline oscillations or wandering of the baseline.

▸ Typically, R waves can be detected at regular intervals within the artifact, but other waves may be more difficult to identify.

▸ To minimize artifact, proper skin preparation (such as brisk rubbing with gauze and alcohol) before electrode placement is recommended.

ECG Waveforms and Intervals

To interpret a rhythm strip, the examiner must be able to distinguish normal ECG patterns from abnormal variations. The normal ECG waveforms and intervals are shown in Figure 6-21. Analysis of rhythm strips is relatively straightforward if a systematic approach is used, as described in Table 6-20. Heart rate can be calculated according to either of the methods illustrated in Figure 6-22. Alternatively, the rate can be measured by using an ECG ruler, which involves placing the reference arrow on an R wave and then counting two or three R-to-R intervals (depending on the design of the specific ruler) and reading the corresponding rate. The characteristics of the various rhythms and arrhythmias are described in the following sections.

Sinus Node Rhythms and Arrhythmias

- Normal sinus rhythm (NSR) (Figure 6-23)
  ▸ Rate: 60 to 100 bpm
  ▸ Rhythm: Regular
  ▸ P waves: Smooth and rounded, positive in lead II, no more than 2.5 mm in height and not more than 0.1 second in duration; all are identical, and each is followed by a QRS

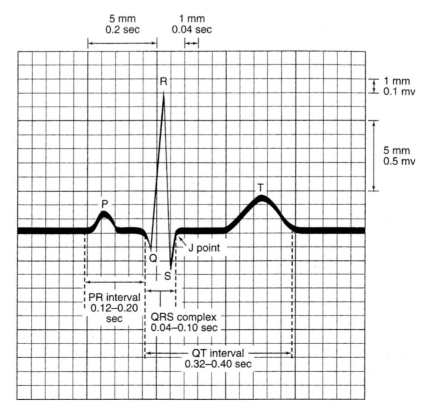

Figure 6-21: Electrocardiogram (ECG) waveforms and intervals. The normal ranges of the various intervals are also included.

TABLE 6-20: Systematic Approach for Analyzing ECG Rhythm Strips

Procedure	Important Observations
Scan rhythm strip to obtain initial impression	Is the rate unusually slow or fast?
	Does the rhythm appear to be regular?
	Are any "funny beats" obvious?
Evaluate rhythm by comparing R-to-R intervals	Are all R-to-R intervals equal or nearly equal (i.e., within 0.04 s)?
	If irregularity is present, is there some kind of pattern or is it totally irregular?
Calculate HR by most appropriate method*	If rhythm is regular, divide 300 by the number of large squares, including fractions of a square, between two consecutive R waves to determine the ventricular rate. If every P wave is not followed by a QRS complex, follow the same process for P waves to obtain the atrial rate
	If rhythm is irregular, obtain an ECG strip representing 6 s (30 large squares, or the distance between three time marks at the top of many ECG papers), count the number of QRS complexes, and multiply by 10 to obtain the ventricular rate per minute. Follow the same process for P waves, if necessary
Look at P waves to see whether sinus node is pacemaker in command	Are P waves present or absent?
	Are P waves all identical, smooth contoured, and upright in leads I, II, and III?
	Is each P wave followed by a QRS complex?
If P waves are present, measure P–R interval to see whether any delay in conduction through AV nodal region exists	Is P–R interval 0.12–0.20 s in duration (i.e., 3.0–5.0 small boxes)?
	Note: P–R interval varies inversely with the HR and is therefore normally lower in infants and children
Examine QRS complexes to determine whether conduction through ventricles is normal	Are the QRS complexes 0.04–0.10 s (i.e., 1.0 to 2.5 boxes) in duration?
	Are the QRS complexes all identical in shape?
Assess ST segment	Is the ST segment at the level of the baseline at 0.08 s after the J point?

AV, Atrioventricular; ECG, electrocardiographic; HR, heart rate.
*See Figure 6-22.

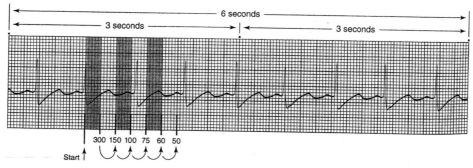

Figure 6-22: Heart rate can be calculated by counting the number of complexes in a 6-second strip and multiplying the result by 10 (particularly useful in very irregular rhythms) or by dividing 300 by the number of large squares between two R waves. To find the specific rate when the second R wave falls between two large squares, determine the difference between the two large squares on either side of the R wave (e.g., in the ECG shown above, $100 - 75 = 25$) and divide this number by 5 (the number of small boxes in a large square); then multiply the result by the number of small boxes between the lesser number and the R wave (e.g., above, $5 \times 3 = 15$) and add this result to the value of the lesser of the two large squares (75), yielding a HR of 90.

▸ P–R interval: Normal (0.12 to 0.20 s)
▸ QRS: Normal (0.04 to 0.10 s)
▸ T wave: Rounded, slightly asymmetrical (the peak occurs after the midpoint of the wave), positive in lead II, less than 5 mm in height
• Sinus bradycardia (Figure 6-24)
  ▸ Rate: Less than 60 bpm

▸ Otherwise the same as NSR
▸ Causes: Seen in many healthy individuals, especially athletes, during rest or sleep, when parasympathetic nervous system is dominant; increased vagal stimulation (gagging, vomiting, tracheal suctioning, and massage of carotid sinus); pain, myocardial ischemia or infarction affecting the right

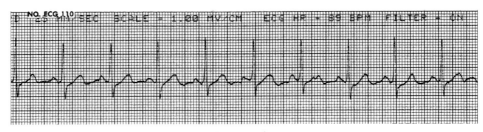

Figure 6-23: Normal sinus rhythm (slight artifact present in some P and T waves).

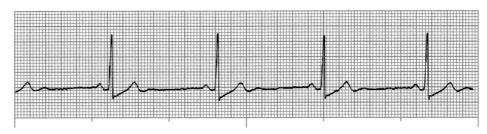

Figure 6-24: Sinus bradycardia (also with ST-segment depression). (From Aehlert B. *ECGs Made Easy.* 3rd ed. St. Louis: Mosby; 2006.)

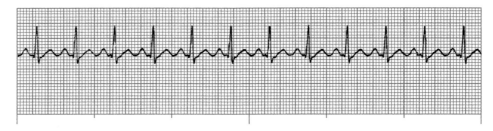

Figure 6-25: Sinus tachycardia. (From Aehlert B. *ECGs Made Easy.* 3rd ed. St. Louis: Mosby; 2006.)

coronary artery (RCA), severe body anoxia, increased intracranial pressure, and certain medications (e.g., digitalis, β-blockers, and verapamil)

▸ Significance: Generally harmless, except as a sign of underlying disorders; if pronounced, cardiac output will drop and the patient may feel dizzy or faint; if myocardial ischemia or any signs and symptoms of cardiac or cerebral hypoxia develop, bradycardia is considered a medical emergency; also, the slow rate may allow time for irritable ectopic sites to take over as pacemaker

• Sinus tachycardia (Figure 6-25)
▸ Rate: 100 to 180 or more bpm
▸ Otherwise the same as NSR
▸ Causes: Compensatory mechanism of body to increase cardiac output under stressful situations (exercise, fear, fever, pain, etc.) and in congestive heart failure (CHF), shock, hyperthyroidism hypoxia, and anemia; certain drugs (e.g., xanthine derivatives: theophylline and aminophylline)

▸ Significance: Minor, except as a signal of other underlying disorders; may have hemodynamic consequences if there is LV dysfunction and the increased workload created by faster HR is not tolerated

• Sinus arrhythmia (Figure 6-26)
▸ Definition: Phasic quickening and slowing of impulse formation, generally coordinated with respiration (increased on inspiration and decreased on expiration)
▸ Otherwise the same as NSR, including P waves
▸ Causes: Alterations in blood flow and pressures due to changes in intrathoracic pressure during respiration; commonly seen in the very young and very old
▸ Significance: None, benign

• Sinus arrest and sinus exit block (Figure 6-27)
▸ Definition: Failure of the sinoatrial (SA) node to initiate or conduct an impulse for one or more cycles, producing a pause in the sinus rhythm in which one or more beats is missing

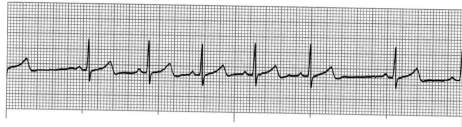

Figure 6-26: Sinus arrhythmia. (From Aehlert B. *ECGs Made Easy.* 3rd ed. St. Louis: Mosby; 2006.)

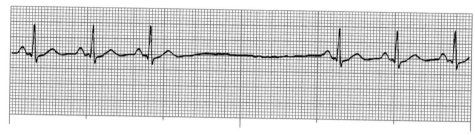

Figure 6-27: Sinus rhythm with an episode of sinus arrest. (From Aehlert B. *ECGs Made Easy.* 3rd ed. St. Louis: Mosby; 2006.)

▸ Characteristics: Abrupt pause in underlying sinus rhythm producing notably long P-to-P distance with complete absence of one or more PQRST sequences

▸ Causes: Digitalis toxicity (most common), SA node disease, and increased vagal influence

▸ Significance: Indicates failure of the SA node as pacemaker; if prolonged or frequent, cardiac output will drop, producing dizziness, near syncope, or syncope

Atrial Dysrrhythmias

• Premature atrial complexes (PACs or APCs) (Figure 6-28)

▸ Definition: An ectopic site in either atrium initiates an impulse before the next impulse is initiated by the SA node; the underlying rhythm is usually NSR, with a PQRST sequence occurring earlier than expected after the preceding PQRST

▸ Rhythm: Irregularly irregular or sometimes regularly irregular

▸ P wave: Noticeably different than normal sinus P waves (configuration depends on the site of impulse formation but is premature and abnormal in size, shape, and direction—commonly small, upright, and pointed, but may be inverted or hidden in preceding T wave, causing distortion of the T wave)

▸ P–R interval: Usually normal but may be prolonged; cannot measure if P is hidden in preceding T wave

▸ QRS: Premature, usually the same as others from SA node, although aberrant conduction may occur (producing a widened QRS complex); on occasion the premature beat occurs early enough that a portion of the conduction system may be refractory, so that the impulse is not conducted and no QRS complex is noted (a blocked PAC, the most common cause of pauses)

▸ Causes: Emotional stress, apprehension, tobacco, coffee, alcohol, and fatigue; hypoxia, myocardial ischemia, CAD, atrial enlargement, chronic lung disease, and sympathomimetic drugs

▸ Significance: Generally benign; if very frequent, may result in decreased cardiac output; may progress to atrial tachycardia, flutter, or fibrillation

• Multifocal PACs (also called wandering atrial pacemaker) (Figure 6-29)

▸ Definition: With the SA being the dominant pacemaker, other impulses arise from various ectopic sites in the atria (sometimes an impulse is aberrantly conducted through the ventricles, as described for PACs)

▸ Rhythm: Irregularly irregular

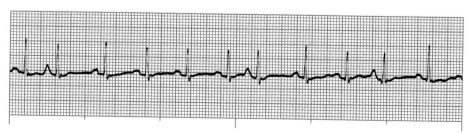

Figure 6-28: Sinus tachycardia with three premature atrial complexes (PACs). Note the taller size of the P waves compared with the sinus beats. (From Aehlert B. *ECGs Made Easy.* 3rd ed. St. Louis: Mosby; 2006.)

Lead II (continuous)

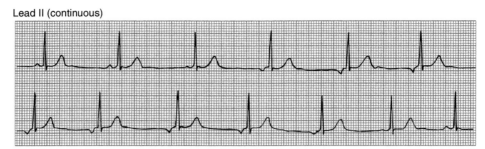

Figure 6-29: Wandering atrial pacemaker shown in a continuous ECG strip using lead II. (From Aehlert B. *ECGs Made Easy.* 3rd ed. St. Louis: Mosby; 2006.)

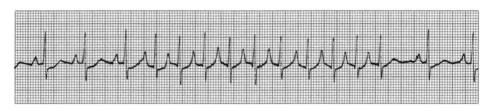

Figure 6-30: Paroxysmal supraventricular tachycardia at a rate of 185 bpm. P waves are merged with the T waves. (From Aehlert B. *ECGs Made Easy.* 3rd ed. St. Louis: Mosby; 2006.)

- ▸ P wave: Different configurations (flattened, peaked, notched, or inverted) in addition to the normal sinus P waves
- ▸ QRS: Premature, usually the same as others from the SA node, although aberrant conduction may occur
- ▸ Causes: CHF, atrial infarction, and idiopathic
- ▸ Significance: Minor, although may lead to atrial flutter or fibrillation
- • Paroxysmal atrial or supraventricular tachycardia (PAT, PSVT) (Figure 6-30)
  - ▸ Definition: Sudden bursts of very rapid atrial or nodal tachycardia
  - ▸ Rate: 150 to 250 bpm
  - ▸ Rhythm: Very regular
  - ▸ P waves: Abnormal and often merged with T wave (thus called PSVT)
  - ▸ QRS: Usually the same as others from the SA node; there may be some degree of block (at very rapid HRs, the atrioventricular [AV] node may not be able to conduct all impulses, so that not every P wave will be followed by a QRS complex)

- ▸ Other: Begins and ends abruptly; may be terminated by vagal stimulation (e.g., carotid sinus massage and coughing)
- ▸ Causes: Digitalis toxicity; seen in coronary artery disease (CAD) and rheumatic heart disease; emotional stress, tobacco, coffee, and alcohol; idiopathic
- ▸ Significance: If rate is extremely rapid, ventricular filling may decrease, resulting in decreased cardiac output and low blood pressure; if poor ventricular function or CAD, the patient may develop chest discomfort, lightheadedness, and possibly CHF
- • Atrial flutter (Figure 6-31)
  - ▸ Definition: Very rapid atrial tachycardia
  - ▸ Rate: 250 to 350 bpm
  - ▸ Rhythm: Absolutely regular
  - ▸ P waves: Characteristic sawtooth pattern in leads II, III, and aVF (called flutter, or F, waves)
  - ▸ P–R interval: Not measurable
  - ▸ QRS: Usually normal with some being blocked
  - ▸ Causes: Organic heart disease (myocardial infarction and valve disease), status post (s/p) cardiac surgery, or idiopathic

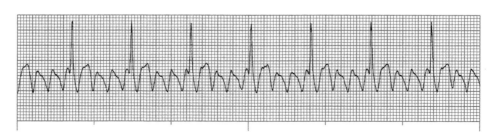

Figure 6-31: Atrial flutter with 4:1 block (the second most common ratio; 2:1 block is the most common ratio). Note the typical sawtoothed F waves. (From Aehlert B. *ECGs Made Easy.* 3rd ed. St. Louis: Mosby; 2006.)

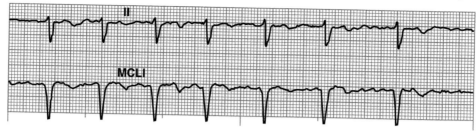

Figure 6-32: Atrial fibrillation shown in leads II and MCL₁. Note the typical, uneven, irregular "f" waves. (From Aehlert B. *ECGs Made Easy*. 3rd ed. St. Louis: Mosby; 2006.)

▸ Significance: Depends on ventricular rate (if very rapid rate cardiac output will decrease or CHF may develop); usually considered serious; may deteriorate into atrial fibrillation
• Atrial fibrillation (Figure 6-32)
  ▸ Definition: Erratic quivering or twitching of the atrial muscle
  ▸ Rhythm: Irregularly irregular
  ▸ Rate: Atrial rate is indeterminate; ventricular rate is highly variable and may be slow, fast, or normal
  ▸ P waves: Absent; instead only a chaotic baseline, called "f" waves
  ▸ QRS: Typical for patient although they occur at irregular intervals
  ▸ Causes: Same as for atrial flutter
  ▸ Significance: Depends on ventricular rate (if very fast or slow rate, cardiac output may drop or CHF may develop); loss of atrial "kick" results in reduced ventricular filling and cardiac output, especially if LV dysfunction exists, and CHF may be provoked even at relatively normal rates; stagnation of blood in atria may lead to thrombus formation and embolization

Nodal/Junctional Arrhythmias

• Premature nodal/junctional complexes (PNCs, PJCs) (Figure 6-33)
  ▸ Definition: Premature impulses arising from the AV node or junctional tissue
  ▸ P waves: Abnormal–inverted; may occur before, during, or after the QRS segment, depending on the site of origin of the impulse
  ▸ P–R interval: Short (<0.10 s)
  ▸ QRS: Premature, same as from SA node

  ▸ Causes: Digitalis toxicity, CAD, decreased automaticity and conduction of the SA node or irritability of the junctional tissue, CHF, and valvular disease
  ▸ Significance: Usually benign unless very frequent, when loss of atrial "kick" may lead to inadequate ventricular filling and reduced cardiac output
• Nodal or junctional rhythm (Figure 6-34)
  ▸ Definition: When the AV node or junctional tissue takes over as pacemaker of the heart
  ▸ Rate: 40 to 60 bpm
  ▸ P waves, P–R interval, QRS: Same as for PNCs
  ▸ Causes: Same as for PNCs/PJCs; trained athletes
  ▸ Significance: Generally well tolerated in normal individuals; in others, may indicate failure of SA node and AV node is unreliable as a pacemaker and may fail; slow rate may allow ectopic foci to fire; in patients with ventricular dysfunction, lack of atrial "kick" may result in signs and symptoms of inadequate cardiac output or CHF (although slow HR often assists in maintaining ventricular filling)
• Accelerated nodal/junctional rhythm (Figure 6-35)
  ▸ Definition: Nodal/junctional rhythm with rate of 70 to 150 bpm, otherwise same as above; rates greater than 100 bpm may be called junctional tachycardia
  ▸ Causes: Organic heart disease, digitalis toxicity, s/p cardiac surgery; idiopathic
  ▸ Significance: Hemodynamic impact depends on HR (if very fast or slow, cardiac output may drop or CHF may develop); otherwise same as for nodal rhythm

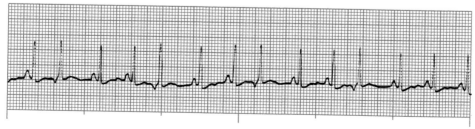

Figure 6-33: Sinus tachycardia with frequent premature nodal/junctional complexes. Note the inverted P waves just before the QRS complex. (From Aehlert B. *ECGs Made Easy*. 3rd ed. St. Louis: Mosby; 2006.)

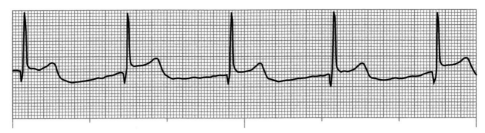

Figure 6-34: Nodal/junctional rhythm with a rate of 44 bpm. No P waves are visible; there are Q waves and ST elevation characteristic of acute myocardial infarction. (From Aehlert B. *ECGs Made Easy.* 3rd ed. St. Louis: Mosby; 2006.)

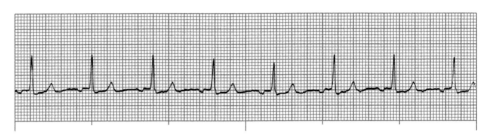

Figure 6-35: Accelerated nodal/junctional rhythm with rate of approximately 75 bpm. Note inverted P waves before the QRS complexes. (From Aehlert B. *ECGs Made Easy.* 3rd ed. St. Louis: Mosby; 2006.)

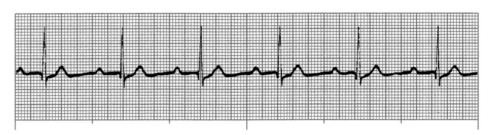

Figure 6-36: First-degree AV block occurring with sinus rhythm at a heart rate of 60 bpm. (From Aehlert B. *ECGs Made Easy.* 3rd ed. St. Louis: Mosby; 2006.)

Heart Blocks

- First-degree AV/heart block (1° AVB) (Figure 6-36)
  - ▸ Definition: Prolongation of conduction through the AV node, and therefore the P–R interval exceeds 0.20 second
  - ▸ P waves: Normal; each is followed by a QRS complex
  - ▸ QRS: Normal, unless another conduction disturbance also exists
  - ▸ Causes: Digitalis toxicity, MI damaging the AV node, and ischemia
  - ▸ Significance: Generally well tolerated but may progress to more serious AV block
- Second-degree AV/heart block (2° AVB)
  - ▸ Definition: Nonconduction of some of the impulses through the AV node
  - ▸ Two types:
    - ⊙ Mobitz I or Wenckebach: Progressive prolongation of the P–R interval until finally one impulse is not conducted (a P

wave without a QRS complex following it); then the cycle repeats (Figure 6-37)
  - ⊙ Mobitz II: PQRST sequences with the same P–R interval (may have 1° AVB) followed by nonconduction of one or more impulses (Figure 6-38)
  - ▸ P waves: Normal; not all are followed by a QRS complex
  - ▸ P–R interval: Variable for Mobitz I, constant for Mobitz II
  - ▸ QRS: Same as for 1° AVB
  - ▸ Causes: Digitalis toxicity; MI or ischemia involving the AV nodal region
  - ▸ Significance: Mobitz I is generally benign; Mobitz II represents a more critical conduction defect. Hemodynamic impact depends on ventricular rate (if rate is very slow, cardiac output may fall); second-degree AV block may progress to third-degree heart block
- Third-degree, or complete, AV/heart block (3° AVB) (Figure 6-39)

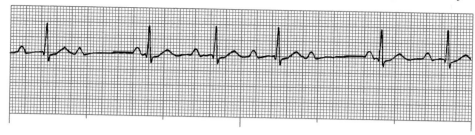

Figure 6-37: Second-degree AV block, Mobitz type I or Wenckebach phenomenon. After the first QRS complex there is a blocked beat, and then three conducted beats with progressively longer P–R intervals and another blocked beat. (From Aehlert B. *ECGs Made Easy.* 3rd ed. St. Louis: Mosby; 2006.)

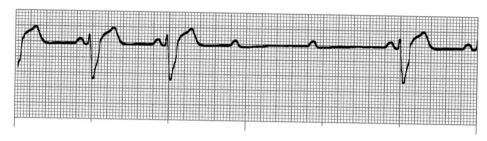

Figure 6-38: Second-degree AV block, Mobitz type II. Two consecutive P–R intervals are the same (and normal) before two dropped beats. Note also the presence of wide QRS complexes and ST elevation. (From Aehlert B. *ECGs Made Easy.* 3rd ed. St. Louis: Mosby; 2006.)

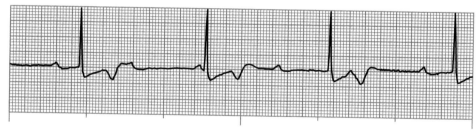

Figure 6-39: Third-degree, or complete, AV block. The P waves and QRS complexes are independent of each other, at a ventricular rate of 37 bpm and an atrial rate of 63 bpm. In addition, ST-segment depression and inverted T waves are present. (From Aehlert B. *ECGs Made Easy.* 3rd ed. St. Louis: Mosby; 2006.)

▸ Definition: All impulses are blocked at the AV node so that none of the impulses from the SA node or atria reach the ventricles; a separate pacemaker for the ventricles must be established or there will be no cardiac output

▸ Rate: Separate atrial and ventricular rates; ventricular rate is usually 30 to 50 bpm

▸ P waves: Usually present, but may be from SA node or atria; can have atrial fibrillation or flutter; no relationship to QRS complexes

▸ QRS: May be either normal or abnormal

▸ Causes: Digitalis toxicity, MI or ischemia of the AV nodal region; other diseases affecting the AV node

▸ Significance: Very unstable rhythm and considered a medical emergency; AV node is unreliable and may fail, so a pacemaker is indicated (if no ventricular pacemaker is established, the individual will die); if the ventricular rate is slow, cardiac output will fall

Arrhythmias Originating From the Ventricles

• Premature ventricular complexes (PVCs, VPCs) (Figure 6-40)

▸ Definition: Impulses originating from an ectopic site in the ventricles earlier than the next expected SA node impulse

▸ Rhythm: Can be regularly irregular (PVCs occurring in a predictable pattern, such as every so-many beats or may be irregularly irregular (occurring at random)

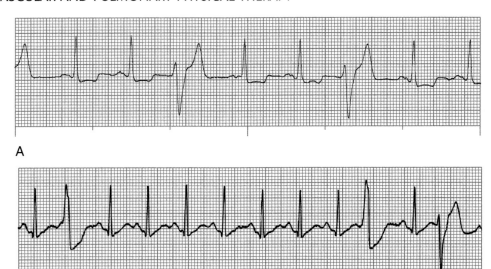

A

B

Figure 6-40: Premature ventricular complexes (PVCs): **A,** PVCs in trigeminy. The PVCs are followed by a full compensatory pause. Note also the wide P waves indicating atrial overload and abnormal ST–T waves. **B,** Multifocal PVCs. Underlying rhythm is sinus tachycardia at a heart rate of 120 bpm. (From Aehlert B. *ECGs Made Easy.* 3rd ed. St. Louis: Mosby; 2006.)

▸ P waves: Usually not seen
▸ QRS: Wide, bizarre looking, usually followed by a complete compensatory pause
▸ Other: Can be isolated versus sequential (e.g., paired/couplets), unifocal versus multifocal, or can occur in a regular pattern:
  ⊙ *Multifocal* PVCs arise from different ectopic foci and thus have different configurations
  ⊙ *Unifocal* PVCs arise from the same ectopic focus and thus have similar configurations
  ⊙ PVCs occurring every other (second) beat is referred to as *bigeminy,* every third beat is *trigeminy,* and every fourth beat is *quadrigeminy*
▸ Causes: Coffee, tobacco, alcohol, and excitement; increased ventricular irritability due to myocardial ischemia or other cardiac disease, acid–base imbalance, electrolyte imbalance, or digitalis toxicity
▸ Significance: Atrial "kick" is lacking and the diastolic filling period is reduced, leading to reduced ventricular filling and decreased stroke volume; increasing frequency of PVCs may indicate increased irritability of the ventricular muscle and cause cardiac output to fall; can progress to ventricular tachycardia or fibrillation
• Ventricular tachycardia (v-tach, VT) (Figure 6-41)
  ▸ Definition: A run of three or more PVCs, usually at a rate of 140 to 250 beats/min
  ▸ P waves: Not seen unless slow rate, and then unrelated to QRS complex
  ▸ QRS: Series of wide, bizarre QRS complexes
  ▸ Causes: Acute MI, CAD, hypertensive heart disease, and digitalis or quinidine toxicity; occasionally seen in athletes during exercise

▸ Significance: Indicates marked ventricular irritability and is usually a medical emergency; lack of atrial contribution to ventricular filling combined with rapid rate results in very low cardiac output and very low blood pressure and possible shock; frequently progresses to ventricular fibrillation and death
• Ventricular fibrillation (v-fib, VF) (Figure 6-42)
  ▸ Definition: Erratic quivering of ventricular muscle
  ▸ PQRST: Waves are absent; grossly irregular up-and-down fluctuations of the baseline; irregular zigzag pattern
  ▸ Causes: Same as for v-tach; may be sequel to v-tach
  ▸ Significance: No effective pumping, no cardiac output, no pulse or BP; patient is clinically dead

Pacemaker Rhythms

Patients who have pacemakers will exhibit an electronic spike immediately preceding the depolarization of the paced chamber for any paced beats, as shown in Figure 6-43.
• An electronic spike is recognized by its extreme brevity.
• With a ventricular pacemaker, the QRS complex begins immediately after the pacemaker spike and is markedly prolonged and bizarre in appearance (due to the altered path of depolarization).
• Multiprogrammable pacemakers may be activated with variable modes of atrial and ventricular stimulation or inhibition depending on patient need (see page 62).

Other Findings

Other ECG changes that can be observed on 12-lead ECGs are sometimes visible on rhythm strips, depending on the lead that is being monitored:
• Bundle branch block (wide QRS complexes)
• Ventricular hypertrophy with or without strain pattern (tall R or deep S waves ± ST changes in opposite direction)

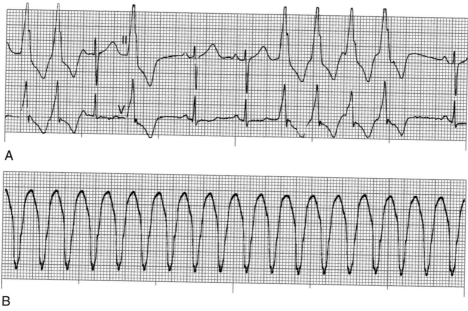

A

B

Figure 6-41: Ventricular tachycardia. **A,** A brief salvo of four beats shown in two leads. There is also a couplet of PVCs and an isolated PVC. **B,** Sustained v-tach is diagnosed when it lasts more than 30 seconds. Here the rate is 180 bpm. (From Aehlert B. *ECGs Made Easy.* 3rd ed. St. Louis: Mosby; 2006.)

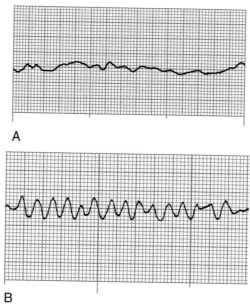

A

B

Figure 6-42: Ventricular fibrillation. **A,** Fine fibrillation. **B,** Coarse fibrillation. (From Aehlert B. *ECGs Made Easy.* 3rd ed. St. Louis: Mosby; 2006.)

- Atrial abnormalities (*P mitrale* or *P pulmonale*)
- Myocardial ischemia or infarction (ST-segment depression or elevation)

ECG Responses to Exercise

Normally there are few if any ECG changes, other than an increase in HR, during exercise.

- The heart should remain in sinus rhythm, developing progressive tachycardia in proportion to the workload but no other dysrhythmias.
- Sometimes trained athletes will have such a slow HR at rest that the AV node becomes the dominant pacemaker (i.e., they are in nodal/junctional rhythm), but as HR increases with exercise, sinus rhythm takes over.

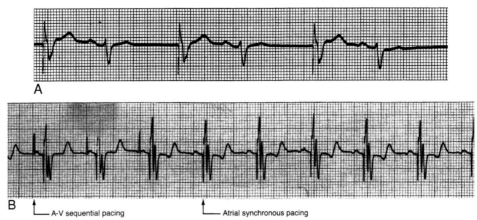

B   └— A-V sequential pacing   └— Atrial synchronous pacing

Figure 6-43: **A,** Electronic pacemaker bigeminy from a ventricular inhibited (VVI) pacemaker with an escape interval of 1.02 seconds, which inhibits activation unless the natural heart rate falls below 58 bpm. **B,** A dual-chamber, dual-sensing, dual-pacing/inhibiting (DDD) pacemaker exhibiting AV sequential and atrial synchronous modes. Note upright atrial pacemaker spike followed by P wave when no atrial activity is sensed within the programmed time period and downward ventricular spike that always produces ventricular depolarization. However, when spontaneous atrial activity (at a rate >76 bpm) is sensed, the DDD pacemaker inhibits atrial pacing and produces only a ventricular stimulus that is synchronized to the atrial activity. (From Phillips RE, Feeney MK. *The Cardiac Rhythms: A Systematic Approach to Interpretation.* 3rd ed. Philadelphia: Saunders; 1990.)

- Individuals who develop myocardial ischemia classically develop ST-segment depression, which may worsen or occur only during recovery, as demonstrated in an exercise test in Figure 6-44. However, ST-segment depression can also result from nonischemic causes, including resting repolarization abnormalities (e.g., LBBB), LVH (e.g., severe aortic stenosis or HTN), digitalis drug effect, cardiomyopathy, hypokalemia, pericardial disorders, mitral valve prolapse, anemia, severe hypoxia, hyperglycemia, and female gender, among others.[2,3,31]

- Exercise-induced arrhythmias are generated by enhanced sympathetic tone and increased myocardial demand and often occur during the period immediately after exercise. Individuals with CAD and those taking diuretics and digitalis are most vulnerable. Increasing PVCs or V-tach with increasing exercise intensity are particularly worrisome in individuals with chest pain syndromes (even without ST-segment depression), cardiomyopathy, valvular heart disease, or a family history of sudden death, because they suggest increasing ventricular irritability and are associated with serious underlying disease and greater risk of mortality.[28,31]

- First-degree AV bock at rest often disappears with exercise because of withdrawal of vagal stimulation.[28]

- On occasion, patients with myocardial ischemia develop conduction disturbances with exercise, including AV, intraventricular, and bundle branch blocks.[28,31]

- On rare occasions, patients develop ST-segment elevation during exercise. When it occurs in leads with abnormal Q waves, exercise-induced ST elevation seems to be related to severe hypokinesis or akinesis in the corresponding segment of myocardium and this may identify an area of myocardial ischemia

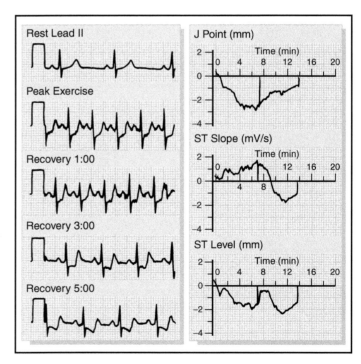

Figure 6-44: Exercise ECG results showing 1.5-mm slow upsloping ST-segment depression at maximal exercise (7.5 min of the Bruce protocol), which becomes horizontal at 3 min of recovery and then downsloping at 5 min of recovery. (From Libby P, Bonow RO, Mann DL, et al.: *Braunwald's Heart Disease: A Textbook of Cardiovascular Medicine.* 8th ed. Philadelphia: Saunders; 2008.)

within infarcted tissue.[28,31] ST elevation may be associated with reciprocal ST-segment depression that simulates myocardial ischemia in other leads. In individuals without abnormal Q waves at rest and no history of previous MI, ST elevation usually indicates severe transmural myocardial ischemia caused by coronary vasospasm or high-grade CAD.

Blood Pressure

The determination of BP is one of the most important clinical measurements performed by PTs and other medical professionals. It not only identifies individuals with hypertension (HTN), it also provides information about cardiac output and total peripheral resistance. However, it is extremely prone to error due to faulty equipment, incorrect technique, and clinician- and patient-related factors, as listed in Table 6-21, which are further compounded during exercise. In addition, cardiac arrhythmias can result in BP inaccuracies because of the wide fluctuations they can create.

- Several different types of devices can be used to measure BP, all of which have advantages and disadvantages.
  - ▸ Mercury sphygmomanometers have always been regarded as the "gold standard" for BP measurement. However, various hospital surveys have found that 20% to 50% of devices had defects that affected their accuracy.[54] Yet, the accuracy of mercury manometers can be easily verified by checking that the upper meniscus of the mercury column is at 0 mm Hg, the glass column is free of dirt, the rubber tubing is without cracks, and the column of mercury rises and falls freely during cuff inflation and deflation. Of note, environmental concerns regarding the toxicity of mercury have resulted in their removal from many clinical practices, and a satisfactory replacement has yet to be identified.
  - ▸ Aneroid sphygmomanometers rely on a mechanical system of metal bellows and a series of levers. Unfortunately, they are prone to problems with maintaining stability, especially with rough handling, and require regular calibration to assure accuracy. In addition, the accuracy of these manometers varies greatly among the different manufacturers, with inaccuracies ranging from 1% to 44%.[54]
  - ▸ Oscillometric BP systems are automated noninvasive measuring devices that use a sphygmomanometer cuff with a sensor to detect the oscillations produced by arterial wall pulsations. Because the oscillations begin well above SBP and continue below diastolic blood pressure (DBP), these devices rely on analysis by a microprocessor and use an empirically derived algorithm to estimate systolic, diastolic, and mean BP. Because the amplitude of the oscillations depends on several factors, particularly the stiffness of the arteries, the mean arterial pressure (MAP), which can be estimated to equal $(SBP + 2 \times DBP)/3$, may be significantly underestimated in older people. In addition, movement artifact makes the use of these devices unreliable for monitoring BP during exercise.[14a]
  - ▸ Hybrid sphygmomanometers combine some of the best features of both electronic and auscultatory devices: they use an electronic pressure gauge like those found in oscillometric devices while the examiner auscultates the Korotkoff sounds with a stethoscope. Thus, they have the potential to become a suitable replacement for the mercury manometer.
  - ▸ The accuracy of the various devices can be checked by connecting the manometer to a mercury column (in good repair) or an electronic testing device with a Y-connector. The needle should rest at the zero point before the cuff is inflated and should register a reading that is within 4 mm Hg of the mercury column or electronic testing device when the cuff is inflated to pressures of 100 and 200 mm Hg, and the needle should return to the zero point after full deflation.
- Numerous surveys have shown that health care professionals rarely follow established guidelines for BP measurement. However, when they are followed, accuracy is greatly enhanced. The proper technique for obtaining BP measurements is as follows[54]:
  - ▸ The individual should be seated comfortably in a chair with the back supported and the legs uncrossed and feet flat on the floor for at least 5 minutes before the first reading is taken. Extraneous and patient-related factors that can produce significant deviations in BP values should be controlled by proper preparation of the individual (see Table 6-21). The person should be instructed to relax and not to talk during the measurement procedure.

TABLE 6-21: Major Sources of Error in the Measurement of Blood Pressure

Source of error	Problem
Faulty equipment	Inaccurate sphygmomanometer (not calibrated)
	Air leak in sphygmomanometer or stethoscope tubing
Extraneous factors	Poor control of room temperature, background noise
Patient-related factors	Full bladder
	Not relaxed, presence of muscle tension
	Talking
Clinician-related factors	Lack of experience
Improper technique	Inadequate patient preparation
	Incorrect cuff size, cuff position
	Improper arm position
	Incorrect stethoscope placement or pressure
	Improper rate and degree of cuff inflation and deflation
Limited accuracy of auscultatory method	Difficulty identifying appropriate Korotkoff sounds (presence of auscultatory gap, lack of phase V sound)
	Poor auditory acuity
	Observer variability
Exercise-induced difficulties	Extraneous noise, mechanical vibration
	Movement artifact

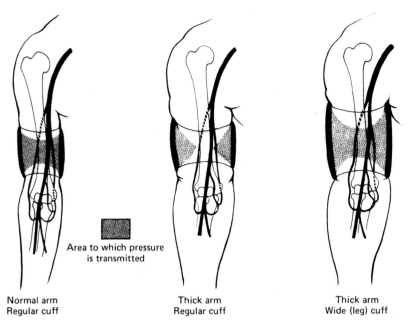

Normal arm
Regular cuff

Thick arm
Regular cuff

Thick arm
Wide (leg) cuff

Area to which pressure
is transmitted

Figure 6-45: Area of pressure transmission by various blood pressure cuffs. Note the inability of the regular, or standard-sized, cuff to transmit adequate pressure to occlude the brachial artery in a person with a thick arm. (From Sokolow M, McIlroy MB. *Clinical Cardiology.* 6th ed. Los Altos, CA: Lange Medical Publications;1993.)

▸ A properly sized cuff should be placed on the patient's arm, 2.5 cm above the antecubital space, with the bladder of the cuff centered over the palpated brachial artery. The bladder of the cuff should be long enough to encircle 80% of the arm and the width of the cuff should be at least 40% of the arm circumference, as shown in Figure 6-45.

  ⊙ The recommended cuff sizes are as follows:
    ☐ "Small adult" size of 12 × 22 cm for arm circumference of 22 to 26 cm
    ☐ "Adult" size of 16 × 30 cm for arm circumference of 27 to 34 cm
    ☐ "Large adult" size of 16 × 36 cm for arm circumference of 35 to 44 cm
    ☐ "Adult thigh" size of 16 × 42 cm for arm circumference of 45 to 52 cm

  ⊙ If the cuff is too short or too narrow, the reading will be erroneously high.
  ⊙ If the cuff is too wide or too long, it will be erroneously low.
  ⊙ When a standard size cuff is too small for the upper arm and a larger cuff is not available or if the arm is so large or its shape cannot accommodate a proper-fitting cuff, the BP should be obtained from a cuff placed on the forearm with auscultation over the radial artery in the wrist.

▸ The BP should be taken in both arms on the initial evaluation unless the patient has an intravenous line in one arm, has had a mastectomy, or has abnormal tone on one side. When there is a consistent interarm difference, the arm with the higher BP should be used for BP monitoring.

▸ With the arm supported so the cuff is at the level of the heart, the cuff should be inflated rapidly to at least 30 mm Hg past the point where the palpated pulse disappears. If the patient's arm is not relaxed or is lower than his/her heart, both the systolic and diastolic values will be erroneously high.

▸ The cuff should be deflated slowly at a rate of 2 to 3 mm/second (or per pulse beat if the HR is very slow) and the reading noted at which the radial pulse is first palpated; then the cuff should be allowed to deflate completely.

▸ Next, the diaphragm of the stethoscope is placed over the brachial artery in the antecubital space and the cuff is reinflated to at least 30 mm Hg past the previously determined level.

▸ The cuff should be deflated slowly while listening with the stethoscope over the brachial artery; the pressure level at which a sound is first heard (Korotkoff phase I) is noted as the SBP and the level where the sound disappears (phase V) should be recorded as the DBP.

  ⊙ Avoid keeping the cuff inflated for more than 30 to 60 seconds, as the discomfort from prolonged inflation will cause the BP to rise.
  ⊙ Always deflate the cuff completely and wait 60 seconds before reinflating it for another measurement.

▸ For baseline resting values, at least two measurements should be taken and the average of the readings should be used. If there is a difference of more than 5 mm Hg between the two readings, additional readings should be obtained and the average of these multiple readings should be used.

▸ When the BP value is recorded, the arm used and the patient's position should be noted.

▸ During exertion, BP should be measured while the patient is actually performing the activity, because BP falls as soon as activity is stopped. If it is not possible to obtain an accurate reading during activity, try taking the BP as the patient marches in place. If this is not successful, the BP should be taken by inflating the BP cuff while the person is still moving and then slowly deflating the cuff as soon as activity is stopped.

- The auscultatory method relies on proper identification of the appropriate Korotkoff sounds: phase I, appearance of clear tapping sounds corresponding to the appearance of a palpable pulse (SBP); phase II, sounds become softer and longer; phase III, sounds become crisper and louder; phase IV, sounds become muffled and softer; and phase V, sounds disappear completely (DBP). However, it is known to have limited accuracy.
  - ▸ The auscultatory method may be unreliable because of poor hearing acuity and observer variability. Automated devices may solve these problems.
  - ▸ Some individuals, particularly those who are older and have a wide pulse pressure, exhibit an auscultatory gap, where there is a temporary disappearance of pulsing sounds lasting up to 40 mm Hg after the initial systolic sounds are heard (Figure 6-46). To avoid false-low SBP determination, it is important to inflate the BP cuff past the point of radial pulse disappearance. On the other hand, erroneously high DBP readings will be obtained, particularly with automatic BP recorders, if the transient loss of Korotkoff sounds is interpreted as the DBP. It is possible to eliminate the auscultatory gap by elevating the arm overhead for 30 seconds before inflating the cuff and then taking the BP with the arm in the usual position (the reduced vascular volume in the limb improves inflow to enhance the Korotkoff sounds).
  - ▸ Sometimes Korotkoff sounds are audible even after complete deflation of the cuff (e.g., pregnancy, aortic insufficiency, and arteriovenous fistula), so it is difficult to determine the DBP.
  - ▸ During exercise, extraneous sounds and body movements increase the difficulty in obtaining accurate BP readings, particularly if the individual is grasping the handrail on a treadmill or the handlebars of a cycle ergometer.
- Normal resting BP values are less than 120 mm Hg for SBP and less than 80 mm Hg for DBP with a pulse pressure (PP = SBP − DBP) of 20 to 59 mm Hg.
  - ▸ Elevated SBP can be due to increases in cardiac output, peripheral vascular resistance (PVR), or both (see page 42).

- ▸ Increased DBP is produced by an increase in PVR, which creates an increased pressure load against which the LV must work to eject blood.
- ▸ Both increased SBP and PP (≥60 mm Hg) are strong predictors of cardiovascular disease (CVD) risk.[19a,22,33,39a]
- The BP response to a controlled expiratory, or Valsalva, maneuver is a simple and valuable test that can be used to distinguish between a heart that is functioning normally and one that is failing.[13]
  - ▸ The intrathoracic pressure changes that occur during the Valsalva maneuver are opposite to those that occur during normal breathing, such that there is an increase (rather than a decrease) in intrathoracic pressure.
  - ▸ A normal response typically shows four distinct phases, as illustrated in Figure 6-47.[13,65]
    - ⊙ Phase 1 consists of an initial rise in SBP and DBP due to transmission of increased intrathoracic pressure to the periphery.
    - ⊙ Phase 2 is characterized by a drop in SBP, DBP, and pulse pressure as venous return is impeded by continued elevation of intrathoracic pressure along with a reflex increase in HR.
    - ⊙ Phase 3 is marked by a sudden drop in all pressures as the strain is released and intrathoracic pressure falls.
    - ⊙ Phase 4 is identified by an overshoot of SBP to above baseline levels with a widened pulse pressure and bradycardia, caused by a transient rise in cardiac output as venous return to the heart increases.
  - ▸ In the failing heart, the typical initial increase in BP (phase 1) and sudden drop in BP when the strain is released (phase 3) occur, but because the heart operates on the flat portion of its Starling curve (see Figure 3-5 on page 43), stroke volume is not affected by the impedance to venous return, so there is no phase 2 drop in BP or increase in HR. In addition, the phase 4 overshoot of BP and bradycardia are also absent. The result is a tracing with a "square-wave" appearance.[65]
  - ▸ Patients with moderate impairment of LV systolic function but not clear failure may exhibit an intermediate response in which there is a phase 2 drop in BP but not a phase 4 overshoot.[65]

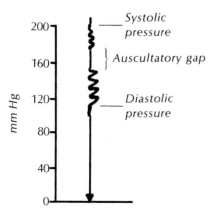

Figure 6-46: An auscultatory gap. (From Bates B. *A Guide to Physical Examination.* 5th ed. Philadelphia: J.B. Lippincott;1991.)

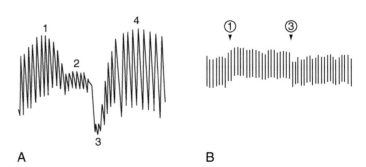

Figure 6-47: Arterial blood pressure responses to the Valsalva maneuver. **A,** Normal response. **B,** Abnormal response. (From DeTurk WE, Cahalin LB. *Cardiovascular and Pulmonary Physical Therapy: An Evidence-based Approach.* New York: McGraw-Hill; 2004.)

- The BP response to a change in body position from supine to standing can also produce a significant challenge to the cardiovascular system. As with the Valsalva maneuver, changing from supine to standing provokes a drop in venous return to the heart, and the resultant changes in SBP and DBP can be helpful in detecting whether the cardiac pump is normal, dysfunctional, or failing.[13] The standing BP must be measured immediately after the change in position.
  - ‣ Normally DBP is lower in the supine position compared with standing because of enhanced venous return and a reduction in peripheral vascular constriction, and a change to the standing position will induce an increase in DBP due to increased vasoconstriction serving to maintain adequate SBP and MAP.
  - ‣ A higher DBP in the supine position compared with standing and a drop in DBP with the move from supine to standing is typical of a failing heart.
  - ‣ In both situations, SBP is maintained during the position change.

BP Responses to Exercise

It is difficult to obtain accurate BP values during exercise because of patient movement, mechanical vibration, artifactual sounds, device limitations, and observer variability.

- It is generally recommended that BP monitoring during exercise be performed with a mercury sphygmomanometer or a recently calibrated aneroid manometer and a stethoscope, because few automated BP devices have been adequately validated during exercise.[2]
- To be meaningful, exertional BPs must be compared with the resting value obtained in the same position or posture (i.e., walking responses should be compared with the standing value and cycling responses should be compared with the sitting value).
- Because BP is the product of cardiac output and PVR, exercise produces different responses in the SBP and DBP, depending on the type of activity performed and the amount of muscle mass involved (Table 6-22).
  - ‣ When exercise is dynamic and involves the large muscles of the body, vasodilation induced by local metabolic effects in the exercising muscles results in a drop in total peripheral resistance so that DBP usually drops slightly or shows little change (a normal DBP response is considered to be ±10 mm Hg). An increase of more than 15 mm Hg in DBP may indicate labile HTN or severe CAD.[3] Because cardiac output increases with exertion, SBP increases in proportion to the workload (typically 10 ± 2 mm Hg per MET with a possible plateau at peak exercise.[3]

TABLE 6-22: Blood Pressure: Normal Values and Responses to Exercise

Normal	Comments
Resting: <120/<80 mm Hg	BP is a factor of cardiac output and total peripheral resistance; increases or decreases in either determinant will cause an ↑ or ↓, respectively, in BP
Dynamic exercise: SBP increases in direct proportion to workload whereas DBP remains within ±10 mm Hg	Normally SBP increases 10 ± 2 mm Hg per MET ↑ in workload during exercise involving large muscles of body, to a peak of 160–200 mm Hg; SBP may plateau at peak exercise
	With exercise involving small muscles of body, DBP increases because of ↑ peripheral vascular resistance due to SNS-mediated vasoconstriction
	During steady state submaximal aerobic exercise, SBP increases for first 2–3 min, and then remains constant or decreases slightly.
	Pulse pressure (SBP–DBP) generally increases in direct proportion to workload
	Abnormal BP responses: Hypertensive response: An excessive ↑ in BP with exercise (>10 mm Hg ↑ in DBP with activity or >12 mm Hg per MET ↑ in SBP or >260 mm Hg) or failure of SBP to level off during sustained submaximal exercise
	Blunted response: Some ↑ in SBP but <8 mm Hg per MET ↑ in workload; may occur in individuals taking β-blockers or other antihypertensive medications as well as nitrates
	Hypotensive response: SBP that fails to rise or falls (>10 mm Hg) with increasing workload; may signify myocardial ischemia and/or LV dysfunction
	Low maximal SBP: A maximal value of <140 mm Hg suggests a poor prognosis
Static/isometric exercise: Progressive ↑ in SBP and DBP proportional to the intensity of contraction	An ↑ in peripheral resistance results in an ↑ in DBP and when an ↑ in cardiac output is superimposed on this, there is a greater ↑ in SBP than with dynamic exercise

↓, Decrease; ↑, increase; BP, blood pressure; bpm, beats per minute; DBP, diastolic blood pressure; ECG, electrocardiographic; HR, heart rate; LV, left ventricular; MET, metabolic equivalent for oxygen consumption (1 MET, 3.5 mL O_2/kg/min); SBP, systolic blood pressure; SNS, sympathetic nervous system.

▸ When activity involves the smaller muscles of the body (e.g., upper extremities), the localized vasodilatory effects are not sufficient to offset the generalized vasoconstriction caused by sympathetic nervous system stimulation, and therefore PVR increases and both SBP and DBP rise. The smaller the exercising muscle mass and the more intense the workload, the higher the SBP and DBP responses will be.

▸ With endurance exercise at a sustained submaximal workload, SBP rises slowly for the first 2 to 3 minutes, and then remains constant or may decrease slightly.

▸ During static/isometric exercise, the strength of the muscle contraction directly affects the blood flow through the muscle and offsets the local metabolic effects that induce vasodilation, so there is a marked progressive increase in DBP. The increase in SBP due to higher cardiac output is superimposed on the elevated DBP, causing a more marked progressive increase in SBP. In patients with LV dysfunction, sustained static contractions may provoke a significant rise in LV end-diastolic pressure with resultant reductions in ejection fraction and cardiac output, so the expected rise in SBP is attenuated, and patients may exhibit other signs and symptoms of exercise intolerance.

• Abnormal BP responses to activity consist of the following:

  ▸ *Hypertensive responses* occur when the SBP increases excessively for the workload (i.e., >12 mm Hg per MET increase), the exertional DBP increases more than 10 mm Hg compared with the resting value, the postexercise DBP remains elevated during recovery, or the SBP fails to level out when the body should be in a steady state condition during sustained submaximal exercise. Exaggerated BP responses are usually due to increased PVR and in normotensive adults increase the likelihood of developing HTN over the next 5 to 15 years by threefold and are associated with an increased risk of later cardiovascular mortality and a greater prevalence of angiographic CAD.[31,44,48]

  ▸ *Hypotensive responses* occur when the SBP fails to rise or falls (>10 mm Hg), sometimes precipitously, with increasing workloads, which is indicative of severe pathological conditions (e.g., moderate to severe aortic stenosis, severe CAD, and/or poor LV function).

  ▸ *Blunted BP responses* are defined as lower than expected SBP increases with increased workloads (<8 mm Hg per MET increase); these are usually due to medications, especially β-blockers.

  ▸ *Postexercise hypotension* occurs when blood pools in the lower extremities because of inadequate cooldown; this can be prevented with 5 to 10 minutes of low-intensity exercise, using the large muscles of the body.

Rate–Pressure Product

A commonly used indirect index of myocardial oxygen demand is the rate–pressure product (RPP), or double product, which is equal to the product of HR and SBP (i.e., RPP = HR × SBP). RPP is determined primarily by intramyocardial wall stress, HR, and contractility and therefore increases progressively with incremental exercise.

• There is a direct relationship between RPP and myocardial oxygen uptake ($M\dot{V}O_2$) and coronary blood flow. Because the heart is dependent on aerobic metabolism with little capacity to generate energy through anaerobic metabolism, it relies on augmented coronary blood flow to meet the demands of increasing activity. Therefore, individuals with obstructive CAD with luminal narrowing of more than 70%, who may have limited ability to increase coronary flow, may develop myocardial ischemia during exercise and their peak RPP values will be reduced. Of note, patients with CAD tend to develop angina or anginal equivalents (see page 106) and ECG changes typical of myocardial ischemia at a consistent RPP, regardless of the type of activity.[2,49] Thus, RPP indicates the degree of functional limitation produced by an individual's heart disease (i.e., the lower the RPP at the time an individual experiences symptoms of exercise intolerance, the more severe the functional limitation). In addition, RPP provides an objective measure to evaluate the effects of various interventions, including exercise training, on cardiac performance.

• Individuals with other types of heart disease may also develop symptoms at lower RPPs due to increased $M\dot{V}O_2$ induced by higher submaximal HRs, ventricular dilation or hypertrophy, and/or elevated intraventricular pressures.

• The RPP is usually expressed as a two-digit number $\times 10^3$. For example, an individual who develops chest discomfort at a HR of 145 bpm and a BP of 160/80 mm Hg during exercise would have an RPP of 145 × 160, or 23×10^3, at this point.

• Most normal individuals achieve peak RPPs of $20–35 \times 10^3$, whereas those with significant CAD have values less than 25×10^3.[18] Therefore, there is significant overlap between those with disease and those without disease rather than a clear cutoff point that can serve as a diagnostic marker to distinguish between the two.

• However, in general, a healthy, physically fit individual will be able to achieve a higher RPP than a healthy, sedentary individual, who will be able to achieve a higher RPP than an individual with heart disease.

• Various cardiovascular medications exert significant influence on RPP by virtue of their lowering effects on HR, SBP, or both, and therefore reduce myocardial oxygen demand and thus the incidence of ischemia and angina.

Respiration

Normally, patients are comfortable at rest with an RR of 12 to 20 breaths per minute, and the actual number of breaths per minute is not necessarily measured by the therapist. However, when there are any signs of increased work of breathing (e.g., recruitment of accessory muscles of respiration, nasal flaring, or pursed-lip breathing), the RR should be measured.

• Because the RR frequently changes when a patient is aware of his/her breathing, the most accurate results are obtained when the patient is unaware that the measurement is being taken. This can best be achieved by observing from a distance or while pretending to do something else, such as palpating the HR.

• The same technique can be used when obtaining the RR during exercise. As an alternative, many clinicians choose to use one of the dyspnea rating scales that are available (see page 283) to document the functional impact of a patient's respiratory limitation instead of measuring the RR.

- The recommended time over which the RR is determined is a full minute, although a 30-second count will offer minimal error if the RR during that period is truly representative of the patient's status.

Respiratory Responses to Exercise

During exercise several factors, both chemical (e.g., central and peripheral chemoreceptor responses to hypoxemia, hypercapnia, and acidemia) and neural (e.g., cortical and peripheral locomotor input, as well as reflexes related to pulmonary blood flow and movement of the lungs and respiratory muscles), influence the respiratory responses to exercise. The result is an increase in minute ventilation ($\dot{V}E$), resulting from increases in tidal volume (V_T) and RR, that is proportional to the workload. Resting $\dot{V}E$ averages 6 L/min and typically increases to 75 L/min during moderate exercise and to 150 L/min during vigorous exercise.[49,62b]

- At lower intensities there is a greater relative increment in V_T than in RR.
- During more strenuous exercise, V_T levels off at its maximum (about 60% of the vital capacity), and further increases in $\dot{V}E$ are due to increasing RR.
- During vigorous exercise (intensities at or exceeding the ventilatory threshold, which is related to the shift to predominantly anaerobic metabolism in the exercising muscles), increasing CO_2 production leads to rising serum CO_2 levels and a drop in pH, which stimulates a disproportionate increase in $\dot{V}E$ and often the sensation of shortness of breath.
- When $\dot{V}E$ exceeds 50 L, the energy cost of breathing becomes progressively greater, increasing from usual values of 3% to 5% of total $\dot{V}O_2$ during moderate exercise to 8% to 10% at maximal exercise. However, in patients with respiratory disease, the work of breathing is elevated so the energy cost may increase to as much as 40% of total $\dot{V}O_2$ in patients with severe disease.[49]
- Ventilation is higher during upper extremity exercise at any given $\dot{V}O_2$ than during lower extremity exercise and results in hyperventilation (i.e., an increase in ventilation that exceeds the oxygen requirements of metabolism).[62b]
- The respiratory system is not usually the limiting factor in exercise tolerance, except when there is significant pulmonary dysfunction due to inadequate ventilation, abnormal perfusion, and/or impaired diffusion (see Table 6-17).
  - ▸ In obstructive disease (e.g., COPD), increased airway resistance, dynamic hyperinflation, and ventilation–perfusion ($\dot{V}/\dot{Q}$) mismatching during exercise lead to worsening of gas exchange and further aggravate the work of breathing. Thus, $\dot{V}E$ is higher at lower workloads.
  - ▸ Restrictive lung dysfunction results in limited ability to increase V_T, and therefore increases in $\dot{V}E$ are dependent predominantly on increasing RR, especially as disease severity progresses.[45a]
- Patients with cardiovascular dysfunction often show abnormal respiratory responses to exercise because of reduced cardiac output.[62a,62b]
  - ▸ Limited cardiac output leads to impaired delivery of oxygen to exercising muscles and an earlier onset of anaerobic metabolism. The resultant hypercapnia and acidemia provoke exaggerated ventilatory responses to exercise at low work rates.

- ▸ In addition, patients with CHF and pulmonary edema develop $\dot{V}/\dot{Q}$ mismatching due to an increase in dead space ventilation relative to V_T, which further provokes dyspnea.

Oxygenation Status

There are two ways to monitor a patient's oxygenation status: through direct sampling of the arterial blood and by indirect assessment of the oxygen saturation of the blood. Lacking either of these measures, the clinician must rely on observation of the signs and symptoms of hypoxemia (refer to Table 6-13 on page 241).

Arterial Blood Gases

Analysis of arterial blood gases provides the best indicator of a patient's level of oxygenation and is described on page 227.

- PaO_2 is normally about 97 mm Hg, although values of at least 80 mm Hg are considered to be within normal limits.
- PaO_2 of 60 to 79 mm Hg corresponds to mild hypoxemia.
- PaO_2 of 40 to 59 mm Hg is considered moderate hypoxemia.
- PaO_2 less than 40 mm Hg represents severe hypoxemia.

Because current technology does not allow continuous monitoring of a patient's oxygenation status, it is critical that PTs recognize the signs and symptoms of hypoxemia during assessment of patients who exhibit reduced tolerance for exercise.

Pulse Oximetry, Oxygen Saturation Monitoring

As described previously, arterial oxygen saturation of hemoglobin (SaO_2) can be estimated via pulse oximetry (SpO_2) (see page 18), which provides a digital readout that is updated every few seconds and therefore is capable of providing immediate feedback regarding the effects of positional change or activity on SaO_2.

Pulse oximeters tend to have an accuracy of ±2% when resting SaO_2 is 80% to 100%, but accuracy may decrease to ±5% during exercise and when oxygen saturation is less than 70% to 80%.[20] Inaccuracies are especially likely to occur during rapid or severe desaturation and in patients requiring intensive care, where patients with an oxygen saturation by ABGs (SaO_2) of 90% were found to have SpO_2 values that varied from 86% to 94%, potentially leading to very different clinical interpretations and interventions.[36] In addition, the accuracy of results can be affected by poor peripheral perfusion (e.g., peripheral arterial disease, vasoconstriction, or low cardiac output) and other factors (see Table 2-8).

- Pulse oximeters that display a pulse waveform derived from the absorption measurements can be helpful in verifying the accuracy of results; the identification of adequate waveforms can also be used to select appropriate monitoring sites and to troubleshoot questionable results.
- In pulse oximeters that display HR, the accuracy of the HR readings, assessed by comparison with the palpated pulse rate or ECG reading, provides an index of the pulse-rate signal detection, which often affects the quality of the oximeter readings. This procedure can also be used to locate the best monitoring sites.
- When a valid HR reading or pulse waveform is not obtained, the accuracy of SpO_2 values should be questioned.
- Because of limitations due to motion artifact and reduced perfusion, SpO_2 values should be used with caution in assessing oxygen requirements during exercise, during which both false

high and low results may occur.[64a] Furthermore, significant measurement errors can occur even when there is adequate pulse-rate signal detection, and reliable data may be provided during exercise even with poor pulse-rate signal detection.[37] When discrepancies are found between the SpO_2 results and the patient's clinical presentation, blood gas analysis is indicated.

- Again, the PT's ability to recognize the clinical manifestations of hypoxemia is important when assessing a patient's responses to exertion.

Assessment of SpO_2 is strongly advised for all patients with an FEV_1 of less than 50% of predicted or a diffusing capacity (D_{LCO}) of less than 60% of predicted, because these patients are likely to exhibit desaturation during activity. SaO_2 is normally greater than 95%.

- SpO_2 values must be interpreted within the context of the patient's respiratory and metabolic status, because shifts of the oxygen–hemoglobin (O_2–Hb) curve will affect the affinity of oxygen and hemoglobin (see Figure 2-5, page 8).
- Because of the shape of the O_2–Hb dissociation curve, small changes in SaO_2 from 96% to 90% represent large decreases in PaO_2 (e.g., at an SaO_2 of 90%, the PaO_2 has dropped from 98 to 60 mm Hg) and should be considered significant. Then, as SaO_2 drops below 90% and the curve becomes steeper, larger decreases in SaO_2 are associated with smaller reductions in PaO_2 (e.g., at an SaO_2 of 75% the PaO_2 is 40, whereas at an SaO_2 of 50% the PaO_2 is 27).
- However, different conditions cause the O_2–Hb curve to shift to the right or left, which changes the ease with which oxygen binds to Hb in the blood and is released to the tissues.
  - ▶ Acute acidosis, hypercapnia, and increased body temperature (all of which occur in the muscle capillaries during vigorous exercise) and increased 2,3-diphosphoglycerate (2,3-DPG) cause a shift of the O_2–Hb curve to the right, so that there is greater release of O_2 to the muscle at lower PaO_2 levels.
  - ▶ Acute alkalosis, hypocapnia, and hypothermia (all of which occur in the lungs during vigorous exercise), as well as decreased 2,3-DPG, cause a shift of the O_2–Hb curve to the left, so that the amount of O_2 that binds with Hb at any given PaO_2 is increased in the lungs.
- Activity should be terminated if the SpO_2 drops to less than 90% in acutely ill patients or to 85% or less in patients with chronic lung disease. Discussion with the physician is warranted regarding a trial of or higher dose of oxygen therapy during activity.

Rating of Perceived Exertion

Rating of perceived exertion (RPE) uses a numerical scale in relation to subjective perception of exertion, taking into account personal fitness level, environmental conditions, and general fatigue levels, to provide an estimate of exercise intensity. Although ratings can be influenced by psychological factors, mood states, environmental conditions, exercise modes, and age, when used correctly they correlate well with exercise HRs and work rates, particularly within individuals.[8] Two RPE scales are commonly used.

- The Category RPE Scale uses numerical ratings of 6 to 20, with the following correlations:
  - ▶ No exertion at all is rated 6
  - ▶ Extremely light exertion is rated 7
  - ▶ Very light exertion is rated 9
  - ▶ Light exertion is rated 11
  - ▶ Somewhat hard exertion is rated 13
  - ▶ Hard or heavy exertion is rated 15
  - ▶ Very hard exertion is rated 17
  - ▶ Extremely hard exertion is rated 19
  - ▶ Maximal exertion is rated 20
- The Category-Ratio RPE Scale uses ratings of 0 to 10 to rate perception of effort, though higher ratings are possible:
  - ▶ Nothing at all is rated 0
  - ▶ Extremely weak or barely noticeable exertion is rated 0.5
  - ▶ Very weak exertion is rated 1
  - ▶ Weak or light exertion is rated 2
  - ▶ Moderate exertion is rated 3
  - ▶ Strong or heavy exertion is rated 5
  - ▶ Very strong exertion is rated 7
  - ▶ Extremely strong or maximal exertion is rated 10
  - ▶ Absolute maximum or highest possible exertion can be rated higher than 10
- During exercise testing, RPE is useful in indicating progress toward maximal exertion and impending fatigue. At maximal exercise most apparently healthy individuals declare ratings of 18 to 19 (very, very hard) on the Borg Category (6 to 20) Scale or 9 to 10 (very, very strong) on the Borg Category-Ratio (0 to 10) Scale.
- RPE is also valuable as a means of monitoring and adjusting exercise intensity during aerobic exercise training.
  - ▶ An RPE of 13 to 14 (somewhat hard) represents about 70% of HR_{max} during exercise on a treadmill or cycle ergometer.[49]
  - ▶ An RPE of 11 to 12 (fairly light to somewhat hard) corresponds to lactate threshold for both trained and untrained individuals.[56]
  - ▶ Most individuals can quickly learn to exercise at a specific RPE.
- It is important to use standardized instructions to avoid problems related to the misinterpretation of RPE. The recommended instructions for using the Borg RPE Category (6 to 20) Scale during exercise testing are as follows[9]:
  - ▶ During the work we want you to rate your perception of exertion, that is, how heavy and strenuous the exercise feels to you and how tired you are. The perception of exertion is mainly felt as strain and fatigue in your muscles and breathlessness or aches in the chest.
  - ▶ Use this scale from 6 to 20, where 6 means "No exertion at all" and 20 means "Maximal exertion."
    - ⊙ 9 is *very light*. As for a healthy person taking a short walk at his or her own pace.
    - ⊙ 13 is *somewhat hard*. It still feels OK to continue.
    - ⊙ 15 is *hard* and tiring, but continuing is not terribly difficult.
    - ⊙ 17 is *very hard*. It is very strenuous. You can still go on, but you really have to push yourself and you are very tired.
    - ⊙ 19 is *extremely hard*. For most people this is the most strenuous exercise they have ever experienced.
  - ▶ Try to appraise your feeling of exertion and fatigue as spontaneously and honestly as possible, without thinking about what the actual physical load is. Try not to underestimate,

nor to overestimate. It is your own feeling of effort and exertion that is important, not how it compares to other people's. Look at the scale and the expressions and then give a number. You can equally well use even as odd numbers.

▸ Any questions?

• The recommended instructions for using the Borg RPE Category-Ratio (0 to 10) Scale during exercise testing are similar but specific to the scale[10]:

▸ Use this rating scale to report how strong your perception is. It can be exertion, pain, or something else. Ten (10) or "Extremely strong"–"Maximal" is a very important intensity level. It serves as the reference point on the scale. This is the most intense perception or feeling (e.g., of exertion) you have ever had. It is, however, possible to experience or imagine something even more intense. That is why we've placed "Absolute maximum" outside and further down on the scale without any corresponding number, just a dot. If your experience is stronger than "10," you can use a larger number.

▸ First look at the verbal expressions. Start with them and then the numbers. If your experience or feeling is "Very weak," you should say "1"; if it is "Moderate," say "3." If the experience is "Strong" or "Heavy" (it feels "Difficult") say "5." Note that "Strong" is about 50 percent, or about half, of "Maximal." If your perception is "Very strong" ("Very intense") choose a number from 6 to 8, depending on how intense it is. Feel free to use half-numbers like "1.5" or "3.5" or decimals like "0.3" or "0.8" or "2.3." It is very important that you report what you actually experience or feel, not what you think you should report. Be as spontaneous and honest as possible and try to avoid under- or overestimating. Look at the verbal descriptors and then choose a number.

▸ When rating perceived exertion give a number that corresponds to your feeling of exertion, that is, how hard and strenuous you perceive the work to be and how tired you are. The perception of exertion is mainly felt as strain and fatigue in your muscles and breathlessness or aches in the chest. It is important that you only think about what you feel, and not about what the actual load is.

⊙ 1: Very light. As for a healthy person taking a short walk at his or her own pace.

⊙ 3: Moderate, or somewhat but not especially hard. It feels good and not too difficult to go on.

⊙ 5: The work is hard and tiring, but continuing isn't terribly difficult. The effort and exertion are about half as intense as "Maximal."

⊙ 7: Quite strenuous. You can still go on, but you really have to push yourself and you are very tired.

⊙ 9: An extremely strenuous level. For most people this is the most strenuous exercise they have ever experienced.

⊙ •: "Absolute maximum," for example, "12" or more.

▸ Any questions?

Other Symptoms and Signs of Exercise Intolerance

In addition to the abnormal physiological responses already discussed, the patient's symptoms must always be considered, as well as some other signs that indicate limited exercise tolerance, such as those listed subsequently. Angina, dyspnea, and fatigue are the most common complaints during exertion. A number of rating scales have been developed through which patients can indicate the level of their discomfort during activity. Some of these are presented; in addition, Borg has created subjective rating scales similar to the category-ratio RPE scale for dyspnea and other symptoms.[8]

When a patient develops abnormal signs or symptoms, exercise intensity should be monitored closely and may need to be reduced during subsequent therapy sessions. The therapist should expect that the patient is likely to progress more slowly with the rehabilitation activities because of tolerance for only gradual increases in duration and intensity.

• A number of abnormal signs and symptoms that may develop during or immediately after exertion are indicative of exercise intolerance:

▸ Anginal discomfort (see description on page 104), which can be subjectively rated as shown in Table 6-23

▸ Dyspnea, which can be rated with subjective and objective scales (see Table 6-24 through Table 6-26) or a visual analog scale (a 100-mm-long vertical line with "No Breathlessness" at the bottom and "Greatest Breathlessness" at the top, along which the individual marks his or her level of breathlessness)[46a]

▸ Excessive fatigue at low workloads[30] (RPE may serve as a good indicator)

▸ Lightheadedness, dizziness

▸ LE claudication, which can be rated subjectively (Table 6-27)

▸ Other abnormal signs and symptoms, as listed in Table 6-28

• Some signs and symptoms that develop later after exertion may also indicate exercise intolerance:

▸ Slow recovery from activity, especially persistent tachycardia lasting more than 5 to 10 minutes after exertion

TABLE 6-23: Angina Scale for Subjective Rating of Intensity

Rating	Description
1	Light, barely noticeable
2	Moderate, bothersome
3	Moderately severe, very uncomfortable
4	Most severe pain or intense pain ever experienced

From American College of Sports Medicine. *Guidelines for Exercise Testing and Prescription.* 7th ed. Philadelphia: Lippincott Williams & Wilkins; 2006.

TABLE 6-24: Dyspnea Scale for Subjective Rating of Intensity

Rating	Description
1	Light, barely noticeable
2	Moderate, bothersome
3	Moderately severe, very uncomfortable
4	Severe difficulty, patient cannot continue

From American College of Sports Medicine. *Guidelines for Exercise Testing and Prescription.* 7th ed. Philadelphia: Lippincott Williams & Wilkins; 2006.

TABLE 6-25: Borg Scale for Rating Breathlessness

Level	Description
0	Nothing at all
0.5	Very, very slight (just noticeable)
1	Very slight
2	Slight
3	Moderate
4	Somewhat severe
5	Severe
6	
7	Very severe
8	
9	Very, very severe (almost maximal)
10	Maximal

From Borg G. Psychophysical bases of perceived exertion. *Med Sci Sports Exerc.* 1982:14:377–381. Used with permission.

TABLE 6-26: Objective Rating of Dyspnea Level*

Level	Description
0	Able to count to 15 easily without taking an additional breath
1	Able to count to 15 but must take one additional breath
2	Must take two additional breaths to count to 15
3	Must take three additional breaths to count to 15
4	Unable to count

From *Physical Therapy Management of Patients with Pulmonary Disease.* Physical Therapy Department, Ranchos Los Amigos Medical Center; Downey, CA,1980. Used with permission.
*The patient is asked to inhale normally and then to count out loud to 15 over a 7.5- to 8-second period. Any shortness of breath can be graded by levels, as shown in the table.

TABLE 6-27: Claudication Pain Scale for Subjective Rating of Intensity

Grade	Description
1	Definite discomfort or pain, but only of initial or modest levels (established but minimal)
2	Moderate discomfort or pain from which the patient's attention can be diverted (e.g., by conversation)
3	Intense pain (short of grade 4) from which patient's attention cannot be diverted
4	Excruciating and unbearable pain

From American College of Sports Medicine. *Guidelines for Exercise Testing and Prescription.* 7th ed. Philadelphia: Lippincott Williams & Wilkins; 2006.

▸ Excessive fatigue lasting more than 1 to 2 hours after exertion
▸ Insomnia
▸ Weight gain due to fluid retention
▸ Orthopnea or paroxysmal nocturnal dyspnea

Exercise Capacity

Exercise, or aerobic, capacity is defined in terms of maximal oxygen consumption ($\dot{V}O_{2\,max}$), or as the greatest volume of oxygen a person can utilize for energy production during dynamic exercise involving the large muscle groups of the body. $\dot{V}O_{2\,max}$ is equal to the product of cardiac output and arteriovenous oxygen difference and therefore is a measure of the functional limits of the cardiovascular system.

- $\dot{V}O_{2\,max}$ can be measured directly via ventilatory gas analysis during maximal exercise testing; more often it is estimated from the maximal workload achieved during exercise testing, using established formulas, which must be based on the same population as the person being tested.
- Exercise capacity is determined by the individual's natural endowment or heredity, fitness level, body size and composition, age, and gender.
- Cardiorespiratory fitness can be classified according to $\dot{V}O_{2\,max}$ relative to body weight, as shown in Table 6-29.
- $\dot{V}O_{2\,max}$, and therefore fitness level, can be increased through aerobic and, to a lesser degree, resistance exercise training, in both healthy individuals and those with various chronic medical problems as described in Chapter 7 (Cardiovascular and Pulmonary Physical Therapy Treatment; see page 301).

◻ 6.6 OTHER ASSESSMENT TOOLS

A number of other assessments are performed by PTs to determine an individual's risk of cardiovascular or other health problems, to evaluate specific cardiopulmonary problems that occur in some patients, and to determine the impact of health problems on quality of life. These include body composition determination or associated risk level, autonomic dysfunction testing, respiratory muscle strength and endurance testing, health and fitness appraisals, and quality of life measures.

BODY COMPOSITION

Because obesity, especially excessive intraabdominal (visceral) fat, is associated with increased morbidity and mortality due to HTN, CAD, stroke, type 2 DM, and other diseases, an assessment of body composition or risk status due to overweight or obesity is often performed by PTs. Although there are neither universally accepted norms for body composition nor a consensus regarding the percentage of body fat that is associated with optimal health risk, the lowest statistical health risk is associated with body fat percentages of 12% to 20% for males and 20% to 30% for females.[1] As described by Gallagher and colleagues, the percentage of body fat associated with elevated health risk varies with age[35]:

- For males, health risk is elevated with body fat values of:
  ▸ 20% to 24% for ages 20–39 years
  ▸ 22% to 27% for ages 40–59 years
  ▸ 25% to 29% in ages 60–79 years

TABLE 6-28: Other Signs and Symptoms of Exercise Intolerance

Abnormal Sign/Symptom	Common Causes
Immediate Responses*	
Angina pectoris	Myocardial ischemia
Dyspnea	Cardiac and pulmonary dysfunction, anemia, peripheral arterial disease, deconditioning, etc.
Excessive fatigue or weakness	Limited cardiac output due to LV dysfunction or arrhythmias; deconditioning, medication side effect, etc.
Lightheadedness or dizziness	Hypotension caused by inadequate cardiac output due to LV dysfunction, arrhythmias, medication side effect, etc.
Near-syncope or syncope	Abrupt drop in cardiac output due to arrhythmia or severe LV outflow obstruction (e.g., aortic stenosis, hypertrophic obstructive cardiomyopathy)
Pallor or cyanosis	Inadequate cardiac output (see preceding entry for fatigue), hypoxemia, anemia
Facial expression of distress	Any type of moderate to severe discomfort
LE claudication	Peripheral arterial disease
Nausea, vomiting	Inadequate cardiac output
Mental confusion, loss of coordination, ataxia	Inadequate cerebral perfusion
Onset of pulmonary crackles	Pulmonary edema
Onset of third heart sound (S_3)	Elevated end-diastolic LV filling pressure induced by myocardial ischemia or LV dysfunction
Delayed Responses	
Slow recovery from activity, especially persistent tachycardia >5 to 10 min after exertion	Increased SNS stimulation due to deconditioning or LV dysfunction
Excessive fatigue lasting >1–2 h after exertion	Overexertion, excessive intensity of exercise relative to condition of individual (deconditioned or impaired cardiac function)
Insomnia	Compensatory SNS stimulation that persists after exercise
Weight gain due to fluid retention	Venous congestion due to ventricular dysfunction
Orthopnea or paroxysmal nocturnal dyspnea	Pulmonary congestion or increased preload due to reabsorption of fluid retention

LE, Lower extremity; LV, left ventricular; SNS, sympathetic nervous system.
*Occurring during or immediately after exercise.

TABLE 6-29: Cardiorespiratory Fitness Classification

Age (yr)	Maximal Oxygen Uptake (mL/kg/min)				
	Low	**Fair**	**Average**	**Good**	**High**
Women					
20–29	<24	24–30	31–37	38–48	49+
30–39	<20	20–27	28–33	34–44	45+
40–49	<17	17–23	24–30	31–41	42+
50–59	<15	15–20	21–27	28–37	38+
60–69	<13	13–17	18–23	24–34	35+
Men					
20–29	<25	25–33	34–42	43–52	53+
30–39	<23	23–30	31–38	39–48	49+
40–49	<20	20–26	27–35	36–44	45+
50–59	<18	18–24	25–33	34–42	43+
60–69	<16	16–22	23–30	31–40	41+

From Committee on Exercise, American Heart Association: *Exercise Testing and Training of Apparently Healthy Individuals: A Handbook for Physicians.* Dallas, Texas: American Heart Association, 1972. Used with permission.

- For males, health risk is high with body fat values of:
  - ▸ 25% or more for ages 20–39 years
  - ▸ 28% or more for ages 40–59 years
  - ▸ 30% or more in ages 60–79 years
- For females, health risk is elevated with body fat values of:
  - ▸ 33% to 38% for ages 20–39 years
  - ▸ 34% to 39% for ages 40–59 years
  - ▸ 36% to 41% in ages 60–79 years
- For females, health risk is high with body fat values of:
  - ▸ 39% or more for ages 20–39 years
  - ▸ 40% or more for ages 40–59 years
  - ▸ 42% or more in ages 60–79 years
- Values below these levels are also associated with physiological dysfunction, as observed in the chronically undernourished. In addition, low levels of lean body mass are associated with a number of abnormalities. Deficient bone mass and density are primary predictors of risk of fractures due to osteoporosis. Low muscle mass and muscle wasting impairs muscle strength and functional ability to perform daily activities and is associated with increased mortality.

Body Composition Measures

Body composition can be assessed by a number of different indirect methods, including hydrodensitometry, measurement of total body potassium, and dual-energy x-ray absorptiometry, which are considered to be reference methods but require cumbersome equipment and are expensive. More commonly employed, because of their low cost and ease of use, are several doubly indirect methods, including anthropometry, bioelectrical impedance, and near-infrared interactance. All these methods have various advantages and disadvantages.

- *Underwater, or hydrostatic, weighing* is considered the "gold standard" for determining percentage body fat and is based on the difference in density between fat and lean tissue (muscle, bone, and fluid), such that an individual with more body fat will displace more water and weigh less in water (i.e., has a lower body density) than a person with greater lean body mass of the same dry weight. Because the amount of air in the lungs also affects underwater weight, the individual must perform a maximal exhalation to reduce the volume to a minimum during weighing, and the residual volume must be determined. The disadvantages of this method include the special equipment that is required, the difficulty in determining an accurate residual volume, and the level of cooperation required and performance of the subject.
- *Dual-energy x-ray absorptiometry (DEXA)* is a scanning technique that measures the differential attenuation between two x-rays as they pass through the body. Serial transverse scans are performed from head to toe at 1.2-cm intervals, and computer analysis provides an indirect measure of bone mineral, fat tissue, and fat-free soft tissue. DEXA is considered to be one of the most useful and reliable methods of body composition, but it requires sophisticated equipment and is costly.[53]
- *Skinfold assessment* relies on the measurement of skinfold thicknesses at selected body sites using skinfold calipers and the calculation of percent body fat via various regression equations. The reliability and validity of this method depend on the proficiency of the tester, the type of caliper, factors related to the subject (e.g., skinfold compressibility, edema, variability of fat pattern and distribution), and the use of an appropriate prediction equation (based on age, gender, ethnicity, and level of physical activity).
- *Bioelectrical impedance analysis (BIA)* employs a single-frequency (50 kHz) low-level electrical current (500 μA), which flows through the intracellular and extracellular fluid, to measure whole body impedance. Because fat-free mass (FFM) contains a much larger amount of water and electrolytes than body fat, the total body impedance is determined primarily by the amount of fluid and muscle mass of the individual. Although BIA is inexpensive and requires a lower degree of technical skill and minimal cooperation on the part of the subject, its accuracy is affected by the BIA instrument used, various subject factors (e.g., fluid status [which is affected by food and fluid intake and prior exercise], fluid distribution, and body temperature), and the use of an appropriate regression equation. Obese individuals have significantly greater extracellular fluid volumes, so BIA tends to overestimate FFM and underestimate fat mass.[53] The reverse is true of the estimated values for lean persons. Multiple-frequency BIA (MFBIA) may eliminate some of the error resulting from hydration status and thus may provide a better estimation of FFM.[3]
- *Near-infrared interactance (NIR)* uses a fiber optic probe to emit an infrared light that passes through both fat and muscle to a depth of 1 cm and is reflected, absorbed, and transmitted according to the tissue composition (fat versus fat-free). A digital analyzer measures the intensity of the light that is reemitted, and prediction equations (based on age, gender, height, weight, frame size, and activity level) are used to calculate percentage body fat. NIR is noninvasive, quick, and inexpensive, but it has large individual variances and tends to underestimate percent body fat increasingly as the degree of adiposity increases.[53]

Risk Status Due to Overweight or Obesity

Instead of using the indirect or doubly indirect methods described previously to estimate percent body fat, clinicians often choose to employ simple body measurements to screen individuals for their relative risk of disease associated with being overweight and obese: body mass index, waist circumference, and waist-to-hip ratio.

Body Mass Index

Body mass index (BMI) is the most commonly used method for assessing risk related to excess body weight. It is calculated by dividing the individual's body weight (in kilograms) by body surface area (in meters squared) and is easily obtainable from charts when the weight and height are known, as depicted in Table 6-30.

- A BMI of 19 to 25 is associated with the lowest statistical health risk.[1]
- A BMI of 25 or more is associated with greater health risk, as shown in Table 6-31.[17a,45]

Waist Circumference

Persons with large waist circumferences have an increased risk of cardiovascular disease and impaired health compared with those

TABLE 6-30: Body Mass Index Calculated From Height in Inches and Weight in Pounds

BMI	19	20	21	22	23	24	25	26	27	28	29	30	31	32	33	34	35	36
Height (in) *							Body Weight (lb)†											
58	91	96	100	105	110	115	119	124	129	134	138	143	148	153	158	162	167	172
59	94	99	104	109	114	119	124	128	133	138	143	148	153	158	163	168	173	178
60	97	102	107	112	118	123	128	133	138	143	148	153	158	163	168	174	179	184
61	100	106	111	116	122	127	132	137	143	148	153	158	164	169	174	180	185	190
62	104	109	115	120	126	131	136	142	147	153	158	164	169	175	180	186	191	196
63	107	113	118	124	130	135	141	146	152	158	163	169	175	180	186	191	197	203
64	110	116	122	128	134	140	145	151	157	163	169	174	180	186	192	197	204	209
65	114	120	126	132	138	144	150	156	162	168	174	180	186	192	198	204	210	216
66	118	124	130	136	142	148	155	161	167	173	179	186	192	198	204	210	216	223
67	121	127	134	140	146	153	159	166	172	178	185	191	198	204	211	217	223	230
68	125	131	138	144	151	158	164	171	177	184	190	197	203	210	216	223	230	236
69	128	135	142	148	155	162	169	176	182	189	196	203	209	216	223	230	236	243
70	132	139	146	153	160	167	174	181	188	195	202	209	216	222	229	236	243	250
71	136	143	150	158	165	172	179	186	193	200	208	215	222	229	236	243	250	257
72	140	147	154	162	169	177	184	191	199	206	213	221	228	235	242	250	258	265
73	144	151	159	166	174	182	189	197	204	212	219	227	235	242	250	257	265	272
74	148	155	163	171	179	186	194	202	210	218	225	233	241	249	256	264	272	280
75	152	160	168	176	184	192	200	208	216	224	232	240	248	256	264	272	279	287
76	156	164	172	180	189	197	205	213	221	230	238	246	254	263	271	279	287	295
BMI	37	38	39	40	41	42	43	44	45	46	47	48	49	50	51	52	53	54
Height (in)							Body Weight (lb)†											
58	177	181	186	191	196	201	205	210	215	220	224	229	234	239	244	248	253	258
59	183	188	193	198	203	208	212	217	222	227	232	237	242	247	252	257	262	267
60	189	194	199	204	209	215	220	225	230	235	240	245	250	255	261	266	271	276
61	195	201	206	211	217	222	227	232	238	243	248	254	259	264	269	275	280	285
62	202	207	213	218	224	229	235	240	246	251	256	262	267	273	278	284	289	295
63	208	214	220	225	231	237	242	248	254	259	265	270	278	282	287	293	299	304
64	215	221	227	232	238	244	250	256	262	267	273	279	285	291	296	302	308	314
65	222	228	234	240	246	252	258	264	270	276	282	288	294	300	306	312	318	324
66	229	235	241	247	253	260	266	272	278	284	291	297	303	309	315	322	328	334
67	236	242	249	255	261	268	274	280	287	293	299	306	312	319	325	331	338	344
68	243	249	256	262	269	276	282	289	295	302	308	315	322	328	335	341	348	354
69	250	257	263	270	277	284	291	297	304	311	318	324	331	338	345	351	358	365
70	257	264	271	278	285	292	299	306	313	320	327	334	341	348	355	362	369	376
71	265	272	279	286	293	301	308	315	322	329	338	343	351	358	365	372	379	386
72	272	279	287	294	302	309	316	324	331	338	346	353	361	368	375	383	390	397
73	280	288	295	302	310	318	325	333	340	348	355	363	371	378	386	393	401	408
74	287	295	303	311	319	326	334	342	350	358	365	373	381	389	396	404	412	420
75	295	303	311	319	327	335	343	351	359	367	375	383	391	399	407	415	423	431
76	304	312	320	328	336	344	353	361	369	377	385	394	402	410	418	426	435	443

Data from North American Association for the Study of Obesity (NAASO), National Heart, Lung, and Blood Institute (NHLBI). *Practical Guide on the Identification, Evaluation, and Treatment of Overweight and Obesity in Adults.* NIH Publication No. 00-4084. Bethesda, MD: National Institutes of Health; 2000. Available at http://www.nhlbi.nih.gov/guidelines/obesity/prctgd_c.pdf (accessed February 2009).
BMI, Body mass index.
*To convert height in centimeters to inches, multiply the height by 0.3937.
†To convert weight in kilograms to pounds, multiply the weight by 2.2.

TABLE 6-31: Classification of Overweight and Obesity by Body Mass Index (BMI) and Associated Disease Risk Relative to BMI and Waist Circumference

	BMI (kg/m²)	Disease Risk Relative to Normal Weight and Waist Circumference	
		M ≤40 in. (102 cm); F ≤35 in. (88 cm)	M >40 in. (102 cm); F >35 in. (88 cm)
Underweight	<18.5	—	—
Normal weight	18.5–24.9	—	—
Overweight	25.0–29.9	Increased	High
Obesity, class			
I	30.0–34.9	High	Very high
II	35.0–39.9	Very high	Very high
III (extreme obesity)	≥40	Extremely high	Extremely high

Data from North American Association for the Study of Obesity (NAASO), National Heart, Lung, and Blood Institute (NHLBI). *Practical Guide on the Identification, Evaluation, and Treatment of Overweight and Obesity in Adults.* NIH Publication No. 00-4084. Bethesda, MD: National Institutes of Health; 2000. Available at http://www.nhlbi.nih.gov/guidelines/obesity/prctgd_c.pdf (accessed February 2009). BMI, Body mass index; F, female; M, male.

with normal waist circumferences within the healthful, overweight, and class I obesity BMI categories.[45]

- The recommended procedure for measuring waist circumference (WC) is to place the measuring tape in a horizontal plane around the abdomen at the level of the iliac crest, ensuring that the tape is snug but does not compress the skin and is parallel to the floor. The reading should be obtained at the end of a normal expiration.[51]

- WC of 35 in. or more (88 cm) for females and 40 in. or more (102 cm) for males is recognized as an indicator of excessive abdominal fat and is associated with increased health risk, including type 2 DM, HTN, and CAD (see Table 6-31).[45] However, more specific criteria have been proposed[11]:
  - ▸ Very low risk: WC less than 28.5 in. (70 cm) for females and less than 31.5 in. (80 cm) for males
  - ▸ Low risk: WC 28.5 to 35.0 in. (70 to 80 cm) for females and 31.5 to 39.0 in. (80 to 99 cm) for males
  - ▸ High risk: WC 35.5 to 43.0 in. (90 to 109 cm) for females and 39.5 to 47.0 in. (100 to 120 cm) for males
  - ▸ Very high risk: WC greater than 43.5 in. (110 cm) for females and greater than 47.0 in. (120 cm) for males

- It is especially important to measure WC in individuals with a BMI less than 35, because increased WC independently defines elevated health risk, particularly for metabolic syndrome.

Waist-to-Hip Ratio

The waist-to-hip (WHR) ratio is an index of abdominal to lower body fat distribution and is obtained by dividing waist circumference (see earlier) by hip circumference at the widest point. Its use led to the recognition of the importance of central obesity as a major risk factor for the diseases associated with obesity. However, simple WC has proved to be as good or better than the WHR as a standard for the measurement of central fat and requires only a single measurement, and therefore WC is now preferred by most clinicians.

- In general, a WHR less than 0.8 for males and less than 0.7 for females is associated with a low health risk.[2]
- However, healthful values for WHR vary with age as well as gender, and thus progressively higher values fall into the low-risk category as an individual ages (e.g., men and women in their 60 s will have a low risk of chronic disease if the WHR is less than 0.91 or 0.76, respectively).

RESPIRATORY MUSCLE STRENGTH AND ENDURANCE

As noted in Chapter 4, respiratory muscle dysfunction occurs in a wide variety of diseases that affect the cardiovascular and pulmonary systems, including COPD, asthma, cystic fibrosis, CHF, neuromuscular and neurologic disorders, myopathies, obesity, connective tissue disorders, other restrictive lung diseases, diabetes mellitus, renal failure, long-term use of corticosteroids, and critically ill patients with infection, sepsis, and shock.[55] In addition, poor nutrition, prolonged deconditioning, and aging are associated with reductions in respiratory muscle strength and endurance. The clinical consequences include dyspnea, reduced exercise tolerance, impaired cough, respiratory insufficiency, and difficulty weaning from mechanical ventilation.

Therefore, assessment of respiratory muscle strength and endurance is valuable for many patients who experience dyspnea on exertion. The findings can be used to clarify the cause of abnormal breathing patterns and direct appropriate treatment interventions and can serve as outcome measures to document their effectiveness.

- Respiratory muscle strength is assessed clinically by several indirect methods:
  - ▸ Manual muscle testing cannot be performed as a direct measure of strength of the diaphragm or other isolated respiratory muscles. Indirect testing using manual resistance added to various palpation techniques (described on page 250) is

sometimes performed, but it tends to be unreliable because of the inability to objectively quantify the findings.

▸ Maximal inspiratory and expiratory pressures (MIP or $P_{I_{max}}$ and MEP or $P_{E_{max}}$, respectively) are commonly determined using a number of commercially available and assembled devices that measure the amount of negative pressure developed during a maximal inspiration and the amount of positive pressure created by a maximal expiration. These values provide estimates of the force produced by all of the inspiratory or expiratory muscles.

⊙ To obtain accurate and reliable data, the patient should be seated with the trunk at 90 degrees to the hips and maintain that posture throughout testing, wear a noseclip, and achieve an adequate seal at the mouthpiece.[14,21]

⊙ For MIP, the patient should expire fully to near residual volume (RV), without leaning forward, and then inspire as forcefully as possible, without extending backward, and maintain the inspiration for at least 1 second; strong verbal encouragement is recommended and visual feedback is also helpful.

⊙ For MEP, the patient should inspire fully to total lung capacity (TLC) and then exhale as forcefully as possible with encouragement.

⊙ Measurements are repeated at least 5 to 10 times (for inexperienced patients, there is a large learning effect between the fifth to ninth trial) with at least 1 minute of rest between measurements. The highest value for MIP and MEP obtained after 1 second of maximal effort are selected as the final measurement.

⊙ Normal predicted values for MIP and MEP, which vary with gender and age and typically have a large standard deviation (as much as ±40%), can be found elsewhere.[14,21,38] Inspiratory muscle weakness is defined as a $P_{I_{max}}$ less than 50% of predicted in the presence of clinical signs of respiratory muscle dysfunction (e.g., dyspnea, impaired cough, orthopnea, or paradoxical breathing pattern).[38]

⊙ Measurement accuracy is effort dependent and is also affected by lung volume, and therefore it is crucial that measurements be taken at known lung volumes. Theoretically, measurements should be taken from functional residual capacity (FRC), at which the elastic recoil of the lungs and thoracic cage balance each other and therefore will not influence the respiratory muscle force produced. However, sophisticated pulmonary function equipment is required to document that the patient is at FRC, and therefore measurements are usually obtained from RV and TLC, as described previously, which may affect validity.

▸ Sniff nasal inspiratory pressure (SNIP), which consists of a rapid inspiratory effort through one nostril while the other one is plugged, also provides a measurement of $P_{I_{max}}$. Although this test also requires patient cooperation, it is a natural maneuver and thus tends to be easier for most patients to perform than the MIP test.

▸ Transdiaphragmatic pressure (the difference between esophageal and abdominal pressures) can be used to provide an indication of diaphragmatic muscle force. It requires the insertion of two balloon-tipped catheters down the esophagus, one into the lower third of the esophagus and one into the stomach, and therefore is not used by most therapists.

▸ It has been reported that single tests, such as MIP, MEP, and SNIP, tend to overdiagnose respiratory muscle weakness and that the use of multiple tests of respiratory strength increases the precision of the diagnosis.[59] The use of MIP and SNIP is said to result in a relative reduction of 19.2% of patients falsely diagnosed with inspiratory muscle weakness.

• Because the inspiratory muscles work repetitively against low-intensity loads without rest, assessment of respiratory muscle endurance may be more informative than estimates of their strength. A variety of tests can be used for this purpose:

▸ Maximal voluntary ventilation (MVV) is a measure of the capacity of an individual to ventilate the lungs as fast and deeply as possible (see Table 2-6 on page 14), which provides an estimate of the functional capacity (and, to a lesser degree, the endurance) of the respiratory muscles. Because it is prone to error, MVV is best measured by experienced personnel in a pulmonary function laboratory with a low-impedance spirometer. Results may be found in the patient's medical record.

▸ "Endurance time" is the most commonly used measure of respiratory muscle endurance, which determines the time to task failure while breathing against a fixed submaximal inspiratory load (typically 60% to 75% of MIP). However, a single simple measurement tends to be of little value, as it is extremely variable when produced by untrained individuals, being influenced by subtle changes in breathing patterns and respiratory muscle recruitment. Much more reproducible is the determination of a "sustainable load," which is derived from an endurance curve produced by a series of endurance times obtained at various loads.

▸ Maximal sustainable ventilatory capacity (MSVC) is the average ventilation that can be maintained over the eighth minute of maximum effort. Using visual feedback, the patient breathes while targeting 70% to 85% of his or her measured MVV, and as fatigue develops and ventilation declines (usually over the first 1 to 3 min), the target ventilation is adjusted up or down to just above the patient's maximal effort until the eighth minute is completed. End-tidal carbon dioxide is usually measured to ensure that the individual does not hyperventilate. Young, asymptomatic persons can usually sustain ventilations of approximately 75% to 85% of MVV, whereas elderly persons can sustain ventilations of about 60% to 65% of MVV, which reflects the ventilatory capacity of both the inspiratory and expiratory muscles.[21]

▸ Maximal sustainable load pressure is determined by using a device that applies an afterload on the inspiratory muscles in order to measure their endurance. The most common is a simple inspiratory resistance device. If this device is attached to a flow-measuring device, such as a disposable incentive spirometer, a targeted flow can be maintained in order to prevent the patient from adjusting his or her flow rate over time to reduce the pressure load; the addition of a metronome can assist in regulating breathing rhythm to increase the accuracy of the resulting endurance time.

Alternatively, a threshold resistor can be used. The individual performs a series of endurance measurements to task failure starting at 90% of MIP and decreasing in 5% increments until the load can be sustained for more than 10 minutes. Untrained individuals can sustain approximately 68% of MIP (SD, ±3%).[21] Another method of applying this test is to use weights on the abdominal area as the pressure load.

▸ Maximal incremental threshold loading involves breathing against progressively increasing resistances, typically beginning at 20% to 30% of MIP and increasing by 10% to 20% every 2 minutes, to determine the highest pressure that can be sustained for 2 minutes. Usually, most nonelderly asymptomatic individuals can sustain a peak pressure of 88% of MIP, whereas elderly persons reach about 80% of MIP.[40]

- It is important to note that one of the most important indicators of respiratory muscle dysfunction is an abnormal breathing pattern. Therefore, careful clinical observation of rib cage and abdominal movements is valuable in distinguishing various forms of respiratory muscle dysfunction and weakness.

▸ Rib cage paradox, in which the rib cage collapses during inspiration, commonly occurs in patients with high cervical spinal cord injury because of an inability to stabilize the thoracic cage as negative intrapleural pressure is generated.

▸ Abdominal paradox is manifested by the inward movement of the abdomen as the rib cage expands, which may be seen in patients with bilateral diaphragmatic paralysis or in patients who are developing respiratory failure and are attempting to optimize the thoracic muscles as a pressure generator.

▸ *Respiratory alternans* refers to the alternating use of various accessory muscles of respiration so that there is alternating paradoxical movement of the abdomen and rib cage. It is thought to occur as a result of the patient trying to shift the workload among the various respiratory muscle groups.

▸ Dyssynchronous or asynchronous breathing results from abnormal patterns of respiratory muscle recruitment, causing there to be a time difference between activation of the diaphragm and other inspiratory muscles. A time lag between the expansion of the thorax and the outward motion of the abdomen is often observed.

▸ Hoover's sign may be noted in patients with COPD and severe lung hyperinflation. When the diaphragm becomes so flattened that the fibers become horizontal, contraction causes the ribs to be pulled inward so that the transverse diameter of the rib cage diminishes during inspiration. These patients become dependent on lifting of the anterior chest wall by the accessory muscles for thoracic expansion and often lean forward to support their shoulders to maximize the efficiency of these muscles.

▸ *Orthopnea* refers to difficulty breathing when lying flat, which is most commonly seen in heart failure. However, it can also occur in patients with diaphragmatic paralysis and severe COPD, as well as morbid obesity. In the supine position, the diaphragm must work against and lift the abdominal contents during contraction, so when the diaphragm is too weak or the load is increased, ventilation is reduced

and dyspnea develops. In severe COPD, the reduction in lung volumes that can occur in the supine position can also limit ventilation, causing distress. These individual learn to sleep sitting in an upright position to avoid orthopnea.

- Finally, the special needs of patients with likely respiratory muscle dysfunction must be considered during the assessment process.

▸ Monitoring of oxygen saturation is important during testing to avoid desaturation in these high-risk patients.

▸ Careful monitoring for any signs or symptoms of respiratory muscle fatigue (see page 243) is also crucial to avoid inducing injury or precipitating ventilatory failure.

AUTONOMIC DYSFUNCTION

Autonomic dysfunction is a common complication of DM, chronic kidney disease (CKD), and spinal cord injury, and it is often present despite a lack of clinical symptoms. Autonomic neuropathy can affect all bodily organs, resulting in a variety of abnormalities, including impaired exercise tolerance; orthostatic hypotension; silent myocardial ischemia; gastrointestinal, genitourinary, and metabolic dysfunction; and impaired thermoregulation.[47,61]

- Cardiovascular autonomic neuropathy (CAN) affects approximately 50% of patients with DM, in whom it appears early and is significantly associated with age, duration of DM, microangiopathy, and peripheral neuropathy, and with obesity in type 2 DM.[60] It usually affects the parasympathetic nervous system (PNS) before the sympathetic nervous system (SNS), so resting HRs are elevated in these patients.

- CAN should be suspected in all individuals with type 2 DM and in those with type 1 DM for more than 5 years. Once established, CAN is associated with significant deterioration in quality of life and increased morbidity and mortality.[47]

- CAN produces abnormalities in HR control and central and peripheral vascular dynamics and thus can be detected by some simple assessment techniques[61]:

▸ The *HR response to deep breathing*, which for the most part is under the control of the PNS and thus is one of the earliest indicators of CAN, can be assessed by measuring the HR variability during paced deep breathing. The patient lies quietly and breathes deeply at a rate of 6 breaths/min (which produces maximal variation in HR) while an ECG monitor records the difference between the maximal and minimal HRs (as determined by the shortest and longest R-to-R [R–R] intervals, respectively). Normally, the HR response to deep breathing is greater than 15 bpm, but individuals with CAN exhibit a blunted response, with less than 10 bpm being defined as abnormal.[61] However, R–R variation is affected by ectopic beats and is age dependent.

▸ The *HR and BP responses to standing* depend on activation of a baroreceptor-initiated, centrally mediated SNS reflex to produce an increase in peripheral vascular resistance and HR.

⊙ The HR response is evaluated with an ECG recording during the change from the horizontal to the vertical position. Normally, there is a characteristic rapid rise in the HR on standing that is maximal at approximately the 15th heart beat after standing, which is followed by a relative bradycardia that is most pronounced at approximately the 30th heart beat after standing. The longest R–R interval during beats 20 to 40 is divided by the shortest R–R interval during beats 5 to 25 to obtain the maximum-to-minimum ratio. Normally, this so-called 30:15 ratio is greater than 1.03.[61] Patients with CAN exhibit a slow rise in HR to standing and therefore have less HR variability and a lower 30:15 ratio.

⊙ BP values are obtained in the supine position and immediately on standing. A normal response is a fall in SBP of less than 10 mm Hg, whereas orthostatic hypotension is defined as a greater than 20- to 30-mm Hg fall in SBP or as a greater than 10-mm Hg fall in DBP (in-between values are considered borderline). Orthostatic hypotension is characterized by lightheadedness, dizziness, and presyncopal symptoms, although weakness, fatigue, visual blurring, and neck pain may also occur. However, many patients are asymptomatic despite a significant drop in BP.

- The *BP and HR responses to the Valsalva maneuver,* as described on page 278, are also affected by CAN. The HR response is blunted (reduced rises in phases 2 and 3) and there is often a reduced decline in BP during strain (phase 2), followed by a slow recovery after release (phase 3). The Valsalva ratio is determined by calculating the ratio of the longest R–R interval after the maneuver (reflecting the bradycardic response to BP overshoot) to the shortest R–R interval during or shortly after the maneuver (reflecting tachycardia as a result of strain), and is normally greater than 1.2.[61]

  ▸ The *HR and BP responses to exercise* are also reduced in CAN because of impaired PNS and SNS responses. The severity of CAN has been shown to correlate inversely with the increase in HR at any time during exercise and with the maximal increase in HR.[61] In addition, there is a reduction in ejection fraction and cardiac output due to systolic and diastolic dysfunction, which leads to exercise intolerance.

- Because CAN lowers the threshold for life-threatening arrhythmias and increases the risk of hemodynamic instability, clinical monitoring during assessment is extremely important in patients with DM and CKD.

QUESTIONNAIRES AND SURVEYS

Various self-administered questionnaires and surveys are available for clinical use to assist in determining such things as a client's activity habits, health status, and potential risk associated with exercise and other physical therapy interventions, and quality of life.

Health and Fitness Appraisals

One means of reducing the risk of adverse events occurring during exercise testing and PT assessments is to have clients complete some form of health or fitness appraisal before performing the evaluation. A few of the common or relevant questionnaires are described here.

- The *modified AHA/ACSM Health/Fitness Facility Preparticipation Screening Questionnaire,* shown in Figure 6-48, is an example of a self-administered survey that can be used as a preliminary screening tool for individuals who are interested in beginning an exercise program (either independent or

supervised).[2] It is designed to identify individuals with cardiovascular risk factors and symptoms as well as a broad scope of chronic diseases that might be aggravated by exercise.

  ▸ A *yes* answer to any item alerts the therapist to the need for physician clearance before participation in an exercise program. Clinical monitoring of exercise responses should be performed once the individual has received medical clearance.

  ▸ If *no* statements are checked, the individual should be safe to begin exercising without medical clearance, although HR and BP monitoring during the initial assessment will provide useful information for creating an exercise prescription and may reveal unknown abnormalities.

- The *Physical Activity Readiness Questionnaire (PAR-Q)* contains seven simple questions that are used to screen individuals aged 15 to 69 years.[15] It is depicted in Table 6-32.

  ▸ Individuals who answer *yes* to one or more questions should talk to her/his physician and may require medical clearance before performing more vigorous physical activity or an exercise test. Physiological monitoring of exercise responses is recommended during PT evaluation of these individuals.

  ▸ Individuals who answer *no* honestly to all questions are unlikely to develop any problems during at least moderate exercise and can begin an exercise program without medical clearance. Because the prevalence of undiagnosed HTN is so high, even in younger adults, blood pressure monitoring is recommended during PT evaluation of all adults.

  ▸ Persons who have acute illnesses should be advised to delay participation in more vigorous exercise until they are feeling better, and pregnant women should discuss appropriate exercise with their physician before initiating a new exercise program.

- The *Duke Activity Status Index (DASI)* is a 12-item questionnaire that aims to provide an indirect measure of functional capacity and an assessment of aspects of quality of life (Table 6-33).[41] The weighted values for various exercise and daily household activities that can be performed by an individual are added together to provide a rough estimate of peak oxygen uptake and MET level.

  ▸ The DASI has been found to be valid and reliable for a variety of different patient populations, including those with heart failure and chronic obstructive pulmonary diseases.[6,16]

  ▸ For patients who can not tolerate a graded exercise test, DASI scores can be used to prescribe exercise activities on the basis of METs, as described in Chapter 7 (see page 307).

  ▸ As shown in the table, repeated DASI can serve as an outcome measure to document the change in status resulting from physical therapy interventions.

Quality of Life Measures

Besides physiological variables, other factors, including level of daily functioning and well-being, are affected by chronic diseases and may be impacted by various treatment interventions and therefore are recognized as important outcomes of medical care. They help determine whether a patient's status is stable, improving, or deteriorating. A number of general health-related quality of life (HRQoL) measures and disease-specific quality of life (QoL) questionnaires have been developed, some of which are presented in the following sections.[22a,24,26,43,64]

Assess your health status by marking all _true_ statements

History
You have had:
——— a heart attack
——— heart surgery
——— cardiac catheterization
——— coronary angioplasty (PTCA)
——— pacemaker/implantable cardiac
   defibrillator/rhythm disturbance
——— heart valve disease
——— heart failure
——— heart transplantation
——— congenital heart disease

Symptoms
——— You experience chest discomfort with exertion.
——— You experience unreasonable breathlessness.
——— You experience dizziness, fainting, or blackouts.
——— You take heart medications.

Other health issues
——— You have diabetes.
——— You have asthma or other lung disease.
——— You have burning or cramping sensation in your lower
   legs when walking short distances.
——— You have musculoskeletal problems that limit your
   physical activity.
——— You have concerns about the safety of exercise.
——— You take prescription medication(s).
——— You are pregnant.

If you marked any of these statements in this section, consult your physician or other appropriate health care provider before engaging in exercise. you may need to use a facility with a **medically qualified staff.**

Cardiovascular risk factors
——— You are a man older than 45 years.
——— You are a woman older than 55 years, have had a
   hysterectomy, or are postmenopausal.
——— You smoke, or quit smoking within the previous 6 months.
——— You blood pressure is >140/90 mm Hg.
——— You do not know your blood pressure.
——— You take blood pressure medication.
——— You blood cholesterol level is >200 mg/dL.
——— You do not your know cholesterol level.
——— You have a close blood relative who had a heart attack or
   heart surgery before age 55 (father or brother) or age 65
   (mother or sister).
——— You are physically inactive (i.e., you get <30 minutes of
   physical activity on at least 3 days per week).
——— You are >20 pounds overweight.

If you marked two or more of the statements in this section you should consult your physician or other appropriate health care provider before engaging in exercise. You might benefit from using a facility with a **professionally qualified exercise staff†** *to guide your exercise program.*

——— None of the above

You should be able to exercise safely without consulting your physician or other appropriate health care provider in a self-guided program or almost any facility that meets your exercise program needs.

*Modified from American College of Sports Medicine and American Heart Association. ACSM/AHA Joint Position Statement: Recommendations for cardiovascular screening, staffing, and emergency policies at health/fitness facilities. Med Sci Sports Exerc 1998:1018.

†Professionally qualified exercise staff refers to appropriately trained individuals who possess academic training, practical and clinical knowledge, skills, and abilities commensurate with the credentials defined in Appendix F.

Figure 6-48: The modified AHA/ACSM Health/Fitness Facility Pre-participation Screening Questionnaire. (From Cardinal BJ, Esters J, Cardinal MK. Evaluation of the revised Physical Activity Readiness Questionnaire in older adults. *Med Sci Sports Exerc.* 1996:28:468–472.)

General Health Measures

By design, general health status instruments are broad in scope and applicability so that they can be used across various patient populations. Although they are not as sensitive in discriminating the range of impairment within disease groups or as responsive to change over time as disease-specific measures, several HRQoL questionnaires have been validated and demonstrate reliability and responsiveness among patients with specific diseases, including COPD, heart disease, or both; among these are the SIP, QWB, and SF-36 (see later).[24,26,43,64]

- The Short Form 36 (SF-36) is probably the most well known and widely used generic health status measure. Developed from the Medical Outcomes Study (MOS) questionnaire, the SF-36 measures subjective heath status in eight domains, including physical and social function, mental health, pain, energy/vitality, health perceptions, and change in health. It offers the advantages of being short, and broad in range of areas adversely affected by illness. However, it sacrifices detail of information and many patients with serious chronic illnesses record the lowest and highest possible values on a number of

TABLE 6-32: Physical Activity Readiness Questionnaire

PAR-Q Question	Yes	No
1. Has your doctor ever said you have a heart condition *and* that you should only do physical activity recommended by a doctor?		
2. Do you feel pain in your chest when you do physical activity?		
3. In the past month, have you had chest pain when you were not doing physical activity?		
4. Do you lose your balance because of dizziness or do you ever lose consciousness?		
5. Do you have a bone or joint problem that could be made worse by a change in your physical activity?		
6. Is your doctor currently prescribing drugs (for example, water pills) for your blood pressure or heart condition?		
7. Do you know of *any other reason* why you should not do physical activity?		
If you answered yes to one or more questions, it's important that you see your health care professional before you begin a new exercise program.		

From Cardinal BJ, Esters J, Cardinal MK: Evaluation of the revised Physical Activity Readiness Questionnaire in older adults, *Med. Sci. Sports Exerc.* 28:468–472, 1996. PAR-Q, Physical Activity Readiness Questionnaire.

TABLE 6-33: Duke Activity Status Index (DASI)

Activity: Can you...	Weight	Pre	Post
Take care of yourself (eating, dressing, bathing, or using the toilet)?	2.75		
Walk indoors, such as around your house?	1.75		
Walk a block or two on level ground?	2.75		
Climb a flight of stairs or walk up a hill?	5.00		
Run a short distance?	8.00		
Do light work around the house like dusting or washing dishes?	2.70		
Do moderate work around the house like vacuuming, sweeping floors, or carrying in groceries?	3.50		
Do heavy work around the house like scrubbing floors or lifting or moving heavy furniture?	8.00		
Do yard work like raking leaves, weeding, or pushing a power mower?	4.50		
Have sexual relations?	5.25		
Participate in moderate recreational activities like golf, bowling, dancing, doubles tennis, or throwing a baseball or football?	6.00		
Participate in strenuous sports like swimming, singles tennis, football, basketball, or skiing?	7.50		
DASI score = sum of positive responses/weights	58.2*		

$\dot{V}O_2$ peak (mL/kg/min) = $[0.43 \times (DASI\ score)] + 9.6$

METs = $\dot{V}O_2$ peak/3.5

From Hlatky MA, Boineau RE, Higginbotham MB, et al. A brief self-administered questionnaire to determine functional capacity (the Duke Activity Status Index). *Am J Cardiol.* 1989:64:651–654.
METs, Metabolic equivalents of energy expenditure (i.e., multiples of resting energy metabolism); $\dot{V}O_2$ = oxygen uptake.
Instructions: Enter weight value for each "yes" answer in the "Pre" column and total column for the DASI score. The "Post" column allows for a repeat measure and ease of comparison after an intervention.
*Maximal possible score = 58.2.

scales, so it may not be sensitive to clinically important changes in status.[43,64]

- The Sickness Impact Profile (SIP) is a generic measure consisting of 136 items that quantify everyday activities in 12 categories: sleep and rest, emotional behavior, body care and movement, home management, mobility, social interaction, ambulation, alertness behavior, communication, work, recreation and pastimes, and eating. Its major disadvantage is the 20 to 30 minutes required to complete the survey.

- The Quality of Well-Being (QWB) Scale is a health status measure that looks at symptoms and level of functioning across three domains (mobility, physical activity, and social activity) over 6 days. Disadvantages include its length and the need for trained interviewers for its administration. However, a self-administered version (QWB-SA) has been developed that includes an expanded list of symptoms and assesses only the 3 previous days, which reduces recall bias and the time it takes to complete (typically about 10 min). Because the QWB looks at actual functional performance and symptoms over specific days rather than functional ability, its results are subject to variations in status produced by acute illness, aggravation of symptoms, and so on, and therefore test–retest evaluations may have little meaning.

- The Duke Health Profile (DUKE) is a 17-item questionnaire that measures functional health status and HRQoL during a 1-week time period. The DUKE is composed of 11 scales, 6 of which measure functional health (physical, mental, social, general, perceived health, and self-esteem) and 5 of which look at dysfunctional health (anxiety, depression, anxiety–depression, pain, and disability). It is easy to understand, with only three simple response options, and usually takes less than 5 minutes to complete.

Respiratory Disease-specific Questionnaires

- The Chronic Respiratory Disease Questionnaire (CRQ), which is available in an interview version and a self-administered version, assesses the physical health status of patients with COPD. It consists of 20 questions that deal with dyspnea, fatigue, emotional function, and mastery. A unique feature of the CRQ is its ability to assess limitations in patient-specific activities (each patient chooses five activities that provoke the greatest shortness of breath); however, this also limits its power to make comparisons between patients.
- The St. George's Respiratory Questionnaire (SGRQ) measures the impact of respiratory disease on overall health, daily life, and perceived well-being in patients with asthma, COPD, and several other chronic pulmonary diseases. It contains 50 self-administered items with 76 weighted responses that address symptomatology (frequency and severity), activity limitations, and psychosocial impact of the disease. It usually takes about 10 to 15 minutes to complete. The SGRQ has been demonstrated to detect decrements in HRQoL among patients with mild disease, to discriminate between patients who have mild-to-severe COPD, to describe the magnitude of the effect of COPD exacerbations on health status, and to document the effects of medications and other interventions.[24]
- The Seattle Obstructive Lung Disease Questionnaire (SOLDQ) is a relatively new self-administered instrument that is designed to assess physical and emotional function, coping skills, and treatment satisfaction in patients with asthma and COPD. It consists of 29 items that can be completed in about 10 to 15 minutes. It has demonstrated predictive validity for all-cause mortality and hospitalizations for COPD and related illness.[24]

Cardiac Disease-specific Questionnaires

- The Minnesota Living with Heart Failure Questionnaire (MLHFQ, or simply LHFQ) consists of 21 questions dealing with the key physical, emotional, social, and mental dimensions of QoL that measure the patient's perception of heart failure and its effects on daily life.[22a] It is self-administered and requires 5 to 10 minutes to complete, and it takes into consideration the side effects of medications, hospital stays, and cost of care. Because many patients score at the very top and very low ends of the instrument, it has limited ability to document change in status.

- The Chronic Heart Failure Questionnaire (CHQ) is an individual-specific health status measure designed to assess CHF, and therefore the number of questions asked varies from patient to patient. As with the CRQ, the CHQ enumerates five activities that provoke the greatest shortness of breath and quantifies the intensity. It also addresses fatigue and emotional function. When applied to patients with CAD, the CHQ (sometimes referred to at the Chronic Heart Disease Questionnaire) asks about activities that induce chest pain/discomfort or shortness of breath. Some studies have found that a number of patients score at the very top and very low ends of some scales of the CHQ, resulting in a limited ability to document change in status in these patients.
- The Kansas City Cardiomyopathy Questionnaire (KCCQ) is a detailed, disease-specific health status measure that contains 23 questions, focusing on fluid retention, and quantifying the associated physical limitations, symptoms, disease severity, change in status over time, self-efficacy, and quality of life. It takes only 4 to 6 minutes to complete.
- The Quality of Life after Myocardial Infarction (QLMI) Questionnaire contains 26 items that assess 5 domains: symptoms, restriction, confidence, self-esteem, and emotion. The revised version, the QLMI-2, consists of 27 items grouped into 3 domains: emotional, physical, and social.
- The Seattle Angina Questionnaire (SAQ) measures five clinically important dimensions of health in patients with CAD: physical limitation, anginal stability, anginal frequency, treatment satisfaction, and disease perception. Although it is described by the authors as a disease-specific functional status measure, 7 of the 19 items address social and emotional issues, and thus it also serves as a disease-specific HRQoL tool.[22a,26] The SAQ has been shown to predict 1-year mortality and admission to the hospital for acute coronary syndrome (ACS).

6.7 ASSESSMENT OF FINDINGS

Throughout the PT evaluation, the therapist constantly assesses the patient's responses and decides how much activity the patient can safely perform versus when it is appropriate to stop. However, once the patient evaluation has been completed, all of the findings must be assessed to define appropriate treatment goals and to develop an effective treatment plan. Although a single abnormal finding can indicate a life-threatening situation, this is generally not the case. Rather, it is the sum of all the clinical data that describes the patient's clinical status. Of particular importance are the HR, BP, Sao_2, ECG (if available), and signs and symptoms of exercise intolerance.

CHEST ASSESSMENT

The various abnormal findings that may be detected on chest assessment should be evaluated together and in relation to each other, for the pattern of abnormalities often reveals the pathological and anatomic disturbances responsible for them, as indicated in Table 6-34.

- By identifying the patient's pathological condition through chest assessment, an appropriate treatment plan can be instituted.
- After treatment, the patient's clinical status is reassessed to document the effectiveness of treatment.

ACTIVITY AND ENDURANCE EVALUATION

Many patients exhibit normal physiological responses to increasing activity without any adverse signs and symptoms and therefore are safe to participate in unrestricted physical therapy treatment programs. However, a significant percentage of patients have some form of diagnosed or undiagnosed cardiopulmonary dysfunction and exhibit abnormal responses to exertion, although these may not be recognized by the therapist if physiological monitoring is not performed.

Sometimes, the only abnormalities are related to orthostatic hypotension, with a drop in BP as the patient moves from supine to sitting to standing, which may result from deconditioning, antihypertension medications, or autonomic dysfunction. Avoidance of quick changes of position is an important treatment modification for these patients in order to prevent falls. Other times, the abnormal signs and symptoms are more extreme and imply marked exercise intolerance (see Table 6-28), in which case the evaluation or treatment session should be terminated and consultation with the referring physician is probably indicated. Finally, the abnormalities may simply indicate deconditioning or low

TABLE 6-34: **Physical Signs Observed in Various Pulmonary Disorders**

Condition	Breath Sounds	Adventitious Sounds	Voice Sounds	Inspection/ Palpation	Tactile Fremitus	Percussion
Normal	nl	None	Muffled, distant, indistinct	Trachea midline, symmetric chest expansion	nl	nl
Asthma, acute moderately severe attack	↓, bronchial, prolonged expiration	Inspiratory plus expiratory wheezes	↓	↑ Use of accessory muscles, tachypnea	↓	nl–↑ reson
Atelectasis	↓ or Ø	Crackles	↓ Or Ø	Trachea deviated to AS, ↓ CWE on AS	↓	↓–↓↓ reson
Bronchiectasis	nl	Crackles	nl	↓ CWE on AS, tachypnea, clubbing	↑ Rhonchal fremitus	nl
Bronchitis	nl, possible prolonged expiration	Crackles, wheezes	nl	Possible ↓ CWE, occasional use of accessory muscles	↓ Bilaterally	↑ Reson bilaterally
COPD	↓–↓↓, prolonged expiration	None versus crackles and wheezes	↓ Or Ø bilaterally	Barrel-shaped chest, moves as a unit, ↑ use of accessory muscles, ↓ CWE bilaterally	↓ Bilaterally	↑ Reson bilaterally
Consolidation	Bronchial	Crackles	↑ Transmission	Trachea midline, ↓ CWE on AS	↑	↓ Reson
Fibrosis						
Localized	↓	Crackles	↓	↓ CWE over area	↓ or Ø	↓ Reson
Generalized	↓	Crackles	↓	↓ CWE bilaterally	↓ or Ø	↓ Reson
Pulmonary edema	nl	Dependent crackles	nl	nl CWE, tachypnea	nl	nl
Pleural effusion (moderate to large)	↓ or Ø,* bronchial†	Possible pleural rub	Ø * or ↑†	↑ RR, trachea deviated to OS, ↓ CWE on AS	↓ or Ø	↓–↓↓
Pneumothorax (>15%)	↓ or Ø	None	↓ or Ø	↓ CWE on AS	↓ or Ø	↑

↓, Decreased; ↓↓, very decreased; ↑, increased; Ø, absent; AS, on affected side; COPD, chronic obstructive pulmonary disease; CWE, chest wall excursion; nl, normal; OS, opposite side; reson, resonance; RR, respiratory rate.
*Absent over the effusion.
†Possible increased transmission above the fluid.

fitness level (see Table 6-29) and the need to monitor exercise intensity and the individual's responses to incremental activity and to progress slowly in the treatment program.

Warning Signs and Symptoms of Limited Exercise Tolerance

- Resting tachycardia
- Lack of HR or BP response to exertion
- Excessive HR or BP response to exertion
- Greater than 10–mm Hg fall in SBP after initial rise with an increase in workload
- Increasing arrhythmias during or immediately after exertion
- Low anginal threshold
- Excessive dyspnea
- Leg claudication or other pain
- Pallor, facial expression of distress
- Lightheadedness, dizziness
- Slow HR recovery from activity
- Excessive fatigue lasting more than 1 to 2 hours after exertion

DEFINING THE PHYSICAL THERAPY PROBLEMS

The purpose of assessing all the evaluative findings is to define the physical therapy problems for each patient and thereby develop appropriate treatment goals and plans that directly address these problems.

- Many individuals can be identified who have elevated risk for cardiovascular disease
- Patients with either cardiac or pulmonary dysfunction may have any of the following physical therapy problems:
  - ▸ Impaired exercise tolerance or deconditioning
  - ▸ Abnormal physiological responses to exertion
  - ▸ Inability to meet the demands of daily living activities
- In addition, patients with pulmonary dysfunction may have one or more of the following specific problems:
  - ▸ Impaired ventilation and gas exchange
  - ▸ Impaired secretion clearance
  - ▸ Impaired ability to protect airway
  - ▸ Increased work of breathing

The physical therapy interventions that are used to treat these problems and restore patients to better function are presented in Chapter 7.

REFERENCES

1. Abernathy RP, Black DR. Healthy body weights: an alternative perspective. *Am J Clin Nutr.* 1996;63(suppl):448S-451S.
2. American College of Sports Medicine. *ASCM's Guidelines for Exercise Testing and Prescription.* 7th ed. Philadelphia: Lippincott Williams & Wilkins; 2006.
3. American College of Sports Medicine. *ASCM's Resource Manual for Guidelines for Exercise Testing and Prescription.* 4th ed. Philadelphia: Lippincott Williams & Wilkins; 2001.
4. American Physical Therapy Association. Guide to Physical Therapist Practice. 2nd ed. *Phys Ther.* 2001;81:9-746.
5. American Thoracic Society. ATS statement: guidelines for the Six-Minute Walk Test. *Am J Respir Crit Care Med.* 2002;166:111-117.
5a. American Thoracic Society/American College of Chest Physicians. ATS/ACCP statement on cardiopulmonary exercise testing. *Am J Respir Crit Care Med.* 2003;167:211-277.
6. Arena R, Humphrey R, Peberdy MA. Using the Duke Activity Status Index in heart failure. *J Cardiopulm Rehabil.* 2002;22:93-95.
7. Baum GL, Wolinsky E, eds. *Textbook of Pulmonary Diseases.* 4th ed. Boston: Little, Brown & Co; 1989.
8. Borg G. *Borg's Perceived Exertion and Pain Scales.* Champaign, IL: Human Kinetics; 1998.
9. Borg G. *Borg's RPE scale.* Copyright Gunnar Borg; 1994.
10. Borg G. *Borg CR10 Scale.* Copyright Gunnar Borg; 1982, 1998, 2003.
11. Bray GA. Don't throw the baby out with the bath water. *Am J Clin Nutr.* 2004;79:347-349.
12. Brooks D, Davis AM, Naglie G. Validity of 3 physical performance measures in inpatient geriatric rehabilitation. *Arch Phys Med Rehabil.* 2006;87:105-110.
13. Cahalin LP. Cardiovascular evaluation. In: DeTurk WE, Cahalin LB, eds. *Cardiovascular and Pulmonary Physical Therapy: An Evidence-Based Approach.* New York: McGraw-Hill; 2004.
14. Cahalin LP. Pulmonary evaluation. In: DeTurk WE, Cahalin LB, eds. *Cardiovascular and Pulmonary Physical Therapy: An Evidence-Based Approach.* New York: McGraw-Hill; 2004.
14a. Cameron J, Stevenson I, Reed EB, et al. Accuracy of automated auscultatory blood pressure measurement during supine exercise and treadmill stress electrocardiogram-testing. *Blood Press Monit.* 2004;9:269-275.
15. Cardinal BJ, Esters J, Cardinal MK. Evaluation of the revised Physical Activity Readiness Questionnaire in older adults. *Med Sci Sports Exerc.* 1996;28:468-472.
16. Carter R, Holiday DB, Grouthues C, et al. Criterion validity of the Duke Activity Status Index for assessing functional capacity in patients with chronic obstructive pulmonary disease. *J Cardiopulm Rehabil.* 2002;22:298-303.
17. Casale PN, Devereux RB, Alonso DR, et al. Improved sex-specific criteria of left ventricular hypertrophy for clinical and computer interpretation of electrocardiograms: Validation with autopsy findings. *Circulation.* 1987;75:565-572.
17a. Celli BR, Cote CG, Marin JM, et al. The body-mass index, airflow obstruction, dyspnea, and exercise capacity index in chronic obstructive pulmonary disease. *N Engl J Med.* 2004;350:1005-1012.
18. Chaitman BR. Exercise stress testing. In: Zipes DP, Libby P, Bonow PO, Braunwald E, eds. *Braunwald's Heart Disease.* 7th ed. Philadelphia: Saunders; 2005.
19. Chimowitz MI, Mancini GBJ. Asymptomatic coronary artery disease in patients with stroke—Prevalence, prognosis, diagnosis, and treatment. *Curr Concepts Cerebrovasc Dis Stroke.* 1991;26:23-27.
19a. Chobanian AV, Bakris GL, Black HR, et al. Seventh Report of the Joint National Committee on Prevention, Detection, Evaluation, and Treatment of High Blood Pressure. *Hypertension.* 2003;42:1206-1252.
20. Christensen CC, Ryg MS, Edvardsen A, et al. Relationship between exercise desaturation and pulmonary haemodynamics in COPD patients. *Eur Respir J.* 2004;24:580-586.
21. Clanton TL, Diaz PT. Clinical assessment of the respiratory muscles. *Phys Ther.* 1995;75:983-995.
22. Cockcroft JR, Wilkinson IB, Evans M, et al. Pulse pressure predicts cardiovascular risk in patients with type 2 diabetes mellitus. *Am J Hypertens.* 2005;18:1463-1467.
22a. Cokkinos DV. The value of questionnaires in assessing physical activity, fitness, and quality of life. *Heart Fail Rev.* 1999;3:305-311.
22b. Cohen M, Michel TH. *Cardiopulmonary Symptoms in Physical Therapy Practice.* New York: Churchill Livingstone; 1988.
23. Crawford MH, DiMarco JP, Paulus WJ. *Cardiology.* 2nd ed. Philadelphia: Mosby; 2004.
24. Curtis JR, Patrick DL. The assessment of health status among patients with COPD. *Eur Respir J.* 2003;21(suppl 41):36s-45s.
25. Decramer M. Hyperinflation and respiratory muscle interaction. *Eur Respir J.* 1997;10:934-941.
26. Dempster M, Donnelly M. Measuring the health related quality of life of people with ischaemic heart disease. *Br Med J.* 2000;83:641-644.
27. de Troyer A. Effect of hyperinflation on the diaphragm. *Eur Respir J.* 1997;10:708-713.
28. Ellestad MH. *Stress Testing: Principles and Practice.* 5th ed. Oxford: Oxford University Press; 2003.

29. Emtner M, Porszasz J, Burns M, et al. Benefits of supplemental oxygen in exercise training in nonhypoxemic chronic obstructive pulmonary disease patients. *Am J Respir Crit Care Med.* 2003;168:1034-1042.

30. Evans WJ, Lambert CP. Physiological basis of fatigue. *Am J Phys Med Rehabil.* 2007;86(suppl):S29-S46.

31. Fletcher GF, Balady GJ, Amsterdam ES, et al. Exercise standards for testing and training: a statement for healthcare professionals from the American Heart Association. *Circulation.* 2001;104:1694-1740.

32. Foster C, Jackson A, Pollock M, et al. Generalized equations for predicting functional capacity from treadmill performance. *Am Heart J.* 1984;107:1229-1234.

33. Franklin SS, Larson MG, Khan SA, et al. Does the relation of blood pressure to coronary heart disease risk change with aging: the Framingham Heart Study. *Circulation.* 2001;103:1245-1249.

34. Fuster V, Alexander RW, O'Rourke RA. *Hurst's The Heart.* 11th ed. New York: McGraw-Hill; 2004.

35. Gallagher D, Heymsfield SB, Heo M, et al. Healthy percentage body fat ranges: an approach for developing guidelines based on body mass index. *Am J Clin Nutr.* 2000;72:694-701.

35a. Gibbons R, Balady GJ, Bricker JT, et al. ACC/AHA 2002 Guideline update for exercise testing: summary article. *Circulation.* 2002;106:1883-1892.

36. Gibson GJ, Geddes DM, Costabel U, et al. *Respiratory Medicine.* 3rd ed. Philadelphia: Saunders; 2003.

37. Goodman CC, Snyder TEK. *Differential Diagnosis for Physical Therapists: Screening for Referral.* St. Louis: Saunders; 2007.

38. Gosselink R, Dal Corso S. Respiratory muscle training. In: Frownfelter D, Dean E, eds. *Cardiovascular and Pulmonary Physical Therapy: Evidence and Practice.* 4th ed. St. Louis: Mosby; 2006.

39. Guyatt GH, Pugsley SO, Sullivan MJ, et al. Effect of encouragement on walking test performance. *Thorax.* 1984;39:818-822.

39a. Haider AW, Larson MG, Franklin SS, et al. Systolic blood pressure, diastolic blood pressure, and pulse pressure as predictors of risk for congestive heart failure in the Framingham heart study. *Ann Intern Med.* 2003;138:10-16.

40. Herster NR, Young JR, Beven EG, et al. Coronary angiography in 506 patients with extracranial cerebrovascular disease. *Arch Int Med.* 1985;145:849-852.

40a. Hillegass E. Assessment procedures. In Hillegass EA, Sadowsky HS, editors. *Essentials of Cardiopulmonary Physical Therapy.* 2nd ed. Philadelphia: Saunders; 2001.

41. Hlatky MA, Boineau RE, Higginbotham MB, et al. A brief self-administered questionnaire to determine functional capacity (the Duke Activity Status Index). *Am J Cardiol.* 1989;64:651-654.

42. Iriberri M, Gáldiz JB, Gorostiza M, et al. Comparison of the distances covered during 3 and 6 min walking test. *Respir Med.* 2002;96:812-816.

43. Kaplan RM, Ganiats TG, Seiber WJ, et al. The Quality of Well-Being Scale: critical similarities and differences with the SF-36. *Int J Qual Health Care.* 1998;10:509-520.

44. Kjeldsen SE, Mundal R, Sandvik L, et al. Supine and exercise systolic blood pressure predict cardiovascular death in middle-aged men. *J Hypertens.* 2001;19:1343.

45. Kushner RF, Blatner DJ. Risk assessment of the overweight and obese. *J Am Diet Assoc.* 2005;105:S53-S62.

45a. Lama VN, Martinez FJ. Resting and exercise physiology in interstitial lung disease. *Clin Chest Med.* 2004;25:435-453.

46. Leung ASY, Chan KK, Sykes K, et al. Reliability, validity, and responsiveness of a 2-min walk test to assess exercise capacity of COPD patients. *Chest.* 2006;130:119-125.

46a. Mahler D, Wells C. Evaluation of clinical methods for rating dyspnea. *Chest.* 1988;93:580-586.

47. Maser RE, Lenhard MJ. Review: cardiovascular autonomic neuropathy due to diabetes mellitus: Clinical manifestations, consequences, and treatment. *J Clin Endocrinol Metab.* 2005;90:5896-5903.

48. Matthews CE, Pate RP, Jackson KL, et al. Exaggerated blood pressure response to dynamic exercise and risk of future hypertension. *J Clin Epidemiol.* 1998;51:29-35.

49. McArdle WD, Katch FI, Katch VL. *Exercise Physiology—Energy, Nutrition, and Human Performance.* 5th ed. Philadelphia: Lea & Febiger; 2001.

50. McConnell T, Clark B. Prediction of maximal oxygen consumption during handrail-supported treadmill exercise. *J Cardiopulm Rehabil.* 1987; 7:324-331.

51. North American Association for the Study of Obesity (NAASO), National Heart, Lung, and Blood Institute (NHLBI). *Practical Guide on the Identification, Evaluation, and Treatment of Overweight and Obesity in Adults.* NIH Publication No. 00-4084. Bethesda, MD: National Institutes of Health; 2000. Available at http://www.nhlbi.nih.gov/guidelines/obesity/prctgd_c.pdf (accessed February 2009).

52. Newman AB, Siscovick DS, Manolio TA, et al. Ankle–arm index as a marker of atherosclerosis in the Cardiovascular Health Study. *Circulation.* 1993;88:837-845.

53. Panotopoulis G, Ruiz JC, Guy-Grand B, et al. Dual x-ray absorptiometry, bioelectrical impedance, and near infrared interactance in obese women. *Med Sci Sports Exerc.* 2000;33:665-670.

54. Pickering TG, Hall JE, Appel LJ, et al. Recommendations for blood pressure measurement in humans and experimental animals. 1. Blood pressure measurement in humans: a statement for professionals from the Subcommittee of Professional and Public Education of the American Heart Association Council on High Blood Pressure Research. *Hypertension.* 2005;45:142-161.

55. Reid WD, Dechman G. Considerations when testing and training the respiratory muscles. *Phys Ther.* 1995;75:971-982.

56. Seip RL, Snead D, Pierce EF, et al. Perceptual responses and blood lactate concentration: Effect of training state. *Med Sci Sports Exerc.* 1991;23:80-87.

57. Skinner JS. *Exercise Testing and Exercise Prescription for Special Cases: Theoretical Basis and Clinical Applications.* 2nd ed. Philadelphia: Lea & Febiger; 1993.

58. Solway S, Brooks D, Lacasse Y, et al. A qualitative systematic overview of the measurement properties of functional walk tests used in the cardiopulmonary domain. *Chest.* 2001;119:256-270.

59. Steier J, Kaul S, Seymour J, et al. The value of multiple tests of respiratory muscle strength. *Thorax.* 2007;62:975-980.

60. Valensi P, Pariès J, Attali JR, et al. Cardiac autonomic neuropathy in diabetic patients: Influence of diabetes duration, obesity, and microangiopathic complications—the French Multicenter Study. *Metabolism.* 2003;52: 815-820.

60a. Van de Louw A, Cracco C, Cerf C, et al. Accuracy of pulse oximetry in the intensive care unit. *Intensive Care Med.* 2001;27:1606-1613.

61. Vinik AI, Maser RE, Mitchell BD, et al. Diabetic autonomic neuropathy. *Diabetes Care.* 2003;26:1553-1579.

62. Wagner GS. *Marriott's Practical Electrocardiography.* 10th ed. Philadelphia: Lippincott Williams & Wilkins; 2001.

62a. Wasserman K. Dyspnea on exertion. Is it the heart or the lungs? *JAMA.* 1982;248:2039-2043.

62b. Weisman IM, Zeballos RJ. An integrative approach ot the interpretation of cardiopulmonary exercise testing. *Prog Respir Res.* 2002;32:300-322.

63. Williams MA. Exercise testing in cardiac rehabilitation: exercise prescription and beyond. *Cardiol Clin.* 2001;19:415-431.

64. Wolinsky FD, Wyrwich KW, Nienaber NA, et al. Generic versus disease-specific health status measures: an example using coronary artery disease and congestive heart failure patients. *Eval Health Prof.* 1998;21:216-243.

64a. Yamaya Y, Bogaard HJ, Wagner PD, et al. Validity of pulse oximetry during maximal exercise in normoxia, hypoxia, and hyperoxia. *J Appl Physiol.* 2002;92:162-168.

65. Zipes DP, Libby P, Bonow PO, Braunwald E, eds. *Braunwald's Heart Disease.* 7th ed. Philadelphia: W.B. Saunders; 2005.

ADDITIONAL READINGS

Anderson J, Fink JB. Assessing signs and symptoms of respiratory dysfunction. In: Fink JB, Hunt GE, eds. *Clinical Practice in Respiratory Care.* Philadelphia: Lippincott Williams & Wilkings; 1999.

Andreoli TE, Carpenter CC, Griggs RC. *Cecil Essentials of Medicine.* 7th ed. Philadelphia: Saunders; 2004.

Bates DW. *Respiratory Function in Disease.* 3rd ed. Philadelphia: Saunders; 1989.

Braunwald E, ed. *Heart Disease—A Textbook of Cardiovascular Medicine.* Philadelphia: Saunders; 1992.

Brewis RAL, Gibson GJ, Geddes DM, eds. *Respiratory Medicine.* London: Bailliére Tindall; 1990.

Cherniack RM, Cherniack L. *Respiration in Health and Disease.* 3rd ed. Philadelphia: Saunders; 1983.

Chung EK, ed. *Quick Reference to Cardiovascular Diseases.* 3rd ed. Baltimore: Williams & Wilkins; 1987.

Cohen M, Michel TH. *Cardiopulmonary Symptoms in Physical Therapy Practice.* New York: Churchill Livingstone; 1988.

de Troyer A. Actions of the respiratory muscles. In: Hamid Q, Shannon J, Martin J, eds. *Physiologic Basis of Respiratory Disease.* Hamilton, Ontario: BC Decker Inc; 2005.

Farzan S. *A Concise Handbook of Respiratory Diseases.* 3rd ed. Norwalk, CT: Appleton & Lange; 1992.

Fink JB, Hunt GE. *Clinical Practice in Respiratory Care.* Philadelphia: Lippincott Williams & Wilkins; 1999.

Flenley DC. *Respiratory Medicine.* 2nd ed. London: Bailliére Tindall; 1990.

Garritan SL. Chronic obstructive pulmonary disease. In: Hillegass EA, Sadowsky HS, eds. *Essentials of Cardiopulmonary Physical Therapy.* 2nd ed. Philadelphia: Saunders; 2001.

Goldman L, Ausiello D, editors-in-chief. *Cecil Textbook of Medicine.* 22nd ed. Philadelphia: Saunders; 2004.

Guyton AC, Hall JE. *Textbook of Medical Physiology.* 10th ed. Philadelphia: Saunders; 2000.

Hammon III WE. History. In: Frownfelter D, Dean E, eds. *Cardiovascular and Pulmonary Physical Therapy – Evidence and Practice* 4th ed. St. Louis: Mosby; 2006.

Hammon WE. Physical therapy for the acutely ill patient in the respiratory intensive care unit. In: Irwin S, Tecklin JS, eds. *Cardiopulmonary Physical Therapy.* 3rd ed. St. Louis: Mosby; 1995.

Hess DR, MacIntyre NR, Mishoe SC, et al., eds. *Respiratory Care: Principles and Practice.* Philadelphia: Saunders; 2002.

Hillegass E. Assessment procedures. In: Hillegass EA, Sadowsky HS, eds. *Essentials of Cardiopulmonary Physical Therapy.* 2nd ed. Philadelphia: Saunders; 2001.

Humberstone N, Tecklin JS. Respiratory evaluation. In: Irwin S, Tecklin JS, eds. *Cardiopulmonary Physical Therapy.* 3rd ed. St. Louis: Mosby; 1995.

Humes HD, editor-in-chief. *Kelley's Textbook of Internal Medicine.* 4th ed. Philadelphia: Lippincott Williams & Wilkins; 2000.

Hurst JW, Schlant RC, Rackley CE, Sonnenblick EH, Wenger NK, eds. *The Heart, Arteries and Veins.* 7th ed. New York: McGraw-Hill Information Services Co.; 1990.

Irwin S, Blessey RL. Patient evaluation. In: Irwin S, Tecklin JS, eds. *Cardiopulmonary Physical Therapy.* 2nd ed. St. Louis: Mosby; 1990.

Kloner RA, ed. *The Guide to Cardiology.* 2nd ed. New York: Le Jacq Communications; 1990.

Marriott HJL. *Practical Electrocardiography.* 5th ed. Baltimore: Williams & Wilkins; 1972.

McNamara SB. Clinical assessment of the cardiopulmonary system. In: Frownfelter D, Dean E, eds. *Cardiovascular and Pulmonary Physical Therapy – Evidence and Practice.* 4th ed. St. Louis: Mosby; 2006.

Murray JF, Nadal JA, editors-in-chief. *Textbook of Respiratory Medicine.* 3rd ed. Philadelphia: Saunders; 2000.

Phillips RE, Feeney MK. *The Cardiac Rhythms—A Systematic Approach to Interpretation.* 3rd ed. Philadelphia: Saunders; 1990.

Ruderman N, Devlin JT, Schneider SH, et al., eds. *Handbook of Exercise in Diabetes.* 2nd ed. Alexandria, VA: American Diabetes Assoc; 2002.

Tecklin JS. Common pulmonary diseases. In: Irwin S, Tecklin JS, eds. *Cardiopulmonary Physical Therapy: A Guide to Practice.* 4th ed. St. Louis: Mosby; 2004.

Wasserman K, Hansen JE, Sue DY, et al. *Principles of Exercise Testing and Interpretation.* Philadelphia: Lea & Febiger; 1987.

Wolfson MR, Shaffer TH. Respiratory muscle: physiology, evaluation, and treatment. In: Irwin S, Tecklin JS, eds. *Cardiopulmonary Physical Therapy.* 3rd ed. St. Louis: Mosby; 1995.

Cardiovascular and Pulmonary Physical Therapy Treatment

Jeffrey Rodrigues, PT, DPT, CCS and Joanne Watchie, PT, CCS

As with all specialty areas, cardiovascular and pulmonary physical therapy treatment techniques can range from the fundamental skills that are performed routinely by many practicing clinicians to those that require the expertise and knowledge of a clinical specialist. These treatment techniques can, and should, be incorporated in the treatment plans of patients with a wide variety of other pathological conditions, as the cardiovascular and pulmonary systems can affect, and are affected by, the other systems in the body. The problem-oriented approach of this chapter is designed to facilitate the physical therapy management of common problems seen in patients with cardiopulmonary diagnoses and dysfunction, as well as patients with other medical and surgical diagnoses, as outlined in the *Guide to Physical Therapist Practice*.[7] Treatment techniques that are available to improve function and well-being are described. Specific recommendations and treatment modifications for particular patient diagnoses are also provided in Chapter 2 (Pulmonology), Chapter 3 (Cardiovascular Medicine), and Chapter 4 (Cardiopulmonary Pathology).

7.1 ELEVATED CARDIOVASCULAR RISK

Among the goals of physical therapy practice are the promotion of optimal physical wellness and fitness and the prevention of onset, symptoms, and progression of impairments and functional limitations that may result from disease. As such, identifying the presence of coronary risk factors and providing guidance regarding lifestyle modifications aimed at reducing their impact are appropriate interventions for physical therapists (physical therapist [PT] preferred practice pattern 6A),[7] especially those who practice through direct access. Table 7-1 lists the major coronary risk factors and some physical therapy interventions designed to address them. The reader is referred to Table 4-7 on page 103 and to other information presented in Chapter 4 on some of these risk factors (hypertension, obesity, metabolic syndrome, and diabetes).

On the basis of a profusion of research documenting the importance of regular physical activity in both preventing and treating many established atherosclerotic risk factors, including hypertension (HTN), insulin resistance and glucose intolerance, elevated triglyceride levels, low levels of high-density lipoprotein (HDL) cholesterol and high levels of low-density lipoprotein (LDL) cholesterol, and obesity, public health recommendations regarding the type and amounts of physical activity needed by adults to reduce the risk of chronic disease, premature mortality, functional limitations, and disability have been published.[41,69] These recommendations along with the key elements of exercise training are described in the next section.

Moreover, these recommendations apply to ourselves as well as the clients we serve. As health professionals, PTs should personally engage in an active lifestyle and participate in regular aerobic and resistance exercise programs, not only to reduce cardiovascular (CV) risk but also to be familiar with the issues involved in maintaining lifelong physical activity habits and to set a positive example for our patients and the public.

Outcome measures that can be used to document reductions in cardiovascular risk include reduction and improved control of blood pressure (BP), improved glucose tolerance and control of blood glucose levels, improved lipid levels, reduction or cessation of smoking, reduced adiposity, reduction of stress, and improved exercise tolerance. Long-term outcomes include reductions in morbidity and mortality.

7.2 IMPAIRED EXERCISE TOLERANCE

The most common problem encountered in patients with CV and pulmonary disease, as well as those with many other chronic diseases or simply chronic inactivity, is progressively reduced activity tolerance or endurance. This leads to a decrease in functional mobility and independence. A downward cycle develops of inactivity leading to reduced muscular inefficiency (i.e., deconditioning) causing increasing symptomatology during exertion and further abatement of activity in order to avoid discomfort and fatigue (Figure 7-1). As the patient continues on this downward cycle, the end result is complete disability with inability to comfortably perform even the most basic activities of daily living (ADLs). Fortunately, most patients receive medical intervention at some point and do not deteriorate fully to this level before death.

Individuals with impaired exercise tolerance usually benefit from aerobic exercise training and resistance exercise, both of which increase exercise tolerance (PT preferred practice pattern 6B).[7] In addition, exercises aimed at increasing flexibility are important for improving mobility and preventing injury, especially in older individuals, and balance training is indicated for those with increased risk of falls; however, these topics are not discussed in this book. This section begins with a brief review of the principles of training that should be considered when prescribing endurance and resistance exercise programs.

PRINCIPLES OF EXERCISE TRAINING

Common to all the components of exercise training are some basic physiological principles: the overload principle, specificity of training, individual variations in training responses, the transient and reversible

TABLE 7-1: Physical Therapy Interventions for Modifying Major Coronary Risk Factors

Coronary Risk Factor	Physical Therapy Interventions
Hypertension	Monitor BP during PT sessions until control has been established
	Inform physician if adequate BP control is not maintained during rehabilitation activities (so medications can be adjusted)
	Encourage compliance with prescribed medications and exercise treatment
	Educate patient regarding benefits of endurance training and provide appropriate exercise prescription (see pages 91–102)
	Monitor progress with exercise program and provide positive encouragement and feedback
Cigarette smoking	Encourage smoking cessation and offer information regarding successful programs
	Recommend exercise as a diversional activity for dealing with the urge to reach for a cigarette
	Prescribe endurance and resistance exercise training programs to counter weight gain and development and progression of CVD
↓HDL cholesterol	Prescribe appropriate endurance and resistance exercise training programs
↑LDL cholesterol	Prescribe appropriate endurance and resistance exercise training programs
	Encourage low-cholesterol, low-fat diet
Diabetes mellitus or glucose intolerance	Educate regarding benefits of endurance and resistance exercise training and provide appropriate exercise prescriptions (see pages 130–135)
	Encourage compliance with prescribed medications and exercise treatment
Sedentary lifestyle	Prescribe appropriate endurance and resistance exercise programs
Stress	Instruct in relaxation exercises, offer biofeedback
	Prescribe appropriate endurance and resistance exercise training programs
Obesity	Prescribe appropriate endurance and resistance exercise training programs (see pages 128–130)
	Encourage low-fat, low-cholesterol, high-fiber diet

↓, Increased; ↑, decreased; BP, blood pressure; CVD, cardiovascular disease; HDL, high-density lipoprotein; LDL, low-density lipoprotein; PT, physical therapy.

nature of training, and the progression of the exercise program. Application of these principles will optimize the effectiveness of an exercise prescription, and educating patients about them will promote better understanding of exercise training and improve the clinical outcome.

Overload Principle

To enhance function and attain a training effect, exercise must create a physiologic overload, which occurs as a result of manipulating the four components of the exercise prescription (frequency, duration, intensity, and mode) in such a way that the demands of the exercise are greater than normal. Most often overload is maintained by progressively increasing the exercise duration and intensity of a particular mode of exercise.

- For resistance exercise, overload is achieved by gradually increasing the weight that is being applied.
- For aerobic exercise training, the initial focus is usually on increasing the exercise duration; once the duration goal is met, the focus is then shifted to increasing the intensity.

Specificity of Training

Training adaptations are highly specific to the type of activity and to the volume and intensity of the exercise performed. For best effect, skeletal muscles must be trained in a manner similar to the task they are being trained for, and the training should relate directly to the individual's goals (e.g., returning to work, enhancing performance of ADLs, exercising in the neighborhood, or training for a particular event).

- The training program should be designed to meet the specific requirements of different movement patterns within the particular task. For example, if the individual wants to return to off-road bicycling for exercise and recreation, training on a stationary or standard cycle would be more appropriate than swimming or jogging. However, it is important to note that varying the training mode can add interest and prevent boredom.
- When evaluating the training effects achieved by an individual, the testing mode should be the same as the training mode whenever possible (e.g., treadmill for walking and running and cycle ergometer for bicycling).

Principle of Individual Differences

Individuals performing the same exercise program may exhibit very different magnitudes of responses and rates of adaptation. Factors that influence an individual's response to training include genetic factors, prior level of fitness, rate of progression, and any treatment modifications required to meet the needs of each individual. Thus, this principle emphasizes the importance of individualizing each exercise prescription.

Transient and Reversible Nature of Training

When an individual stops exercising, decrements in physiological function and performance (i.e., detraining) occur. There are significant reductions in both metabolic and exercise capacity within

EFFECTS OF INACTIVITY

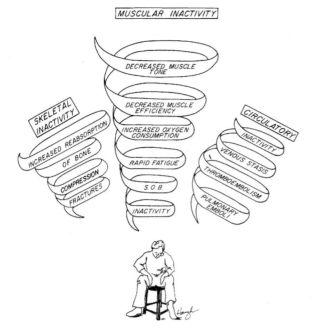

Figure 7-1: A downward cycle of inactivity leading to deconditioning, with its deleterious effects on bone, muscle, and circulation, causing increasing symptomatology during exertion. This leads to further abatement of physical activity in order to avoid these symptoms. SOB, shortness of breath. (From Frownfelter DL. *Chest Physical Therapy and Pulmonary Rehabilitation: An Interdisciplinary Approach.* 2nd ed. Chicago: Year Book Medical Publishers; 1987.)

2 weeks of inactivity, as listed in Table 7-2. A loss of 50% of initial improvement in maximal oxygen uptake occurs after 4 to 12 weeks of detraining, and there is a return to pretraining levels after 10 weeks to 8 months, with those who have performed aerobic training for years declining at the slower rates.[74] Thus, even among highly trained athletes, the beneficial effects of exercise training are transient and reversible. Of note, a much lower volume of training is required to maintain training effects than is needed to achieve them. For example, cardiorespiratory endurance can be maintained with a frequency of 2 days/wk if training duration and intensity are held constant, and muscle strength and power can be maintained with continued training one or two times per week.[60,74]

Rate of Progression

Much of the progression of an individual's exercise program relates to his or her goals, functional exercise capacity, adaptations to the exercise program, health status, and activity preferences. There are three stages that an individual progresses through during the training process.[4]

- The initial stage allows the patient to become accustomed to low-level exercise while minimizing the risk of orthopedic injuries. It may be broken down into two phases. The first phase consists of interval training performed two or three times per day, in which the intervals gradually increase in duration and

TABLE 7-2: Adverse Effects of Prolonged Inactivity

System	Effects
Cardiovascular system	↓ Resting and submaximal SV
	↑ Resting and submaximal HR
	↓ Maximal HR
	↓ Maximal CO
	↓ Maximal $\dot{V}o_2$
	↓ Cardiac size
	↓ Total blood volume
	↓ Hemoglobin concentration
	↑ Risk of venous thrombosis
	Orthostatic hypotension
Pulmonary system	↓ Vital capacity
	↓ Residual volume
	↓ Ventilatory muscle endurance
	↓ Pao_2
	↓ Ability to clear secretions
	↑ Ventilation/perfusion mismatch
Musculoskeletal system	↓ Muscle mass
	↓ Muscle capillary density
	↓ Muscle strength and power
	↓ Muscle endurance
	↓ Oxidative enzymes
	↓ Muscle glycogen
	↓ Flexibility
Central nervous system	↓ Intellectual function
	Emotional and behavioral disturbances
	Altered sensation
Metabolic system	Hypercalcemia
	Osteoporosis

↓, Decreased; ↑, increased; CO, cardiac output; HR, heart rate; Pao_2, partial pressure of arterial oxygen; SV, stroke volume; $\dot{V}o_2$, oxygen consumption.

fewer rests are required. Once the individual can tolerate a continuous exercise program, he/she then progresses to the second phase, during which the exercise duration gradually increases to 20 to 30 minutes per session, 3 to 5 days/wk, (see text, page 302) at an intensity of 40% to 60% of heart rate reserve (HRR). This stage generally lasts about 4 to 6 weeks.

- The improvement stage aims to intensify the training stimulus by increasing both duration and intensity of exercise. Exercise duration is increased to a minimum of 30 minutes at a frequency of 4 or 5 days/wk (see discussion on page 302 for public health recommendations), while intensity gradually rises to 50% to 85% of HRR. Increases in duration and frequency should precede an increase in intensity. This stage produces significant improvement in aerobic fitness and usually lasts 4 to 8 months.

- The maintenance stage commences once the individual's fitness goals have been achieved and is designed to sustain the gains made during the improvement stage, thus avoiding detraining. The individual continues to exercise three to five times per week (see discussion, page 302) for 20 to 60 minutes at an intensity of 70% to 85% of HRR. Varying intensity inversely with duration and performing different modes of exercise help keep the exercise interesting and avoid boredom.

COMPLIANCE

Achieving compliance with an exercise training program is one of the greatest challenges faced by PTs and other professionals. The typical compliance rates with supervised exercise programs is 50% at best and even lower for independent programs.[27]

- To optimize compliance with any exercise prescription, it is important to recognize the major barriers to increasing physical activity, as listed in Box 7-1, so that these can be addressed with each individual and effective strategies worked out in advance.
- Success is highly associated with the performance of activities that the individual finds enjoyable![78] Therefore, it is important to ask questions regarding each patient's interests, abilities, limitations, motivations, and lifestyle preferences. The PT must carefully listen to both what the person says and does not say. In addition, it is important to determine the mode of learning that best suits the individual and to provide verbal, written, and/or illustrated instructions. Patience is required, for the individual may have little prior experience with regular exercise and may not know what will work best without some trial and error.
- Other strategies that increase compliance with exercise training include the following[69a]:
  - ▸ Identify convenient times and locations.
  - ▸ Use cues and prompts to stimulate the desired behavior (e.g., exercise diary posted on the refrigerator).
  - ▸ Establish short- and long-term goals.
  - ▸ Set up behavioral contracts.

BOX 7-1: **Major Barriers to Increasing Physical Activity**

- Lack of time due to work, family, and/or other commitments
- Cost of equipment or gym membership
- Poor weather, pollution
- Lack of nearby facilities
- Concerns for personal safety when exercising outdoors alone
- Disability or injury, age
- Too tired
- Enjoyment of sedentary behaviors (TV viewing, socializing, reading, using computer)

Data from Ries AL, Bauldoff GS, Casaburi R, et al.: Pulmonary rehabilitation: Joint AACP/AACVPR evidence-based clinical practice guidelines, *Chest* 131:4S–42S, 2007.

- ▸ Maintain a record of exercise performed.
- ▸ Allow rewards for reaching goals.
- ▸ Receive positive reinforcement from others.
- ▸ Make exercising as social as possible by involving friends, family members, or others with similar medical/health conditions, so it becomes more difficult to cancel planned workouts.
- Various authors have demonstrated higher compliance in obese and middle- to older-aged individuals when low-intensity rather than moderate intensity exercise is prescribed, and intermittent exercise is often prefered.[5,27,43]

COMPONENTS OF AN EXERCISE TRAINING SESSION

To maximize safety and effectiveness, the format of each exercise session should include warm-up, conditioning, and cooldown periods. A comprehensive exercise program includes both aerobic and resistance training, flexibility exercises, and guidance about recreational activities.

Warm-Up

A warm-up period of 5 to 10 minutes of low-intensity large muscle activity, such as low-intensity calisthenic-type exercise or aerobic activity and gentle stretching, facilitates the transition from rest to exercise, increasing heart rate (HR), augmenting blood flow, increasing oxygen uptake, and warming up muscles. Warm-up may reduce the risk of musculoskeletal injury by increasing connective tissue distensibility, improving joint range of motion and function, and enhancing muscular performance.[74] Of note, patients with heart disease may exhibit delayed adaptive circulatory responses to the onset of exercise, the magnitude of which is probably related to the degree of left ventricular dysfunction, and thus may require longer warm-up periods.

Conditioning

The conditioning phase includes endurance, resistance, and flexibility exercises, parts of which may be performed on different days. Each of these types of exercise will be discussed in more detail in future sections.

Cooldown

A cooldown period of 5 to 10 minutes provides for gradual physiological recovery after aerobic exercise, which allows HR and BP to return to near-resting values, maintains adequate venous return, facilitates the dissipation of body heat and removal of lactic acid, and attenuates the postexercise rise in plasma catecholamines (which may induce ventricular arrhythmias). Cooldown is critical for exercise safety for both healthy individuals and those with disease, as it reduces the risk of postexercise hypotension and myocardial ischemia. Low-intensity exercise (e.g., slow walking or cycling) and stretching are typical modes of cooldown exercise.

AEROBIC EXERCISE TRAINING

There is an abundance of research touting the adverse health consequences of physical inactivity and poor fitness level and expounding the beneficial effects of aerobic exercise on CV function, risk reduction and disease management, and overall health.

- In many practice settings, PTs encounter patients who have experienced prolonged bed rest or limited physical activity as they recover from acute illnesses, surgery, or disabling events. The adverse physiological effects of this inactivity, listed in Table 7-2, must be taken into account when designing appropriate therapy programs for these patients.

- There are also many long-term effects of poor fitness level and physical inactivity resulting from low levels of job-related and leisure time exertion, even in healthy individuals, including increased incidences of obesity, HTN, glucose intolerance, metabolic syndrome, type 2 diabetes mellitus (DM), CV disease (including nonfatal and fatal coronary artery disease events and thromboembolic stroke), osteoporosis, some cancers (breast and colon), anxiety and depression, and all-cause mortality.[41]

- On the other hand, regular physical activity and aerobic exercise are associated with many health and fitness benefits (Box 7-2), which appear to occur in proportion to exercise dose (the combination of exercise intensity, duration, and frequency, or the amount of energy expended), such that people who have the highest levels of physical activity and fitness have the lowest risk of morbidity and premature mortality.[30,83,90] In general, aerobic capacity increases 15% to 25% with training, with the biggest gains occurring in the most sedentary individuals, who may actually achieve improvements of up to 50%.[60]

- It is important to recognize that health benefits can be derived from physical activity of lower intensities than that required to improve maximal oxygen uptake if duration and frequency are increased appropriately. In fact, many significant health benefits are achieved simply by going from a sedentary lifestyle to one with a minimal level of physical activity.[30,74] However, far greater advantage is gained with exercise doses that are sufficient to produce fitness gains.

Therefore, it is essential to include aerobic exercise training in the PT treatment plan for almost every patient who is not already engaged in such a program. Notably, such training usually facilitates the other components of the physical therapy program. Effective training programs generally incorporate one or more modes of exercise performed at the appropriate duration, intensity, and frequency for each individual. Classically, this has consisted of exercise involving the large muscles of the body, which is sustained continuously for at least 20 to 30 minutes at sufficient intensity to stress the CV system and performed at least 3 days/wk.

However, recommendations for physical activity and public health by the American College of Sports Medicine (ACSM) and the American Heart Association (AHA) now advise higher exercise doses in order to optimize health-related benefits, including reduced risk of chronic disease, premature mortality, functional limitations, and disability[41,69]:

- Healthy adults, ages 18 to 65 years, should perform a minimum of 30 minutes of moderate-intensity aerobic physical activity performed at least 5 (preferably 7) days/wk, or a minimum of 20 minutes of vigorous-intensity aerobic activity performed at least 3 days/wk, or a combination of the two.[41]

  ▸ Physical activity is classified as moderate intensity if its estimated energy expenditure is 3.0 to 6.0 METs (1 MET is the amount of energy the body uses at rest per kilogram of body weight per minute, approximately 3.5 mL O_2/kg/min) or the exercise HR is 64% to 76% of the predicted maximal heart rate (HR_{max}) (e.g., brisk walking).

  ▸ Vigorous intensity is defined as more than 6 METs or at least 77% of HR_{max} (e.g., jogging or running).

BOX 7-2: Health Benefits of Regular Physical Activity and Exercise Training

Reduces cardiovascular risk factors:
- Hypertension
- Dyslipidemias (↓ LDL and ↑ HDL cholesterol, ↓ triglycerides)
- Excess body fat, intraabdominal fat
- Insulin resistance, glucose intolerance, type 2 DM
- Blood platelet adhesiveness and aggregation
- Sedentary lifestyle

Reduces risk of developing:
- CVD (HTN, CAD, stroke, peripheral artery disease)
- Obesity
- Type 2 DM
- Osteoporosis (must be weight-bearing exercise)
- Certain cancers (colon, breast)

Primary prevention of:
- Premature death of any cause
- Morbidity and mortality due to CVD, type 2 DM, osteoporotic fractures, colon and breast cancer, and gallbladder disease

Secondary prevention (attenuates or reverses disease progression in those with established disease) of:
- Cardiovascular and all-cause mortality (in post-MI patients who participate in a cardiac rehabilitation program)
- Type 2 DM or high risk for its development

Improves:
- Energy level and endurance
- Respiratory efficiency
- Muscle strength and functional level, risk of falls
- Joint mobility and alleviates symptoms of arthritis
- Weight management (in combination with balanced diet)
- Psychological well-being (relieves stress, anxiety, depression)
- Sleep quality
- Quality of life

CAD, Coronary artery disease; CVD, cardiovascular disease; DM, diabetes mellitus; HDL, high-density lipoprotein; HTN, hypertension; LDL, low-density lipoprotein; MI, myocardial infarction.

▸ The duration of moderate intensity activity can be divided into multiple intervals of at least 10 minutes that total at least 30 min/day.

▸ This recommended amount of aerobic activity is in addition to routine activities of daily living of light intensity (e.g., self-care, cooking, casual walking or shopping) or lasting less than 10 minutes in duration (e.g., walking around the home or office or walking from the parking lot).

▸ The new physical activity recommendation also includes resistance training targeting the major muscle groups at least twice per week (see page 308).

• Older persons (aged 65+ years) and adults aged 50 to 64 years with clinically significant chronic conditions or functional limitations that affect movement ability, fitness, or physical activity follow similar recommendations as other adults.[69]

▸ However, in these individuals it is critical that the level of effort be established relative to each individual's level of aerobic fitness, so that moderate intensity activity rates a 5 or 6 on a 10-point scale (where sitting is 0 and all-out effort is 10) and produces noticeable increases in HR and breathing, while vigorous-intensity activity rates a 7 or 8 out of 10 and produces large increases in HR and breathing.

▸ Thus, for some older adults a moderate-intensity walk translates into a slow walk whereas for others it might be a brisk walk.

▸ Recommendations for resistance exercise, flexibility activities, and balance training are also offered.

• Both resistance and aerobic exercise training result in improvements in many important health and disease risk measures, as listed in Table 7-3.[13a,89,92] Because performance of aerobic and muscle-strengthening activities above the minimally recommended amounts provides additional health benefits and results in higher gains in aerobic capacity, all adults are encouraged to exceed the previously stated minimums if they have no conditions that preclude the increased amount of activity.[41,69]

Aerobic Exercise Prescription

The starting place for the aerobic exercise prescription is an exercise test or the endurance evaluation described in the previous chapter (see page 257). This consists of a low-level submaximal exercise assessment designed to define a patient's physiological responses to increasing workloads, including the patient's upper limit of comfortable tolerance. The results provide information about appropriate exercise intensity, duration, and indirectly, frequency.

This section presents guidelines for prescribing exercise training programs that aim to increase exercise tolerance and improve health status with specific applications to various patient populations. As will become apparent, there are relationships between intensity, frequency, and duration so that a limitation in one of these can be compensated for by adjustments in the others. The recommended intensity, duration, and frequency are in keeping with the latest public health guidelines, a summary of which is presented in Table 7-4.

Mode

For aerobic exercise training, the mode is defined as any exercise activity that will improve cardiopulmonary physical fitness. Acceptable modes of exercise use the large muscles of the body; are aerobic, dynamic, and rhythmic in nature; can be performed

TABLE 7-3: Effects of Resistance and Aerobic Exercise Training on Health and Disease Risk Measures

Measure	Aerobic Exercise	Resistance Exercise
Strength	↔	↑↑↑
Glucose metabolism		
Insulin response to glucose challenge	↓↓	↓↓
Basal insulin levels	↓	↓
Insulin sensitivity	↑↑	↑↑
GLUT-4 transporter number	↑↑	↑
Serum lipids		
HDL cholesterol	↑↑	↑↔
LDL cholesterol	↓↓	↓↔
Systemic inflammation (TNF-α, CRP, IL-6)	↓	↓
Homocysteine	↑↔	↓
Antioxidant enzyme activity	↑↑	↑
Lipid peroxidation	↓↓	↓↓
Resting heart rate	↓↓	↔
Stroke volume	↑↑	↔
Blood pressure at rest		
Systolic	↓↓	↔
Diastolic	↓↓	↓↔
Blood pressure during exertion		
Aerobic exercise	↓↓	↓↓
Anaerobic exercise	↓	↓↓
$\dot{V}O_{2\ max}$	↑↑↑	↑
Endurance time	↑↑↑	↑↑
Physical function	↑↑	↑↑↑
Basal metabolism	↑	↑↑
Body composition		
Percent fat	↓↓	↓
Lean body mass	↔	↑↑
Abdominal adipose tissue		
Visceral	↓↓	↓
Subcutaneous	↓↓	↓
Intraabdominal	↓↓	↓↓
Bone mineral density	↑	↑↑

From Vincent KR, Vincent HK. Resistance training for individuals with cardiovascular disease. *J Cardiopulm Rehabil.* 2006;26:2007–2016.
↓, Decrease; ↑, increase; ↔, unchanged; CRP, C-reactive protein; GLUT-4, glucose facilitated transporter-4; HDL, high-density lipoprotein; IL-6, interleukin-6; LDL, low-density lipoprotein; TNF-α, tumor necrosis factor-α; $\dot{V}O_{2\ max}$, maximal oxygen consumption.

in a continuous manner; and, most importantly of all, should be enjoyable for the individual. The most commonly used modes of aerobic exercise include walking and/or jogging (track or treadmill), bicycling (stationary, recumbent, or road/trail), swimming,

TABLE 7-4: Summary of Guidelines for Components of an Endurance Exercise Prescription

Component	Guidelines
Mode	Any activity involving the large muscles of the body that is dynamic in nature and can be performed in a continuous manner (e.g., walking, jogging, bicycling, dancing, aerobics, swimming, cross-country skiing, rowing, stair climbing)
Intensity	Depends on fitness level, health status, and goals of program: • For healthy, sedentary-to-active individuals, intensity is commonly based on percentage of age-predicted or true maximal HR (e.g., 70%–85% of HR_{max} or 60%–80% of HRR), with the percentage being determined by the individual's exercise tolerance • For older patients and adults with chronic disease or taking medications that affect HR, intensity is based on the results of an endurance evaluation (i.e., the defined upper limit of comfortable tolerance) • If the patient's goals are to reduce body fat, control hypertension, or relieve intermittent claudication, lower intensity, longer duration exercise is recommended, although the incorporation of some higher intensity exercise may be beneficial for weight control
Duration	Depends on the individual's level of fitness initially, then the intensity: • For very deconditioned individuals, start with short intervals according to tolerance with brief (1–2 min) rests interposed between them, and then increase the length of each interval (usually by about 1 min/d) and decrease the number of rest periods • For typical, sedentary-to-active individuals, start with duration of tolerance (when onset of fatigue or discomfort appears), and then increase by 1–2 min every day • Goal should be at least 30 min of total, combined exercise time at a moderate intensity, or 40–60 min of exercise at low intensity, or minimum of 20 min of vigorous exercise (>6 METS or ≥77% of HR_{max}) • On days when sufficient time is not available, any amount of exercise is better than none; if possible try to incorporate a number of 10-min periods throughout the day • Longer duration, lower intensity exercise is recommended for those trying to control weight, hypertension, or intermittent claudication

Frequency	Depends on the duration and intensity:
	• If continuous exercise duration is <15–20 min, frequency should be two or three times per day
	• If continuous exercise duration is >20 min, frequency is once daily, most days of the week, depending on intensity:
	  ▸ If low-to-moderate intensity, program should be performed at least 5 d/wk (preferably 7)
	  ▸ If higher intensity program, frequency of at least 3 d/wk is acceptable

HR, Heart rate; HR_{max}, maximal heart rate; HRR, heart rate reserve.

aerobics (chair, low impact, step, etc.), dancing, skating, cross-country skiing (snow or machine), stair stepping, elliptical training, and rowing machines.

- For the acute inpatient, ambulating around the nursing unit or using a stationary bicycle or treadmill can provide the aerobic component of an exercise program, and using an elastic band (e.g., *Thera-Band;* Hygenic, Akron, OH) for upper and lower body exercises can provide the strengthening component.

- Participants in an outpatient cardiac or pulmonary rehabilitation program usually have the opportunity to work out using several different exercise modes in an interval fashion. Typically, these programs include walking and jogging, stationary cycling, and/or rowing machine. In addition, many offer arm ergometry and four extremity modalities (e.g., Schwinn Airdyne, cross-country ski machine, and elliptical trainer; Nautilus, Vancouver, WA) whereas others may offer an aquatics program (swimming and water aerobics). Resistance training to improve musculoskeletal strength and endurance may use calisthenics, hand weights, or elastic bands. Such variety enhances patient motivation and minimizes the potential for injury.

- Defining a practical yet enjoyable mode is a most challenging task when working with clients who are exercising independently at home. Walking or jogging is the simplest as far as equipment requirements are concerned but can pose problems in patients with joint disease and those living in unsafe neighborhoods. In addition, environmental factors such as extremes of weather, poor air quality, or living in a hilly community may present complications. Thus, it is advisable to investigate facilities in the community with controlled environments, such as shopping malls that open their doors early, which may be available as alternative walking sites. A local high school or college track may be an appropriate site, as it provides a level surface that has a measured distance. The more information and alternatives that can be offered to patients, the easier it becomes for them to comply with the program.

- One suggestion for individuals who are interested in purchasing some type of home exercise equipment is to encourage them to try out various machines at places such as fitness stores, friends' houses, and health clubs. Once they identify their favorite(s), they can then look for bargains through community want-ads, garage sales, or on the Internet at sites such as eBay or craigslist. Exercise equipment purchased through these means, more often than not, has been used only a handful of times, if at all, and costs much less than brand new equipment.

- Because of the specificity of exercise training, cross-training that emphasizes the use of a variety of large muscle groups, utilizing different modes of exercise, may be advantageous for achieving greater physical function.

$$HR_{max} = 208 - 0.7(\text{patient's age})$$

Figure 7-2: Formula for predicting maximal heart rate (HR_{max}), used as an alternative method for patients at the extremes of the age range.

Intensity

There are several different ways to prescribe exercise intensity. An important consideration is that the intensity and duration of the exercise are inversely related. As the intensity of the exercise increases, the duration can be shortened in order to achieve the desired level of aerobic fitness gains. This approach will also help to reduce the potential for injury.

- The exercise intensity that has traditionally been recommended on the basis of research documenting fitness increments is 65% to 80% of HR_{max}, which corresponds to 50% to 70% of maximal oxygen consumption ($\dot{V}O_{2\ max}$). HR_{max} is determined either by performance of a maximal exercise stress test or by calculation based on age ($HR_{max} = 220 - $ age). However, improvements in aerobic capacity are also known to occur at lower levels in persons with very low fitness, that is, as low as 55% HR_{max}, or 40% of $\dot{V}O_2$ reserve ($\dot{V}O_2R$) (see Table 7-5).[74]
- An alternative formula for calculating maximum HR is shown in Figure 7-2. This method tends to be more accurate and appropriate for patients at the extremes of the age range.
- Another method of prescribing exercise intensity uses a percentage of the HRR, which takes into account the resting HR and more accurately relates to oxygen consumption. This calculation, called *Karvonen's formula*, is shown in Figure 7-3. Using this method for training, 60% to 80% of the HRR is equivalent to 60% to 80% of $\dot{V}O_{2\ max}$. However, the accuracy of this relationship is not maintained at the lower end of the intensity scale but can be improved by relating HRR to oxygen

$$Target\ HR = (MHR - RHR)(\%) + RHR$$

Figure 7-3: Karvonen's formula for calculating training heart rate (HR) based on the HR reserve, or difference between maximal and resting HR (MHR and RHR, respectively).

consumption reserve ($\dot{V}O_2R$), which is the difference between maximal and resting $\dot{V}O_2$.[4]

- Using any of these methods, a training HR zone is defined within which the intensity of exercise is adequate to achieve a training effect, as shown in Figure 7-4. The ACSM recommends exercising at an intensity of 64% to 93% of HR_{max}, which corresponds to 40% to 84% of HHR and $\dot{V}O_2R$.[4] Using these values, the exercise intensity is moderate and can be sustained by most individuals for a prolonged period with little or no discomfort.
  ▸ When starting an untrained individual on an exercise program, it is appropriate to start with HR values at the lower end of the training zone, whereas more fit persons require intensities at the upper end of the range to achieve benefits.
  ▸ The use of formulas based on maximal predicted HR is inappropriate for many individuals with chronic diseases and those taking medications that affect HR (e.g., β-blockers). A training program based on an age-predicted maximal HR would be excessively intense for these individuals, and they would be unlikely to comply with it. However, these formulas are often appropriate when based on the actual HR_{max}

TABLE 7-5: **Classification of Physical Activity Relative Intensity**

	Aerobic Exercise			**Resistance Exercise***
Intensity	**$\dot{V}O_{2\ max}$ (%)**	**Maximal HR (%)**	**RPE[†]**	**Maximal Voluntary Contraction (%)**
Very light	<20	<50	<10	<30
Light	20–39	50–63	10–11	30–49
Moderate	40–59	64–76	12–13	50–69
Hard (vigorous)	60–84	77–93	14–16	70–84
Very hard	≥85	≥94	17–19	≥85
Maximal[‡]	100	100	20	100

Modified from Fletcher GF, Balady GJ, Amsterdam EA, et al.: Exercise standards for testing and training: A statement for healthcare professionals from the American Heart Association. *Circulation* 104:1694–1740, 2001.
HR, Heart rate; RPE, Rating of Perceived Exertion Scale; $\dot{V}O_{2\ max}$, maximal oxygen consumption.
*On the basis of 8 to 12 repetitions for persons under 50 to 60 years of age and 10 to 15 repetitions for persons aged 50 to 60 years and older.
[†]Borg Rating of Perceived Exertion 6–20 Scale.
[‡]Maximal values are mean values achieved during maximal exercise by healthy adults.

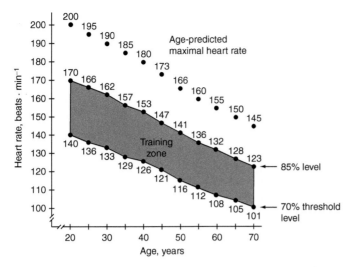

Figure 7-4: Maximal heart rates and training zones, using a lower level of 70% and an upper level of 85% of maximal heart rate, according to age.

achieved during a symptom-limited exercise stress test performed while taking their current medications (i.e., peak HR).

- A practical alternative is to define the intensity by using a rating of perceived exertion (RPE) scale, according to the procedures described for the endurance evaluation (see page 281). Given proper instruction, RPE is a valid and reliable indicator of the level of physical exertion during steady state exercise, and thus can serve as an effective means of monitoring exercise intensity during endurance training.[12] The RPE is also an appropriate method of determining intensity for those individuals who have chronic diseases or are taking HR-altering medications. Using the 15-point scale (ranging from 6 to 20), a rating of 12 to 13 corresponds to approximately 60% of HR_{max}, and a rating of 16 corresponds to approximately 85% of HR_{max}. Studies suggest that most people prefer to exercise at an intensity of 60% to 65% of $\dot{V}O_{2\ max}$, which corresponds to an RPE of 12 or 13, or "somewhat hard" on the 15-point scale, or 3 or 4 when using the 11-point scale (ranging from 0 to 10).[74]

- Another method of prescribing exercise intensity relies on metabolic equivalents of energy expenditure, or METs. One MET is the amount of energy the body uses at rest per kilogram of body weight per minute, which is approximately 3.5 mL $O_2/$kg/min. The energy cost of various activities can be compared by determining their MET level. For example, walking 2.0 miles per hour (mph) on level ground usually uses about twice as much energy as sitting rest, or about 2 METs (actually ≈2.5 METs), and walking 3.0 mph consumes about three times as much oxygen, or about 3 METs (actually ≈3.3 METs).
  - ▸ To establish a range for prescribing exercise activities on the basis of METs, the therapist calculates the energy expenditure during a graded submaximal exercise test or endurance evaluation and extrapolates the maximal MET level from the results. For individuals who cannot tolerate a graded exercise test, the Duke Activity Status Index (DASI) questionnaire, described in Table 6-33 (see page 292), can be used.[1,6,19,44]
  - ▸ To prescribe exercise on the basis of METs, the desired range of energy expenditure is determined, which is typically 50% to 85% of the maximal level. The therapist then prescribes

activities that are known to require energy expenditures within the range.
  - ▸ The energy costs of various recreational and household activities are listed in Table 7-6. Note that a range of METs is provided, because an individual's energy cost for any activity varies with level of fitness, experience, and metabolic efficiency (it differs from person to person and can even vary at different times in the same individual).

- Finally, the individual's goals for engaging in an endurance training program are taken into consideration when prescribing exercise intensity. For example, research has shown that lower intensity, longer duration exercise is more successful in promoting weight loss, controlling BP, and relieving lower extremity claudication.[4,34,39,43,81] On the other hand, if a person's goals include competition, higher intensity exercise is required. In addition, higher intensity training appears to be more effective in achieving glycemic control in patients with DM, if they can tolerate it.[12a,75a] Furthermore, it may be that higher levels of energy expended through a combination of moderate- and vigorous-intensity activities may confer even greater health and fitness benefits.[41,50,82]

Duration

Duration is defined as the amount of time spent during the exercise activity while at the desired target training HR (intensity) to elicit cardiopulmonary adaptations. The initial duration of the exercise program will be determined by the individual's prior level of fitness, results of an exercise stress test, if performed, and medical history, as well as the exercise intensity and frequency.

- Patients who are extremely deconditioned may be restricted to low-level household ambulation and activities initially in order to avoid excessive dyspnea or other symptoms of intolerance (these activities would be moderate in intensity relative to the individual's aerobic fitness level). Such patients benefit significantly from interval training, which incorporates two or three short bouts of exercise, often starting at 3 to 5 minutes, with brief rest periods of 1 to 2 minutes in-between intervals. Although these brief intervals are too short to be truly aerobic in nature, patients typically can add 1 minute to one or more of the intervals each day. Using the interval training principle, patients who may have been limited to 5 minutes of ambulating at the onset of training may be able to progress to intervals of at least 10 minutes by the end of the first week, thus doubling their exercise time.

- Healthy sedentary individuals can typically tolerate 10 to 20 minutes of moderate continuous exercise before peripheral muscle fatigue or cardiopulmonary limitations cause them to stop. Using a conservative approach to duration and intensity at the start of an exercise program can prevent excessive musculoskeletal fatigue, distress, and possible injury while allowing the cardiopulmonary system to adapt to the increased physiological demands. These individuals often progress at a fairly quick pace, typically adding 1 to 2 min/day.

- The goal is to gradually increase exercise duration to at least 30 minutes of continuous exercise without injury or signs or symptoms of exercise intolerance (see page 284), before increasing the intensity of exercise. Depending on the patient's goals, time constraints, and eagerness to progress, as well as the intensity of exercise, the duration of continuous activity can be increased to

TABLE 7-6: Energy Cost of Various Activities, in Metabolic Equivalents of Energy Expenditure

Activity	Mean METs	Range	Activity	Mean METs	Range
Backpacking	7.0	5–11	Rope jumping: 60–80 skips/min	8.0	7–10
Badminton	4.5	3.5–9+	120–140 skips/min	12.0	11–123
Basketball (nongame)	6.0	3–9	Running		
Gameplay	8.3	7–12+	5 mph (12 min/mile)	8.0	6–11
Bowling	3.0	2–4	6 mph (10 min/mile)	10.0	8–13
Canoeing, rowing, kayaking	—	3–12	7.5 mph (8 min/mile)	12.5	10–15
Calisthenic exercises	4.5	3–8+	10 mph (6 min/mile)	16.0	14–19
Climbing hills	7.0	5–10+	Cross-country	9.0	7.5–11+
Cycling <10 mph	4.0	3–8+	Sailing	3.0	2–5
10.0–11.9 mph	6.0	4.5–9	Self-care (washing, dressing, shaving, etc.)	—	1.5–4
14.0–15.9 mph	10.0	8–13	Shoveling dirt, digging	—	6–9
Stationary	7.0	3–13	Shoveling snow	6.0	5–7
Dancing (social, square, tap)	4.5	3.0–7.5	Skating (ice and roller)	7.0	5–9+
Dancing (aerobic)	6.5	5–9	Skiing: Downhill	7.0	4–10
Fishing (from bank or boat)	—	2–5	Cross-country	8.0	6–12+
Wading in stream	6.0	5–7	Cross-country machine	7.0	5–10
Flexibility exercises	2.5	2.0–5	Soccer	7.0	5–12+
Football (touch)	8.0	6–10	Stair climbing	—	4–8
Gardening (light to moderate)	—	3–6	Stair step ergometer	9.0	6–12+
Golf (power cart)	3.5	2–3	Step aerobics	8.5	7–12
Walking (carrying bag or pulling cart)	4.5	4–7	Swimming	—	5–12+
Handball	12.0	8–14	Table tennis	4.0	3–5
Hiking (cross-country)	6.0	3–8	Tennis	7.0	4–9+
Home repair	—	3–8	Volleyball	4.0	3–9+
Horseshoe pitching	3.0	2–4	Walking		
Housework: Light to moderate	—	2–4	2 mph (30 min/mi)	2.5	2–3
Moderate to vigorous	—	4–8+	3 mph (20 min/mi)	3.3	3–4
Jogging on minitrampoline	4.5	—	4 mph (15 min/mi)	5.0	4.5–7
Judo, karate, kick boxing	10.0	8–14	With braces + crutches	6.5	5.5–7.5
Lifting items continuously (10–20 lb)	4.0	3–5.5	Water aerobics	4.0	3–6
Mountain climbing	8.0	5–10+	Water jogging	8.0	6–10
Music playing	—	1.8–4	Water skiing	6.0	5–7
Paddlebal, racquetball	6.5	5–12	Weight lifting	—	3–8+

Data from Ainsworth BE, Haskell WL, White MC, et al. Compendium of physical activities: an update of activity codes and MET intensities. *Med Sci Sports Exerc.* 2000; 32:S498–S516; McArdle WD, Katch FI, Katch VL: *Exercise Physiology—Energy, Nutrition, and Human Performance,* 5th ed. Philadelphia, Lea & Febiger, 2001; Wilmore JH, Costill DL. *Physiology of Sport and Exercise,* 2nd ed. Champaign, IL, Human Kinetics, 1999.
MET, The amount of energy the body uses at rest per kilogram of body weight per minute; 1 MET is approximately 3.5 mL O_2/kg/min.

45 to 60 minutes. For example, if the individual's goal is to reduce body fat and weight, the exercise duration ideally should be 45 to 60 minutes of moderate- to high-intensity exercise, accumulating a total of at least 150 minutes, if not 200 to 300 minutes (3.3–5 h), of exercise per week.[4]

• Of course, an individual's lifestyle and time schedule may impose constraints on the exercise duration. Some days (or weeks) may not be able to accommodate 30 to 40 minutes of continuous exercise. In this case, any amount of exercise is better than none. Three exercise bouts of at least 10 minutes throughout the day at moderate intensity have the same effect on aerobic fitness as one 30-minute session bout,[4] and the shorter bouts may offer advantages for increasing bone density and flexibility.[11]

Frequency

Frequency is defined as the number of days per week that the person participates in an exercise program. This may vary with exercise duration and intensity, as well as the individual's prior activity level and exercise tolerance.

- Very deconditioned patients (functional capacity of <3 METs), should perform multiple short bouts every day, and deconditioned individuals with a functional capacity of 3 to 5 METs should perform one to two short exercise sessions at least 5 days/wk. with the goal of increasing duration to 20 minutes of continuous exercise.
- When the individual can perform 20 minutes of low-intensity, continuous aerobic exercise, the frequency can be reduced to once daily, at least 5 days/wk. More frequent training may be more effective when training at a lower intensity.[34]
- To improve aerobic fitness, an individual must perform moderate-intensity aerobic exercise a minimum of 30 min/day on three to five nonconsecutive days per week or higher intensity exercise ($\geq$77% of HR_{max}) for at least 20 min/day on 3 to 5 days/wk.
- To maintain a given level of aerobic fitness, individuals performing moderate-intensity aerobic exercise can get by with 30 min/day on three nonconsecutive days per week whereas those performing higher intensity exercise can manage with at least 20 min/day twice per week.[2]
- However, once again, the recommendations for optimizing health benefits must be kept in mind, as stated on page 302.[41,69]

Summary

The four elements of an aerobic exercise prescription include the mode of exercise, intensity, duration, and frequency. It is the task of the PT to incorporate the patient's medical history, functional capacity, physical limitations, interests, abilities, motivations, and lifestyle preferences when designing an individualized exercise program that optimizes successful participation in terms of safety, effectiveness, and compliance. If the patient is attending a formalized rehabilitation program, the presence of trained staff should provide for safe and effective training, and the novelty of the process and socialization with other participants may provide enough interest and motivation to maintain the patient's compliance. However, an entirely different situation exists when the patient is being seen just before discharge from the hospital, or as a home patient or outpatient, and will be performing the program independently with only occasional, if any, supervision and reinforcement.

Even patients with significant physiological and functional limitations can gradually improve exercise tolerance with an appropriate individualized exercise prescription and attention to the basic principles of exercise training.[47,72]

As shown in Table 7-7, individuals with cardiac disease achieve many of the same physiological adaptations as healthy individuals with aerobic training. However, to obtain the greatest benefits, exercise training should be combined with other positive lifestyle modifications and in many cases with appropriate medical therapy to reduce CV risk factors.

Outcome measures that are useful in documenting the effects of aerobic exercise training include improvements in exercise test or functional timed walk test performance, health-related quality of life, and return to role function (home, leisure, work).

RESISTANCE EXERCISE TRAINING

Although resistance training elicits only modest increases in $\dot{V}O_2$ max it offers many of the other benefits of aerobic exercise, and it has greater effect on muscular strength and endurance, fat-free body mass, and physical function and for maintaining bone mineral density (see Table 7-3).[89,92] These benefits are particularly important for older individuals and those with COPD, HTN, CVD, CHF, metabolic syndrome, DM, and chronic kidney disease, as well as individuals who are overweight or obese.[4,13a,42,77,83,89,89a,92,93]

- Resistance training (using weight-bearing calisthenics, hand weights, elastic bands, commercial exercise machines, etc.) should be performed through full range of motion (ROM) for maximal benefit.
- Muscle strength and endurance are developed by progressive overload (increasing resistance, number of repetitions, or frequency).
  - Muscle strength is increased best by using heavier weights with fewer repetitions.
  - Muscle endurance is increased best by performing more repetitions with lighter weights.
- To elicit improvements in both muscular strength and endurance, the latest public health guidelines recommend[41,69] the following:
  - Performing 8 to 10 exercises that target the major muscle groups of the body
  - Using resistance that causes substantial fatigue after 8 to 12 repetitions of each exercise for healthy adults, or
  - Using resistance that elicits moderate to high effort for 10 to 15 repetitions (moderate-intensity effort rates a 5 or 6 out of 10 [where no effort is 0 and maximal effort is 10] and high-intensity effort rates a 7 or 8) for older persons and adults aged 50 to 64 years with clinically significant chronic conditions or functional limitations that affect exercise tolerance
  - Exercising for strength gains on two or three nonconsecutive days per week

FLEXIBILITY EXERCISE

Limited flexibility is commonly seen with advancing age and often leads to impaired musculoskeletal function. Thus, flexibility exercises designed to maintain adequate range of motion for all the major joints are important to include in each individual's PT treatment plan. These exercises should be performed in a slow, controlled manner with a gradual progression to greater ranges of motion, as follows:

- Begin with warmup activities to elevate muscle temperature.
- Perform slow static muscle stretches of all major joints, paying particular attention to those that have reduced range of motion.
- Stretch each joint to the end of its range of motion to the point of tightness, avoiding discomfort that will elicit protective activation of the muscle(s).
- Hold each stretch for at least 15 to 30 seconds.
- Repeat each stretch two to four times.
- Perform the stretching routine at least 2 to 3 days/wk, preferably 5 to 7 days/wk.

TABLE 7-7: Cardiovascular Effects of Endurance Training in Healthy Individuals and Cardiac Patients

		Changes With Endurance Training	
Variable	**Units**	**Healthy Adults**	**Cardiac Patients**
Maximal Values			
Oxygen uptake	mL/kg/min	↑	↑
Cardiac output	L/min	↑	↔*
Heart rate	bpm	↔–↓	↔
Stroke volume	mL	↑	↔–↑*
Arteriovenous O_2 difference	mL O_2/dL blood	↑	↑
Systolic BP	mm Hg	↔	↔?*
Rate–pressure product	bpm × mm Hg × 10^3	↔	↔?*
Endurance	Sec	↑[†]	↑[†]
Ejection fraction	%	↑[‡]	↔–↓*[‡]
Submaximal Values[§]			
Oxygen uptake	mL/kg/min	↔–↓	↔–↓
Cardiac output	L/min	↔–↓	↔–↓
Heart rate	bpm	↔–↓	↔
Stroke volume	mL	↑	↑
Systolic BP	mm Hg	↓	↓
Rate–pressure product	bpm × mm Hg × 10^3	↓	↓
Resting Values			
Oxygen uptake	mL/kg/min	↔	↔
Heart rate	bpm	↓	↓
Systolic BP	mm Hg	↔–↓	↔–↓
Diastolic BP	mm Hg	↔–↓	↔–↓
Rate–pressure product	bpm × mm Hg × 10^3	↓	↓

Modified from Pollock ML, Wilmore JH: *Exercise in Health and Disease,* 2nd Ed. Philadelphia, Saunders, 1990.
↓, Decrease; ↑, increase; ↔, unchanged; BP, blood pressure.
*These values may increase in some patients with high-intensity training.
[†]The performance will improve, that is, performance at a given distance will decrease, and performance time on a treadmill or cycle ergometer will increase.
[‡]Ejection fraction determined as a change from rest to exercise.
[§]Same absolute workload.

CARDIAC AND PULMONARY REHABILITATION PROGRAMS

Participation in a comprehensive cardiac or pulmonary rehabilitation program offers major advantages to patients in the scope and effectiveness of care received because of the involvement of an interdisciplinary team with a wider variety of expertise and the ability to more thoroughly address the other lifestyle modifications and medical therapies that may reduce each patient's risk of morbidity and mortality.

Cardiac rehabilitation is an individually tailored, multidisciplinary program of care for patients with cardiovascular disease (CVD) that is designed to optimize physical, psychological, and social function.[2,54] The goals are to stabilize, slow, or possibly reverse disease progression and thus reduce morbidity and mortality. The components of a comprehensive cardiac rehabilitation program include the following:

- Patient assessment
- Patient and family education regarding the disease process, risk factors and reduction strategies, and treatment interventions
- Individually prescribed, medically supervised exercise training (aerobic, resistance, and flexibility)
- Aggressive risk factor reduction (smoking, dyslipidemia, HTN, overweight and obesity, glucose intolerance, and DM)
- Cardioprotective medications for secondary prevention
- Nutrition counseling
- Behavioral/psychosocial counseling
- Vocational counseling

Pulmonary rehabilitation is an individually tailored, multidisciplinary program of care for patients with chronic respiratory impairment that is designed to optimize physical and social performance and autonomy and aims to control and alleviate symptoms, reduce disability, improve physical function and health-related quality of life, and possibly reduce overall health care services utilization.[3,77] The components of a pulmonary rehabilitation program include the following:

- Patient assessment
- Patient and family education and training regarding the disease process, exacerbating factors and management strategies (smoking cessation, proper nutrition for weight loss or gain, stress management, environmental modifications, and flu and pneumonia immunizations), symptom management, and treatment interventions
- Optimal disease management (medications, bronchial hygiene treatments, and supplemental oxygen)
- Individually prescribed, medically supervised aerobic and resistance exercise training, flexibility exercises
- Nutrition counseling
- Psychosocial support and counseling
- Promotion of long-term adherence

7.3 ABNORMAL PHYSIOLOGICAL RESPONSES TO EXERTION

Patients with many acute and chronic medical problems may exhibit abnormal physiological responses to increasing activity, frequently as a result of CV or pulmonary dysfunction (PT preferred practice patterns 6A–6G).[7] Common abnormalities include excessive increases, decreases or blunted responses in HR and BP, increasing irregularity of the pulse or arrhythmias on electrocardiogram (ECG), excessive respiratory rate (RR), dyspnea, chest discomfort, oxygen desaturation, and other signs and symptoms of exercise intolerance, as discussed in Chapter 6 (Cardiopulmonary Assessment).

- Whenever possible the cause of an abnormality should be identified and appropriate therapy instituted (e.g., prescription of or adjustments in medications, volume replacement for dehydration, and supplemental oxygen for desaturation). Sometimes the cause is simply deconditioning due to prolonged illness and inactivity, with resulting tachycardia and orthostatic hypotension.
- The appropriate PT intervention is continued clinical monitoring consisting of HR, BP, oxygen saturation, RR, ECG, and RPE, depending on available equipment as the patient performs gradually increasing physical activity. These vital signs should be monitored with the patient at rest, at regular intervals during activity, and during postexercise recovery. The goal is to allow as much activity as possible while optimizing patient safety to avoid adverse reactions.
- Close monitoring of clinical signs and symptoms, using the techniques described in the previous chapter, allows the therapist to optimize both treatment and safety and to institute treatment modifications, as indicated, that reduce the physiological stress of rehabilitation activities (Box 7-3).
- It is important for PTs to note the medications currently being taken, as they may have a significant effect on the patient's HR, BP, oxygen saturation, and ECG response during exercise (see Table 5-22, page 216). In addition, it may also be necessary to identify the time of day when the patient takes certain medications, and if needed, to schedule therapy sessions to avoid adverse affects (e.g., insulin).

BOX 7-3: Physical Therapy Treatment Modifications for Patients With Limited Tolerance

- Avoid scheduling therapy sessions during the hour after meals so that the demands of rehabilitation will not be superimposed on the extra work of digestion.
- Schedule appointments so that the patient has some rest time between the various rehabilitation services appointments.
- Schedule appointments around timing of patient medications so as to avoid times when the dose is initially high (starting to take effect) or low, which may affect the patient's exercise response or outcomes.
- Interject frequent brief rests while performing more strenuous rehabilitation activities, such as those involving the upper extremities, especially above shoulder level, and those performed in the quadruped position.
- Monitor the patient's physiological responses to activity to determine which activities cause problems and what modifications are effective in ameliorating them.
- Use the Rating of Perceived Exertion Scale (see page 281) along with the patient's signs and symptoms to monitor exercise intensity and rate of progression.
- Encourage coordination of breathing with activity to avoid the deleterious effects of breath holding and the Valsalva maneuver.

- A critical element of the PT treatment plan is patient education in self-monitoring of exercise intensity using HR and rhythm, RPE, and/or symptoms of intolerance. As confidence is gained in the individual's self-monitoring skills, he/she can progress to increasing levels of independence in the exercise program. Even patients who are at high risk for morbidity and mortality after acute myocardial infarction and others who continue to exhibit abnormal responses to exercise should be encouraged to achieve independence in self-monitoring in order to maximize safety during home and work activities.

Outcome measures that can be used to show effectiveness of PT interventions include improved hemodynamic and symptomatic responses to activity, compliance with exercise prescription parameters, and quality of life scores.

7.4 INABILITY TO MEET THE DEMANDS OF DAILY LIVING ACTIVITIES

Some individuals with chronic diseases, such as congestive heart failure (PT preferred practice pattern 6D)[7] or chronic lung disease with ventilatory limitation (PT preferred practice pattern 6E) become so debilitated that they are unable to meet the physical demands of essential activities of daily living independently. The patient and family are then faced with decisions regarding changing needs and circumstances, level of safety, and appropriate living arrangements. Fortunately, PT interventions can often improve the patient's functional status and level of independence.

FUNCTIONAL TRAINING

Functional activity and mobility training teaches debilitated patients how to function more effectively in their environment. The therapist helps identify the specific difficulties each patient is having and devises adaptations of the environment, task performance, or both, that enable the individual to deal with these problems. Efforts are directed toward optimizing patient function in bed mobility, transfers (in the home, to/from the car, and in the community), and ambulation.

EXERCISE TRAINING

Exercise training is essential for improving functional strength and endurance, as described in Section 7.2, including in patients with chronic cardiopulmonary dysfunction and other chronic diseases.[47,72] Benefits occur even in patients who are unable to achieve physiological gains in cardiac and pulmonary function, largely through improvements in peripheral skeletal muscle energy utilization.

- Aerobic exercise training is designed to increase functional capacity and endurance, allowing the patient to perform more activities with reduced energy demand.
- Resistance training is valuable for increasing muscular strength and endurance, which is essential for greater independence in activities of daily living.

ENERGY CONSERVATION/WORK SIMPLIFICATION TECHNIQUES

Instruction in energy conservation and work simplification techniques can allow patients to perform many activities that they find difficult. Simplifying tasks helps reduce the energy cost of various activities and increases the efficiency of effort that is expended.

- Work simplification involves five basic steps:
  - ▸ *Plan* the day in the morning, on wakening (or the evening before):
    - ⊙ Consider the best time of day for each activity.
    - ⊙ Alternate more demanding tasks with light work throughout the day.
    - ⊙ Set priorities.
  - ▸ *Organize* time both on a daily and weekly basis to conserve energy:
    - ⊙ Create a written plan of action; this is often the most practical way to organize.
    - ⊙ Avoid fatigue by allowing plenty of time so that there is no need to rush.
    - ⊙ Pace activities.
  - ▸ *Modify* or change some activities, if needed, in order to continue doing them:
    - ⊙ Do as much work as possible while sitting down. It takes twice as much energy to do an activity while standing than it does while seated.
    - ⊙ Replace heavy dishware and utensils with lighter, modern labor-saving devices.
  - ▸ *Eliminate* unnecessary steps:
    - ⊙ Let dishes air dry.
    - ⊙ Soak pots and pans to eliminate scrubbing.
    - ⊙ In cooking, use "one bowl" method recipes, prepared mixes, or frozen foods.
    - ⊙ Acquire multipurpose energy-saving equipment.
  - ▸ *Analyze* methods of doing things and question details to be sure the most energy-efficient method is being used:
    - ⊙ Is it necessary? Why?
    - ⊙ When should it be done? How often?
    - ⊙ Where should it be done? Is there a better place?
    - ⊙ How is the best way for me to do it?
- General considerations for energy conservation and work simplification include the following:
  - ▸ Do not waste energy on unnecessary tasks.
  - ▸ Plan activities so rest breaks can be taken when necessary and *before* fatigue sets in.
  - ▸ Realize that activities using the arms, especially when working above shoulder height, are more demanding than those using the legs. Push—don't pull! Slide—don't lift and carry!
  - ▸ Delegate work whenever possible.
  - ▸ Make the work environment more comfortable through the use of good ventilation, proper lighting, comfortable clothing, and soft music.
  - ▸ Use good posture to prevent fatigue.
  - ▸ Store objects where they are the most convenient. If an item is frequently used in more than one location, consider buying duplicates to keep in each area in order to minimize unnecessary trips.
  - ▸ Specific suggestions are summarized in Tables 7-8 and 7-9.

OTHER INTERVENTIONS

Physical therapists often assist debilitated patients and their families with self-management in other ways also:

- A home visit can identify potential safety hazards and assist with creative problem solving to deal with specific difficulties the patient is having.
- Therapists can initiate a referral for social service or case management consultations when warranted.

Outcome measures that are useful in documenting improvements in an individual's ability to meet the demands of daily living activities include quality of life and activity status indices, functional health status questionnaires, and functional timed walk tests.

7.5 IMPAIRED VENTILATION AND GAS EXCHANGE

Impaired ventilation, or hypoventilation, is manifested by elevated arterial carbon dioxide tension ($Paco_2$ or Pco_2) and low arterial oxygen tension (Pao_2 or Po_2). The causes include respiratory muscle weakness or paralysis; reduced respiratory muscle endurance; impaired ventilatory drive; restricted lung or thoracic compliance, including that which occurs with aging; retained secretions; and increased dead space ventilation. Physical therapy interventions for impaired ventilation and gas exchange vary with the cause, although there is considerable overlap (PT preferred practice patterns 6D-6G).[7,23a] Techniques designed to improve respiratory muscle strength and endurance, improve thoracic mobility, and reduce dead space ventilation are presented in this section. Refer to Section 7.6 for techniques used to treat excessive pulmonary secretions.

TABLE 7-8: Energy Conservation/Work Simplification Techniques

Technique	Examples
Establish a routine	Plan each day to include only what you can realistically accomplish Leave enough time for each task Allow a 30 to 60-min rest period after each meal and after any particularly strenuous activity (e.g., your exercise program, showering/bathing) Do several different kinds of activities each day Include personal time for hobbies, going outside, reading, or other relaxing pursuits, as well as exercise time and time for daily tasks Avoid making multiple trips up and down the stairs (if you live in a multistory home): Plan your day to do all your activities on one level, and then go to the next level and do your activities there
Pace yourself	Allow ample time to complete each task so you don't have to rush Take your time with tasks and rest before you become really tired Alter your pace depending on the task, temperature, and time of day Work to music with a slower beat
Sit whenever possible	Facing the task, sit in a chair or stool large enough to support your weight evenly, support your lower back, and allow placement of your feet flat on the floor Upper extremities should be supported
Eliminate unnecessary tasks	Plan ahead and assemble all supplies for a task to minimize extra trips Use paper plates and cups when you want to save time and energy Straighten covers while still in bed to make bed making easier Let dishes air dry Cut hair short and/or get a permanent wave Delegate tasks to others when necessary
Avoid strenuous arm activities	Avoid straining or vigorous activities using arm motions: vacuuming, scrubbing, heavy carpentry, washing walls or windows, heavy gardening, painting walls, digging, etc. Pace yourself during other arm activities, such as setting hair or strenuous clapping after a performance Seek consultation from an occupational therapist regarding adaptations to reduce the energy cost of favorite activities requiring arm work
Keep cool	Perform more physically stressful activities during the cooler part of the day or evening Do your exercise program in a comfortable environment (e.g., an air-conditioned mall or church hall) Avoid excessively hot baths, showers, Jacuzzis Make slow transitions with temperatures, such as moving from an air-conditioned building to the hot, humid outdoors, or diving into cool water on a hot day
Watch what you eat	Avoid stimulants (e.g., caffeine, nicotine, over-the-counter drugs) Pay attention to the sodium content in foods, over-the-counter drugs, etc.
Increase your activity level gradually	Start easy, with low-level activities at first, taking frequent rest breaks as needed As you continue to feel better, add a little more each day Include one or two new activities per day as you improve Gradually increase the duration of your activity periods and shorten your rest periods
Avoid lifting	Avoid lifting chairs or other furniture, heavy grocery bags or laundry baskets, children, the corner of a mattress when making beds, etc. Transport items on a wheeled cart if possible. If a wheeled cart is not available, slide objects rather than lifting and carrying Divide groceries and laundry into small, easily handled parcels
Organize your work areas	Keep items that are used most often within easy reach Store items where they are used most. This does not mean cleaning out all of your drawers and closets; it usually means clearing out one or two easily accessible drawers or cabinets and moving a few frequently used items
Avoid isometric contractions	Avoid pushing, pulling, or lifting heavy items Avoid breath holding during dressing or other activities requiring concentration Avoid using the Valsalva maneuver

Continued

TABLE 7-8: Energy Conservation/Work Simplification Techniques—Cont'd

Technique	Examples
Use assistive devices	Use a shower chair Use long-handled lower extremity bathing and dressing aids Use long-handled tools to avoid bending and reaching (e.g., reacher, long-handled dust pan, long-handled sponge)
Adjust work heights	The best work height for a table top is about 2 in. below your bent elbow
Avoid sustained positions	Change your posture, work height, and placement of objects used in an activity so that you are not required to maintain any one position for a prolonged period of time Otherwise, take frequent short rest periods to ease the stress on your body

From Foderaro D. *Energy Conservation and Work Simplification Techniques.* Occupational Therapy Department: Santa Clara Valley Medical Center, San Jose, CA.

TABLE 7-9: Energy Conservation Techniques for Self-Care Activities

Technique	Examples
Bathing and hygiene	Use a chair or stool to sit while showering Sit to undress, bathe, dry, and dress Have a towel or robe nearby; use a terry-cloth robe to eliminate the need for drying off with towels Use a long-handled scrub brush or sponge to wash your back and feet to avoid overreaching and bending When bathing, wash in head-to-toe order Avoid overexerting by taking rest periods
Dressing	Set up clothes the night before and place where they can be easily reached Sit to dress Avoid tight clothing For lower body dressing, minimize bending by crossing one leg over the other while sitting to put on socks, underwear, pants, and shoes. Put on underwear and pants at the same time—pull up to knees while sitting, then stand and pull both underwear and pants to waist
Grooming	Sit whenever possible Avoid aerosols and strong scents Wash hair in shower Have hair done professionally Support your elbows on the table or sink when tasks take longer than 5 min
Cleaning and laundry	Pace yourself—clean one or two rooms per day rather than the entire house. Finish cleaning each room before going on to the next Eliminate unnecessary clutter and dust catchers Don't move furniture when you clean; have someone else move it Use a long-handled feather duster or vacuum for high and low dusting Working with your arms above shoulder height is harder than working with them below your shoulders. Have someone rearrange your cabinets so those things you use most often are in front. Avoid washing windows, dusting high areas, hanging clothes on the line, and reaching for things above your shoulders Make up one side of the bed completely before going to the other side so that you minimize the number of times you walk around the bed Sit on the edge of the tub and use a long-handled brush or sponge when cleaning Avoid washing large loads of laundry Sit down when folding laundry If it is necessary to iron, sit and lower the ironing board. Use a lightweight iron with gliding motions rather than lifting it on and off garments

From UCLA Healthcare Physical and Occupational Therapy, Los Angeles, CA, 2004.

FUNCTIONAL MOBILITY TRAINING

One of the most important interventions PTs perform that serves to improve ventilation and gas exchange is functional mobility training, whereby the patient is instructed and assisted in bed mobility and progressive mobilization out of bed and ambulation. Confinement to bed because of serious illness or surgery has profound physiological effects, as described on page 300. In addition, the effects of anesthesia and surgical incisions of the chest or abdomen interfere with normal pulmonary function, decreasing tidal volume, air flow rates, and respiratory muscle force production and increasing pulmonary shunt and the risk of atelectasis. Early mobility training can reverse or prevent these abnormalities.

- Functional mobility training begins with bed mobility. Patients learn the importance of frequent position changes while in bed and techniques for rolling to side-lying and scooting up in bed. Patients advance to sitting at the side of the bed to standing to transfers to a bedside chair to walking.
  - ▸ The rate at which patients advance through these steps varies considerably, with many succeeding within the first treatment session and some requiring numerous sessions.
  - ▸ Clinical monitoring of physiological responses to increasing activity provides guidance about a particular patient's readiness to proceed through these steps.
  - ▸ Coordination of breathing with exertion and supportive coughing maneuvers are also beneficial.
- Patients who are receiving mechanical ventilatory assistance can also participate in functional mobility training, including ambulation.
  - ▸ Early mobilization of patients receiving mechanical ventilation helps avert deconditioning and further weakening of the respiratory and peripheral muscles and improves functional outcomes.[23]
  - ▸ Close monitoring of vital signs is important to ensure patient safety and to avoid adverse responses to activity.
  - ▸ Before the initiation of ambulation, patients may require increased emphasis on sit-to-stand activities, balance training, functional transfer training, and walking in place.
  - ▸ During gait training the patient is ventilated with manual rescusitator bag or portable ventilator, which is usually managed by a respiratory therapist or intensive care unit nurse.
  - ▸ Some precautions to note when working with patients receiving mechanical ventilation include the following:
    - ⊙ Before moving the patient, any water in the ventilator tubing should be emptied according to the appropriate procedure so that it is not poured unintentionally back into the patient's airways.
    - ⊙ Before turning the patient or performing upper extremity exercise, the therapist should ensure adequate clearance of the ventilator tubing to prevent it from becoming compressed or disconnected during activity.
    - ⊙ Mobilization of a patient receiving mechanical ventilation invariably causes ventilator alarms to sound; the cause of all alarm soundings should be investigated (see page 29). The first course of action is to determine whether the patient is receiving adequate ventilation (no signs of distress, appropriate rise and fall of the chest with each ventilatory cycle,

adequate pulse oximeter values, etc.) and to initiate appropriate interventions if there is a problem (begin manual ventilation with a self-inflating bag, alert the nurse, etc.).
    - ⊙ Excessive resistance during strengthening exercise should be avoided in order to prevent breath holding or the Valsalva maneuver, which will cause the ventilator to deliver breaths at a higher pressure.
  - ▸ For patients who have required prolonged mechanical ventilation, weaning is usually both physiologically and psychologically stressful. PTs can assist the process by instructing patient in body positioning and relaxation exercises, as well as providing emotional support, to reduce these stresses. Physical activity should be minimized immediately before, during, and after weaning periods, especially initially.
- Because most normal daily activities and a number of job-related and recreational activities involve some static muscle work, some attention should be directed at assessing the physiological responses to predominantly static activities and performing some functional training activities with appropriate modifications to minimize adverse responses.

AEROBIC EXERCISE

Any form of aerobic exercise of moderate to high intensity serves as a stimulus to increase respiratory muscle strength and endurance. Thus, an endurance training program prescribed to increase fitness level will also improve respiratory muscle function (see Section 7.2).

- Patients who have more severe impairment usually require an individualized exercise program that begins with interval training with frequent rest periods. A gradual rate of progression guided by frequent monitoring of the patient's subjective and objective responses is recommended.
- Patients who are receiving mechanical ventilation can also perform aerobic exercise, including ambulation and stationary cycling. To be appropriate for training, the patient should be hemodynamically stable, on not more than 5 cm of positive end-expiratory pressure, and tolerating a weaning mode of ventilation.
  - ▸ Therapeutic exercises for all extremities and the trunk are performed to increase peripheral and respiratory muscular strength and endurance.
  - ▸ Ambulation away from the bedside requires ventilation with a manual rescusitator bag or portable ventilator. A stationary bike can usually be positioned within reach of the patient's ventilator so that exercise training is less complicated.
  - ▸ Because of the specificity of training, progressive ambulation is important to optimize the patient's level of functional independence when ventilatory assistance is no longer required.

BREATHING EXERCISES

There are several forms of breathing exercises that can improve ventilation and gas exchange.

Breathing Retraining

A number of breathing retraining techniques are used to relieve and control dyspnea in patients with COPD and asthma. PTs often teach diaphragmatic breathing and pursed-lip breathing to improve ventilation, ventilatory efficiency, and gas exchange. In addition, patients may benefit from Buteyko or Papworth breathing techniques and yoga training. Although none of these breathing techniques provide consistent improvements in all patients, specific techniques may provide benefits for individual patients.

Diaphragmatic Breathing Exercises

Diaphragmatic breathing (DB) exercises are traditionally performed to improve ventilation, decrease the work of breathing, mitigate dyspnea, normalize breathing pattern, and reduce the incidence of postoperative pulmonary complications.[62] Yet, there is some controversy as to whether teaching diaphragmatic breathing exercises actually achieves any of these goals.[18]

One review of the literature regarding the efficacy of DB reports that there are both beneficial and detrimental effects of DB in patients with COPD.[18] Potential beneficial effects include improvements in tidal volume, abdominal motion, pulmonary function, respiratory rate, and arterial blood gases. Potential deleterious effects of DB consist of paradoxical chest wall motion, decreased efficiency of breathing, and increased dyspnea. The following conclusions are offered:

- ▸ It is possible that persons with moderate to severe COPD and marked hyperinflation of the lungs without diaphragmatic motion or change in tidal volume during DB may be poor candidates for instruction in DB.
- ▸ Conversely, persons with COPD who have faster respiratory rates, low tidal volumes that increase during DB, and abnormal arterial blood gases with adequate diaphragmatic movement may benefit from DB.
- ▸ The development of an abdominal paradoxical breathing pattern and worsening dyspnea and fatigue during or after DB indicates that DB should be modified (e.g., use of more upright body positions or trunk flexion) or discontinued.
- • The techniques for teaching diaphragmatic breathing exercises are as follows:
  - ▸ Have the patient assume a comfortable position that optimizes DB (e.g., sitting supported, semi-Fowler position). In patients with COPD with marked hyperinflation of the lungs and a paradoxical breathing pattern, sitting with trunk flexion is recommended.[18,79] In addition, it has been suggested that a posterior pelvic tilt may facilitate DB and that internal rotation and adduction of the upper extremities may inhibit upper chest motion.[31,33]
  - ▸ Explain the purpose and goals of the exercise and demonstrate the desired result.
  - ▸ Provide tactile stimulation by placing one hand on the patient's abdomen over the umbilicus and the other on the upper chest while asking the patient to breathe slowly and comfortably. Follow the patient's breathing with the hands and note the movement of the abdomen versus the upper chest. Normally, the lower hand will rise with inspiration as the diaphragm pushes the abdominal contents down and fall with expiration as the diaphragm returns to its relaxed position; motion of the upper chest should be minimal.
  - ▸ Visual stimulation can be added by having the patient observe increased motion of the hand over the abdomen and decreased motion of the hand over the upper chest,

while auditory stimulation can be provided by the therapist through the provision of loud inspiratory and expiratory sounds corresponding to the patient's respiratory cycle.
- ▸ Monitor several respiratory cycles. As the patient completes an exhalation, instruct the patient to breathe more deeply with verbal cues such as "fill my hand with air" or "take a breath into my hand." Notice the expansion under the lower hand. Instruct the patient to exhale normally.
- ▸ If the patient has difficulty with diaphragmatic breathing, instruct him or her to "sniff" first to promote a diaphragmatic contraction and then to breathe as described previously, or apply a firm quick-stretch, using the hand on the abdomen just before inspiration. The counterpressure caused by the quick-stretch will facilitate the muscular response. Using the verbal commands as noted previously readies the patient for action.
- ▸ Some practitioners recommend the use of abdominal muscle contraction at end expiration in order to lengthen the diaphragm and increase its force-generating capacity (termed abdominal–diaphragmatic breathing).[55]
- ▸ Have the patient continue practicing the exercise until s/he can perform it correctly without manual stretch assistance.
- ▸ Then have the patient place her/his own hands on the abdomen and upper chest and repeat the same procedure while following the verbal cues from the therapist.
- ▸ Continue practicing until the patient can demonstrate competency in DB (e.g., doubling of abdominal tidal excursion with reduced upper chest excursion and increased tidal volume during DB).
- • In breathing retraining, diaphragmatic breathing exercises can be progressed to higher levels of difficulty by having the patient perform the exercise while sitting unsupported, standing, and then walking, with cues initially and then sequentially removing the various cues.

Breathing Control

Breathing control is a variation of diaphragmatic breathing that acknowledges the altered lung mechanics that occur with obstructive lung disease, when the diaphragm is often flattened and at a mechanical disadvantage favoring the use of accessory muscles. It involves normal tidal volume breathing using the lower chest and, if needed, the accessory muscles with the goal of decreasing the work of breathing and improving air flow.

Pursed-lips Breathing

Another technique that can be effective in improving gas exchange is pursed-lips breathing (PLB), which aims to slow the rate of expiration, increase the volume of expired air, and limit dynamic hyperinflation during periods of increased ventilatory demand, including daily activities and exercise. PLB has been shown to decrease the respiratory rate and minute ventilation, improve gas exchange (both oxygen and carbon dioxide), increase tidal volume, and reduce the work of breathing, thus relieving dyspnea and increasing exercise tolerance.[26,68] However, not all patients with airflow limitation experience benefits with this technique; some studies have failed to demonstrate a reduction in dyspnea, and others have shown increased breathlessness at rest and during exercise.[36]

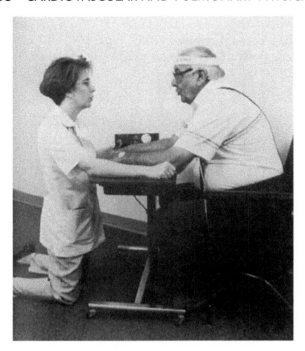

Figure 7-5: A physical therapist instructs a patient in the use of pursed-lip breathing and forward leaning posture in sitting to relieve dyspnea. (From Barr RN. Pulmonary rehabilitation. In Hillegass EA, Sadowsky HS, editors. *Essentials of Cardiopulmonary Physical Therapy,* 2nd ed. Philadelphia: Saunders; 2001.)

- Pursed-lips breathing is often used spontaneously by patients with COPD to relieve dyspnea, or the technique may require instruction by the physical therapist, as illustrated in Figure 7-5.
  ‣ The patient should assume a comfortable position as the therapist describes and demonstrates the technique for PLB and explains its expected benefits.
  ‣ With a hand on the patient's midabdominal muscles, the therapist instructs the patient to inhale slowly through the nose.
  ‣ The patient is then told to let the air escape gently through the pursed lips, avoiding excessive use of the abdominal muscles. Giving the patient a verbal cue, such as "imagine you want to make the flame flicker on a candle that is being held at arm's length from you," will enhance the patient's understanding and performance.
  ‣ The patient is directed to stop exhaling when abdominal contraction is detected.
  ‣ When able to perform PLB without cues, the patient substitutes his/her own hand for the therapist's.
- In breathing retraining, PLB can be progressed in difficulty by eliminating the tactile feedback of the hand on the abdomen, advancing to standing, and finally proceeding to other activities such as ambulating or riding a stationary bicycle while continuing to use the technique.

Other Breathing Retraining Techniques

Patients with asthma often complain of respiratory symptoms (dyspnea and chest tightness) as well as anxiety, lightheadedness, and fatigue as a result of dysfunctional breathing, despite pharmacologic treatment. It has been documented that 30% of survey responders pursue breathing techniques to relieve persistent symptoms.[75] Several breathing techniques have shown promise in improving various outcome measures (subjective symptoms, medication requirements, peak flow, airway reactivity, and exercise time), but reliable conclusions were limited by small sample sizes and by methodologic problems.

- The Buteyko technique is a series of breathing exercises that focus on slow nasal breathing, breath-holding (controlled pauses), and relaxation. Reductions in medication use and symptoms have been reported.[15]
- The Papworth method is a multicomponent program of breathing and relaxation exercises that are designed to reduce rapid shallow breathing during times of stress. It emphasizes relaxed deep diaphragmatic nose-breathing and has been shown to ameliorate respiratory symptoms and improve quality of life in a general practice population of patients with mild to moderate asthma.[45]
- Yoga breathing training includes a number of rhythmic breathing techniques accompanied by simple hand and body movements. Prayanama uses prolonged expiration, abdominal/diaphragmatic breathing, resisted inspiration and expiration, and yogasanas and chanting maneuvers. Other yoga breathing techniques that slow breathing without voluntary breath-holding include Nadishuddhi, Sitkari, and Bhramari. Improvements in peak flow, medication requirements, and frequency of exacerbations have been observed.[75]

Segmental Breathing Exercises

Segmental breathing exercises (also called localized expansion breathing exercises or thoracic expansion exercises, TEE) are used to preferentially augment localized lung expansion. The goals are to increase and redistribute ventilation, improve gas exchange, aid in reexpansion of air spaces, mobilize the thoracic cage, and increase the strength, endurance, and efficiency of the respiratory muscles. Although evidence supporting the effects of segmental breathing exercises on regional ventilation is lacking, these exercises appear to be beneficial for the other goals mentioned.[84]

- Segmental breathing exercises use manual pressure as proprioceptive input to encourage expansion of specific areas of the chest. Hand placements (unilateral or bilateral) commonly used by therapists are listed in Table 7-10.
  ‣ After identifying the area of treatment, the therapist's hand(s) are placed on the appropriate part of the patient's chest, applying firm pressure at the end of expiration.
  ‣ The therapist then instructs the patient to take a slow, deep breath in through the nose "to fill my [the therapist's] hand with air" while applying gradually diminishing resistance to permit full range of motion (ROM).
  ‣ Maximal inspiration is sustained for 2 to 3 seconds and then the patient exhales, which is sometimes assisted by the PT's manual pressure.
  ‣ Once the patient demonstrates understanding of the previous steps, s/he can be instructed to perform the exercise with her/his own hands or a towel or belt. The patient places a towel/belt over the area of treatment, grasps the ends with her/his hands, and applies firm pressure at the end of

TABLE 7-10: Hand Placement by Therapist for Segmental Breathing Exercises

Hand Location for the Therapist	Focal Area of Lung Being Emphasized
Subclavicular areas	Upper lobes
Anterior midchest	Right middle lobe and lingula
Anterior lower ribs	Anterior basal segments of the lower lobes
Lower lateral costal area	Lateral basal segments of the lower lobes
Posterior lower chest	Posterior basal segments of the lower lobes
Posterior midchest (with scapulae abducted)	Superior segments of the lower lobes

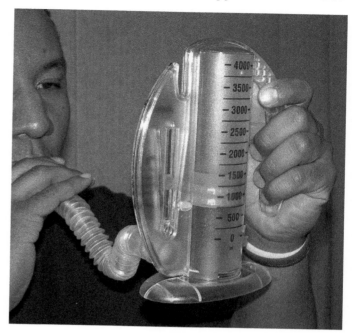

Figure 7-6: Patient using an incentive spirometer.

expiration. As the patient is taking a slow, deep breath in through the nose, s/he is applying gradually diminishing resistance through the towel/belt, adjusting to allow full ROM. Maximal inspiration is sustained for 2 to 3 seconds and then the patient exhales, which may be assisted manually or with the towel/belt.

- In addition, *proprioceptive neuromuscular facilitation (PNF) techniques,* using patterns involving the upper extremities and trunk coordinated with inspiration and expiration, can be performed by the PT for patients with neurologic deficits.[59]
  - ▸ With the therapist's hands placed so that the fingers are aligned with the contracting muscle fibers, a quick-stretch is applied just before inspiration in order to increase the force of muscle contraction.
  - ▸ Then, at the end of a deep inspiration, repeated stretches are applied as the patient is asked to breathe in more, more, more (as in "ah-ah-ah-ah-choo!") in order to increase chest expansion.

Incentive Spirometry

Incentive spirometry (IS) involves the use of a visual or auditory feedback device to encourage reproducible slow, deep inspirations (Figure 7-6). IS is commonly performed by postoperative patients in order to reduce the incidence of pulmonary complications associated with surgery-related shallow breathing, bed rest, diaphragmatic dysfunction, pain, and impaired mucociliary clearance.[52]

- Two types of incentive spirometers are commonly used:
  - ▸ A flow IS typically consists of one or more chambers containing table tennis–like ball(s) that are elevated by sufficient inspiratory air flow.
  - ▸ A volume IS consists of bellows or pistons that register the volume inspired and can indicate whether a preset volume goal is achieved.
- Instruction in proper technique is critical to the effectiveness of IS, especially with flow devices: a rapid inspiratory rate will elevate the ball(s) to the top of the chamber(s) with a relatively low-volume breath; or a deep breath at a slow flow rate may achieve a high volume without moving the ball(s).

- ▸ With the patient in a sitting, semi-Fowler, or supine position (with the head of the bed raised 10 to 15 degrees, to relieve diaphragmatic resistance applied by the abdominal contents), the patient is instructed to take three or four slow, easy breaths with normal exhalations in between.
- ▸ After these breaths, the patient exhales slowly but completely, places the mouthpiece in the mouth, forming a tight seal with the lips, and then performs a slow, deep diaphragmatic breath, minimizing any upper chest movement, in order to elicit the visual cue(s) of the apparatus (plunger/balls rising, lights flashing, etc.).
- ▸ The inspiration is sustained as long as possible (to allow collateral ventilation of the well-aerated alveoli with those that are poorly ventilated) before the mouthpiece is removed and the patient relaxes to allow expiration.
- ▸ This procedure is typically performed 10 times every hour while awake.

Diaphragm-strengthening Exercises

For patients with less than normal diaphragmatic strength without respiratory muscle fatigue, diaphragmatic strengthening exercises are beneficial. As with all skeletal muscle, initial muscle strength determines the technique used for strengthening.

- Progressive resistive exercise can be used for greater than "fair" diaphragm strength. Resistance can be applied with weights, manual pressure, positioning, or incentive spirometry.
  - ▸ Weights are applied over the epigastric area with the patient in the supine position, thus providing resistance to diaphragmatic descent. Cuff weights tend to be the most comfortable and have less chance of falling off the patient with the breathing movement. The proper starting weight should permit full diaphragmatic excursion (i.e., full epigastric rise) using a coordinated, unaltered breathing pattern (no signs of accessory muscle contraction) for 15 minutes. As strength improves

additional weight can be added until the patient demonstrates normal strength. The therapist must take care that the weights do not topple off the patient's abdomen at peak inspiration.

▸ As an alternative, progressively increasing manual resistance can be applied in a similar manner. Once the patient is comfortable with this technique, family members, a significant other, or friends can be taught how to apply manual resistance to assist the patient.

▸ Another option is to use positioning so that the force of the abdominal contents provides resistance to diaphragmatic contraction. This is accomplished by placing the patient in a gentle Trendelenburg position (a 15-degree head down tilt results in approximately 10 lb of force against the diaphragm) and having the patient perform several series of three to five slow sustained deep diaphragmatic breaths with interposed rest periods. Be aware of any contraindications to using the Trendelenburg position (see page 329).

• When diaphragm strength is "fair" or less (manifested as just normal or less than normal diaphragmatic excursion, or epigastric rise, in the supine position), IS and inspiratory, or ventilatory, muscle training are often used to increase strength and endurance. Of import, care must be taken not to overstress the muscle, causing fatigue, because the diaphragm must continue to function throughout the day.

▸ IS is performed with the patient in a supine position with the head of the bed raised 10 to 15 degrees, as described in the previous section.

▸ Respiratory muscle training is detailed in the next section.

• For patients with "poor" diaphragm strength, the emphasis is on breathing retraining emphasizing proper technique and timing of diaphragmatic or lower chest breathing. In these patients, ventilation is usually most comfortable when the patient is in the supine position because of the mechanical advantage of the abdominal contents holding the diaphragm in a more normal resting position. In addition, both the diaphragm and the accessory muscles are in a gravity-eliminated position in this position. In contrast, when the patient is in the upright position, as in sitting, the abdominal contents shift inferiorly (and anteriorly if the abdominal muscles are weak), pulling the diaphragm into a more horizontal position, where its mechanical function is at an extreme disadvantage.

▸ In patients with quadriplegia, lower chest expansion can actually become negative during inspiration (as demonstrated by a reduction of chest circumference of 0.5 to 1 in. as measured at the xiphoid process).[33] Therefore, the use of an abdominal corset is recommended in patients with weak abdominal muscles to support the intestines and to maintain the diaphragm in a more functional position, as illustrated in Figure 7-7.[40]

▸ In patients with completely flaccid abdominal muscles, a body jacket may provide better postural and respiratory function. It consists of a rigid trunk support with an anterior abdominal cutout to allow diaphragmatic movement.

Respiratory Muscle Training

Specific exercise training can be performed to increase the strength and endurance of the inspiratory and expiratory muscles. Typically, strength training is accomplished by performing a

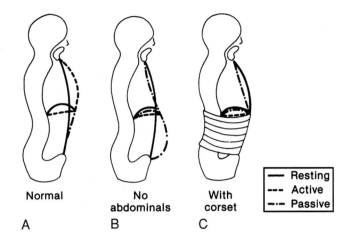

—	Resting
---	Active
-·-	Passive

Normal	No abdominals	With corset
A	B	C

Figure 7-7: The advantage of an abdominal corset in patients with poor abdominal strength. **A,** Normal diaphragm position. **B,** Weak abdominal muscles allow gravity to pull the diaphragm into a horizontal position. **C,** Corset application supports optimal diaphragm positioning. (From Alvarez SE, Peterson M, Lunsford BR. Respiratory treatment of the adult patient with spinal cord injury. *Phys Ther.* 1980;61:1737–1745.)

maximal static maneuver (either inspiratory or expiratory) against a closed glottis or a nearly closed occluded resistance valve, whereas endurance training entails breathing through a variable resistor at a predetermined percentage of maximal capacity for a specific period of time. Interestingly, increases in strength of both the inspiratory and expiratory muscles occurred regardless of the muscle group targeted and also with other, nonrespiratory strength-training programs.[38]

It is important to note that weakened respiratory muscles benefit from resistive muscle training, whereas fatigued muscles do not (see page 243). The performance of respiratory muscle training in the presence of fatigue is likely to provoke respiratory failure, and thus the appropriate treatment is rest, usually by means of ventilatory assistance. As the respiratory muscles begin to recover, training can be initiated with careful monitoring.

Outcome measures that are useful in documenting the effects of respiratory muscle training include the change in maximal voluntary ventilation for respiratory muscle endurance and changes in maximal inspiratory and expiratory pressures and peak flow measures for respiratory muscle strength.

Inspiratory Muscle Training

Inspiratory, or ventilatory, muscle training is indicated for patients who are limited by inspiratory muscle weakness or diminished endurance, as occurs with COPD, stroke, spinal cord injury, muscular dystrophy, amyotrophic lateral sclerosis, Guillain-Barré syndrome, and many other neurological and neuromuscular disorders and myopathies. Respiratory muscle dysfunction has also been observed in some restrictive lung disorders, chronic heart failure, and end-stage renal disease.

Ventilatory muscle training can be performed by several methods, all of which aim to improve inspiratory muscle strength and endurance and to reduce dyspnea.

• Unloaded hyperpnea involves breathing at respiratory rates of 45 to 60 breaths per minute against normal resistance.

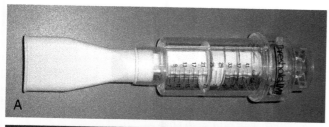

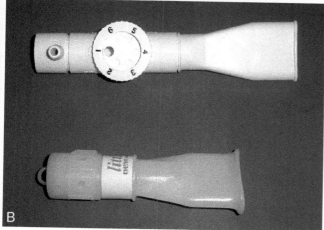

Figure 7-8: Two handheld resistive breathing training devices. **A,** A threshold-type inspiratory muscle training device. **B,** Two non-threshold-type inspiratory muscle training devices. (From Irwin S, Tecklin JS. *Cardiopulmonary Physical Therapy: A Guide to Practice,* 4th ed. St. Louis: Mosby; 2004.)

- Normocapnic hyperpnea requires the patient to breathe at a high proportion (>60%) of her/his maximal voluntary ventilation (MVV) using a partial rebreathing training system for 15 to 20 minutes.
- Inspiratory resistive training entails the patient breathing through a device with adjustable resistance settings (progressively narrower airways) at a normal respiratory rate (usually 15 breaths per minute). Several such devices are commercially available, as shown in Figure 7-8.
  - ▶ Typically, patients begin using the device at a resistance setting of approximately 25% to 35% of the maximal negative inspiratory pressure measured at functional residual volume (or at an arbitrarily chosen low resistance that does not cause dyspnea, fatigue, or oxygen desaturation).
  - ▶ The device is used twice daily for 15 to 30 minutes. When the patient can comfortably complete two 15- to 30-minute sessions per day at a particular setting, the resistance is increased to the next higher setting.
  - ▶ Although this device is simple to use, its resistance is flow dependent.
- Threshold loading uses a valve that opens at a critical pressure, and thus is independent of inspiratory flow rate. Although this device requires the development of adequate negative pressure before flow is initiated, it offers the advantages of enhancing the velocity of inspiratory muscle shortening, reducing inspiratory time, and increasing the time available for expiration and relaxation.

- In addition, an isometric exercise can be performed by having the patient exert a maximal inspiratory effort using a device with a closed shutter, which is held for 4 seconds and repeated every 20 seconds.
- Also effective, particularly in children, are some entertaining computer-based games that rely on respiratory effort.

Most of the research evaluating ventilatory muscle training has involved patients with chronic obstructive pulmonary disease (COPD),[42,56,70,76] and it has also been used with success with patients being weaned from prolonged mechanical ventilation and in those with a wide variety of other conditions, including quadriplegia, neuromuscular diseases, and chronic heart failure (CHF).[71] Patients with restricted thoracic expansion have also been studied.[16,86] Significant improvements in inspiratory muscle function have been demonstrated, and there have often been increased exercise tolerance, decreased dyspnea, and improved maximal work capacity and quality of life, although these benefits were not always statistically significant.

Patients whose respiratory muscles are prone to fatigue may benefit from the addition of nocturnal ventilatory assistance, such as continuous positive airway pressure (CPAP), which provides the respiratory muscles with an opportunity to rest. Thus, gains in strength and endurance are maximized while inefficient muscle function due to fatigue is avoided.[8]

Expiratory Muscle Training

Expiratory muscle training has been used to increase the strength and endurance of the expiratory muscles (abdominals and internal intercostals) in patients with glucose-6-phosphate dehydrogenase (C6PD) deficiency, spinal cord injury, and other neuromuscular diseases, as well as in the elderly.[49,91] In patients with COPD, expiratory muscle weakness and fatigue are features of the generalized myopathy that occurs in this population and may contribute to reduced exercise tolerance and quality of life as well as reduced cough efficacy.[91] Expiratory muscle training can be achieved through the use of a handheld device that provides resistance on exhalation, via threshold loading or repeated Valsalva maneuvers.

Glossopharyngeal Breathing

Patients with high-level quadriplegia are often instructed in glossopharyngeal breathing (GPB), in which the patient swallows air into the lungs in order to increase vital capacity. GPB is used to augment cough effectiveness, provide internal mobilization of the chest wall, and improve quality of life by allowing periods of ventilator or phrenic nerve stimulator independence and more effective phonation.[59]

- The patient creates a pocket of negative pressure within the mouth by dropping the tongue to maximize the internal space, thereby causing air to be sucked in.
- The patient then closes off his lips and forces the air back and down his throat with a stroking maneuver of the tongue, pharynx, and larynx.

THORACIC MOBILIZATION

Impaired ventilation due to inefficient ventilatory patterns can also result from thoracic pump dysfunction inhibiting chest wall expansion. Thoracic mobility exercises and mobilization techniques serve to improve thoracic expansion and thus allow freer breathing patterns.

Thoracic Mobility Exercises

Any exercise that affects the shoulders or trunk will help mobilize the chest. In addition, patients can be instructed in specific breathing exercises to increase chest expansion, segmentally and regionally. Finally, manual stretching and facilitation techniques can also be employed.

- A variety of *total body motions* can be used to increase chest mobility:
  - ▸ While sitting in a chair, the patient exhales while bending forward to touch the floor with the arms crossing at the feet. Then the patient extends up while taking a deep inspiration and lifts the arms up and out into a "V" above the head.
  - ▸ While sitting in a chair with the right hand holding the left wrist, the patient exhales while bending and rotates to touch the floor lateral to the right ankle with the left hand. The patient then inspires while extending upward and rotates the left arm and hand up over the head while rotating the trunk to the left. The procedure is then performed in a similar manner while holding the right wrist. As an alternative, this exercise can be performed with a cane or wand.
  - ▸ With the patient lying in the supine position and the hips and knees flexed, the patient can perform modified sit-ups, or pelvic tilt with head lift, to strengthen the abdominal muscles. To add more thoracic mobility, the patient may stretch both arms overhead on inspiration and then reach past the knees on exhalation; or the patient may stretch the right hand up over the head and out to the right (160 degrees of abduction) during inspiration, then exhale while bringing the extended arm over and across the body, lifting the shoulders and head to reach past the left hip. If the patient needs more than one breath to complete the move, s/he can take an extra breath at the completion of each arc. S/he should rest for a few breaths before repeating the move with the opposite side.
  - ▸ On hands and knees, the patient can rock forward during inspiration and then backward to heel sitting with chin tucked during expiration. This move should be slow, relaxed, and rhythmic, pausing in the heel-sitting position for an additional breath or two. As a variation, starting from the heel-sitting position, rock forward during inspiration, drop one elbow down to touch the floor on expiration, push back onto hands and knees on inspiration, and rock back to heel sitting on expiration.
- In addition, exercises emphasizing shoulder and trunk mobility will mobilize the chest:
  - ▸ Standing with hands on a wall at shoulder height, the patient performs a modified push-up. The patient exhales while bending the elbows and lowering the body to the wall. The patient then inhales while pushing away from the wall, returning to an erect position while extending the arms. As strength improves, difficulty can be increased by having the patient use a high counter or sink instead of the wall. Careful monitoring to ensure avoidance of the Valsalva maneuver is important.
  - ▸ A variation of the preceding exercise involves the patient performing a corner stretch. The patient stands facing a corner with their arms flexed to 90 degrees at the elbow and the shoulder flexed to 90 degrees. The forearms or hands are placed on the wall. The patient is instructed to exhale while leaning their chest toward the corner. The patient then inhales while returning to the starting position.
  - ▸ Sitting with arms extended at the sides, the patient inspires while forward flexing both arms up and over the head and expires while returning them to the sides (can also be done with a cane or wand).
  - ▸ Sitting with arms extended at the sides, the patient inhales while abducting both arms up and over the head and exhales while returning them to the sides. The patient can also sit with both arms forward flexed to 90 degrees and inhale while spreading the arms apart (horizontal abduction) and exhale as the arms come together again.
  - ▸ Sitting with hands holding opposite forearms and resting on top of the head, the patient rotates the trunk to look past the right elbow, holds the position while taking two slow deep breaths, then repeats to the opposite side (can also be done with a cane or wand held overhead).
  - ▸ Sitting in a chair with arms at the sides, the patient abducts one arm out and over the head during inspiration and then continues the motion into a side bend toward the opposite side during expiration. The patient inhales while returning to an upright position and exhales while returning the arm to the side. Repeat on other side.
  - ▸ Sitting in a chair with hands behind the head, the patient inhales while extending up as tall as possible and pressing the elbows back. The patient then exhales while flexing forward and brings the elbows toward each other in front.
  - ▸ Sitting in a chair, the patient inhales while lifting the hands up in front and toward the ceiling. The patient then exhales while reaching way behind the head, leading with bent elbows, and lowers the hands behind the body. Another inhalation/exhalation cycle is used to return to the starting position.
  - ▸ Sitting in a chair with both hands held together and resting on the patient's right knee, the patient inhales while raising the hands above the left shoulder and rotating to the left. The patient then exhales while returning the hands to the right knee. The process is repeated on the other side. The motion should look similar to someone chopping wood.
  - ▸ Sitting in a chair with both hands held at shoulder height, the patient inhales and then exhales while reaching forward in a punching motion during exhalation. The right hand should reach for a target that is to the left of the patient, across the midline of their body, in order to rotate the trunk to the left. The process is repeated toward the right side.
- *Segmental breathing exercises,* as previously described on pages 316 to 317, also serve to mobilize the thoracic cage.

Thoracic Mobilization Techniques

Thoracic mobilization techniques can be used in patients with rib cage restrictions or decreased intercostal strength to maintain or increase chest wall mobility. The following interventions using positioning or manual techniques can be used to mobilize the thoracic cage:

- Positioning to open up the chest wall[33]:
  - ▸ Place a rolled towel or a pillow under the patient's spine when supine to open up the anterior chest wall.

▶ Place one or more towel rolls or pillows under the dependent chest wall (ribs 8–10) in the side-lying position to open up the contralateral chest wall. This creates a gentle stretch to the focal area.

▶ The therapist can then instruct the patient in the segmental, or localized, breathing exercises already described.

• The addition of breathing-coordinated active, or active-assisted, range of motion with the arms going overhead via shoulder flexion or abduction while positioned as described previously: Having the patient watch her/his hands during these motions further enhances inspiratory and expiratory volumes.

• Manual chest wall stretching can be used to maintain thoracic cage mobility in patients with significant intercostal weakness or paralysis, as illustrated in Figure 7-9.

▶ The chest wall is stretched by placing one hand under the ribs, with the tips of the fingers of one hand on the transverse processes, and the other hand on top of the chest with the heel of the lateral palmar area to the sternum; the hands are then brought together in a wringing motion to create the stretch.

▶ Care is given not to apply force directly on the edges of the ribs or sternum.

▶ Pressure is distributed evenly over the entire surface of the hands.

▶ The stretches are applied progressively up the chest, alternating hands.

• Counterrotation of the trunk can be used to increase thoracic mobility and to reduce high neuromuscular tone.[33]

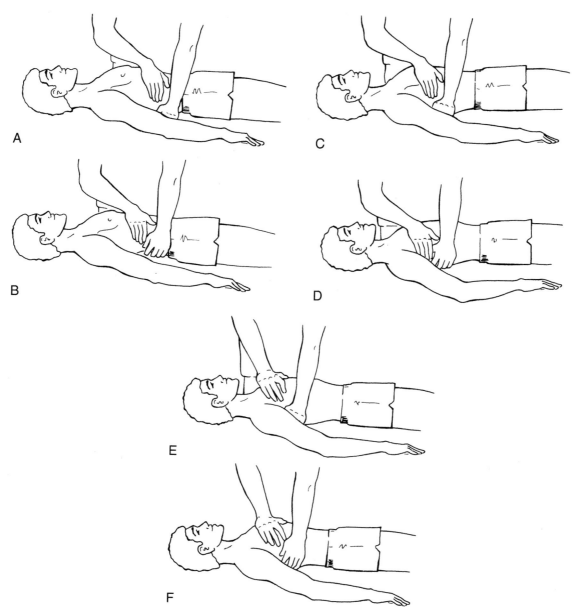

Figure 7-9: Manual chest stretching for lower (**A,** beginning position; **B,** stretching motion), middle (**C,** beginning position; **D,** stretching motion), and upper chest (**E,** beginning position; **F,** stretching motion); see text for explanation. (From Irwin S, Tecklin JS. *Cardiopulmonary Physical Therapy: A Guide to Practice.* 4th ed. St. Louis: Mosby; 2004.)

- ▸ The therapist works in a diagonal pattern while positioned behind the patient.
- ▸ The therapist places a hand (the same hand as the side the patient is lying on) over the patient's shoulder region. When going into the flexed position, the PT will move the hand on top of the shoulder and pull toward the hip. When going into the extended position, the PT will move the hand over the scapula and push out toward the shoulder.
- ▸ The therapist places the other hand over the lateral hip region. When going into the flexed position, the PT will move the hand to the gluteal fossa and push up toward the shoulder. When going into the extended position, the PT will move the hand over the iliac crest and pull down and away from the patient's trunk.
- ▸ In the first phase, the PT initially follows along with the patient's respiratory cycle with the hands on the appropriate regions, which allows assessment of the patient's breathing rate and rhythm as well as neuromuscular tone.
- ▸ In the second phase the therapist assists the patient with her/his breathing pattern, using the previously mentioned hand placements. During inspiration the chest is expanded by the PT gently pulling the patient into the extended position. During expiration the chest is compressed as the PT gently places the patient into the flexed position. To facilitate a stronger response, the PT can give a quick-stretch just before the initiation of inspiration. This maneuver is performed for three to five breathing cycles in order to achieve good ventilation of all lung segments.
- ▸ At first, the PT coordinates timing with the patient's respiratory cycle, but as the technique induces a reduction in the patient's tone and an improvement in ventilation, the PT gradually slows the rate of rotation, giving the patient auditory breathing cues to further facilitate a slowing of her/his breathing rate.
- ▸ The PT can advance this technique by decreasing the manual input and later by eliminating the auditory cues.
- Specific manual therapy techniques can be applied to mobilize the thoracic spine and rib cage (refer to appropriate orthopedic textbooks for descriptions of these techniques).
- Myofascial release techniques and soft tissue massage can be used to loosen connective tissue and muscle tissue around the chest wall.

POSITIONING

Body positioning can have a significant effect on ventilation and other components of the oxygen transport system. Consequently, various body positions and frequent positioning changes can be used to improve the distribution of ventilation, ventilation–perfusion ($\dot{V}/\dot{Q}$) matching, and gas exchange. The specific positions required to optimize ventilation and $\dot{V}/\dot{Q}$ matching depend on the patient's pulmonary condition as well as on such factors as age and body weight.[84]

- Acutely ill and postoperative hospitalized patients tend to assume the recumbent supine position and reduce their physical activity, which diminishes alveolar volume, functional residual capacity (FRC), and lung compliance; interferes with the distribution of ventilation, respiratory muscle efficiency, and gas exchange; and promotes airway closure. In addition, secretions pool in the dependent posterior aspects of the lungs. All these factors impair oxygen transport and elevate the work of breathing, and lead to an increased risk of pulmonary complications, especially in smokers, older adults, obese individuals, and patients receiving mechanical ventilation

- Cardiopulmonary function is optimized when patients are in the upright position and moving because ventilation and perfusion are most uniform and lung volumes and capacities (except closing volume) are expanded.[25]

- The effects of side-lying positions on lung compliance, respiratory muscle efficiency, FRC, and work of breathing are intermediate between those of the supine and upright positions. When side-lying, the volume of the dependent lung is reduced and ventilation is enhanced, but the inspiratory volume and FRC are reduced.[57a] The same is true of the lower, dependent regions of the upper lung. Perfusion is increased in the lower, dependent lung and the lower, dependent regions of the upper lung. Optimal $\dot{V}/\dot{Q}$ matching occurs in the upper one third of each lung field in the side-lying positions, and oxygenation is enhanced compared with the supine position. In patients who have undergone thoracotomy and those with unilateral lung pathology, lying with the good lung down usually improves oxygenation, whereas lying on the affected side is often detrimental to gas exchange.[25,31] In patients with bilateral lung disease, gas exchange is often improved when patients lie on the right side rather than on the left. Clinical monitoring will reveal the effects of side-lying positioning for individual patients.

- Research involving both adults and neonates has documented the efficacy of prone positioning in improving ventilation and oxygenation and in reducing the work of breathing.[9,14,64] The prone position is particularly beneficial for those with acute respiratory distress syndrome (ARDS) and those with diaphragm paralysis in whom the added abdominal wall support and assistance during the respiratory cycle enhances pulmonary function.

- The Trendelenburg position improves pulmonary mechanics in patients with COPD and flattened diaphragms and in those with pathology in the lung bases. It also promotes drainage of secretion from the lower lobes of the lungs. However, the head-down position is associated with detrimental effects in many patients, as detailed on page 329, and therefore it is no longer recommended in many treatment centers.

- Patients who are having difficulty breathing often lean forward at the hips with hands or forearms placed on a fixed object, such as the thighs, a front-wheeled walker or shopping cart, or the wall. This position stabilizes the shoulders, freeing the accessory muscles of respiration to increase ventilation more effectively (see page 337 regarding dyspnea relief positions).

- Some patients with COPD and low, flattened diaphragms obtain relief from dyspnea by lying supine, because, again, the diaphragm is pushed up into a lengthened, more advantageous position.

- Care must be taken when positioning patients with abdominal or thoracic incisions, described in Table 7-11 (see also Figure 2-21 on page 34) during physical therapy activities. Log rolling, similar to that used for patients who have recently had spinal surgery, tends to be the most comfortable technique

TABLE 7-11: Common Incisions for Thoracic Surgeries

Type of Incision	Commonly Associated With:
Median sternotomy: From the sternal notch through the sternum and xiphoid process	Most open heart surgeries including: Coronary artery bypass, valve repair or replacement, aortic root repair, heart transplant
Thoracotomy: Along the lateral wall of the chest in the intercostal space; occasionally a segment of the rib will be removed, usually 15–30 cm	Single lung transplant Lung volume reduction Heart valve repair or replacement
Minimal thoracotomy: In the intercostal space; varies as to the area being operated on (commonly used with younger patients for cosmetic reasons), usually 10–12 cm	Heart valve repair or replacement
Double thoracotomy ("clamshell"): Bilateral thoracotomy incisions that are joined anteriorly across the distal end of the sternum	Double lung transplant
Minimally invasive approach: From two to four small incisions (4–8 cm) made in the intercostal spaces; varies as to the area being operated on	Minimally invasive coronary bypass surgery Heart valve repair

for mobilizing these patients into a side-lying position. From there the patient can move to sitting on the edge of the bed, and functional mobility can be advanced. The technique is reversed when returning the patient to bed.

• Potentially deleterious positions to be used with caution or avoided entirely include lying on the side affected by unilateral lung disease and left side-lying in those with bilateral lung disease, as these positions may cause significant decreases in oxygenation.

Outcome measures that may be used to document the effects of treatment interventions aimed at improving ventilation and gas exchange include auscultation of breath sounds, observation of breathing pattern/dynamics, measurement of thoracic excursions, performance on incentive spirometer, changes in maximal voluntary ventilation and peak inspiratory and expiratory pressures, analysis of arterial blood gases, particularly during exercise, and quality of life and activity status indices.

🔲 7.6 IMPAIRED SECRETION CLEARANCE

Secretion clearance problems can be caused by excessive secretion production, inadequate mucociliary function, or impaired cough force. Excessive secretions are typically seen in chronic bronchitis, asthma, bronchiectasis, cystic fibrosis, and sometimes infection

such as pneumonia. Mucociliary transport may be hindered by cigarette smoking, anesthetics and analgesics, hypoxia or hypercapnia, dehydration, electrolyte imbalance, inhalation of dry gases or pollutants, and a cuffed endotracheal tube. Cough force may be impaired by pain, weak or paralyzed respiratory muscles or those subject to abnormal tone, or structural chest abnormalities.

A variety of techniques are available to facilitate the mobilization and expulsion of secretions, including coughing, physical exercise, and airway clearance techniques (PT preferred practice pattern 6C).[7,23a] Among the most important of these are forced expirations (huffing) and coughing.[85]

COUGHING

A cough serves as an important defense mechanism of the lungs and the primary means of clearing the first six to seven generations of airways of excess secretions and foreign material.[32] Furthermore, directed cough is considered the most effective and important part of conventional chest physical therapy (CPT) treatments (i.e., postural drainage, percussion, and vibration or shaking, or PDPV for short).[85] Coughs can be initiated voluntarily or can occur spontaneously, being triggered reflexively by mechanical stimulation of the larynx or by increased mucociliary stimulation by excessive secretions.[20,66]

An effective cough consists of a deep inspiration followed by closure of the glottis and a momentary hold during which contraction of the abdominal muscles increases intrathoracic and intraabdominal pressures. The glottis then opens and forceful abdominal contraction produces expulsion of the trapped air. In addition to mobilizing and expelling secretions, the high pressures generated during a cough may be an important factor in reexpanding poorly ventilated lung tissue.[32]

If any of the cough maneuvers is deficient (i.e., inadequate inspiratory volume, insufficient glottal closure, reduced expiratory force, or decreased maximal expiratory flow rate), the cough force will be diminished. Common causes of ineffective cough include respiratory muscle weakness or paralysis, uncoordinated muscular effort, pain, abnormal thoracic configuration reducing mechanical efficiency (e.g., COPD and thoracic deformity), and depression of the central nervous system. An impaired cough results in retained secretions and bronchial obstruction which can lead to atelectasis or pneumonia and other problems.

• Various cough techniques are described in Table 7-12.
  ▸ Surgical patients, particularly those with thoracic or abdominal incisions, should be taught how to splint the incision with a towel or pillow, etc., before coughing.
  ▸ Huffing, also called *forced expiration,* is an effective alternative for many patients who are unable to cough well.
    ⊙ It can be performed at various lung volumes: a huff from mid- to low lung volume will help mobilize more peripheral secretions, whereas one from mid- to high lung volume will mobilize secretions from the larger, more proximal airways.[63]
    ⊙ A huff from total lung capacity (TLC) increases the peak expiratory flow rate from 0.66 to 7.76 L/sec, which is nearly that produced by a cough (8.14 L/s).[61]
    ⊙ Huffing produces less airway compression than coughing and therefore is safer for patients with unstable airways.

TABLE 7-12: Various Cough Techniques

Cough Technique	Description
Double cough	After a deep inspiration, the patient performs two coughs in one breath; the second is usually more forceful than the first
Controlled cough	The patient takes three deep breaths, exhaling normally after the first two and then coughing firmly on the third; the first two breaths are believed to decrease atelectasis and increase the volume of the cough
Series of three coughs	The patient takes a small breath and gives a fair cough, then takes a bigger breath and gives a harder cough, and finally takes a really deep breath and gives a forceful cough; this technique allows patients to work their way up to a forceful cough
Huffing	The patient takes a deep inspiration and then air is forcefully exhaled as in coughing except that the mouth is kept open (less stressful on the patient and more effective than constant forced coughing, especially in patients who tend to prolong the expiratory phase of a cough almost into a wheeze, such as asthmatics and others with COPD). The patient makes a sound similar to "huff"
Pump coughing	The patient takes a deep breath and then gives three short easy coughs followed by three huffs (facilitates secretion clearance in patients with air trapping)

COPD, Chronic obstructive pulmonary disease.

⊙ In patients with respiratory muscle weakness, manual support can be added to huffing to increase the expiratory force.
- The *forced expiratory technique (FET)* refers to the combination of huffing with controlled breathing. The patient performs one or two huffs from middle to low lung volumes followed by a period of relaxed, controlled, deep diaphragmatic or lower chest breathing. The process is then repeated.
- *Directed cough* refers to a standard cough that is assisted by a care provider coaching the patient to take some deep slow breaths before the cough and assisting the cough effort with abdominal or thoracic compression during exhalation. More recently, directed cough has been redefined by some to include techniques such as FET and the active cycle of breathing technique.[29]
- Regular doses of pain medication should be encouraged if the patient's pain is limiting cough effectiveness.
- Most patients will cough better when sitting and possibly leaning forward slightly, although those with sternotomy incisions often do well with a high side-lying position because of the chest stabilization provided. Patients with quadriplegia usually cough better with the head of the bed flat and often in a side-lying position.
- Extra hydration is indicated if secretions are extremely thick. If fluid intake is not restricted, the patient should be encouraged to increase the consumption of liquids during the day. Ultrasonic nebulizer or aerosol treatments can also help thin the secretions if administered before coughing exercises.
- Patients with impaired cough frequently benefit from the following modifications:
  ▸ In patients with inadequate inspiration, inspiratory volumes can be increased through the use of:
    ⊙ Verbal cues during each of the four stages of a cough
    ⊙ Trunk extension, upward eye glaze, and flexion of arms overhead during inspiration
    ⊙ Stacked breaths, in which the patient voluntarily or with the use of a valve takes a series of deep breaths without allowing full expiration between breaths

⊙ Diaphragmatic or lateral costal breathing
⊙ Intermittent positive-pressure breathing treatment or a manual resuscitation bag for those with limited ventilatory muscle strength
▸ The force of expiration can be augmented with trunk flexion and downward eye gaze, the use of an abdominal binder to support the abdominal wall, and manual assistance (see the next section).
▸ Huffing and pump coughing (Table 7-12) are helpful for many patients, especially those prone to bronchospasm.
▸ Use of the series of three coughs (Table 7-12) is particularly effective in postoperative patients.
▸ The addition of an inspiratory hold for several seconds at maximal inspiration is thought to enable air to move distal to secretions so they can be mobilized during the expiratory phase.
▸ Patients with COPD with hyperinflation can avoid further air trapping by using controlled small or medium-sized breaths followed by huffs or a small series of coughs. Other effective alternatives include the active cycle of breathing and forced expiratory pressure techniques.
▸ Patients with quadriplegia can use glossopharyngeal breathing (see page 319) to increase vital capacity and thus cough effectiveness. The use of a pillow on the lap to increase abdominal compression can also increase cough force.
- The effectiveness of any of these cough techniques can be assessed by observing changes in oxygen saturation, improvements in breath sounds, increases in expiratory flow rates, and reductions in the patient's level of dyspnea.

Assistive Cough Techniques

If the patient's cough remains ineffective despite appropriate instruction and modifications, a number of assisted and self-assisted cough techniques or mechanical cough augmentation can be used.[38,59]

Manual Assisted Techniques

Therapists can provide manual assistance during coughing, using a variety of techniques to enhance expiratory force.

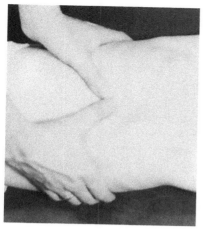

Figure 7-10: Hand placement for costophrenic assisted cough technique. (From Frownfelter D, Massery M. Facilitating airway clearance with coughing techniques. In Frownfelter D, Dean E editors. *Cardiovascular and Pulmonary Physical Therapy: Evidence and Practice.* 4th ed. St. Louis: Mosby; 2006.)

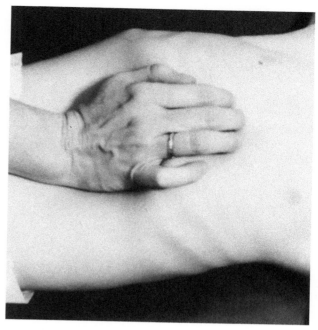

Figure 7-11: Hand placement for Heimlich-type assisted cough technique. (From Frownfelter D, Massery M. Facilitating airway clearance with coughing techniques. In Frownfelter D, Dean E editors. *Cardiovascular and Pulmonary Physical Therapy: Evidence and Practice.* 4th ed. St. Louis: Mosby; 2006.)

Costophrenic Assist

The costophrenic assist can be used in both the supine and side-lying positions.

- With the patient in the supine position, the therapist places the hands on the costophrenic angles of the patient's rib cage (see Figure 7-10). At the end of expiration the therapist applies a quick stretch down and in on the patient's lower chest to facilitate a stronger diaphragmatic and intercostal muscle contraction.
  - ▸ During the patient's inspiration, the therapist applies a series of three PNF repeated quick-stretch contractions down and in to encourage maximal inspiration. The patient is asked to hold the deep inspiration for a few seconds.
  - ▸ While instructing the patient to cough, the therapist applies strong pressure through the hands in toward the central tendon of the patient's diaphragm.
- The technique can be performed unilaterally (on the upper side only) while the patient is in the side-lying position. This produces an asymmetric cough which can be beneficial for unilateral atelectasis.
- The patient who has limited bed mobility may benefit the most from this assisted cough technique.

Heimlich-type Assist

The Heimlich-type assist can be used in both the supine and side-lying positions.

- With the patient in the supine position, the therapist places the heel of one hand inferior to the patient's xiphoid process and below the patient's lower ribs, as shown in Figure 7-11.
  - ▸ The patient is instructed to take in a deep breath and hold it. Then, just as the patient is instructed to cough, the therapist applies a quick push up and in under the diaphragm with the heel of the hand.
  - ▸ Patients with low neuromuscular tone or flaccid abdominal muscles tolerate this procedure the best.

- In patients with increased neuromuscular tone, this technique is more effective when performed in the side-lying position, following the same procedure.
- Because this technique can be uncomfortable for the patient, it should be used only when other techniques are not effective and the need to cough is great.

Combination of Heimlich-type Assist and Costophrenic Assist

The combination of Heimlich-type assist and costophrenic assist can be used only when the patient is in the side-lying position.

- The therapist uses one hand to assist lateral compression of the chest (costophrenic assist), while the other hand performs a Heimlich-type assist, pushing up and in.
- Because it uses more planes of respiration, the combined technique is more effective at clearing secretions than either technique used alone.

Anterior Chest Compression Assist

The anterior chest compression assist technique can be used only when the patient is in the supine position.

- The therapist puts one arm across the patient's pectoral region to stabilize or compress the upper chest while the other arm is placed either parallel on the lower chest or abdomen or is placed as in the Heimlich-type technique, below the xiphoid process.
- Inspiration is facilitated by the pressure on anterior chest, followed by a "hold."
- Just as the patient is instructed to cough, the therapist applies a quick force with both arms: down and back on the upper chest and up and back on the lower chest or abdomen.

Massery Counterrotation Assist

The Massery counterrotation assist is performed in patients with neurological disorders and spinal stability. The patient is positioned on his or her side, with the knees bent and arms out in front of the head or shoulders.

- The technique is performed as described on page 321 for counterrotation of the trunk to increase ventilation.
- The cough assist is then performed by first giving an accentuated end-expiratory quick compression of the chest (patient into the flexed position) and then shifting hands quickly to perform the extension move as the patient takes a deep breath, which is held briefly at maximum. Finally the therapist shifts hands quickly back to the flexion position to perform a quick and forceful chest compression as the patient gives a strong cough.
- This technique is extremely effective even in patients who are incoherent or unresponsive.

Self-assisted Cough Techniques

There are a number of techniques that patients can be taught to augment their own coughing efforts.

Prone-on-elbows Head-flexion Self-assisted Cough

The prone-on-elbows head-flexion self-assisted cough technique is performed with the patient prone on elbows. Although this technique produces a weaker cough due to inhibition of the diaphragm and lower anterior chest movement, it is one that quadriplegics who have good head and neck control and who can roll independently can perform on their own.

- The patient learns to take in a maximal inspiration while extending the head and neck up and back as far as possible.
- The patient then coughs as forcefully as possible while throwing the head forward and down.
- The pattern can be assisted initially by the therapist to establish the desired moves and gradually progressed to a resisted pattern to strengthen the accessory muscles.

Long-sitting Self-assisted Cough for the Patient With Quadriplegia

The patient performs a self-assisted cough while positioned in a long-sitting posture with arm support. The patient extends the head and body backward while taking a maximal inspiration and then coughs forcefully while throwing the head and upper body forward into a flexed position (Figure 7-12).

Long-sitting Self-assisted Cough for the Patient With Paraplegia

The long-sitting self-assist for the patient with paraplegia is similar to that for the patient with quadriplegia. The exception is that the patient's hands may be placed on the back of the head in a butterfly position and the patient throws the body forward onto the legs during the cough/flexion phase, thereby using both the upper and lower chest. The patient must have good control of the trunk musculature in order to properly and safely perform this technique (Figure 7-13).

Short-sitting Self-assisted Cough

The patient is placed in a short-sitting position (e.g., in a wheelchair or at the side of the bed), with one wrist over the other or grasping each wrist while placing them in their lap. The patient extends the head and trunk backward while taking in a deep breath and then flexes forward and pulls the hands up and under the diaphragm while coughing forcefully (Figure 7-14).

Hands-and-knees Rocking Cough

The patient is on hands and knees and rocks all the way forward while looking up and taking a deep breath. Then the patient coughs with a flexed head while rocking backward to the heels (Figure 7-15).

Standing Self-assisted Coughs

Patients with adequate standing balance and upper extremity support can perform any of the previously described techniques in the standing position using any combination of trunk, head, and extremity movement during the cough and with appropriate modifications for the standing posture.

Mechanical Insufflator–Exsufflator

Mechanical insufflation–exsufflation (MI-E) involves a mechanical device (the CoughAssist insufflator–exsufflator; Respironics, Murrysville, PA) that assists patients in clearing bronchial secretions by mimicking the physiological effects of a cough through

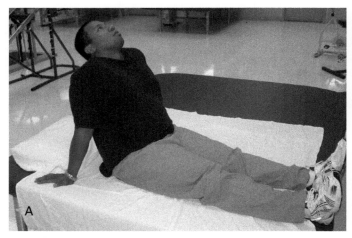
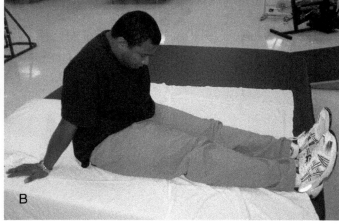

Figure 7-12: Long-sitting self-assisted cough for the patient with quadriplegia. **A,** Inspiration phase. **B,** Expiration, or cough, phase.

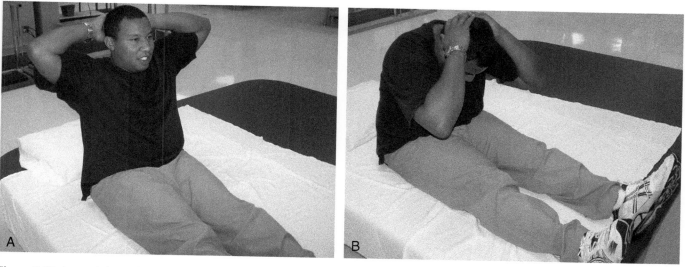

Figure 7-13: Long-sitting self-assisted cough for the patient with paraplegia. **A,** Inspiration phase. **B,** Expiration, or cough, phase.

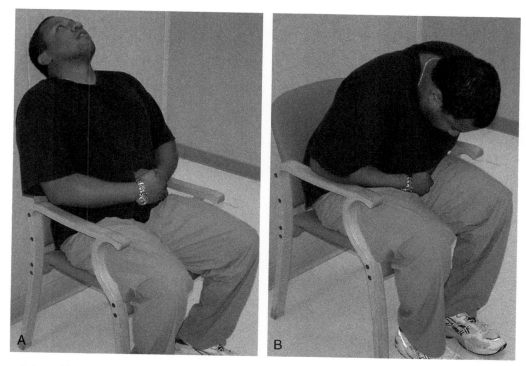

Figure 7-14: Short-sitting self-assisted cough. **A,** Inspiration phase. **B,** Expiration, or cough, phase.

increased peak cough flow.[22] Positive air pressure is delivered into the airways (most often via a face or oronasal mask or connection to an artificial airway), gradually providing a deep inspiration. This is followed by an immediate and abrupt change to negative pressure, which provokes a rapid expiration. The expiratory flow created by the device is usually strong enough to elicit a powerful cough.[37]

- Commonly used in conjunction with other airway clearance techniques in patients with neuromuscular disease and muscle weakness due to central nervous system injury, MI-E treatments consist of about five positive-to-negative pressure cycles followed by 20 to 30 seconds of normal or ventilator breathing. The series is repeated five or more times per session.

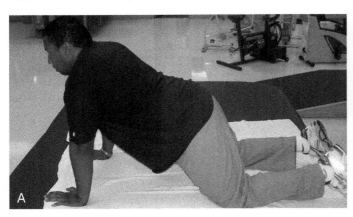 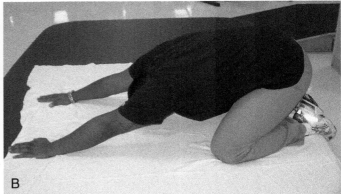

Figure 7-15: Rocking self-assisted cough. **A,** Inspiration phase. **B,** Expiration, or cough, phase.

- During upper respiratory tract infection, patients often perform three or more sessions per day.

MI-E has demonstrated efficacy in mobilizing secretions in patients with neuromuscular disorders, reducing the incidence of nasotracheal suctioning, tracheotomy and invasive mechanical ventilation, and hospitalization, and increasing survival time.[38,46,65,88] It can be safely administered by trained nonprofessional caregivers.

Complications associated with the use of MI-E are rare. They include gastric and abdominal distension (which can be avoided by reducing the insufflation pressure to achieve an inspired volume that is less than the inspiratory reserve volume), aggravation of gastroesophageal reflux, hemoptysis, chest and abdominal discomfort, acute CV effects, and pneumothorax.

EXERCISE FOR AIRWAY CLEARANCE

One of the most effective means of improving secretion clearance is by increasing physical activity. Exercise provokes increases in expiratory flow and minute volume, as well as sympathetic activity, which can lead to an increase in mucociliary clearance. On the basis of improvements in pulmonary function, many practitioners have suggested that exercise of sufficient intensity and duration to increase ventilatory demand may be a substitute for postural drainage and percussion (PD&P) in patients with chronic lung disease, but studies in patients with cystic fibrosis (CF) have not supported this idea.[13,63,85] However, the addition of exercise to other airway clearance techniques significantly increases the amount of sputum that is expectorated and offers other health and quality of life benefits as well.

- In acute care patients, frequent positional changes in bed, sitting at the bedside, out-of-bed activities, and progressive ambulation serve to increase tidal volume, mobilize secretions, and improve cough force. Once patients can tolerate increased activity, they can participate in other rehabilitation activities.
- Hospitalized patients limited to in-room activity only (because of monitors, multiple lines, medications, infection precautions, protective isolation, etc.) can benefit from aerobic training modalities that can be brought to the bedside, such as a stationary bicycle, upper extremity ergometer, or a bedside treadmill, and a variety of resistance training activities.
- Healthier patients at home (those with FEV_1 [forced expiratory volume in 1 s] exceeding 50%–60%, who can walk >250–350 ft in 6 min, and have ≤2/4 dyspnea [see page 283] can follow

the standard recommendations regarding aerobic exercise training previously described (see pages 303–308).
- More limited patients benefit from referral to a pulmonary rehabilitation program.

AIRWAY CLEARANCE TECHNIQUES

A variety of techniques and devices can be used to assist with the mobilization and expulsion of bronchial secretions. Patients most likely to benefit from secretion clearance methods are those with objective signs of secretion retention (e.g., persistent crackles or decreased breath sounds) or subjective signs of difficulty in expectorating secretions, and those with progression of disease that might be due to secretion retention (e.g., recurrent exacerbations or infections or a rapid decline in pulmonary function).[85] Figure 7-16 shows a proposed algorithm for choosing airway clearance techniques.

Conventional chest physical therapy treatments consisting of postural drainage, percussion, and vibration or shaking (again, PDPV for short) have been the most widely used intervention in patients with airway disease and have been shown to be effective in increasing mucus transport and sputum expectoration in appropriate patients, although there are conflicting data.[13,23a,35,63,85] More recently, PDPV has been replaced by alternative airway clearance techniques, many of which can be performed independently by the patient.

Analyses of the research evaluating the various techniques for airway clearance are limited by inadequate sample sizes; in addition, the few studies that have been done involved different patient populations (making the data difficult to compare), and were often poorly designed. Thus the level of evidence for all modalities tends to be low, and studies have failed to identify clearly significant efficacy of one particular technique over the others.[13,63,85] However, it is likely that specific techniques may be more effective in certain circumstances, and future research should focus on this issue.

At present, the best way to measure the clinical effectiveness of an airway clearance technique or combination of techniques is by assessing the patient's subjective preference and the amount of expectorated sputum. This entails an "*n* of 1" study using the various airway clearance modalities to determine which, if any, provide the greatest benefit for each patient.

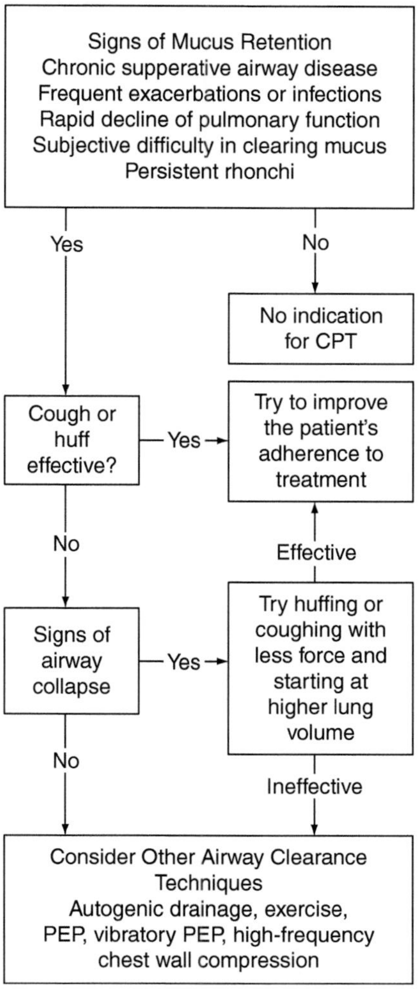

Figure 7-16: Algorithm for choosing airway clearance interventions. Conventional chest physical therapy (postural drainage, percussion, and vibration/shaking) is another airway clearance intervention that can be performed. (From van der Schans CP. Conventional chest physical therapy for obstructive lung disease. *Respir Care* 2007;52:1198–1206.)

Bronchial/Postural Drainage

Bronchial, or postural, drainage consists of positioning the patient according to bronchopulmonary anatomy so that each distinct lung segment is placed with its bronchus perpendicular to gravity. The goal is to facilitate drainage of secretions into the segmental bronchus, from which they can be removed by coughing or suctioning.

- The positions for bronchial drainage of the various segments of the upper, middle, and lower lobes are illustrated in Figure 7-17.
  - However, on the basis of studies documenting detrimental effects of head-down, or Trendelenburg, positions in patients with CF, including hypoxic episodes, aggravation of gastroesophageal reflux, and decreased maximal expiratory pressures and peak expiratory flow rates, many experts recommend modifying PD to eliminate the head-down positions.[13]
  - Fortunately, a study assessing the effects of using these modified positions over a 5-year period in patients with CF has demonstrated improved outcomes.[17]

- Some specific precautions and contraindications related to bronchial drainage are as follows:
  - The head-down position is definitely contraindicated in patients with pulmonary edema, increased intracranial pressure, unstable CV status, aortic aneurysm, recent esophageal anastomosis, untreated pneumothorax, poor diaphragmatic strength, hemoptysis, large pleural effusion, morbid obesity, and ascites and in any patient who becomes agitated or anxious during treatment. However, these patients can often tolerate modified positions with the bed flat or nearly flat and the lower body elevated as tolerated.
  - Caution is also indicated when positioning patients who are recovering from orthopedic surgery, such as total hip replacement or laminectomy, for whom certain movements or positions are to be avoided.
- The procedures involved in positioning patients for bronchial drainage include the following:
  - Explain the treatment to the patient and ask the patient to loosen any tight or binding clothing.
  - Observe any tubes or other equipment connected to the patient, making sure everything has enough slack to allow the positional change without pulling taut or dislodging. Make any required adjustments.
  - Check the pulse, BP, oxygen saturation, respiratory rate, and pain level, as able, before positioning any patient who is critically ill or possibly unstable. Monitor the patient during treatment.
  - If the patient has excessive secretions, have her/him cough or perform suctioning before positioning. Simply moving the patient into the postural drainage position may induce a productive cough.
  - Place the patient in the proper, or modified, position, with assistance from other staff if necessary. Watch for any signs of intolerance.
  - Maintain position for 5 to 20 minutes, depending on the quantity and tenacity of secretions and patient tolerance.
  - Have the patient cough or perform suctioning before changing positions.
  - If several positions are being used, it is best to limit total treatment time to 30 to 40 minutes because of the stress placed on the patient. Always treat the most critical areas first.
  - Encourage the patient to cough periodically after treatment, as some secretions may take 30 to 60 minutes to clear.
- Patients should never be left in the head-down position unsupervised unless they are alert and independent in functional mobility, so that they can reposition themselves or call for assistance if needed.
- Manual techniques, such as percussion and vibration, are usually applied during bronchial drainage to facilitate the mobilization of secretions.

Percussion

Percussion is a treatment technique that consists of rhythmically and alternately striking the chest wall with cupped hands to mechanically jar and dislodge retained secretions in underlying lung segments. The therapist molds her/his hand(s) to fit the contour of the area being treated and applies a force that is appropriate to the individual patient. The hand should be cupped with the

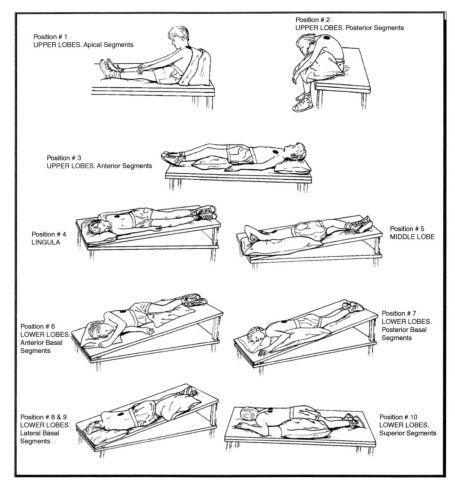

Figure 7-17: Bronchial drainage positions with treatment areas marked for percussion, if provided. (From Cystic Fibrosis Foundation. *Consumer Fact Sheet: An Introduction to Postural Drainage & Percussion,* Figure 4, page 4. Bethesda, Md: Cystic Fibrosis Foundation; 2005.)

fingers and thumb adducted (Figure 7-18) so that a hollow "popping" sound is produced. It is important to keep the wrists "loose" and flexible during the procedure to allow more comfort for both the patient and the therapist.

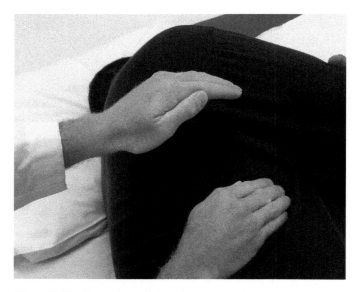

Figure 7-18: Cupped hands for chest percussion.

- Percussion should be performed over a layer of thin cloth such as a hospital gown or T-shirt. A towel will damper most of the force of percussion and drastically reduce the effectiveness of cupping.
- If percussion is painful for the patient, the therapist should ensure proper technique and decrease the amount of force being used so that it is not uncomfortable. Factors that influence the amount of force used are the patient's age and tolerance, condition of the chest, presence of pain, secretion density and amount, and anatomic site. It is not the force but the cupping that is effective.
- Percussion is performed with the patient in the appropriate bronchial drainage position for each segment, although modified positions may be indicated, as stated in the previous section.
  - ▸ Upper lobes
    - ⊙ Apical segments: The patient sits and leans back on pillows against a chair or the therapist at a 60-degree angle; percuss between the clavicle and the top of the scapula on each side.
    - ⊙ Posterior segment of left upper lobe: The patient leans forward over pillows or table at a 30-degree angle; percuss over the upper back on the left.
    - ⊙ Anterior segment of left upper lobe: The patient lies on the back with the head elevated at a 30-degree angle; percuss between the clavicle and the nipple on the left side.

⊙ Anterior segment of right upper lobe: The patient lies flat on the back with the knees on a pillow; percuss between the clavicle and the nipple on the right side.

⊙ Posterior segment of right upper lobe: With the bed flat, the patient lies on the left side, then rolls the right shoulder 45 degrees forward with pillows placed for comfort; percuss over the upper back on the right side.

▶ Right middle lobe and lingula

⊙ Right middle lobe: The patient lies on the left side with the head 15 degrees lower than the hips; the patient then rolls the right shoulder back 45 degrees onto a pillow; percuss over the right nipple area (or just above it on a female).

⊙ Lingular segment of left upper lobe: The patient lies on the right side with the head 15 degrees lower than the hips; the patient then rolls the left shoulder back 45 degrees onto a pillow; percuss over the left nipple area (or just above it on a female).

▶ Lower lobes

⊙ Superior, or apical, segments: The patient lies in a prone flat position with pillow under the hips and ankles for comfort; percuss over mid-back just below the scapula on each side.

⊙ Anterior segments: The patient lies in a supine position with the head 30 degrees lower than the hips; percuss over the lower ribs of each side.

⊙ Lateral segment of right lower lobe: The patient lies on the left side with a pillow between the knees for comfort and the head 30 degrees lower than the hips; percuss over the upper portion of lower ribs on the right side.

⊙ Posterior segments: The patient lies in a prone position with a pillow under the hips and ankles for comfort and the head 30 degrees lower than the hips; percuss over the lower ribs on each side.

⊙ Lateral segment of left lower lobe: The patient lies on the right side with a pillow between the knees for comfort and the head 30 degrees lower than the hips; percuss over the upper portion of the lower ribs on the left side.

- Percussion should be continued for 2 to 5 minutes per lung segment followed by vibration and coughing or suctioning. When chest radiography or clinical assessment reveals a new atelectasis, treatment is continued with repeating cycles of percussion, vibration, and coughing/suction until resolution is clinically apparent (e.g., improved breath sounds, resolution of crackles, return of normal midline position of the trachea) and coughing/suctioning is no longer productive.

- Precautions and contraindications for percussion include the following:

  ▶ Rib fractures or flail chest
  ▶ Osteoporosis
  ▶ Avoidance of bony prominences (clavicle, spine of scapula, spinous processes of the vertebrae) and breast tissue
  ▶ Metastatic cancer to the ribs
  ▶ Recent spinal fusion
  ▶ Unstable cardiovascular status
  ▶ Subcutaneous emphysema of the neck and thorax
  ▶ Fresh burns, open wounds, skin infection in the thoracic area
  ▶ Untreated pneumothorax

  ▶ Resectable tumor
  ▶ Pulmonary embolism
  ▶ Low platelet count ($20–40 \times 10^3/mm^3$, depending on the policies of the physicians and/or facilities) or if excessive erythema is noticed under the area percussed
  ▶ Poor tolerance to the treatment

- Premedication for pain is important in postsurgical patients and others in whom ventilation and cough are limited by discomfort. Allow at least 20 to 30 minutes for analgesics to take effect before initiating treatment. Incisional pain may be reduced by having the patient hold a pillow or rolled towel over the painful site during percussion.

- The therapist should monitor the patient's oxygen saturation, as it may fall during percussion. This can be eliminated by implementing thoracic mobility exercises (as described earlier in this chapter) and pausing for breathing control.[28]

- For patients in whom percussion is contraindicated or poorly tolerated, vibration can usually be used effectively.

Vibration/Shaking/Rib Springing

Vibration consists of gentle, high-frequency oscillations combined with compression of the chest wall produced by tensing all muscles in the upper extremities in co-contraction. Shaking involves more pronounced bouncing chest compressions. A more vigorous form of shaking is termed *rib springing,* in which the ribs are "pumped" in a springing fashion three or four times during exhalation.

Performed during exhalation only, these techniques are purported to achieve more rapid and efficient mobilization of secretions by moving the secretions that were dislodged during percussion toward the larger airways in the bronchial tree, from which they can be expectorated.[28] Vibration increases peak expiratory flow rates (PEFRs) by 50% relative to relaxed expiration, which is greater than that achieved through chest wall compression or chest wall oscillation alone, and can effect a decrease in the viscoelastic properties of mucus.[61]

- The therapist's hand can be placed on both sides of the patient's chest or one hand can be placed on top of the other, depending on therapist preference (Figure 7-19).

- The patient is instructed to take a deep inspiration and then chest compression with vibration/shaking/rib springing is performed throughout exhalation, following the movement of the chest wall. This procedure is repeated for six to eight breaths. For patients with rapid respiratory rates, these maneuvers can be performed on alternate breaths, which may help reduce the breathing rate and allow better therapist coordination with exhalation.

- Patients unable to take a deep breath can be assisted with intermittent positive-pressure breathing or a manual resuscitation bag.

- Caution is indicated when performing vibration and shaking in patients with a stiff, inelastic chest wall or a history of osteoporosis, as the risk of rib fracture is increased with these techniques. Rib springing is contraindicated in these patients as well as in those with rib or spinal fractures, other bone abnormalities involving the chest, or with pain.

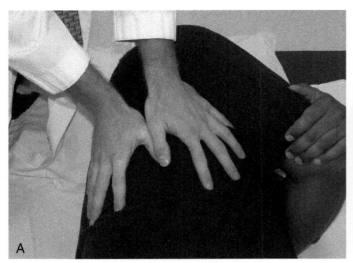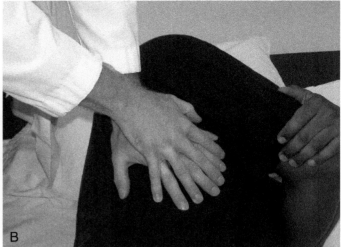

Figure 7-19: Chest vibration with hands positioned on both sides of the chest **(A)** and with one hand placed on top of the other **(B)**.

Manual Hyperinflation

Manual hyperinflation (MH) is a technique used to mobilize pulmonary secretions, reinflate atelectatic alveoli, and increase alveolar oxygenation in patients receiving ventilatory support or who have a tracheostomy. A manual resuscitation bag is used to deliver the MH breaths by one care provider while a second care provider performs vibration or shaking. There are several important factors involved in performing effective MH.[28,57]

- Premedication for pain will improve patient tolerance.
- A larger-than-normal tidal volume (at least 50% greater than baseline tidal volume) should be delivered with a peak inspiratory pressure of 20 to 40 cm H_2O.
- In spontaneously breathing patients, "bag squeezing" should be coordinated with the patient's inspiratory efforts.
- Slow inspiratory flow rates should be used to allow for proper alveolar expansion without excessive peak inspiratory pressure.
- An inspiratory hold should be maintained for 3 to 5 seconds to improve the distribution of ventilation and to promote inflation of atelectatic alveoli.
- A pressure manometer should be used to assist in maintaining proper pressure gradients and to avoid barotrauma due to excessive inspiratory pressures.
- The MH technique is repeated until the patient is able to cough the secretions up through the endotracheal tube or the secretions are sufficiently mobilized that they can be suctioned from the tube (see page 336).
- MH is contraindicated in patients with unstable hemodynamics, pulmonary edema, air leak, and severe bronchospasm

The use of MH has been shown to significantly increase sputum production and peak expiratory flow rates in patients who are intubated and receiving ventilator support.[10]

Active Cycle of Breathing

The active cycle of breathing technique (ACBT) is an airway clearance technique that can be performed independently by the patient after appropriate instruction. It involves a combination of breathing control, thoracic expansion exercises, and FET performed in series and repeated for several cycles.[28,29,63] The patient is instructed to inhale through the nose and exhale through the mouth for each phase. Positioning may be used in order to treat a specific lung region, or the treatment can be performed in the upright sitting position.

- The first phase is the breathing control phase, which consists of relaxed breathing at tidal volume with emphasis on diaphragmatic and lower rib cage expansion. The patient is encouraged to relax the upper chest and shoulders until s/he is relaxed and ready for the next phases, usually 5 to 10 seconds.
- The second phase is the thoracic expansion phase, during which the emphasis is on the patient increasing inspiration up to the inspiratory reserve volume (a maximal inspiration). Expiration is passive and relaxed. The patient should perform three or four deep breaths which may or may not include a 3-second inspiratory hold or a sniff to encourage collateral ventilation for the reexpansion of atelectatic alveoli. In addition, the patient or a care provider can perform percussion or vibration/shaking to the area being treated during expiration to help mobilize secretions.
- The first and second phases are repeated, and then the first phase is repeated once again before advancing to the third phase.
- The third phase consists of the forced expiration technique, which consists of huffing alternating with breathing control (i.e., FET). Huffing is performed at two different volumes: first the patient performs one or two medium-volume huffs to mobilize secretions from the peripheral airways followed by a period of breathing control, and then the patient does a high-volume huff to clear secretions that have reached the larger, proximal airways.
- The cycles are continued until the patient can demonstrate a nonproductive, dry huff from a medium-sized inspiration for two cycles in a row.

ACBT can be performed in cycles that vary in composition according to each patient's specific condition, as illustrated in Figure 7-20. For example, patients with high volumes of mucus production, but without much airway hyperreactivity, atelectasis, or plugging, may benefit from simple ACBT (A), while a patient with significant bronchospasm may require longer periods of

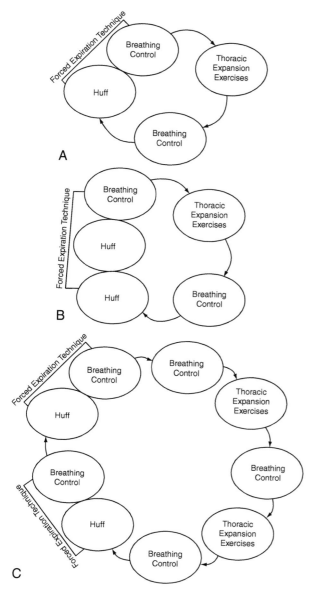

Figure 7-20: Three possible active cycle of breathing routines. See text for explanation of their indications. (From Fink JB. Forced expiratory technique, directed cough, and autogenic drainage. *Respir Care* 2007;52:1210–1221. Discussion 1221–1223.)

breathing control (B), and patients with airway plugging, atelectasis, and some reactive airway disease may benefit more from additional breathing control and thoracic expansion exercises (C).

Several studies have demonstrated that ACBT is as effective as PDPV in improving pulmonary function and airway clearance and is less likely to cause oxygen desaturation.[29,63] In addition, it has been shown to be at least as effective as positive expiratory pressure (PEP), oscillating PEP (Flutter [Axcan Pharma, Mont-Saint-Hilaire, PQ, Canada] or Acapella [Smiths Medical, St. Paul, MN]), and high-frequency chest compressions (HFCCs).[29,73]

Autogenic Drainage

Autogenic drainage (AD) is another form of self-treatment that uses a series of progressive breathing phases to maximize expiratory flow with minimal airway closure, starting with the small

airways and moving secretions from smaller to larger airways in three phases: unsticking, collection, and evacuation.[28,29,51,63] The patient inhales a deep breath through the nose, performs a 2- to 4-second breath hold to allow for collateral ventilation, and then moves mucus by a relaxed sighing exhalation through the mouth, regulating airflow and velocity with the use of the expiratory muscles to avoid unnecessary expiratory resistance. The aim is to maximize expiratory flow.

AD requires intensive training and a great deal of patient cooperation. It should be performed in a quiet room with a minimum of distraction. The patient must learn to determine (through proprioceptive, sensory, and auditory signals) when bronchial secretions are present in the smaller, medium, or larger airways and also how to breathe at low, medium, and high lung volumes for the purpose of mobilizing secretions in those airways, while suppressing the urge to cough in order to avoid collapse of airways.

In performing AD, the patient performs staged breathing at different lung volumes (Figure 7-21):

• The first phase is also known as the unsticking phase. After a brief period of relaxed diaphragmatic or lower chest breathing (inspiring slowly through the nose followed by an inspiratory hold, and then exhaling slowly through the mouth), the patient exhales deeply through the mouth to a low lung volume (within the expiratory reserve volume) and then breathes at a normal low tidal volume at the low lung volume, using the same diaphragmatic breathing pattern except that the abdominal muscles will contract on expiration. This is continued until the patient becomes aware of secretions in the smaller airways (by sensing vibrations through a hand placed on the upper chest and listening for the sound of secretions in the airways at the beginning of expiration), which usually takes 1 to 3 minutes.

• The patient then moves into the second phase, known as the collection phase. Using the same diaphragmatic breathing pattern, the patient slowly increases the depth of inspiration to midlung volume (both inspiratory and expiratory volumes increase) so that secretions are mobilized proximally into the

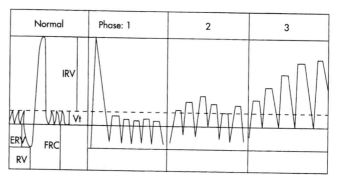

Figure 7-21: Phases of autogenic drainage shown on a spirogram of a normal person. Phase 1, unsticking; phase 2, collection; phase 3, evacuation. ERV, expiratory reserve volume; FRC, functional residual capacity; IRV, inspiratory reserve volume; RV, residual volume; Vᴛ, tidal volume; IRV + Vᴛ + ERV, vital capacity. [From Schoni MH. Autogenic drainage: A modern approach to physiotherapy in cystic fibrosis. *J R Soc Med.* 1989;82(Suppl. 16):32–37.]

medium-sized airways. This is repeated several times until the sound and feel of mucus decrease or move to a more central position, indicating that the secretions have moved into the central airways. This usually takes 2 to 3 minutes.

- At this point the patient enters the third phase, the evacuation phase, during which s/he increases breathing to higher lung volumes (within the inspiratory reserve volume), approaching maximal inspiration. This continues until the secretions move into the trachea and are ready to be expectorated by a stronger exhalation or a high-volume huff. Repeat huffs until no more secretions can be expectorated. This phase typically takes 2 to 3 minutes and completes one cycle of AD totaling 6 to 9 minutes.
- After a 1- to 2-minute break, using relaxed diaphragmatic breathing, the cycles are repeated until all mucus has been cleared.
- Important points to note regarding AD include the following:
- The velocity of the airflow must be controlled at each phase so that it is as high as possible without being so high as to provoke airway collapse or coughing. If wheezing develops, the expiratory flow rate should be reduced. If coughing becomes unavoidable, the patient should perform two or three huffs.
- The duration of each phase of AD depends on the location of the patient's secretions.
- AD is usually performed twice per day, with each session taking an average of 30 to 45 minutes, depending on the total amount and viscosity of the secretions.

AD is reported to be at least as effective as PDPV and PEP with respect to sputum production and has a low risk of oxygen desaturation or bronchospasm.[29,63,85] AD is also as effective as PDPV at maintaining pulmonary function over a 1-year period, and many patients prefer it to PDPV. Studies comparing AD with ACBT have shown conflicting results, with some stating the superiority of AD and others finding no significant difference.[29,63]

Positive Expiratory Pressure

Positive expiratory pressure (PEP) therapy entails breathing through a mouthpiece or face mask fitted with an expiratory resistor and a manometer.[29,51,67] The patient breathes through the one-way valve with inspiration unimpeded and exhales against a back pressure, which is adjusted to the desired level with the manometer. During the long exhalation against positive pressure, peripheral airways are stabilized while collateral ventilation is promoted distal to retained secretions and aids in their mobilization into larger airways.

PEP can be performed against low or high pressure. Low-PEP involves tidal volume inspirations and slightly active expirations against pressures of 5 to 20 cm H_2O, whereas high-PEP uses high lung volumes and forced expiratory maneuvers against much higher pressure (producing an FVC greater than that produced with no PEP, usually 26–102 cm H_2O).[67] The commercially available standard PEP device is TheraPEP (Smiths Medical), although it is possible to construct a bubble PEP device, which is particularly useful when treating children (see reference 28).

- For PEP therapy the patient sits upright with arms resting on a table. S/he begins with normal tidal volume diaphragmatic or lower chest breaths through the PEP device with a 2- to 4-second

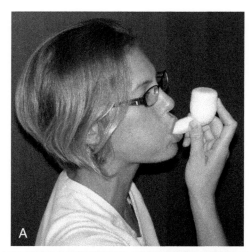

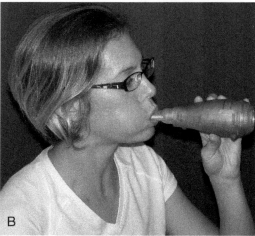

Figure 7-22: Patient using oscillatory positive expiratory pressure (PEP) devices. **A,** The Flutter; **B,** the Acapella.

inspiratory hold. Aerosolized medications can be administered during this portion of the PEP cycle.
- For low-PEP, the patient then takes in a larger than normal breath (but not to total lung capacity) and performs a slightly active exhalation (using abdominals but not forced) through the PEP device, which lasts three to four times as long as inspiration. The patient performs 10 to 15 of these breaths at a normal respiratory rate.
- For high-PEP, the patient breathes in and out through the device at tidal volume for 6 to 10 breaths and then takes in a maximal inspiration followed by a forced expiratory maneuver.
- The PEP device is then removed and the patient performs several huffs and/or coughs to mobilize and remove secretions.
- The cycle should be repeated four to six times so that the entire session takes 10 to 20 minutes. It is recommended that the patient perform at least two PEP sessions per day, or more during acute exacerbations.

Oscillatory, or *vibratory, PEP (OPEP)* combines the benefits of PEP with airway vibrations or oscillations, which reportedly reduce the viscoelastic properties of mucus so that it is easier to mobilize and create short bursts of increased expiratory airflow that assist in mobilizing secretions up the airways.

There are three commercially available OPEP devices: the Acapella, Flutter, and Quake (Thayer Medical, Tucson, AZ). However, all studies evaluating OPEP have used the Flutter valve.

- The Flutter is a handheld device shaped like a pipe, which contains a high-density steel ball that sits in a circular cone inside the bowl of the "pipe" (Figure 7-22). The cover over the ball has perforations that allow expiratory airflow to pass through the device, causing the ball to rise and fall within the cone. This creates an intermittent PEP of 5 to 35 cm H_2O and airflow pulsations throughout the airways. The pressure and frequency of the oscillations can be altered by changing the angle of the device: Tilting the Flutter upward increases the pressure and frequency whereas tilting the device downward results in lower pressure and frequency. Palpation of the chest can provide feedback regarding the optimal angle of the device (that which generates the greatest amount of airway vibration).

- The Acapella uses a counterweighted plug and magnet to create airflow oscillations during expiration and comes in three models (see Figure 7-22). Its operation is not affected by gravity, and therefore it can be used more easily in nonupright positions.

- The Quake device has a manually operated rotating handle that creates the oscillations, with the oscillation frequency being determined by how quickly the handle is turned. Rotating the handle slowly creates low-frequency oscillations and a higher pulsatile expiratory pressure, whereas rotating the handle quickly provides faster oscillations and a lower pulsatile expiratory pressure. Usually the handle is rotated at a steady rate of one to two turns per second during exhalation.

OPEP is performed in a similar manner as PEP:

- The Flutter is used while taking 5 to 15 deep (but not maximal) inspirations with an inspiratory hold followed by long, "mucus-mobilizing" exhalations (reasonably fast but not too forceful speed and not fully emptying the lungs) through the device, during which any coughing is suppressed. The patient then performs two forceful "mucus-removing" expirations through the Flutter, with cough allowed as the urge arises.

- The Acapella protocol recommends 10 to 20 breaths as described for the Flutter, before the device is removed for high-volume huffs and/or coughs.

Analyses of the research evaluating PEP and OPEP are limited by relatively small sample sizes and the small number of studies that involved different patient populations. However, the general consensus is that both PEP and OPEP appear to improve pulmonary function status and facilitate secretion removal to a similar degree as PDPV and other airway clearance techniques, with high-PEP possibly being more effective than low-PEP.[13,23b,51,67,85] There does not appear to be any difference between PEP and OPEP in terms of patient outcomes, with the possible exception of transient blood gas changes.[67] Patients tend to prefer PEP to PDPV because of its convenience and shorter treatment time.

High-frequency Chest Wall Compression

High-frequency chest wall compression (HFCWC) is another form of self-administered airway clearance therapy that is accomplished by encasing the chest in an inflatable vest, which is attached by hoses to an air-pulse generator, as shown in Figure 7-23. Small

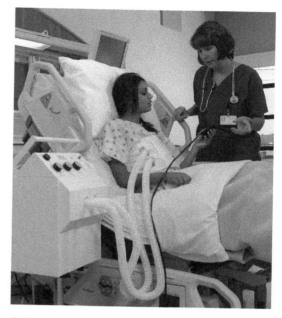

Figure 7-23: Patient using The Vest Airway Clearance System for high-frequency chest wall compression (HFCWC). (Courtesy Hill-Rom, Batesville, IN.)

amounts of air/gas are injected and withdrawn at a rapid rate, and the resultant repeated pressure pulses loosen secretions and move them from the peripheral to the central airways to be expectorated.[21,28,38,51] Popular HFCWC systems currently on the market include The Vest airway clearance system (formerly the ThAIRapy vest) (Hill-Rom, Batesville, IN), and the MedPulse respiratory vest system (Electromed, New Prague, MN).

- The patient sits upright in a chair with the HFCWC vest fitted comfortably around the chest and connected to the air-pulse generator. The patient turns the device on and off by a hand or foot control.

- The patient progresses from low (5 to 10 Hz) to medium (10 to 14 Hz) and then high (15 to 20 Hz) frequencies, spending 5 to 10 minutes at each frequency with the time periods varying on the basis of patient tolerance and amount of secretions. The total treatment time is usually about 30 minutes.

- After the 5- to 10-minute treatment time at each frequency, the patient is instructed to breathe deeply and huff and/or cough to clear loosened secretions.

HFCWC has been shown to be at least as effective, if not more so, than PDPV in mobilizing secretions and maintaining pulmonary function in patients with CF, although the level of evidence is low (as with all the other airway clearance techniques).[21,38,51,85] Its disadvantages include the size and significant cost of the equipment.

High-frequency chest wall oscillation (HFCWO) involves the use of a rigid chest cuirass, rather than an inflatable vest, connected to an air compressor that can deliver both positive and negative pressures to the chest wall. This allows greater control over inspiratory and expiratory flow ratios, which is theorized to optimize mucus clearance.[21] The only HFCWO device available is the Hayek RTX biphasic cuirass ventilatory system (United Hayek Medical, London, UK), but its efficacy for airway clearance has yet to be documented.

Intrapulmonary Percussive Ventilation

Intrapulmonary percussive ventilation (IPV) is a patient-controlled, pneumatic, oscillating-pressure breathing device that loosens secretions by internally percussing the airways with high-frequency bursts of gas at 100 to 300 cycles/min delivered through a mouthpiece.[21,28,38,51] During inspiration these high-frequency gas pulses, which oscillate between 5 and 35 cm H_2O, expand the lungs, vibrate and enlarge the airways, and deliver gas into distal lung units beyond retained secretions. Available devices include the Percussionator (Percussionaire Corp, Sandpoint, ID), the Breas IMP2 (Breas Medical, Mölnlycke, Sweden), and the PercussiveNeb (also known as the P-Neb; VORTRAN Medical Technology, Sacramento, CA), the first two of which can be used with a ventilator. Aerosolized bronchodilators and mucolytics can be delivered in line during IPV treatment.

- The patient breathes through the mouthpiece or face mask at a comfortable rate, receiving aerosolized medications if prescribed.
- The patient then presses the thumb control to trigger 15 to 25 high-frequency pulses of gas during a passive prolonged inspiration lasting 5 to 10 seconds.
- At the end of inspiration, the patient releases the thumb control to allow passive expiration through the device.
- When the patient feels the need to cough, the patient releases the control to stop the percussion and removes the mouthpiece or mask to expectorate mucus.
- The patient gradually increases the percussive amplitude during the treatment to raise the mobilized secretions.
- Treatment usually takes 15 to 20 minutes.

IPV appears to be as effective as PDPV and HFCWC in patients with CF and has been used effectively in burn centers where PDPV may not be appropriate.[38] One study has shown that treatment with IPV is successful in significantly increasing Pao_2 and decreasing respiratory rate, $Paco_2$, and length of stay in patients with an acute exacerbation of COPD.[87]

Suctioning

Suctioning is indicated if a patient is unable to clear secretions through coughing or other maneuvers. Because it is an invasive procedure with significant risk, suctioning must be performed with care and caution. Suctioning should be performed under the supervision of an experienced clinician until competency is developed.

- Preparation
  - Check that the suction apparatus is connected and functioning properly. When the suction is turned on the vacuum level should be set between 80 and 150 mm Hg.[24]
  - Make sure the oxygen flow is connected properly, turned on, and attached to the self-inflating breathing bag.
  - Position the patient properly unless contraindicated: Nasotracheal and pharyngeal suctioning are usually performed with the patient in the semi-Fowler position with the patient's neck hyperextended; patients with a tracheostomy or endotracheal tube are suctioned in the supine position.
  - Have water-soluble lubricant available if performing nasotracheal suctioning.
  - Lay out the sterile field containing gloves, catheter, and container for sterile water. Put on protective eyewear.

- Fill the container with sterile water and attach the catheter to suction. Squeeze out lubricant onto the sterile field, if needed. Put on the gloves, using sterile technique.
- Preoxygenation
  - Hyperventilate the patient with 100% oxygen, using a self-inflating breathing bag attached to a mask or artificial airway connector. If the patient is receiving mechanical ventilation the nurse or respiratory therapist can increase the fraction of inspired oxygen (Fio_2) to 100% for the patient. This should be performed for 1 minute before suctioning.
- Lavage (optional)
  - Introduce 5 mL of sterile normal saline solution (NaCl) directly into the endotracheal or tracheostomy tube. The saline solution will make the secretions less viscous and therefore easier to extract. This step is best used on patients who are sedated or have a weak voluntary cough.
- Suction (using sterile technique throughout):
  - Wet the catheter in the sterile water or with the water-soluble lubricant as appropriate.
  - Using the "sterile" hand, insert the catheter (with no suction applied) into the airway until resistance is met or until a reflex cough is triggered. Caution should be used when nasotracheal suctioning is being performed; the potential for trauma to the nasal passage is significant and should be performed only if there is no other way to suction the patient.
  - Pull the catheter back slightly and then withdraw the catheter in a twirling motion while applying suction with the "nonsterile" hand. This should not take longer than 5 to 10 seconds. Be sure to keep the "sterile" hand on the part of the catheter that is passed into the patient and the "nonsterile" hand on the equipment that is external to the patient.
  - Closely monitor the patient and maintain oxygen saturation at 90% or more during the procedure. If the oxygen saturation drops below 90% the patient will need to be reoxygenated before continuing.
  - Reoxygenate the patient with 100% oxygen after suctioning.
  - Clean secretions from the catheter by suctioning some of the sterile water.
  - Repeat the process as necessary until there are no more secretions.
  - Suction the nasal and/or oral pharynges.
- Postsuction
  - The patient should be reassured and positioned comfortably.
  - If open system suctioning is performed, the patient should be reconnected to the ventilator or previous level of equipment.
  - Potential complications associated with suctioning include significant hypoxia, arrhythmias, hypotension, and tissue trauma. Proper technique minimizes the risk of morbidity.

Outcome measures that are useful in documenting the effects of treatment techniques aimed at improving secretion clearance include measurement of sputum production and changes in pulmonary function, chest x-ray, arterial blood gases, breath sounds, and ventilator settings.

7.7 IMPAIRED ABILITY TO PROTECT AIRWAY

Patients with altered level of consciousness or bulbar muscle weakness or paralysis frequently develop pulmonary complications as a result of aspiration. In patients with a high risk of aspiration, airway clearance techniques are often used prophylactically (PT preferred practice pattern 6C).[7] Oral suctioning may be used in patients who have had a stroke as they are more prone to dysphagia, or difficulty swallowing, and will exhibit a cough as a defense mechanism to remove any aspirated contents.[58] These patients should be referred to a speech therapist and placed on a swallowing program to teach them the proper swallowing mechanisms and thus improve cognition of the process and retrain the musculature.[53] Patients with repeated episodes of aspiration pneumonia often require a tracheostomy.

7.8 INCREASED WORK OF BREATHING

All the previously presented pulmonary problems serve to increase the work of breathing (PT preferred practice pattern 6C–6F).[7] The physical therapy techniques already described will succeed in reducing the work of breathing if they are effective in treating the causative problem(s). Other treatment options include instruction in controlling the breathing pattern (i.e., breathing retraining), dyspnea positioning, and relaxation techniques, as well as energy conservation/work simplification techniques (see Tables 7-8 and 7-9).

BREATHING PATTERN CONTROL

Patients with increased work of breathing will benefit from learning to maintain an uninterrupted breathing pattern, particularly during exertion or episodes of dyspnea. Prevention of overbreathing is especially important in patients with asthma and COPD. Avoidance of breath holding or the Valsalva maneuver and unnecessary talking is also important.

Breathing retraining teaches patients specific breathing strategies (see Diaphragmatic Breathing Exercises and Pursed-lip Breathing on pages 315 and 316) that can be used to help them regain control of their breathing and reduce its energy cost. It is postulated that by slowing the respiratory rate and eliminating excessive accessory muscle activity, especially during exertion, the oxygen available to other tissues can be increased. This procedure, however, is controversial in many circumstances, because it has been documented that patients with both obstructive and restrictive lung disease naturally assume a breathing pattern that requires the least energy and delays respiratory muscle fatigue.[48]

Instruction in the *coordination of breathing* with various activities is helpful for patients:

- Inspiration should be performed with trunk extension, shoulder flexion, abduction, and external rotation movements, and with an upward eye gaze.
- Expiration should occur with trunk flexion, shoulder extension, adduction, and internal rotation movements, and with a downward eye gaze.
- Each patient's natural patterns of movements should be assessed during dynamic activities, such as rolling, coming to sit from supine, and dressing, to determine whether s/he tends to move with trunk extension or flexion, and then the appropriate breathing coordination should be reinforced with the patient.
- Coming to stand typically involves both flexion and extension. The initial rocking motions provide a great opportunity to teach breath control, with expiration during the forward rock and inspiration during the backward rock. Then, as the patient extends to stand, the patient takes in a good deep breath while extending the neck and gazing upward. Returning to sit should be coordinated with a slow, controlled exhalation, such as with pursed lips or while counting out loud.
- By teaching and reinforcing these patterns of coordinated breathing, breath holding and the Valsalva maneuver are avoided.

Paced breathing is the volitional coordination of breathing with activity, which is often taught to patients with COPD as they master diaphragmatic breathing or pursed-lip breathing. As patients perform rhythmic activities, they learn to coordinate their breathing rhythm with the rhythm of the activity, thus discouraging breath holding and encouraging a more optimal inspiratory-to-expiratory ratio (typically 1:2 or 1:4 as expiration is prolonged). Alternatively, paced breathing during nonrhythmic activities usually refers to the coordination of breathing with activity by having the patient inhale just before movement and then exhaling during exertion.

The goal is to increase the patient's control over breathing, through slowing of the respiratory rate, and thereby decrease the work of breathing and level of dyspnea, as well as the level of anxiety when dyspnea occurs. It is hoped that the patient will then be less fearful of activity. Theoretically, a conscious slowing of breathing during paced breathing should allow sufficient time for lung deflation before the next inspiration is initiated, thereby reducing the dynamic hyperinflation that often occurs during activity in these patients.

POSITIONING TO RELIEVE DYSPNEA

Patients with severe COPD often have flattened diaphragms and stiff, barrel-shaped chests, whereas patients with severe restrictive lung dysfunction have reduced pulmonary compliance. In both cases their pathologies lead to ventilatory impairments that adversely affect gas exchange. To compensate, they exert more effort toward breathing, often by recruiting their accessory muscles, and are more likely to experience dyspnea, especially during activity.

The "professorial position" is a common position assumed by patients who are experiencing difficulty breathing. The patient leans forward at the hips with hands or forearms placed on a fixed object (similar to a professor standing and leaning forward on a lectern during a lecture). Such positions serve to fix the distal attachments of the pectoralis major muscles so that they work in "reverse" action to lift the upper chest and thus increase ventilation and reduce the cost of breathing. In addition, leaning forward in the sitting position or while upright further assists the patient with COPD by increasing the intraabdominal pressure and pushing the diaphragm up into the thorax for a more optimal position for contraction.[80] Positions that incorporate one or both of these strategies are illustrated in Figure 7-24 and include the following:

- Sitting and leaning forward with the elbows and upper body supported on a table (Figure 7-24, *A*)
- Sitting and leaning forward so that the elbows or forearms are supported by the knees or thighs (Figure 7-24, *B*)

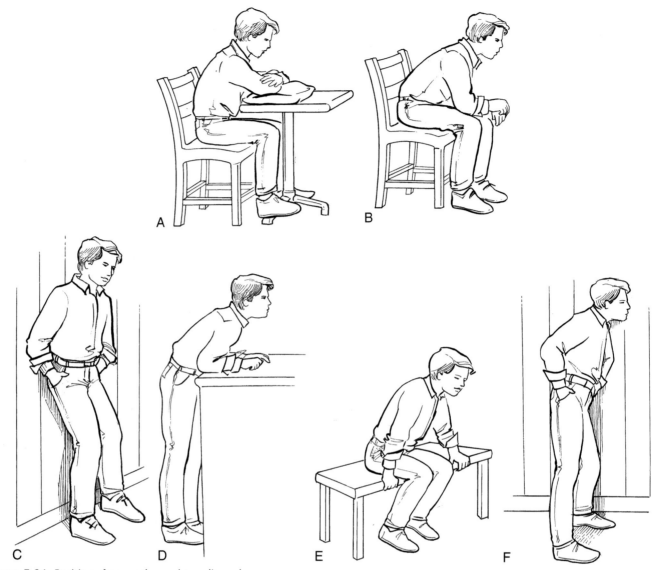

Figure 7-24: Positions frequently used to relieve dyspnea.

- Standing and leaning forward with the arms supported on a countertop, table, or other structure (i.e., the "professorial position") or on a wall (Figure 7-24, *C* and *D*)
- Leaning back against a wall or other structure with the spine straight and supported so that the neck and shoulders are relaxed and the hips are slightly flexed; in addition, hands can be placed in pockets or hooked into the waistband or belt loops to support the upper extremities (Figure 7-24, *E*)
- Resting the forearms on a shopping cart or a tall wheeled walker during ambulation (Figure 7-24, *F*)

ENERGY CONSERVATION/WORK SIMPLIFICATION TECHNIQUES

Patients with increased work of breathing benefit from instruction in energy conservation and work simplification techniques. Simplifying tasks helps to reduce the energy cost of various activities and increases the efficiency of effort that is expended, as previously described on page 311.

RELAXATION TECHNIQUES

Patients with severe lung disease tend to be anxious and tense and often worry about their next breath. Unfortunately, this tension compounds their respiratory problems by tightening the chest wall and spine and increasing their energy expenditure. Several techniques are available that can help patients achieve a more relaxed state: Jacobsen's progressive relaxation, biofeedback, yoga, transcendental meditation, hypnosis, Benson's relaxation response, chest mobilization, and guided imagery or visualization. All include relaxed positioning in a quiet, comfortable atmosphere.

- Jacobsen's progressive relaxation exercises consist of sequentially tightening the various groups of muscles as strongly as possible and then completely releasing the tension. In applying these techniques to pulmonary patients, attention is specifically focused on the upper chest, neck, shoulder, and abdominal muscles in order to improve ventilation.
- Biofeedback uses physiological measurements to train voluntary control of autonomic responses such as HR, BP, and

muscle tension. For pulmonary patients the electrical activity of the muscles of the upper chest, neck, shoulders, and abdomen is selected for monitoring in order to teach individuals to recognize their activity and gain control over them.

- Yoga is a form of exercise consisting of slow stretching and bending into different positions without strain or discomfort, and then holding that position for a period of time before releasing it as slowly as it was assumed. Breathing exercises are also included to increase the relaxation response.
- Transcendental meditation (TM) is an advanced form of autogenic relaxation in which concentration on a specific word or phrase, called a *mantra,* is silently repeated to quiet the body and still the mind. TM is usually performed for 15 to 20 minutes twice a day.
- Hypnosis involves the use of a somewhat altered level of consciousness to achieve a relaxed state. In addition, patients can be given suggestions that help them accomplish specific goals, such as smoking cessation.
- Benson's relaxation response is elicited by four important elements: a quiet environment, a mental device as a constant stimulus (e.g., a repeated word), a passive attitude, and decreased muscle tone related to a comfortable position that requires minimal work to maintain.
- Chest mobilization through rhythmic exercise involving the arms, trunk, and the lower extremities can also serve to promote relaxation. Soft flowing music can be used to increase the sense of relaxation.
- Finally, guided imagery, or visualization, is a process that evokes mentally many senses to create detailed images, or daydreams, that assist an individual to relax. One of the more common images is one of walking to a beautiful, happy, and peaceful spot that becomes synonymous with a relaxing and rejuvenating escape, where all of an individual's worries and tensions are let go and the individual feels free.

Outcome measures that can be used to document the efficacy of techniques for reducing the work of breathing include improved pattern or control of breathing, respiratory rate, dyspnea scores, vocalization, quality of life and activity status measures, functional health status questionnaires, and functional timed walk tests.

 ## 7.9 SUMMARY

This chapter has presented the various interventions used by physical therapists in the treatment of patients with CV and pulmonary dysfunction. A problem-oriented approach was employed so that PTs can use appropriate treatment techniques for any patient experiencing one or more of the described problems, regardless of the referral diagnosis. Some are so simple that any clinician can address them, given an awareness of need (e.g., encouraging cough following changes of position and rehabilitation activities), and others are routinely used by therapists in all areas of practice (e.g., endurance exercise training). PTs should attempt to incorporate an evidence-based approach so that treatment interventions are more likely to be successful. The most important points are reviewed here:

- Impaired exercise tolerance is a common problem of patients with a wide variety of chronic diseases. Endurance exercise training becomes an important component of their treatment

programs because of its effectiveness in increasing exercise tolerance, improving respiratory muscle strength and endurance, facilitating relaxation, and complementing other treatment interventions.

- ▶ To be effective, safe, and enjoyable, careful attention must be directed toward creating an appropriate, individualized exercise prescription, including the proper mode(s), duration, frequency, and intensity. The various principles of training, rate of progression, and compliance factors must also be considered.
- ▶ Patient education regarding the components of their exercise prescription, principles of training, warning signs for overexertion, safe methods of progressing exercise, and compliance factors is important to ensure successful outcomes when treating patients with cardiopulmonary dysfunctions.
- ▶ The individual's physiological responses to exercise should be monitored at least initially to maximize both safety and effectiveness. The goal is for the individual to become independent in self-monitoring techniques.
- ▶ Rating of perceived exertion is a simple yet reliable means of monitoring exercise intensity and is effective for many individuals, particularly those with chronic diseases or who take medications that affect HR.
- ▶ Physiological benefits of exercise training have been documented for both healthy individuals and those with cardiac disease (see Table 7-4) and other chronic medical problems.
- Some individuals are so debilitated that it is difficult for them to perform the daily activities required for independent living.
- ▶ In addition to functional training and aerobic and resistance exercise, these individuals benefit from instruction in energy conservation and work simplification techniques.
- ▶ For patients receiving treatment in a rehabilitation center, some physical therapy activities may be too demanding for their level of tolerance and therefore require modification. Recommended treatment modifications are listed in Box 7-3.
- Patients with pulmonary disease may require a number of other physical therapy treatment interventions to improve ventilation (e.g., breathing exercises, thoracic mobility exercises, respiratory muscle training, and airway clearance techniques), oxygenation (e.g., pursed-lip breathing), and secretion clearance (e.g., coughing, physical exercise, airway clearance techniques, and suctioning), and to reduce the work of breathing (e.g., breathing retraining, positioning, relaxation techniques, and energy conservation and work simplification training).

REFERENCES

1. Alonso J, Permanyer-Miralda G, Cascant P, et al. Measuring functional status of chronic coronary patients: reliability, validity and responsiveness to clinical change of the reduced version of the Duke Activity Status Index (DASI). *Eur Heart J.* 1997;18(3):414-419.
2. American Association of Cardiovascular and Pulmonary Rehabilitation. *Guidelines for Cardiac Rehabilitation and Secondary Prevention Programs.* 4th ed. Champaign, IL: Human Kinetics; 2004.
3. American Association of Cardiovascular and Pulmonary Rehabilitation. *Guidelines for Pulmonary Rehabilitation Prevention Programs.* 3rd ed. Champaign, IL: Human Kinetics; 2004.
4. American College of Sports Medicine. *ACSM's Guidelines for Exercise Testing and Prescription.* 7th ed. Philadelphia: Lippincott Williams & Williams; 2006.

5. American College of Sports Medicine. Position stand. Appropriate intervention strategies for weight loss and prevention of weight regain for adults. *Med Sci Sports Exerc.* 2001;33:2145-2156.

6. Arena R, Humphrey R, Peberdy MA. Using the Duke Activity Status Index in heart failure. *J Cardiopulm Rehab.* 2002;22:93-95.

7. American Physical Therapy Association preferred practice patterns: Cardiovascular/pulmonary. In *Guide to Physical Therapist Practice.* 2nd ed. *Phys Ther.* 2001;81:S463-S520.

8. Barr RN. Pulmonary rehabilitation. In: Hillegass EA, Sadowsky HS, eds. *Essentials of Cardiopulmonary Physical Therapy.* 2nd ed. Philadelphia: W.B. Saunders; 2001.

9. Balaguer A, Escribano J, Roqué M. Infant position in neonates receiving mechanical ventilation. *Cochrane Database Syst Rev.* 2006;4:CD003668.

10. Berney S, Denehy L, Pretto J. Head-down tilt and manual hyperinflation enhance sputum clearance in patients who are intubated and ventilated. *Austr J Physiother.* 2004;50:9-14.

11. Blair SN, Kohl HW, Paffenbarger RS, et al. Physical fitness and all-cause mortality: a prospective study of healthy men and women. *JAMA.* 1989;262:2395-2401.

12. Borg GA. Psychophysical bases of perceived exertion. *Med Sci Sports Exerc.* 1982;14:377-387.

12a. Boulé NG, Kenny GP, Hadad E, et al. Meta-analysis of the effect of structured exercise training on cardiorespiratory fitness in Type 2 diabetes mellitus. *Diabetologia.* 2003;1071-1081.

13. Bradley JM, Moran FM, Elborn JS. Evidence for physical therapies (airway clearance and physical training) in cystic fibrosis: an overview of five Cochrane systematic reviews. *Respir Med.* 2006;100:191-201.

13a. Braith RW, Stewart KJ. Resistance exercise training: its role in the prevention of cardiovascular disease. *Circulation.* 2006;113:2642-2650.

14. Breiburg AN, Aitken L, Reaby L, et al. Efficacy and safety of prone positioning for patients with acute respiratory distress syndrome. *J Adv Nurs.* 2000;32:922-929.

15. Bruton A, Lewith GT. The Buteyko breathing technique for asthma: a review. *Complement Ther Med.* 2005;13:41-46.

16. Budweiser S, Moertl M, Jörres RA, et al. Respiratory muscle training in restrictive thoracic disease: a randomized controlled trial. *Arch Phys Med Rehabil.* 2006;87:1559-1565.

17. Button BM, Heine RG, Catto-Smith AG, et al. Chest physiotherapy in infants with cystic fibrosis. *Arch Dis Child.* 1997;76:148-150.

18. Cahalin LP, Braga M, Matsuo Y, et al. Efficacy of diaphragmatic breathing in persons with chronic obstructive pulmonary disease: a review of the literature. *J Cardiopulm Rehab.* 2002;22:7-21.

19. Carter R, Holiday DB, Grouthues C, et al. Criterion validity of the Duke Activity Status Index for assessing functional capacity in patients with chronic obstructive pulmonary disease. *J Cardiopulm Rehab.* 2002;22: 298-303.

20. Chang AB. Cough, cough receptors, and asthma in children. *Pediatr Pulmonol.* 1999;28(1):59-70.

21. Chatburn RL. High-frequency assisted airway clearance. *Respir Care.* 2007;52:1224-1235.

22. Chatwin M, Ross E, Hart N, et al. Cough augmentation with mechanical insufflation/exsufflation in patients with neuromuscular weakness. *Eur Respir J.* 2003;21:502-508.

23. Chiang LL, Wang LY, Wu CP, et al. Effects of physical training on functional status in patients with prolonged mechanical ventilation. *Phys Ther.* 2006;86:1271-1281.

23a. Ciesla ND. Chest physical therapy for patients in the intensive care unit. *Phys Ther.* 1996;76:609-625.

23b. Darbee JC, Ohtake PJ, Grant BJB, et al. Physiologic evidence for the efficacy of positive expiratory pressure as an airway clearance technique in patients with cystic fibrosis. *Phys Ther.* 2004;84:524-537.

24. Day T, Farnell S, Haynes S, et al. Tracheal suctioning: an exploration of nurses' knowledge and competence in acute and high dependency ward areas. *J Adv Nurs.* 2002;39(1):35-45.

25. Dean E. Body positioning. In: Frownfelter D, Dean E, eds. *Cardiovascular and Pulmonary Physical Therapy: Evidence and Practice.* 4th ed. St. Louis: Mosby; 2006.

26. Dechman G, Wilson CR. Evidence underlying breathing retraining in people with stable chronic obstructive pulmonary disease. *Phys Ther.* 2004; 84(12):1189-1197.

27. Dishman RK. *Exercise Adherence: Its Impact on Public Health.* Champaign, IL: Human Kinetics; 1988.

28. Downs AM. Clinical application of airway clearance techniques. In: Frownfelter D, Dean E, eds. *Cardiovascular and Pulmonary Physical Therapy: Evidence and Practice.* 4th ed. St. Louis: Mosby; 2006.

29. Fink JB. Forced expiratory technique, directed cough, and autogenic drainage. *Respir Care.* 2007;52:1210-1221, Discussion 1221-1223.

30. Fletcher GF, Balady GJ, Amsterdam ES, et al. Exercise standards for testing and training: a statement for healthcare professionals from the American Heart Association. *Circulation.* 2001;104:1694-1740.

31. Frownfelter D, Massery M. Body mechanics—the art of positioning and moving patients. In: Frownfelter D, Dean E, eds. *Cardiovascular and Pulmonary Physical Therapy: Evidence and Practice.* 4th ed. St. Louis: Mosby; 2006.

32. Frownfelter D, Massery M. Facilitating airway clearance with coughing techniques. In: Frownfelter D, Dean E, eds. *Cardiovascular and Pulmonary Physical Therapy: Evidence and Practice.* 4th ed. St. Louis: Mosby; 2006.

33. Frownfelter D, Massery M. Facilitating ventilation patterns and breathing strategies. In: Frownfelter D, Dean E, eds. *Cardiovascular and Pulmonary Physical Therapy: Evidence and Practice.* 4th ed. St. Louis: Mosby; 2006.

34. Gardner AW, Montgomery PS, Flinn WR, et al. The effect of exercise intensity on the response to exercise rehabilitation in patients with intermittent claudication. *J Vasc Surg.* 2005;2(4):702-709.

35. Garrod R, Lasserson T. Role of physiotherapy in the management of chronic lung diseases: an overview of systematic reviews. *Respir Med.* 2007;101:2429-2436.

36. Gigliotti F, Romagnoli I, Scano G. Breathing retraining and exercise conditioning in patients with chronic obstructive pulmonary disease (DOPD): a physiological approach. Review. *Respir Med.* 2003;97:197-204.

37. Gomez-Merino E, Sancho J, Marin J, et al. Mechanical insufflation-exsufflation: pressure, volume and flow relationships and the adequacy of the manufacturer's guidelines. *Am J Phys Med Rehabil.* 2002;81(8):579-583.

38. Haas CF, Loik PF, Gay SE. Airway clearance applications in the elderly and in patients with neurologic or neuromuscular compromise. *Respir Care.* 2007;52:1362-1381.

39. Hagberg JM, Mountain SJ, Martin WH, et al. Effects of exercise training on 60–69 year old essential hypertensives. *Am J Cardiol.* 1989;64: 348-353.

40. Hart N, Laffont I, Perez de La Sota A, et al. Respiratory effects of combined truncal and abdominal support in patients with spinal cord injury. *Arch Phys Med Rehabil.* 2005;86(7):1447-1451.

41. Haskell WL, Lee I-M, Pate RL, et al. Physical activity and public health: updated recommendation for adults from the American College of Sports Medicine and the American Heart Association. *Med Sci Sports Exerc.* 2007;39(8):1423-1434.

42. Hill K, Jenkins SC, Phillippe DL, et al. High-intensity muscle training in COPD. *Eur Respir J.* 2006;27(6):1119-1128.

43. Hills AP, Byrne NM. Physical activity in the management of obesity. *Clin Dermatol.* 2004;22:315-318.

44. Hlatky MA, Boineau RE, Higginbotham MB, et al. A brief self-administered questionnaire to determine functional capacity (the Duke Activity Status Index). *Am J Cardiol.* 1989;64:651-654.

45. Holloway EA, West RJ. Integrated breathing and relaxation training (the Papworth method) for adults with asthma in primary care: a randomized controlled trial. *Thorax.* 2007;62:1039-1042.

46. Homnick DN. Mechanical insufflation–exsufflation for airway mucus clearance. *Respir Care.* 2007;52:1296-1305.

47. Jewell DV. The role of fitness in physical therapy patient management: applications across the continuum of care. *Cardiopulm Phys Ther.* 2006;17(2):47-62.

48. Jones AYM, Dean E, Chow CCS. Comparison of the oxygen cost of breathing exercises and spontaneous breathing in patients with stable chronic obstructive pulmonary disease. *Phys Ther.* 2003;83(5):424-431.

49. Kim J, Sapienza CM. Implications of expiratory muscle strength training for rehabilitation of the elderly: tutorial. *J Rehabil Res Dev.* 2005;42: 211-224.

50. Klem ML, Wing RR, McGuire MT, et al. A descriptive study of individuals successful at long-term maintenance of substantial weight loss. *Am J Clin Nutr.* 1997;66:239-246.

51. Langenderfer B. Alternatives to percussion and postural drainage: a review of mucus clearance therapies: percussion and postural drainage, autogenic drainage, positive expiratory pressure, flutter valve, intrapulmonary percussive ventilation and high-frequency chest compression with the thairapy vest. *J Cardiopulm Rehabil.* 1998;18(4):283-289.

52. Lawrence VA, Cornell JE, Smetana GW. Strategies to reduce postoperative pulmonary complications after noncardiothoracic surgery: systematic review for the American College of Physicians. *Ann Intern Med.* 2006;144:596-608.

53. Leder SB, Espinosa JFL. Aspiration risk after acute stroke: comparison of clinical examination and fiberoptic endoscopic evaluation of swallowing. *Dysphagia.* 2002;17(3):214-218.

54. Leon AS, Franklin BA, Costa F, et al. Cardiac rehabilitation and secondary prevention of coronary heart disease. An American Heart Association scientific statement from the Council on Clinical Cardiology (Subcommittee on Exercise, Cardiac Rehabilitation, and Prevention) and the Council on Nutrition, Physical Activity), in collaboration with the American Association of Cardiovascular and Pulmonary Rehabilitation. *Circulation.* 2005;111:369-376.

55. Levenson CR. Breathing exercises. In Zadai CC, ed. *Pulmonary Management in Physical Therapy.* Philadelphia: Saunders; 1992.

56. Lötters F, van Tol B, Kwakkel G, et al. Effects of controlled inspiratory muscle training in patients with COPD: a meta-analysis. *Eur Respir J.* 2002;20:570-576.

57. Maa SH, Hung TJ, Hsu KH, et al. Manual hyperinflation improves alveolar recruitment in difficult-to-wean patients. *Chest.* 2005;128:2714-2721.

57a. Manning F, Dean E, Ross J, et al. Effects of side lying on lung function in older individuals. *Phys Ther.* 1999;79:456-466.

58. Marik PE. Aspiration pneumonitis and aspiration pneumonia. *N Engl J Med.* 2001;344(9):665-671.

59. Massery M. Respiratory rehabilitation secondary to neurological deficits: treatment techniques. In: Frownfelter DL, ed. *Chest Physical Therapy and Pulmonary Rehabilitation: An Interdisciplinary Approach.* 2nd ed. Chicago: Year Book Medical Publishers; 1987.

60. McArdle WD, Katch FI, Katch VL. *Exercise Physiology: Energy, Nutrition, and Human Performance.* 5th ed. Philadelphia: Lea & Febiger; 2001.

61. McCarren B, Alison JA, Herbert RD. Vibration and its effect on the respiratory system. *Austr J Physiother.* 2006;52:39-43.

62. McConnell TR, Mandak JS, Sykes JS, et al. Exercise training for heart failure patients improves respiratory muscle endurance, exercise tolerance, breathlessness, and quality of life. *J Cardiopulm Rehab.* 2003;23(1):10-16.

63. McIlwaine M. Chest physical therapy, breathing techniques and exercise in children with CF. *Paediatr Respir Rev.* 2007;8:8-16.

64. Michaels AJ, Wanek SM, Dreifuss BA, et al. A protocolized approach to pulmonary failure and the role of intermittent prone positioning. *J Trauma.* 2002;52:1037-1047.

65. Miske LJ, Hickey EM, Kolb SM, et al. Use of the mechanical in-exsufflator in pediatric patients with neuromuscular disease and impaired cough. *Chest.* 2004;125(4):1406-1412.

66. Morice AH, Fontana GA, et al. The diagnosis and management of chronic cough. *Eur Respir J.* 2004;24(3):481-492.

67. Myers TR. Positive expiratory pressure and oscillatory positive expiratory pressure therapies. *Respir Care.* 2007;52:1308-1326.

68. Nield MA, Soo Hoo GW, Roper JM, et al. Efficacy of pursed-lips breathing: a breathing pattern retraining strategy for dyspnea reduction. *J Cardiopulm Rehabil Prevent.* 2007;27:237-244.

69. Nelson ME, Rejeski WJ, Blair SN, et al. Physical activity and public health in older adults: recommendation from the American College of Sports Medicine and the American Heart Association. *Med Sci Sports Exerc.* 2007;39(8):1435-1445.

69a. Oldridge NB, Donner A, Buck CW, et al. Predictive indices for drop-out: the Ontario Exercise Heart Collaborative Experience. *Am J Cardiol.* 1983;51:70-74.

70. Padula CA, Yeaw E. Inspiratory muscle training: integrative review. *Res Theory Nurs Pract.* 2006;20:291-304.

71. Padula CA, Yeaw E. Inspiratory muscle training: integrative review of use in conditions other than COPD. *Res Theory Nurs Pract.* 2007;21:98-118.

72. Pedersen BK, Saltin B. Evidence for prescribing exercise as therapy for chronic disease [review]. *Scand J Med Sci Sports.* 2006;16(suppl 1):3-63.

73. Phillips GE, Pike SE, Jaffe A, et al. Comparison of active cycle of breathing and high-frequency oscillation jacket in children with cystic fibrosis. *Pediatr Pulmonol.* 2004;37:71-75.

74. Pollock ML, Gaesser GA, Butcher JD. ACSM position stand: the recommended quantity and quality of exercise for developing and maintaining cardiorespiratory and muscular fitness, and flexibility in healthy adults. *Med Sci Sports Exerc.* 1998;30(6):975-991.

75. Ram FSF, Holloway EA, Jones PW. Breathing retraining for asthma. *Respir Med.* 2003;97:501-507.

75a. Ridell MC, Perkins BA. Type 1 diabetes and vigorous exercise: applications of exercise physiology to patient management. *Can J Diabetes.* 2006;30:63-71.

76. Riera HS, Rubio TM, Ruiz FO, et al. Inspiratory muscle training in patients with COPD: effect on dyspnea, exercise performance, and quality of life. *Chest.* 2001;120(3):748-756.

77. Ries AL, Bauldoff GS, Casaburi R, et al. Pulmonary rehabilitation: a joint AACP/AACVPR evidence-based clinical practice guidelines. *Chest.* 2007; 131:4S-42S.

78. Salmon J, Owen N, Crawford D, et al. Physical activity and sedentary behaviour: a population-based study of barriers, enjoyment, and preference. *Health Psychol.* 2003;22(2):178-188.

79. Sciaky A, Stockford J, Nixon E. Treatment of acute cardiopulmonary conditions. In: Hillegass EA, Sadowsky HS, eds. *Essentials of Cardiopulmonary Physical Therapy.* 2nd ed. Philadelphia: Saunders; 2001.

80. Sharp JT, Drutz WS, Moisan T, et al. Postural relief of dyspnea in severe chronic obstructive pulmonary disease. *Am Rev Respir Dis.* 1980;122: 201-211.

81. Stewart KJ, Hiatt WR, Regensteiner JG, et al. Exercise training for claudication. *N Engl J Med.* 2002;347(24):1941-1951.

82. Swain DP, Franklin BA. Comparison of cardioprotective benefits of vigorous versus moderate intensity aerobic exercise. *Am J Cardiol.* 2006;97: 141-147.

83. Taylor AH, Cable NT, Faulkner G, et al. Physical activity and older adults: a review of health benefits and the effectiveness of interventions. *J Sports Sci.* 2003;22:703-725.

84. Tucker B, Jenkins S. The effect of breathing exercises with body positioning on regional lung ventilation. *Aust J Physiother.* 1996;42:219-227.

85. van der Schans CP. Conventional chest physical therapy for obstructive lung disease. *Respir Care.* 2007;52:1198-1209.

86. Van Houtte S, Vanlandewijck Y, Gosselink R. Respiratory training in persons with spinal cord injury: a systematic review. *Respir Med.* 2006; 100:1886-1895.

87. Vargas F, Bui HN, Boyer A, et al. Intrapulmonary percussive ventilation in acute exacerbations of COPD patients with mild respiratory acidosis: a randomized controlled trial. *Crit Care.* 2005;9(4):R382-R389.

88. Vianello A, Corrado A, Arcaro G, et al. Mechanical insufflation–exsufflation improves outcomes for neuromuscular disease patients with respiratory tract infections. *Am J Phys Med Rehabil.* 2005;84:83-88.

89. Vincent KR, Vincent HK. Resistance training for individuals with cardiovascular disease. *J Cardiopulm Rehabil.* 2006;26:207-216.

89a. Volaklis KA, Tokmakidis SP. Resistance exercise training in patients with heart failure. *Sports Med.* 2005;35:1085-1103.

90. Warburton DER, Nicol CW, Bredin SSD. Health benefits of physical activity: the evidence. *CMAJ.* 2006;174:801-809.

91. Weiner P, McConnell A. Respiratory muscle training in chronic obstructive pulmonary disease: inspiratory, expiratory, or both? *Curr Opin Pulm Med.* 2005;11:140-144.

92. Williams MA, Haskell WL, Ades PA, et al. Resistance exercise in individuals with and without cardiovascular disease (2007 update): a scientific statement from the American Heart Association Council on Clinical Cardiology and Council on Nutrition, Physical Activity, and Metabolism. *Circulation.* 2007;116:572-584.

93. Winett RA, Carpinelli RN. Potential health-related benefits of resistance training [review]. *Prevent Med.* 2001;33:503-513.

ADDITIONAL READINGS

Humberstone N, Tecklin JS. Respiratory treatment. In: Irwin S, Tecklin JS, eds. *Cardiopulmonary Physical Therapy.* 3rd ed. St. Louis: Mosby; 1995.

Skinner JS. *Exercise Testing and Exercise Prescription for Special Cases. Theoretical Basis and Clinical Applications.* 2nd ed. Philadelphia: Lea & Febiger; 1993.

Tecklin JS. The patient with airway clearance dysfunction – preferred practice pattern 6C. In: Irwin S, Tecklin JS, eds. *Cardiopulmonary Physical Therapy – A Guide to Practice.* 4th ed. St. Louis, MO: Mosby; 2004.

Tecklin JS. The patient with ventilatory pump dysfunction/failure – preferred practice pattern 6E. In: Irwin S, Tecklin JS, eds. *Cardiopulmonary Physical Therapy – A Guide to Practice.* 4th ed. St. Louis, MO: Mosby; 2004.

CHAPTER 8

Pediatrics

Robin J. Winn, PT, MS, PCS and Joanne Watchie, PT, MA, CCS

This chapter provides review of the normal embryologic development of the cardiopulmonary system and its growth and development through childhood and adolescence. It seeks to highlight differences between pediatric and adult systems and presents several of the more frequently encountered pulmonary and cardiovascular pathologies that occur in the pediatric population. More common secondary impairments of the cardiopulmonary system resulting from disorders affecting other systems are also included. In addition, assessment and treatment modifications recommended for use with infants and children are provided.

8.1 NORMAL DEVELOPMENT OF THE CARDIOPULMONARY SYSTEM

An understanding of the normal development and maturation of the cardiopulmonary system (and related musculoskeletal components) is essential to appreciating the abnormalities that may occur and to the application of safe and effective interventions in the pediatric population. This section aims to review normal embryologic development of both the heart and lungs, identify changes that occur at birth and during childhood, examine normal development of the chest wall and mechanics of breathing, and highlight differences between pediatric and adult systems.

DEVELOPMENT OF THE HEART

The cardiovascular system begins development at approximately 19 days of gestation and by the end of neonatal development the number of myocardial cells is finite. Further growth of the myocardium occurs via hypertrophy of existing cells.[93] For the sake of simplicity, development of the human heart can be broken down into several grossly distinct phases that are outlined in Table 8-1. In the human embryo, the circulatory system is the first organ system to become functional.

Fetal Circulation

- The fetus is dependent on the maternal circulation for nutrition and gas exchange. Fetal circulation delivers more highly oxygenated blood to more active, vital organs while deoxygenated blood is routed to less active tissues and back to the placenta for the elimination of metabolites. This is accomplished using parallel circulations, intracardiac shunting, and preferential streaming. Fetal circulation is characterized by high pulmonary vascular resistance (PVR) and relatively low cardiac output. In addition, fetal hemoglobin, which has a higher affinity for oxygen and is present in higher concentration than adult hemoglobin, helps to facilitate gas exchange in the placenta.[123] The fetal circulatory pattern is detailed in Figure 8-1:
  ‣ Oxygenated blood from the placenta reaches the fetus via the umbilical vein and enters the ductus venosus, mainly

bypassing the liver to join the inferior vena cava (IVC), which carries the blood to the right atrium (RA).
  ‣ Preferential streaming of the umbilical blood (versus the deoxygenated blood returning from the lower body of the fetus) through the IVC across the foramen ovale delivers oxygenated blood directly to the left atrium (LA).
  ‣ Blood entering the RA from the superior vena cava (from the upper extremities, head, and neck) combines with unshunted venous return from the IVC and the drainage from the coronary sinus (from the myocardium) and flows into the right ventricle (RV).
  ‣ Blood from the RV is ejected into the pulmonary trunk, where a small amount flows to the high-resistance, unexpanded lungs and most flows through the ductus arteriosus to the descending aorta, which carries blood to the umbilical–placental circulation and to the lower body.
  ‣ Thus, delivery of more highly oxygenated blood to the left side of the heart is accomplished through (1) shunting of the most highly oxygenated blood from the placenta across the ductus venosus and (2) preferential streaming of this blood across the foramen ovale.[93,123] This blood mixes with the scant, deoxygenated pulmonary return and empties into the left ventricle (LV).
  ‣ Blood ejected from the LV to the ascending aorta provides blood flow to the coronary circulation, head and neck, and upper extremities.
- Fetal ventricular output is sometimes referred to as *combined ventricular output (CVO)* because the blood reaching the body and the placenta is derived from the systemic and umbilical venous return with the ventricles effectively acting in parallel. Approximately 55% to 65% of the CVO comes from the RV whereas 35% to 45% comes from the LV.[30,117]
- Because the fetal heart contains relatively more noncontractile mass than the more mature heart, it is less compliant and therefore unable to increase stroke volume, as the adult heart does, when an increase in cardiac output is needed (see page 42). Because cardiac output is a product of stroke volume (SV) and heart rate (HR), CVO is dependent on an increase in HR. This explains why bradycardia is so poorly tolerated by the fetus and neonate.[117] On the other hand, tachycardia can also precipitate rapid congestive heart failure (CHF).

DEVELOPMENT OF THE LUNGS

The lungs begin their development at about 21 days of gestation, with the bronchial structure of the lung forming by week 16 of gestation and the associated vascular structures by week 24. The first primitive alveoli appear between 28 and 32 weeks and alveolar proliferation continues into childhood so that the full complement is achieved

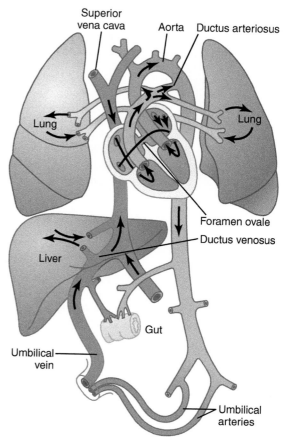

TABLE 8-1: Gross Stages of Embryologic Development of the Heart

Gestational Age (d)	Embryologic Development
≈19	Mesenchymal cells arising from mesoderm proliferate, forming parallel solid cords
≈22–23	Cords canalize to form two endocardial tubes that fold and fuse to form the primordial heart tube; subsequent division results in the left and right horns of the sinus venosus, the atrium, the ventricle, and the bulbus cordis
≈24	Primordial heart tube folds on itself, forming the bulboventricular loop
≈25–49	Partitioning of the major structures occurs:
≈25–28	Enlargement of the endocardial cushions divides the atrioventricular canal into right and left canals
≈29–39	Separation of the atria begins via fusion of the septum primum with the endocardial cushions. The parallel septum secundum forms shortly thereafter and completes atrial division with right/left communication preserved via the foramen ovale
≈37–48	Growth of the interventricular septum toward the endocardial cushions divides the ventricle into two chambers, which communicate until complete closure of the interventricular foramen
≈49	Formation of the aortopulmonary septum divides the bulbus cordis and the truncus arteriosus into the aorta and pulmonary trunk
≈50	Complete development of the four-chambered heart

Figure 8-1: Schematic illustration of the fetal circulation. Three shunts permit most of the fetus's blood to bypass the liver and lungs: the ductus venosus, the foramen ovale, and the ductus arteriosus (see text). The poorly oxygenated blood returns to the placenta for oxygen and nutrients through the umbilical arteries. (Modified from Arey LB. *Developmental Anatomy: A Textbook and Laboratory Manual of Embryology.* 7th ed. Philadelphia: Saunders; 1974.)

by age 4.[19] The phases of embryologic development are described briefly in Table 8-2 and, as indicated, are not without overlap.

CARDIOPULMONARY ADJUSTMENTS AT BIRTH

With the first neonatal breaths, the lungs expand and the pulmonary arterioles dilate so that the transition from placental oxygenation to neonatal lung ventilation and perfusion occurs within minutes to hours after birth. PVR drops rapidly; within the first 24 hours of life, pulmonary artery (PA) pressures decrease to approximately one half of aortic pressures.[123] Simultaneously, clamping of the umbilical cord (or its natural constriction after birth) provokes other major circulatory adjustments that enable the lungs and other organs to function independently. In contrast to fetal circulation, neonatal circulation is characterized by a series circulation, absence of intracardiac shunts, low PVR, and relatively high cardiac output.

- Asphyxia stimulates activation of the respiratory centers in the brainstem. At the onset of breathing, fluid in the lungs is replaced by air, resulting in an increase in blood oxygen and a marked reduction in PVR.
- The drop in PVR results in a dramatic rise in pulmonary blood flow, which occurs within minutes to hours after birth, and allows the transition from placental oxygenation to neonatal lung gas exchange. By age 6 to 8 weeks of life, PVR is at the level of an adult.[93]
- At the same time, cessation of umbilical venous flow and constriction of the ductus venosus that bypasses the liver lead to a fall in IVC flow and RA pressure, while increasing blood flow to the lungs increases LA volume and pressure; this pressure differential between the LA and RA prompts closure of the foramen ovale.
- Gradual closure of the ductus arteriosus likely occurs in response to exposure to increased oxygen levels and a decrease in prostaglandin E_2 (PGE_2), which was produced by the placenta. Thus, a series circulation is established (from the systemic venous system to the right heart to the pulmonary circulation to the left heart and finally to the systemic arterial system and capillaries).

TABLE 8-2: Phases of Development of the Respiratory System

Gestational Age	Phase(s)	Embryologic Development
≈21–28 days	Embryonic	Development of primordial lungs; budding of pulmonary arteries and veins; formation of major bronchi
≈5–12 wk	Pseudoglandular	Separation of the trachea from the esophagus; formation of the larynx; rapid growth and preacinar branching of the bronchi
≈12–17 wk		Distinction of lung lobes with complete adult airway branching pattern; formation of bronchial arteries
≈16–26 wk	Canalicular	Development of airway epithelium and submucosal glands; formation of preacinar pattern of blood supply; initial appearance of alveolar ducts occurring at end of phase
≈24–44+ wk	Saccular/ Alveolar	Rapid proliferation of the alveoli; increasing airway diameter and length, vessel size and number, cartilage mass, and gland growth

- Loss of the low-resistance placental circulation leads to an increase in systemic vascular resistance (SVR), which induces myocardial hypertrophy of the LV; conversely the drop in PVR results in gradual regression of RV wall thickness.
- Cardiac output from the LV increases immediately after birth to meet the augmented oxygen consumption of the newborn infant, who begins to perform independent thermoregulatory and cardiorespiratory functions.

EFFECTS OF PREMATURITY

Premature infants are especially vulnerable to pulmonary disorders because of structural immaturity, lack of surfactant, and the presence of intracardiac shunting. Specific pulmonary disorders experienced by premature infants are presented in Section 8.2.

The cardiovascular system is also affected when birth is premature. First, the ductus arteriosus is likely to remain open because of immature ductal muscle (which is unable to produce the same constriction response when exposed to oxygen as more mature muscle) and persistently elevated PGE_2 levels that exert a continued dilatory effect on the ductus. Second, the fall in PVR after birth occurs more quickly in premature infants than in term infants because of immaturity of the smooth muscle in the pulmonary vasculature, which results in the early onset of left-to-right shunting and CHF.

CHANGES DURING INFANCY, CHILDHOOD, AND ADOLESCENCE

The cardiovascular and pulmonary systems continue to undergo changes as an individual grows through infancy, childhood, and adolescence, which are manifested to some degree by alterations in resting HR, blood pressure (BP), and respiratory rate as a function of age (Table 8-3).

Cardiovascular Changes

The rate of development of the circulatory system slows after the perinatal period. Changes during childhood and adolescence occur in relation to increase in body size, change in body configuration, and in response to exertion.[93] Some of the changes in cardiovascular function that occur during maturation include the following:

- Increasing systemic arterial BP as body size increases
- Progressively decreasing resting HR and respiratory rate with increasing age
- Augmented stroke volume in association with body growth
- Increasing SVR when related to body surface area
- Increasing cardiac output (CO) in proportion to body surface area over the whole age spectrum (CO is not directly related to body weight because of the disparity between body weight and body surface area)
- Slowly decreasing cardiac index (CI) from 3.5 L/min/m^2 in childhood/adolescence[93] to 3.0 L/min/m^2 in adulthood
- Decreasing oxygen consumption, normalized to body surface area or weight, with increasing age because of the diminished

TABLE 8-3: Changes in Vital Signs as a Function of Age

Age	Mean HR (bpm) ± 2 SD	Mean BP (mm Hg)	Mean RR (breaths/ min)
Premature neonate	125 ± 50	35-56 systolic (birth to 7 days)	40–60
Full-term neonate	140 ± 50	75/50	30–40
Infant			
1–6 mo	130 ± 45	80/46	30–40
6–12 mo	115 ± 40	96/65	30
Preschool			
1–2 yr	110 ± 40	99/65	25–30
2–6 yr	105 ± 35	100/60	25
School			
6–8 yr	95 ± 30	105/60	20–25
8–12 yr	95 ± 30	110/60	20
Adolescence			
12–14 yr	82 ± 25	118/60	16–20
14–18 yr	82 ± 25	120/65	14–18
Adult	72 ± 25	127/76	12–15

Bpm, Beats per minute; BP, blood pressure; HR, heart rate; RR, respiratory rate.

surface area-to-body weight ratio and lower energy requirements for growth with aging.[55]

Other important differences between the pediatric and adult heart have been identified:

- At birth, the infant's RV is thicker than the LV, but by 1 month the weight of the LV exceeds that of the RV, and by 6 months of age the ratio of LV weight to RV weight is approximately 2:1. The electrocardiogram (ECG) at birth reflects the normal RV dominance of the newborn with right axis deviation and large rightward and/or anterior QRS forces (i.e., dominant R waves in the right precordial leads).[84] By the age of 3, the ECG resembles that of a young adult.
- Fewer contractile myofibrils in neonatal myocardium results in lower ventricular compliance compared with that of the adult, necessitating an elevation of HR to increase CO in the infant.
- Newborn myocardium is more sensitive to calcium than is adult myocardium because of differences in sarcoplasmic reticulum stores.[123] Therefore, the newborn's inotropic state and CO are affected by alterations in serum calcium levels and by calcium channel–blocking medications.

Pulmonary Changes

Whereas normal development of the human lung is fairly well understood through the saccular stage, less detail is agreed on regarding alveolarization, and vascular growth and development has not been well studied.

- Structural lung development is fairly complete by the end of normal gestation, with the exception of alveolar number. At birth it is estimated that between one third and one half of the adult number of alveoli are present.[48] Although the majority of mature alveoli are formed by 2 years, they continue to proliferate through age 4.[19]
- The surface area of gas-exchange units undergoes an approximate 20-fold increase between birth and adulthood. Growth of the lungs continues through puberty, but the increase in lung volume is achieved primarily through increase in size of all structures, not through proliferation of new alveoli.[19]
- During gestation, vascular growth of the lungs occurs via formation of completely new vessels from endothelial cells and via sprouting of preexisting vessels.[7] At birth the vascular branching pattern is the same as in the adult.[48] Ongoing growth and remodeling occur during infancy and into childhood and are essential to normal adult lung structure.
- Differences in lung function within children of the same age (and for the same child over her/his growth phase) relate to differences in body size, which is reflective of skeletal dimensions and body composition, and in habitual activity.
- Elastic recoil of the lungs increases progressively throughout childhood as ventilatory mechanisms mature.[66]
- Because full lung maturation is not complete until age 18 in females and age 20 in males,[47] exposure to secondhand smoke and air pollution during childhood can have chronic, adverse affects on pulmonary development, as measured by the changes in forced expiratory volumes and flows.[33]

Normal Differences Between Infant and Adult Respiratory Systems

There are a number of anatomic and physiologic differences between the respiratory system of full-term infants and that of older children and adults, which increase the infant's susceptibility to respiratory dysfunction. Some of these differences may be more evident in premature infants and may lead to their greater risk for pulmonary dysfunction.

- Anatomic differences that affect pulmonary function in infants are described in Table 8-4.
- Physiologic differences affecting pulmonary function in infants are described in Table 8-5.

Normal Development of the Chest Wall and Muscles of Respiration

The work of Massery details normal development of the chest wall and muscles of respiration.[68] These trends are listed in Table 8-6.

- The elasticity and alignment of the newborn ribcage, combined with the immaturity of the thoracic musculature, limit the ability of the young infant to expand the thorax effectively against gravity, producing the characteristic belly excursion and nasal-dominant pattern of breathing.

TABLE 8-4: **Anatomic Differences Affecting Pulmonary Function in Infants and Younger Children Compared With Adults**

Anatomic Difference	Effect(s)
High larynx	Allows infant to breathe and swallow simultaneously; may contribute to predominant nasal breathing pattern, in which case any narrowing of the nasal passageways will result in ↑ work of breathing
Enlarged lymphatic tissue (e.g., tonsils); relatively large tongue	↑ Possibility of upper airway obstruction (lymphatic tissue grows quickly until age 6 yr)
Alveolar surface area equals approximately 5% of adult's*	Gas exchange surface area continues to develop through puberty or later; this protective difference allows any early disease-related lung damage to become less significant over time
↓ Airway diameter and structural support	↑ Risk of airway obstruction and collapse
Poorly developed collateral ventilation channels	↑ Incidence of right middle and upper lobe atelectasis in neonates
Cartilaginous sternum and ribs; horizontal configuration of the rib cage; relatively short neck	↓ Efficiency of ventilation compared with adult, ↑ distortion of rib cage; ↑ dependence on diaphragmatic breathing. Accessory muscles of respiration contribute primarily to chest wall stability and are relatively nonfunctional in supporting ventilation

↑, Increased; ↓, decreased.
*From Cotes JE, Chinn DJ, Miller MR: *Lung Function: Physiology, Measurement and Application in Medicine,* Boston, Blackwell, 2006.

TABLE 8-5: Physiological Differences Affecting Pulmonary Function in Infants and Younger Children Compared With Adults

Physiological Difference	Effect(s)
↓ Lung compliance in neonate	Need for ↑ inflation pressures → ↑ work of breathing; worsened if lack of surfactant
↑ Chest wall compliance in infants	↑ Tendency of small peripheral airways to close during tidal breathing → impaired gas exchange. When combined with small size of airways → ↑ risk of airway obstruction in infants and small children
↑ Irregularity of respiratory pattern (↑ sensitivity of respiratory mechanoreceptors and immaturity of carotid bodies in newborn)	↑ Risk of apnea and subsequent bradycardia, desaturation
Respiratory compensation via ↑ rate rather than ↑ depth	↓ Efficiency of ventilation → ↑ work of breathing
↓ Pulmonary reserve	↑ Risk of serious pulmonary dysfunction with any situation calling for ↑ cardiac output; respond to increased demand with ↑ RR
↓ Percentage of type I, high-oxidative fibers in diaphragm	↑ Vulnerability to respiratory muscle fatigue secondary to reliance on diaphragm
↑ Time spent in sleep state overall and REM sleep	↑↑ Work of breathing secondary to ↑ respiratory rate, loss of tonic activity of respiratory muscles* while in REM sleep

*From Lopes J, Muller NL, Bryan MH, et al. Importance of inspiratory muscle tone in maintenance of FRC in the newborn. *J Appl Physiol.* 1981;51:830–834.
↑, Increased; ↑↑, much increased; ↓, decreased; →, leads to; REM, rapid eye movement; RR, respiratory rate.

- The horizontal alignment of the ribs and the activity of the intercostals, internal and external obliques, and the rectus and transversus abdominis musculature combine to stabilize the thorax, enabling the diaphragm to function as the primary muscle of respiration during early infancy. Owing to its attachments, the diaphragm lies more horizontally during infancy with its dome shape increasing as the lower ribs rotate downward over time.[68]
- Although the scalenes and sternocleidomastoids contribute significantly to the stability of the immature thorax, these muscle groups are relatively nonfunctional as accessory muscles of respiration during infancy and early childhood.
- With the development of mature, upright postural control, biomechanical and functional relationships within the musculoskeletal system shift, resulting in the bucket-handle movement seen in efficient adult respiration.

TABLE 8-6: Trends of Normal Chest Wall Development from Infancy Through Childhood

Chest	Infant	Adult
Size	Thorax occupies one third of trunk cavity	Thorax occupies more than half of trunk cavity
Shape	Triangular frontal plane, circular A-P plane	Rectangular frontal plane, elliptical A-P plane
Upper chest	Narrow, flat apex	Wide, convex apex
Lower chest	Circular, flared lower ribs	Elliptical, lower ribs integrated with abdominals
Ribs	Evenly horizontal	Rotated downward, especially inferiorly
Intercostal spacing	Narrow, limits movement of thoracic spine and trunk	Wide, allows for individual movement of ribs and spine
Diaphragm	Adequate, minimal dome shape	Adequate, large dome shape
Accessory muscles	Nonfunctional	Functional

From Massery M. Multisystem consequences of impaired breathing mechanics and/or postural control. In Frownfelter D, Dean E, editors. *Cardiovascular and Pulmonary Physical Therapy: Evidence and Practice.* 4th ed. St. Louis: Mosby; 2006.
A-P, Anteroposterior.

For a more thorough explanation of the mechanics of respiration, refer to page 4. If, for any reason, the thorax and its musculature do not interact with gravity in a way that enables the development of effective, upright postural control, the development of the pulmonary system in turn will also likely be affected, resulting not only in impaired pulmonary function but also potential rib cage deformities over time.

Effects of Gravity and Self-initiated Movement

As explained by Massery, the effect that gravity has on the normal musculoskeletal development of the thorax and respiratory system, in particular, cannot be underestimated. Muscles essential for postural activation and control are also critical for efficient patterns of respiration.[69] The developmental interaction that occurs between the two is essential for normal maturation of the thorax,[68] and evolution of the neonatal respiratory system toward the biomechanically more efficient adult system is dependent on the complex interplay of skeletal, muscular, and motivational components that are experienced by the infant during the first year of life.

- Simply stated, changes in the mobility of the spine and rib cage combine with passive elongation and active contraction of a variety of spinal and torso muscle groups to produce significant changes in both alignment and muscular control of the head and trunk. Dynamic experience in different positions including supine, side-lying, and prone as well as transitional movements performed by the infant (e.g., rolling) contribute to the occurrence of such changes.

- As the child develops more upright postural control and assumes independent sitting positions, the effects of gravity and the influence of the abdominals become more significant and result in greater downward rotation of the ribs and further movement of the rib cage in a caudal direction.
- As more sophisticated transitional movements emerge involving increased weight shifting, upper extremity weight bearing, and rotation of the trunk, a corresponding increase in the mobility of the rib cage is seen that is made possible by the dynamic stability provided to it by the shoulder girdles, neck, and abdominals.

These changes are necessary for the trunk and its musculature to assume a more active role in respiration and in the development of upright postural control. The infant's innate motivation to explore and move through its immediate environment plays an important role in the evolution of all systems, and the respiratory system is no exception. In conditions in which motor control is decreased or absent, as well as when cognitive or motivational impairments are present, both the musculoskeletal alignment and the mechanics of breathing will remain immature and less efficient as the child grows. These effects will become more evident over time unless addressed.

8.2 PEDIATRIC PULMONARY DISEASE

As detailed in the previous section, a number of known anatomic and physiologic developmental differences predispose the pediatric population to compromise of the respiratory system. Increasing social and environmental interaction also exposes the immature immune system to greater risk of infection during this time period. Respiratory disorders are relatively common in children and may result from immaturity (e.g., respiratory distress syndrome), genetics (e.g., cystic fibrosis), congenital anomalies (e.g., pulmonary, cardiac, and abdominal wall defects), immunologic abnormalities, iatrogenic causes (e.g., oxygen toxicity), and aspiration (e.g., accidental or incidental). The more common disorders encountered by physical therapists are presented in this section.

NEONATAL RESPIRATORY DISORDERS

Neonates are particularly vulnerable to pulmonary dysfunction, and premature birth adds to the predisposition to complications and some specific disorders.

Respiratory Distress Syndrome

Respiratory distress syndrome (RDS) is the most common cause of respiratory distress in premature infants and, by definition, develops during the first few hours after birth and lasts longer than 24 hours. It occurs most commonly in infants born at less than 28 weeks of gestation, affects about one third of infants born at 28 to 34 weeks, and less than 5% of those born after 34 weeks.[46] The severity of symptoms is inversely related to both gestational age and birth weight; infants born before 26 weeks of gestational age may present with apnea at birth. Advances in exogenous surfactant therapy and prenatal corticosteroids have resulted in

decreasing rates of RDS, but supplemental oxygen, positive airway pressure support, and/or mechanical ventilation are still frequently required when it presents.

RDS remains the primary cause of morbidity and mortality in preterm infants, with males more likely to both develop and die from RDS than females. Factors that predispose an infant to the development of RDS include prematurity, cesarean section, asphyxia, and maternal diabetes. Factors have also been identified that protect the infant against RDS, including intrauterine stress, female gender, antenatal corticosteroids, and non-Caucasian ethnicity.[43]

Pathophysiology

- Structural immaturity of the lungs combined with an inadequate amount and quality of surfactant results in alveolar collapse, especially at end-expiration, which leads to progressive atelectasis, decreased lung volume, and reduced lung compliance.
- Attempts at reinflation (spontaneous or mechanical) create shear forces that damage lung epithelium and result in bronchiolar necrosis and influx of protein into the airways, which further compromise endogenous surfactant production.[2] Hyaline membranes, the classic lesion of prematurity, form as a result of the disruption to the epithelial–endothelial integrity. Although the term *hyaline membrane disease (HMD)* has been used interchangeably with RDS, it is important to note that hyaline membrane formation is not exclusive to RDS, and respiratory distress may occur in the absence of hyaline membrane formation.
- These abnormalities lead to reduced lung compliance, ventilation–perfusion mismatch, and impaired gas exchange, all of which increase the work of breathing.
- Repair begins approximately 24 hours after injury and if uncomplicated may be completed within 7 days. However, in infants treated with positive-pressure ventilation, the repair process is often impaired, resulting in progressive scarring and fibrosis of the airways and eventual chronic restrictive lung disease of varying degrees.[43]
- If there is a persistent patent ductus arteriosus (PDA), intracardiac left-to-right shunting increases pulmonary blood flow and pressures, which may lead to pulmonary edema and further interference with surfactant production.
- Of note, the pathology of RDS reflects both the underlying disease and the effects of mechanical ventilation and supplemental oxygen required for treatment.

Common Complications

RDS is associated with a number of complications, which may result from premature birth, the pulmonary defects, and/or its treatment.

- Intraventricular hemorrhage (IVH) and/or periventricular leukomalacia (PVL)
- Sepsis
- Pneumonia
- Air leaks
- Pulmonary hemorrhage
- Persistent patency of the ductus arteriosus
- Retinopathy of prematurity (ROP)
- Bronchopulmonary dysplasia (BPD)

Clinical Manifestations

- Signs and symptoms of respiratory distress (Table 8-7)
- Tachycardia (>160 beats/min [bpm]) in severe RDS
- Decreased activity/lethargy (reflecting hypoxia or attempt at energy conservation); or increased irritability
- Difficulty feeding and failure to thrive
- Reduced lung compliance and functional residual capacity
- Abnormal gas exchange (hypoxemia, hypercapnia, and cyanosis) requiring supplemental oxygen or positive-pressure support for more than 24 hours
- Abnormal chest x-ray showing fine reticulogranular pattern with possible air bronchograms

Management

- Primary prevention of prematurity
- Prenatal corticosteroids (betamethasone) to the mother before delivery to boost the production of surfactant in the fetus
- Exogenous surfactant therapy
- Supportive care
  - ▶ Neutral thermal environment
  - ▶ Supplemental nutrition, hyperalimentation
  - ▶ Fluid and electrolyte replacement
  - ▶ Supplemental oxygen
  - ▶ Nasal prong continuous positive airway pressure (NCPAP), conventional mechanical ventilation with pressure support, or high-frequency oscillating ventilation (HFOV).

- Airway clearance techniques for secretion management (or treatment of collapse not caused by lack of surfactant): positioning, percussion, vibration, and suctioning, as indicated, with attention to precautions/contraindications specific to neonates (described on pages 385–389).

Bronchopulmonary Dysplasia

Bronchopulmonary dysplasia (BPD) is a chronic obstructive lung disease (see page 72) manifested as recurrent wheezing and chronic cough that develops in approximately 20% of premature infants born weighing less than 1500 g.[10] It most often develops in infants with RDS who have received prolonged treatment with high concentrations of oxygen and positive-pressure ventilation. BPD is present if there is a need for supplemental oxygen for at least 28 days after birth, and its severity is graded according to the oxygen requirements: mild BPD involves a fraction of inspired oxygen (FIO_2) of 0.21, moderate disease necessitates an FIO_2 of 0.22 to 0.29, and severe RDS requires an FIO_2 of at least 0.30 or continuous positive airway pressure or mechanical ventilation.[10]

Fortunately, advances in the management of RDS, including prenatal steroids and surfactant therapy, have enabled the use of lower airway pressures and oxygen concentrations to manage symptoms and this, in turn, has led to less severe lung pathology in BPD. However, many infants with RDS still develop increasing oxygen requirements over time and radiographic changes

TABLE 8-7: **Clinical Manifestations of Respiratory Distress in Infants**

Observation	Comments
Tachypnea	>60 breaths per minute in attempt to increase oxygenation and eliminate excessive CO_2
Intercostal, suprasternal, subcostal, or substernal retractions	Reflects increased work of breathing in more compliant rib cage with poorly developed intercostal muscles; severe retractions limit anteroposterior chest expansion and effective ventilation
Nasal flaring	Serves to reduce airway resistance in the nasal passages
Expiratory grunting	Expiration through a partially closed glottis attempts to produce physiological PEEP to prevent alveolar and small airway collapse and improve ventilation
Stridor	Crowing sound associated with upper airway obstruction
Head bobbing	Occurs in infants who are attempting to use accessory muscles of inspiration to improve ventilation, but have poor head control; hypertrophy of accessory muscles suggests chronic dyspnea
Pallor, mottling, or webbing of skin	Occurs in distressed infants and may be associated with hypoxemia and anemia, among other problems
Cyanosis (central, peripheral, or differential)	Central cyanosis occurring in the lips, mucous membranes, and tongue denotes arterial hypoxemia; peripheral cyanosis in the absence of central cyanosis indicates poor perfusion or vasoconstriction; differential cyanosis affecting the upper or lower body only indicates serious heart disease
Hypoxemia, oxygen desaturation	Occurs in pulmonary disease and congenital heart defects with right-to-left shunting
Apnea	Respiratory pause >20 s or any pause accompanied by bradycardia and cyanosis or oxygen desaturation; may occur due to hypoxemia or respiratory muscle fatigue
Difficulty feeding	Shortness of breath interferes with sucking and swallowing
Irritability, lethargy	Distressed infants are often irritable and exhibit exaggerated physiological responses to stimulation; hypoxemic infants may be lethargic and hypotonic

PEEP, Positive end-expiratory pressure.

consistent with BPD, and there is increasing evidence to support that inflammation plays a role in the pathogenesis of BPD.[88]

Risk factors associated with the development of BPD include anatomic immaturity of the lung structures, surfactant deficiency, prolonged treatment with high concentrations of oxygen and positive-pressure ventilation, family history of reactive airway disease, and chorioamnionitis.

BPD is associated with adverse neurodevelopmental outcome due to recurrent hypoxia, intraventricular hemorrhage (IVH), periventricular leukomalacia (PVL), poor nutrition during periods of critical brain development, and prolonged hospitalization.[34]

Pathophysiology

- BPD begins with the clinical manifestations and pathophysiology found in RDS (see the previous section), which progress within 1 month (due to further inflammatory reaction induced by barotrauma and oxygen toxicity) to those of chronic lung disease, including mucosal metaplasia, obliterative bronchiolitis with peribronchiolar smooth muscle hypertrophy, atelectasis, and emphysema.
- Ventilatory impairment leads to ventilation–perfusion mismatching, impaired gas exchange, and increased work of breathing.
- Recurrent bacterial or viral infections provoke frequent respiratory relapses.
- Infants requiring chronic ventilatory assistance often have difficulty with secretion management and may suffer from chronic hypercapnia, persistent atelectasis, lobar hyperinflation, and tracheomalacia, bronchomalacia, or both.
- Predisposition to gastroesophageal reflux increases the risk of aspiration.
- The increased work of breathing interferes with feeding and leads to poor growth of the infant.
- Severe BPD can result in pulmonary hypertension (HTN) and right heart failure.
- The sequelae of BPD tend to decrease over the preschool and early childhood years as alveoli and gas-exchange surface area continue to develop.

Clinical Manifestations

- Signs and symptoms of chronic respiratory distress:
- Those listed in Table 8-7 plus:
  - ▶ Carbon dioxide (CO_2) retention and compensated respiratory acidosis
  - ▶ Failure to thrive
- Wheezing (due to reactive airway bronchoconstriction)
- Oxygen dependence
- Abnormal chest radiograph consistent with chronic lung disease
- Signs and symptoms of cor pulmonale (see page 95)
- BPD spells (episodes of spontaneous hypoxemia occurring more often in older infants)
- Other problems associated with BPD[65]:
  - ▶ Behavioral and socialization problems
  - ▶ Gross and fine motor difficulties

Management

- Supportive care
  - ▶ Supplemental nutrition including vitamin A
  - ▶ Diuretics for fluid retention

- ▶ Supplemental oxygenation at lowest possible concentration to achieve oxygen saturation levels of at least 92%
- ▶ Nasal prong continuous positive airway pressure (NCPAP) or mechanical ventilation with minimum peak inspiratory pressures necessary for adequate ventilation
- Bronchodilators for airflow limitation
- Corticosteroids to reduce inflammatory reactions
- Management of BPD spells (by minimizing exposure to hypoxemia)
- Airway clearance techniques for retained secretions due to infection: positioning, percussion, vibration, and suctioning, as indicated, with attention to precautions/contraindications specific to neonates (see Table 8-14 and Box 8-4 on pages 386 and 387). If wheezing and airway collapse are present, pretreatment with bronchodilators may be beneficial.

Meconium Aspiration Syndrome

Meconium aspiration syndrome (MAS) results from the aspiration of meconium (dark, viscous, sterile fetal bowel content) into the fetal or newborn lung either in utero or during the first breaths after birth. Approximately 12% of all term deliveries in the United States produce meconium-stained amniotic fluid, and 5% of these develop MAS.[1] Meconium is rarely passed before 32 weeks of gestation and most infants are at least 37 weeks gestational age; postterm deliveries carry the highest risk, with up to 30% to 40% of infants having meconium-stained amniotic fluid.[115a]

Pathophysiology

- Aspiration of meconium causes mechanical obstruction of the small airways; partial obstruction can produce a ball–valve effect with alveolar air trapping and possible hyperexpansion with air leaks (see the next section), and complete obstruction leads to atelectasis. The end result is ventilation–perfusion mismatch and impaired gas exchange.
- In addition to mechanical blockage, aspiration of meconium leads to pulmonary parenchymal and alveolar injury via inflammatory reactions, disruption of surfactant production and function and resultant reduction in lung compliance, increased airway resistance, ventilation–perfusion abnormalities, hypoxia, and increased work of breathing.
- If MAS is severe or prolonged, pulmonary hypertension develops (>50% of cases of persistent pulmonary hypertension of the newborn [PPHN] are associated with MAS).
- Approximately half of infants affected by MAS require mechanical ventilation, and a small percentage of infants succumb to the respiratory complications.

Clinical Manifestations

- Meconium-stained amniotic fluid noted at birth
- Central nervous system depression at birth (if severe asphyxia has occurred); possible hypotonia, coma, and seizures
- Signs and symptoms of respiratory distress (see Table 8-7)

Management

- As per the September 2007 guidelines from the American College of Obstetricians and Gynecologists (ACOG) Committee on Obstetric Practice: immediate postpartum intubation for direct tracheal suctioning should be performed on infants with meconium-stained amniotic fluid and depressed level of functioning.[17] Intrapartum suctioning is no longer recommended. No intervention is required if the neonate is vigorous (having strong respiratory efforts, good muscle tone, and HR greater than 100 bpm).

- Airway clearance techniques, including postural drainage and percussion, are initiated as soon as possible.
- Supportive care
  - ▸ Supplemental oxygen
  - ▸ Mechanical ventilation
  - ▸ Consideration of surfactant and/or corticosteroids
  - ▸ Diuretics
  - ▸ Supplemental nutrition
- Extracorporeal membrane oxygenation (ECMO)
- Inhaled nitric oxide (iNO)

Air Leak Syndromes

In neonates, overdistension of alveolar sacs and terminal airways caused by positive-pressure ventilation, partial airway obstruction with ball–valve effect, and failure to wean after surfactant replacement therapy, among other things, can result in airway tissue rupture and air leaks that track through various tissues in the chest.

The types of air leaks that are seen in neonates include the following:

- Pneumothorax (air in the pleural space due to rupture of the mediastinal pleura, occurring spontaneously or as a complication of other respiratory disorders or their treatment; see page 89)
- Pulmonary interstitial emphysema (air tracking through the perivascular adventitia to the interstitial spaces), seen mainly in preterm infants
- Pneumomediastinum (air in the mediastinal space due to dissection along vascular sheaths toward the hilum; usually associated with birth trauma or MAS)
- Pneumopericardium (alveolar rupture followed by dissection of air into the pericardium)
- Pneumoperitoneum (mediastinal air tracking downward to the extraperitoneal fascial planes and eventually rupturing into the peritoneal cavity)
- Pulmonary gas embolism and subcutaneous emphysema (rare)

Apnea

Most newborns display self-limiting apnea without bradycardia associated with swallowing, startles, or defecation; however, some exhibit more prolonged episodes of apnea. The American Academy of Pediatrics Task Force on Prolonged Apnea defines clinically significant apnea as prolonged pauses in respiration lasting at least 20 seconds and pauses for shorter periods of time if accompanied by bradycardia, cyanosis, or pallor.[5]

- Apnea must be distinguished from *periodic breathing* which is a benign respiratory pattern of the preterm or young infant in which there are respiratory pauses of less than 10 seconds with normal respirations in between.[38,91a]
- *Apnea of prematurity* is most commonly a central apnea, in which there is complete absence of respiratory effort, occurring in premature infants born at less than 36 weeks of gestation.
- Apnea has been associated with neck flexion in the preterm infant.[108] Therefore, infants in the neonatal intensive care unit (NICU) are typically positioned with the neck in neutral or slightly extended.

- *Obstructive apnea*, when an infant breathes but no airflow occurs because of upper airway obstruction (most commonly at the pharyngeal level), may be the causative factor when neck flexion is not present.[76a]
- In the absence of underlying pathology, apnea generally decreases with maturity.

Congenital Diaphragmatic Hernia

A congenital diaphragmatic hernia (CDH) is an opening between the pleural and peritoneal cavities, which results in herniation of abdominal viscera (intestine, spleen, and occasionally stomach and liver) into the chest cavity, which inhibits lung development. CDH occurs more frequently in the left hemidiaphragm with resultant ipsilateral hypoplasia, but larger defects and defects causing mediastinal shift may also affect development of the contralateral lung. The more severe the compression of the developing lungs, the more significant the resultant pulmonary hypoplasia. Pulmonary hypertension is often present, likely because of the higher concentration of arteries in the periphery of the hypoplastic lung provoking increased pulmonary vascular resistance. CDH may be diagnosed via prenatal ultrasound and confirmed by chest x-ray after birth.

Management includes immediate stabilization and preoperative preparation including mechanical ventilation and placement of a naso- or orogastric tube to decompress the stomach and reduce passage of air through the gastrointestinal tract. Primary closure of the defect is performed, often requiring hospitalization for several weeks while respiratory, gastrointestinal, and feeding issues are addressed. Management of severe respiratory distress may include ECMO. Surfactant replacement therapy may be helpful. Suctioning, postural drainage positions, and/or percussion techniques are often used to mobilize and clear secretions.

Abdominal Wall Defects

Abdominal wall defects are surgical emergencies in the newborn and frequently produce respiratory sequelae.

- *Gastroschisis* is the herniation of unprotected intestinal contents (usually small bowel and a portion of stomach and colon) through a defect in the abdominal wall located to the right of the umbilical cord. It can be diagnosed via prenatal ultrasound.
  - ▸ Exposure of bowel tissue (unprotected by peritoneal sac) to irritating amniotic fluid in utero causes it to be edematous, indurated, and foreshortened at birth.
  - ▸ After birth evaporative fluid loss and rapid cooling of core temperature occurs, requiring immediate, appropriate wrapping to preserve fluids and temperature before prompt surgical intervention.
  - ▸ Primary closure is done via manual stretching of the abdominal wall and reinsertion of the intestinal contents into the abdomen. If the external organs are too voluminous to fit within the abdominal cavity, a prosthetic silo is constructed for temporary "storage" of the contents while awaiting adequate growth, and full closure is performed in stages.
  - ▸ When the tissues are placed back into the abdominal cavity, the diaphragm is pressed up into an elevated position, causing restricted diaphragmatic movement during inspiration. As a result of both postsurgical biomechanics and an attempt to seek out a position that facilitates comfort and ease of

breathing, the baby typically assumes a posture that includes increased neck and trunk extension, anterior pelvic tilt with lower extremity external rotation, and upper extremity elevation and retraction. This atypical postural alignment is not supportive of respiratory or developmental goals, as it encourages extensor muscle activity of the neck and trunk and decreased overall activity, especially of the legs.

- ▸ Total parenteral nutrition (TPN) is provided via a central venous line (CVL) and oral feedings are initially withheld and then limited, resulting in reduced oral stimulation. Sometimes an ostomy is required if intestinal atresia is present.

- ▸ At a minimum, infants and their families spend 3 to 4 weeks in the hospital tolerating intermittent positional restrictions. The severity of illness, inability to take food by mouth, and positional restrictions imposed may limit parental ability to hold their infant, which sometimes results in delayed bonding with the infant.

- *Omphalocele* is a defect in the abdominal wall resulting in herniation of the abdominal viscera within a protective sac through the base of the umbilical cord. If mild, only a small loop of intestines is visible outside the abdomen, but a large or giant omphalocele contains the liver and spleen in addition to intestines, in which case the peritoneal cavity is very small.

- ▸ Management of an intact omphalocele is similar to that of gastroschisis but without concern for evaporative loss and core cooling, and therefore closure is not emergent. The timing of surgery is determined by the dimensions of the defect, size of the infant, and presence of other anomalies (≈25%–40% of infants have other significant congenital anomalies, including chromosomal abnormalities, CDH, and a variety of cardiac defects).[38] Surgical reduction may be difficult to achieve with large or giant defects, even when performed in stages over a prolonged period.

- ▸ If the protective sac ruptures during delivery, the omphalocele presents more like a gastroschisis and must be treated emergently.

- ▸ The mortality rate is higher than for gastroschisis because of complications associated with other anomalies.

- ▸ Infants with omphalocele often acquire atypical postures and movement patterns similar to those described for infants with gastroschisis repair (see earlier).

Although postural drainage and percussion are sometimes used to assist with the management of secretions (with awareness of appropriate precautions) in both conditions, positioning to decrease the work of breathing (on an incline) is also clinically important (see page 384). Any technique that increases intraabdominal pressure such as vibration should be avoided, and manual hyperinflation is contraindicated for both defects. Supportive positioning to minimize neck and trunk extension and gentle activation of flexor musculature, as tolerated, are also recommended.

Esophageal Atresia and Tracheoesophageal Fistula

Abnormal partitioning of the esophagus and trachea early in fetal development may result in incomplete development of the esophagus and a persistent fistula. In the most commonly occurring

variant (≈85% of cases), the esophagus ends distally in a blind pouch about 10 to 12 cm from the nares and the distal portion arising from the stomach through the diaphragm communicates with the trachea via a tracheoesophageal fistula (TEF).[38] Diagnosis is made with x-ray and via attempted passage of an oro- or nasogastric tube.

Specific clinical symptoms vary with the type of defect and may include excessive salivation, aspiration of saliva, reflux of gastric contents into the trachea, and abdominal distension. Aspiration from the pouch into the larynx and main bronchi results in consolidation and atelectasis.

Immediate surgical repair is performed for infants who are clinically stable and involves division of the distal end of the fistula, closure of the trachea, and construction of an end-to-end anastomosis to the proximal esophagus via thoracotomy. Growth time may be allowed for the ends to more closely approximate one another. A temporary gastrostomy may be necessary for staged procedures to ensure that nutritional needs are met. Hospitalization time varies depending on the individual defect and related complications.

Because these infants experience atypical feedings, oral stimulation is reduced and delayed bonding with the family may also occur. The pain and discomfort that occur as a result of reflux, aspiration, and difficulty breathing sometimes give rise to atypical postures in an attempt to decrease the work of breathing, as described for gastroschisis. Care should be taken to avoid hyperextension of the neck in order to protect the surgical anastomosis from excessive tension during initial healing. In addition, suctioning of both the oro- and nasopharyngeal regions must be done with caution after the repair is made.

CLINICAL IMPLICATIONS FOR PHYSICAL THERAPY IN NEONATAL RESPIRATORY DISORDERS

- Neonates with respiratory problems are usually found in the NICU. Although initially overwhelming, this environment is the safest place to evaluate and treat any patient because of the constant monitoring provided and the availability of trained personnel.

- ▸ Always check with the infant's nurse before initiating intervention to ensure knowledge of the most current information about the infant's status, recent events and procedures (see Section 8.5), and appropriateness for physical therapy (PT) assessment and intervention.

- ▸ Some situations that may indicate the need to delay PT intervention include very recent extubation, untreated pneumothorax, immediately after placement of a chest tube (before chest radiograph results), unstable blood gases, recent feeding (unless stomach is bypassed), and intolerance to handling (e.g., increased apnea, bradycardia, and skin color changes).

- Direct handling of infants in the NICU is not appropriate for student physical therapists, physical therapist assistants, or aides and should be reserved for those with advanced training and mentorship.[107]

- Neonates who suffer from pulmonary dysfunction are also at risk for the breadth of other complications that are associated with premature birth (see page 347).

- Neonates are at risk for hypothermia (associated with apnea) and hypoxemia, but exposure to both lower *and* higher temperatures may result in increased oxygen consumption. Because of their inability to effectively self-regulate body temperature, PT intervention for neonates is often provided through portals in an incubator or with special attention to providing radiant warmth or adequate draping, wrapping, or swaddling.
- Physiological monitoring is extremely important for these infants because of their lack of tolerance for increased activity, which further stresses their cardiorespiratory system, and includes the following:
  ‣ HR
  ‣ BP (typically via arterial line)
  ‣ Respiratory rate and pattern (neonates compensate for respiratory insufficiency by increasing their rate of breathing)
  ‣ Skin color changes
  ‣ ECG (see page 263)
  ‣ Transcutaneous or pulse oximetry (see page 18)
- A neonate may tolerate PT intervention better if the dose of supplemental oxygen is increased, which requires a physician's order. Once the infant is stable after treatment, the oxygen must be turned back down to baseline level.
- Positioning can affect ventilation–perfusion relationships and airway clearance, as well as patterns of muscle activation and subsequent movement.
  ‣ Prone positioning is the optimal position for ventilation in an infant with normal tone but requires attention to secure appropriate positional aids in patients with umbilical vein lines, enlarged abdomens, or decreased tone.
  ‣ As with adults, the uppermost lung segments, as related to the infant's position in space, are preferentially ventilated.
  ‣ Careful monitoring of the infant is essential while attempting new positions and with positional changes.
  ‣ Positioning should be used to reinforce cardiopulmonary PT goals as well as to support developmental goals.
- Because of their medical fragility and overall physiological instability, neonates should receive airway clearance techniques (other than positioning) only when there is a clear indication. While the infant is in the acute stages of pulmonary compromise, percussion, vibration, positioning, and/or suctioning may be indicated to help mobilize and clear secretions. Supportive positioning to facilitate neurobehavioral regulation, decrease the work of breathing, and promote functional, flexor-biased movement patterns is always indicated for neonates and infants and should be instituted according to tolerance.

PEDIATRIC PULMONARY DISORDERS

Some pulmonary disorders affecting infants and children result from genetic disorders (e.g., cystic fibrosis and immotile cilia syndrome); most of the others are due to infection, asthma, or accidental ingestion of foreign objects.

Cystic Fibrosis

Cystic fibrosis (CF) is an autosomal recessive disorder resulting from a defect of chromosome 7. More than 1000 mutations of the gene that causes CF have been identified, but the majority of cases are attributed to the ΔF508 mutation. Abnormalities of the CF transmembrane conductance regulator (CFTR) protein cause abnormal ion transport, which results in endocrine dysfunction and hyperviscous secretions. Involvement of other organ systems varies between individuals, but pulmonary and pancreatic clinical manifestations are most common.

Infants may present with meconium ileus (failure to pass meconium after birth), salty tasting skin, failure to thrive despite a voracious appetite, and/or fatty, foul-smelling stools. Normal growth and development are affected by malabsorption. Diagnosis is usually confirmed via two positive sweat tests (chloride content ≥ 60 mEq/L, using pilocarpine iontophoresis) in the presence of family history or clinical symptoms.[92]

In 2006, the predicted mean survival for a person with CF was 36.9 years and approximately 40% of people living with CF were 18 years of age or older, which represents a significant improvement over prior decades.[20] These improvements reflect advances in the management of CF, so that it is no longer a disease only of childhood and adolescence. Today, some adults with CF are surviving into their fifties.

Pulmonary Pathophysiology

- Lung structure and function are normal at birth.
- After birth, in the majority of patients, abnormal bronchial mucous glands produce excessive amounts of hyperviscous mucus, which obstructs the airways and interferes with mucociliary transport. Retention of secretions results in secondary infections (most often *Pseudomonas aeruginosa, Staphylococcus aureus, Haemophilus influenzae,* methicillin-resistant *Staphylococcus aureus* (MRSA), *Staphylococcus maltophilia,* or *Burkholderia cepacia* complex) that usually present as bronchiolitis, bronchitis, or pneumonia. Initial episodes of pulmonary involvement are usually reversible if treated.
- Once chronic infection is present, obstructive pulmonary disease develops over time, leading to suppurative bronchiectasis. Ventilation–perfusion matching becomes increasingly more problematic, inducing arterial hypoxemia, pulmonary hypertension, and eventually cor pulmonale (see pages 72 to 77 and 95). Abnormal gas exchange produces hypercapnia and respiratory acidosis.
- In addition, the markedly elevated work of breathing (especially during acute infections) increases the possibility of respiratory muscle fatigue and respiratory failure (see page 95).

Pulmonary Clinical Manifestations

- Early signs and symptoms include the following:
  ‣ Tachypnea
  ‣ Dyspnea
  ‣ Increased sputum production
  ‣ Cough
  ‣ Mottling of the skin, pallor or cyanosis, especially during crying spells or exertion
  ‣ Acute respiratory infection with fever, productive cough, increased respiratory rate, and increased work of breathing
- Once there is chronic pulmonary infection, signs and symptoms progress to include the following:
  ‣ Chronic, productive cough
  ‣ Decreased breath sounds with prolonged expiration, wheezes, and localized or generalized crackles

- Frequent upper respiratory and sinus infections; possible nasal polyps
- Development of barrel-chest deformity (increased anteroposterior diameter)
- Chest pain (musculoskeletal or pleuritic)
- Increased use of accessory muscles of respiration, even at rest
- Increasing fatigue, decreased exercise tolerance
- Later stages of chronic infection may result in:
  - Blood-streaked mucus, hemoptysis, darkened color of secretions
  - Clubbing of the digits
  - Hypoxemia, possible hypercapnia, and respiratory acidosis
  - Possible signs and symptoms of pulmonary HTN, right ventricular hypertrophy (RVH), cor pulmonale, and/or respiratory failure (see pages 95 and 96)

Management

- Usually coordinated by a regional cystic fibrosis specialty care center
- PT interventions, including airway clearance techniques, exercise prescription, and postural education. The majority of airway clearance techniques described for adults can be used in the pediatric population with modifications (see Section 8.6) as appropriate; techniques that require sequenced breathing patterns (e.g., autogenic drainage, active cycle of breathing technique, Acapella [Smiths Medical, St. Paul, MN], and Flutter [Axcan Pharma, Mont-Saint-Hilaire, PQ, Canada]) are difficult to use in younger children.
- Pharmacologic therapy may include a number of different medications:
  - Bronchodilators
  - Mucolytic aerosols
  - Corticosteroids, inhaled or oral
  - Antibiotics
  - Antifungals
  - Oxygen, diuretics for cor pulmonale
- Nutrition
  - Pancreatic enzymes
  - Supplemental nutrition
  - Monitoring for CF-related diabetes
- Pulmonary function testing to help track the progression of the disease and the effectiveness of interventions
- Lung transplantation for end-stage disease

Clinical Implications for Physical Therapy

- Because bronchial hygiene is a critical part of the successful management of CF, airway clearance techniques must be incorporated into the daily lives of patients and their families and evolve to meet the changing needs associated with age and different life stages. Patient and parent education are extremely important.
  - Early education seeks to develop airway clearance habits that will be maintained throughout the life span, playing a more critical role as pulmonary symptoms progress.
  - It is not unusual for children and families to be familiar with and use more than one type of airway clearance technique.
  - Refer to pages 385 to 389 for descriptions of various treatment techniques.

- Exercise is a critical component of treatment for patients with CF:
  - Aerobic activity is important at all ages to increase cardiopulmonary fitness.
    - ⊙ Older children and adolescents may benefit from formal exercise prescription including treadmill, bicycle, stepper, elliptical trainer, and so on.
    - ⊙ Parents of younger children should be encouraged to stimulate interest in more active recreational activities (e.g., swimming and martial arts) and participation of parent and child together should be supported.
    - ⊙ Pediatric-sized cardiovascular equipment is available including treadmills, upright and recumbent bicycles, steppers, and elliptical trainers.
  - Strengthening exercises in general, and particularly of the postural muscles, is important, as are active and manual interventions to maintain or increase chest wall mobility.
  - Breathing exercises may be used to improve respiratory muscle strength and endurance and to reduce dyspnea.
  - Functional activities (activities of daily living and play-, school-, or job-related activities) should also be incorporated and recommendations offered for modification/adaptation, as needed.
  - Regular physical exercise offers a variety of health benefits, including psychological well-being and improved quality of life (see Table 7-4 on page 304). It may also contribute to the development of self-esteem.
  - Yoga and pilates techniques are being used increasingly for the patients with CF to target postural strengthening and mobility, breath control and support, and improve focus and concentration.
- As the disease progresses, treatment modifications are often required:
  - Supplemental oxygen for desaturation with exercise
  - Slower progression of exercise program because of increasing dyspnea and exercise intolerance, as well as poor nutrition
  - Specific modifications indicated for coexisting medical conditions (e.g., diabetes mellitus, osteoporosis)
  - Support groups for diminished sense of well-being and quality of life

Asthma

Asthma is described on page 78. In 2004, 9 million American children under 18 years of age (12%) had been diagnosed with asthma at some point in time.[12] It was more common in boys (15% in boys compared with 9% in girls) and in very low income families (14%). The prevalence of asthma has increased significantly in a way that parallels that of obesity. Because clinical presentation varies from child to child, asthma may be diagnosed at any age. Asthma may be triggered by both intrinsic and extrinsic factors, and risk factors for asthma include familial predisposition, allergy, past medical history of respiratory syncytial virus infection (see following section), BPD (see page 348), and very low birth weight prematurity.

- As airway diameter increases with growth, children may become less symptomatic during adolescence and early adulthood, but often continue to have measurable spirometric abnormalities and airway hyperreactivity at a subclinical level.[105]

- Asthma severity is widely variable among children (as with adults).
  - Mild symptoms include occasional wheezing in response to a respiratory tract infection.
  - More severe symptoms include daily symptoms of bronchial hyperreactivity, which may range from mild to continuous bronchospasm.
  - In severe disease airway obstruction and chronic hyperinflation are present.
  - Status asthmaticus warrants admission to the hospital for further management, and sometimes requires intensive care.
- Adolescents with asthma pose additional challenges to management because of the developmental, emotional, psychological, and social changes they are dealing with, as well as their fluctuating hormones. They have a greater risk of persistent symptoms, underdiagnosis, and undertreatment of their disease.[20a]
- Exercise-induced asthma (EIA) is common in children and adolescents and occurs in 70% to 90% of those with asthma.[119] It is usually characterized by coughing, dyspnea, wheezing, and chest tightness during or after exercise, and is associated with airflow limitation after exercise, especially in cold air. Some children exhibit atypical symptoms, such as cramps, stomach pain, headache, fatigue, or dizziness.[103]
  - Use of a bronchodilator before exercise is recommended and education in their use is often provided by PTs.
  - Individuals with asthma also benefit from advice regarding the types of exercise that are less likely to provoke bronchoconstriction (e.g., intermittent exercise or team games, swimming, exercise in warm, humid air, and exercise that avoids high pollen [in allergic asthma] or polluted air) versus those that are more likely to cause asthma (continuous, strenuous exercise, such as running, and exercise in cold environments or polluted air, during pollen season, or during upper or lower respiratory infection).[103]
  - Persons with EIA fare better by performing warm-up exercise to 80% to 90% of their maximal workload before beginning the actual workout.
  - Patients with chronic persistent EIA (i.e., forced expiratory volume in 1 s [FEV$_1$] <80% of predicted and symptoms occurring more than twice per week) are usually advised to take daily controller medications.
- Regular exercise is beneficial for children with asthma.
  - Aerobic training has been shown to improve breathing reserve, oxygen pulse (the volume of oxygen extracted from the peripheral tissues per heart beat or the volume of oxygen added to the pulmonary blood per heart beat), and HR reserve at peak exercise and to reduce ventilation and HR at any given workload. These adaptations are likely to result in an increased physiological reserve to respond to a bout of asthma or EIA and may reduce the occurrence of EIA episodes.[119] A number of studies have also reported improvements in quality of life measures, including psychological indices.
  - Swimming is highly recommended and has been shown to be less likely to provoke exacerbations than running (both on ground and on treadmill) and cycling, although some individuals are sensitive to the chlorine fumes in indoor pools.[63,119]

- Yoga and pilates techniques are valuable forms of exercise for patients with asthma because of their beneficial effects an posture, breath control and support, and enhanced focus and concentration, which can be used to help cope with acute asthma attacks.
  - Postural education and breathing specific exercises may be indicated for some patients.
- If mucus plugging or overproduction is present, airway clearance techniques may be indicated.

Bronchiolitis and Respiratory Syncytial Virus Infection

In the pediatric population, bronchiolitis is most frequently caused by respiratory syncytial virus (RSV) infection but may be linked with parainfluenza, influenza, and adenoviruses. RSV is a potentially dangerous threat to infants and children, particularly those less than 2 years old and those with underlying congenital heart disease or history of prematurity. Clinical manifestations of RSV infection may range from those of mild upper respiratory tract infection to bronchiolitis and interstitial pneumonia.

- Bronchiolitis results in bronchiolar edema, necrosis and shedding of the epithelial cells, and increased mucous secretion, which leads to airway obstruction. The result is gross hyperinflation of the lungs along with localized areas of atelectasis.
- Apnea is common in both premature and full-term newborns, and severe symptoms may require intubation and assisted ventilation.
- Most infants and children recover completely and the mortality rate is low.
- Treatment includes supportive care, specifically hydration and oxygenation, supplemental nutrition, and corticosteroids (if complicated by reactive airway disease). Antibiotics may be used if secondary bacterial infection is suspected. Bronchodilators are usually of limited clinical value. ECMO may be necessary if conventional ventilation fails. The use of airway clearance techniques is controversial but may be indicated if mucus plugging is suspected.

Primary Ciliary Dyskinesia

Primary ciliary dyskinesia is an autosomal recessive disorder in which ciliary abnormalities result in the accumulation of secretions in the airways with subsequent chronic upper and lower respiratory tract infections. Variations include absence of cilia, abnormal cilia, or structurally normal cilia with abnormal function. Primary ciliary dyskinesia is present in approximately 25% of cases of situs inversus.[98] Both upper and lower airways are affected, and symptoms include sinusitis, chronic rhinitis, recurrent bronchitis, bronchiectasis, and fertility issues (due to fallopian tube ciliary dysfunction in women and abnormal sperm motility in men). Bronchiectasis is common by early adulthood.

Appropriate medical therapy has been shown to prevent deterioration of lung function,[14] and daily prophylactic airway clearance treatments (including postural drainage, percussion, vibration, active cycle of breathing technique, Acapella, positive expiratory pressure, and high-frequency chest wall compression; see pages 385 to 389) are a major component of this management. The lower lobes and lingua are at risk for collection of secretions because of their dependent position, but in the presence of situs inversus the middle lobe may be more affected than the lingula. Increased frequency of treatments is necessary during acute exacerbations. In addition, regular aerobic exercise is recommended to assist with airway clearance and to improve cardiorespiratory fitness.

Aspiration Syndromes

Aspiration of substances or objects into the respiratory systems of children is not uncommon. Accidental aspiration of small objects into the airways is usually the unfortunate result of innate curiosity and oral exploration, so parents must take precautions to screen immediate environments for toys and other small objects that may be tempting to the young child.

Aspiration pneumonia is the term used to describe the aspiration of gastric contents or mucous secretions of the upper airway into the respiratory system. Severe gastroesophageal reflux with recurrent aspiration can result in chronic pulmonary disease and ultimately bronchiectasis. Aspiration of water into the lungs may occur during accidental drowning.

The outcomes of aspiration range from asymptomatic to fatal. Aspiration of various materials results in a number of patholophysiological responses, including physical obstruction, inflammation, secondary infection (particularly with organic materials), or chemical injury. Ventilation–perfusion abnormalities and pulmonary edema may develop in severe cases. Because the right main stem bronchus is a more direct continuation of the trachea, aspiration tends to involve the right lung more often than the left.

- Clinical manifestations include unilateral absence of breath sounds and/or localized wheezing, stridor, bloody sputum, and possible respiratory distress.
- Foreign bodies must be removed by rigid bronchoscopy whereas other aspiration syndromes may require supportive care and antibiotics. Percussion is not effective in trying to facilitate removal and is contraindicated.
- Gastroesophageal reflux leading to aspiration pneumonia must be identified as quickly as possible and addressed via positioning after feeding, thickening of feeds, and medications. Fundoplication may be required, especially in the setting of BPD or postcongenital diaphragmatic hernia repair.
- Education of parents and other caregivers may help in primary prevention of both foreign body aspiration and aspiration pneumonia.

CLINICAL IMPLICATIONS FOR PHYSICAL THERAPY

Specific clinical implications have already been provided for patients with CF and asthma, so general clinical implications for pediatric patients with lung disease are provided here.

- Physiological monitoring of responses to stimulation and activity in infants and younger children and in response to exercise in older children with secondary cardiopulmonary dysfunction is indicated and consists of:
  - HR
  - BP
  - Respiratory rate and pattern
  - Transcutaneous or pulse oximetry (see page 18)
  - ECG (see page 263)
  - Skin color changes
  - Rating of perceived exertion (see page 281)
- Positioning, described on pages 384 and 387, is beneficial for promoting:
  - Decreased work of breathing
  - Increased ventilation (uppermost lung segments, as related to the infant's position in space, benefit most in infants)
  - Prevention of aspiration in patients with gastroesophageal reflux
  - Neurodevelopmental goals
- Airway clearance techniques, including percussion, vibration, positioning, suctioning, and breathing exercises (see pages 385–389), may be indicated for patients with excessive secretions or impaired ability to mobilize them.
  - Older children often prefer treatment methods such as oscillatory positive expiratory pressure and high-frequency chest wall compression systems.
  - Games and activities involving coordination of breathing patterns and increased ventilation are recommended to improve the efficiency of ventilation.
- Regular physical activity and exercise training is important for patients with pulmonary disease to optimize functional capacity and prevent complications associated with a sedentary lifestyle. Regular exercise may also enhance psychological well-being, quality of life, and self-esteem.
  - Aerobic exercise and recreational activities promote cardiopulmonary fitness.
  - Activities such as yoga and pilates have beneficial effects on posture, strength and flexibility, as well as breath control and support and focus and concentration.
  - Strengthening exercises are also valuable, especially those targeting postural muscles.

8.3 PEDIATRIC CARDIOVASCULAR DISEASE

Whereas most cases of pediatric heart disease result from congenital cardiac lesions, acquired heart disease is not rare. This section identifies the more common acyanotic and a cyanotic congenital heart defects and several noncardiac diagnoses that are frequently associated with cardiovascular dysfunction. The clinical manifestations of heart disease in infants are listed in Box 8-1 and more specifically under each diagnosis. The clinical implications for PT intervention when working with these patients and their families are also presented.

CONGENITAL HEART DISEASE

Congenital heart disease (CHD) has been defined as "a gross structural abnormality of the heart or intrathoracic great vessels that is actually or potentially of functional significance" to the cardiovascular system.[78] Approximately 0.8% of live births are associated with some type of congenital cardiovascular malformation, with moderate to severe CHD occurring in almost 0.6% of live births.[50] CHD forms the core of most pediatric cardiology practices.

BOX 8-1: Clinical Manifestations of Cardiac Disease in Infants

Difficulty feeding; failure to thrive

Irritability, lethargy

Signs and symptoms of respiratory distress (see Table 8-7)

Signs and symptoms of CHF:

- Dyspnea, tachypnea, respiratory distress
- Tachycardia
- Jugular venous distension (may be difficult to appreciate because of short neck)
- Forehead diaphoresis (especially with feeding)
- Pallor
- Lethargy
- Hepatomegaly
- Failure to thrive
- Pulmonary crackles or pleural effusions

Signs of peripheral hypoperfusion:

- Weak, thready peripheral pulses
- Peripheral vasoconstriction
- Slow capillary refill
- Oliguria
- Metabolic acidosis

Precordial bulge (due to cardiomegaly)

Hyperactive pericardium, prominent pulsations or thrills on palpation, according to specific defect(s)

Abnormal cardiac sounds according to specific defect(s) (see page 44)

Bounding pulses (if aortic run-off lesions, such as PDA, AR)

Bradycardia if hypoxemia, heart block, digitalis toxicity, and so on.

AR, Aortic regurgitation; CHF, congestive heart failure; PDA, patent ductus arteriosus.

Congenital heart defects result from disturbances during the complex embryologic development of the heart that either alter the development of a normally occurring structure or hinder further evolution of a normally formed structure during later stages of formation.[117] They are believed to be influenced by genetics, the environment, or an interaction between the two.[36]

Lesions may occur in isolation, in combination, and as components of syndromes affecting multiple systems. Table 8-8 highlights some syndromes that have associated congenital cardiac defects, particularly those that are more frequently encountered by the pediatric physical therapist. It has been estimated that 0.3% of live births require cardiac catheterization or surgery in early infancy to either minimize complications or to prevent death due to CHD.[31] Because of the intimate relationship between the heart and lungs, cardiac dysfunction occurring in infants with CHD often results in increased work of breathing and impaired gas exchange.

This chapter categorizes CHD into cyanotic and acyanotic cardiac defects and presents prevalence, pathophysiology, clinical manifestations and natural history, and management for each lesion presented. Most congenital lesions are compatible with fetal circulation, and it is not until birth that physiological complications arise. Given the significant effects they have on the infant, the majority of complex congenital lesions will be diagnosed during the neonatal period. Less serious lesions may manifest themselves in later years. For this, and other reasons, it is believed that the prevalence of many congenital defects is underestimated.

Surgical procedures performed for the palliation of congenital heart disease are listed in Table 8-9 and those performed for correction are recorded in Table 8-10. Patients who undergo corrective procedures for simple congenital defects tend to do well for years after surgery, but may develop late complications, such as arrhythmias and ventricular dysfunction. Children with corrected complex congenital heart defects are more likely to be troubled by residual defects or shunts, pulmonary HTN, ventricular

dysfunction, tachyarrhythmias, and the need for reoperation. In addition, an increasing number of patients with CHD and previous palliation who later develop ventricular failure are successfully undergoing cardiac transplantation.[57]

Although regular physical exercise has been shown to provide long-term physical, psychological, and social benefits in patients with CHD, a large number of patients remain physically inactive.[49,91] Many factors may contribute to this trend, including habitual poor participation, fear (on the part of the child or parent/caregiver) of increasing physical activity, and/or lack of education regarding the benefits of regular physical activity. The resulting inactive lifestyle leads to diminished aerobic capacity and increases the risk for early development of cardiovascular disease and other illnesses associated with a sedentary lifestyle.

There are few contraindications for exercise for patients with both stable unoperated and operated CHD, especially if asymptomatic, and the risk of complications due to exercise is low.[40,91] Individuals who are suspected of having elevated pulmonary arterial pressure (PAP) should undergo evaluation by echocardiography or cardiac catheterization before being cleared for more vigorous physical exercise. Those with pulmonary HTN and CHD are at risk for sudden death during sports activities, and although most patients self-limit their activity, they should not participate in competitive athletics.

Exercise recommendations and restrictions for participation in competitive athletics for patients with CHD are presented in Table 8-11, and the classification of sports is shown in Table 8-12. This classification is based on peak static and dynamic components achieved during competition, although higher values may be reached during training. In general, static exercise creates a more pronounced pressure overload, the intensity of which is more difficult to control, and therefore it may be less suitable for patients with CHD. Only patients who are New York Heart Association (NYHA) functional class I (see page 223) are appropriate for unrestricted participation in competitive sports.

TABLE 8-8: Congenital Syndromes and Associated Congenital Heart Defects and Extracardiovascular Features Frequently Encountered by Pediatric Physical Therapists

Syndrome	Cardiovascular Features	Most Significant Extracardiovascular Features
Trisomy 21 (Down syndrome)	Endocardial cushion defect (AV canal), ASD, VSD, TOF	Hypotonia, hyperextensible joints, brachycephaly, characteristic facies including epicanthal folds, simian palmar crease, increased space between first and second toes, mental retardation
Trisomy 18 (Edward's syndrome)	VSD, PS, other valvular defects, PDA	SGA and subsequent growth deficiency, clenched hands with overriding second on third and fifth on fourth digits, short sternum, rocker bottom feet, small pelvis, mental retardation
XO (Turner's syndrome)	Coarctation of aorta, bicuspid aortic valve, aortic dilatation; HLHS	Short female, triangular facies, shield chest, congenital lymphedema of hands and feet, webbed neck, perceptual and right–left disorientation
Marfan syndrome	Mitral regurgitation, aortic dilatation and dissection	Arachnodactyly with hyperextensibility, lens subluxation
Ehlers-Danlos syndrome	Arterial dilatation and rupture, mitral regurgitation	Hyperextensible joints, hyperelastic and friable skin
Osteogenesis imperfecta	Aortic incompetence	Fragile bones, blue sclerae
DiGeorge syndrome, a.k.a. CATCH-22 (cardiac defect, abnormal facies, thymic hypoplasia, cleft palate, and hypocalcemia)	Interrupted aortic arch, PDA, TOF, truncus arteriosus	Thymic hypoplasia or aplasia, parathyroid hypoplasia or aplasia, characteristic facies
Holt-Oram syndrome	ASD, VSD	Skeletal upper limb and shoulder girdle defects, phocomelia, small stature
Noonan syndrome	PS (valvular dysplasia), hypertrophic cardiomyopathy	Characteristic facies including broad forehead, ptosis, hypertelorism, webbed neck, shield chest, short stature, cryptorchidism (males), atlantoaxial instability
CHARGE association (coloboma, heart, atresia choanae, retardation, genital and ear anomalies)	TOF, PDA, endocardial cushion defect, VSD, ASD	Coloboma, choanal atresia, mental and growth deficiencies, genital and ear anomalies, hearing loss
VATER (a.k.a. VACTERL) association (vertebral, anal, cardiac, tracheoesophageal, radial/renal, limb anomalies)	VSD	Vertebral and limb anomalies, anal atresia, tracheoesophageal fistula, radial and renal anomalies
Williams syndrome	Supravalvular AS, PS, VSD, ASD	SGA, failure to thrive, characteristic facies, friendly personality, hoarse voice, mental deficiency
Klippel-Feil syndrome	VSD, dextrocardia	Short neck, limited cervical rotation, cervical anomalies
Friedreich's ataxia	Cardiomyopathy, conduction defects	Ataxia, speech defect, degeneration of spinal cord dorsal columns
Pompe disease	Glycogen storage disease of the heart	Acid maltase deficiency, muscle weakness
Fetal alcohol syndrome	VSD, ASD	Microcephaly, growth and mental deficiency, characteristic facies
Maternal lupus during pregnancy	Complete heart block	Intrauterine growth retardation, neonatal lupus

Data from Berg BO. Chromosomal abnormalities and neurocutaneous disorders. In Goetz CG, editor. *Textbook of Clinical Neurology.* 2nd ed. Philadelphia: Saunders; 2003; Marino BS, Wernovsky G. General principles—preoperative care. In Chang AC, Hanley FL, Wernovsky G, Wessel DL, editors. *Pediatric Cardiac Intensive Care.* Baltimore, MD: Lippincott Williams & Wilkins; 1998; Pyeritz RE. Genetics and cardiovascular disease. In Zipes DP, Libby P, Bonow RO, Braunwald E, editors. *Braunwald's Heart Disease: A Textbook of Cardiovascular Medicine.* 7th ed. Philadelphia: Saunders; 2005; and Webb GD, Smallhorn, JF, Therien, J, et al. Congenital heart disease. In Zipes DP, Libby P, Bonow RO, Braunwald E, editors. *Braunwald's Heart Disease: A Textbook of Cardiovascular Medicine.* 7th ed. Philadelphia: Saunders; 2005.

a.k.a., Also known as; AS, aortic stenosis; ASD, atrial septal defect; AV, atrioventricular; HLHS, hypoplastic left heart syndrome; PDA, patent ductus arteriosus; PS, pulmonary stenosis; SGA, small for gestational age; TOF, tetralogy of Fallot; VSD, ventricular septal defect.

TABLE 8-9: Palliative Procedures for Congenital Heart Disease in Children

Procedures	Lesion	Comments
BT shunt (subclavian artery to ipsilateral pulmonary artery anastomosis)	TOF, pulmonary valve atresia	Improves pulmonary blood flow
Modified BT shunt (subclavian artery to ipsilateral pulmonary artery graft)	TOF	Improves pulmonary blood flow; graft is easier to eliminate than in BT shunt when open repair is performed
Balloon atrial septostomy	D-TGA, tricuspid atresia	Enlarges the foramen ovale to increase atrial mixing
Blalock-Hanlon procedure	D-TGA	Creates an ASD to improve atrial mixing
Balloon valvuloplasty, balloon angioplasty	Pulmonary valve stenosis, aortic valve stenosis, coarctation of the aorta	Increases patency of valve or aortic coarctation
Surgical valvotomy	Pulmonary valve stenosis, aortic valve stenosis	Increases valve patency; resultant pulmonary valve insufficiency enhances RV growth
PGE_1 infusion	Pulmonary atresia, tricuspid atresia, TOF, coarctation of aorta, interrupted aortic arch	Maintains/reopens ductus arteriosus to increase pulmonary blood flow
PA banding	Endocardial cushion defects, single ventricle	Decreases pulmonary blood flow, prevents PVOD. Followed by bidirectional Glenn or Complete Fontan
	TGA (both dextro- and levo-)	Increases afterload to train low-pressure LV in preparation for arterial switch operation

ASD, Atrial septal defect; BT, Blalock-Taussig; D-TGA, dextro-transposition of the great arteries; PA, pulmonary artery; PGE_1, prostaglandin E_1; PVOD, pulmonary vascular obstructive disease; RV, right ventricle; TOF, tetralogy of Fallot.

TABLE 8-10: Corrective Procedures for Congenital Heart Disease in Children

Procedure	Lesion	Effect/Comments
Repair of septal defects (suture, patching)	ASD, VSD, endocardial cushion defects	Complete repair
Ross procedure (transfer of PV to the aortic position with placement of pulmonary homograft in PV position)	AS, especially subvalvular	Procedure of choice for aortic valve replacement in children because of potential for growth; eliminates complications associated with prosthetic valves
Valve replacement (mechanical valve or bioprosthesis)	Aortic, mitral, or pulmonic stenosis; Ebstein's anomaly	Repair via mechanical prosthesis carries lifelong need for anticoagulation; repair via bioprosthesis not recommended in children given fast degradation rate
Surgical coarctectomies, arch repairs (patch aortoplasty, end-to-end anastomosis, subclavian flap aortoplasty)	Interrupted arch, coarctation of aorta	Repair with prosthetic patch carries risk of bulging; subclavian flap allows autogenous patch with potential for growth; anastomosis carries higher risk of restenosis
Total correction via open heart surgery	TOF, anomalous venous return, PDA	Complete repair
Atrial baffle operations (atrial switch via Mustard or Senning procedure)	D-TGA	Physiological correction; RV remains systemic ventricle
Jatene procedure (arterial switch operation)	D-TGA	Full anatomic correction
Staged arterial switch operations (REV, Nikaidoh, and Damus-Kaye-Stansel procedures)	D-TGA with VSD + severe PS	Full anatomic correction
Rastelli procedure (redirection of pulmonary and systemic venous blood at the ventricular level)	D-TGA with VSD + severe PS	Anatomic correction; requires reoperations for conduit replacement as child grows

Continued

TABLE 8-10: Corrective Procedures for Congenital Heart Disease in Children—Cont'd

Procedure	Lesion	Effect/Comments
Norwood procedure (connects pulmonary trunk to ascending aorta via patch; creates systemic-to-pulmonary shunt)	HLHS: Stage I repair	Improves functional ability of RV to serve as combined ventricle; provides pressure/volume-controlled PA blood flow
Bidirectional Glenn procedure (end-to-side SVC to PA anastomosis)	HLHS: Stage II repair	Partially separates systemic and pulmonary circuits to reduce load on RV
Hemi-Fontan operation (incorporation of the roof of the atrium into PA anastomosis)	HLHS: Stage II repair	Partially separates systemic and pulmonary circuits to reduced load on RV
Fontan procedure (channels IVC and hepatic flow into PAs via extracardiac conduit, completely excluding the atrium)	HLHS: Stage III repair, tricuspid atresia, double-inlet ventricle, heterotaxy syndrome (right or left isomerism)	Restores an in-series pulmonary-to-systemic circulation; decreases chronic volume load from systemic ventricle
Heart transplant	HLHS	Normal heart with associated transplant risks; availability of donors limited

ASD, Atrial septal defect; AS, aortic stenosis; D-TGA, transposition of the great arteries; HLHS, hypoplastic left heart syndrome; IVC, inferior vena cava; PA, pulmonary artery; PDA, patent ductus arteriosus; PS, pulmonary stenosis; PV, pulmonary valve; REV, réparation à l'étage ventriculaire; RV, right ventricle; SVC, superior vena cava; TOF, tetralogy of Fallot; VSD, ventricular septal defect.

TABLE 8-11: Exercise Recommendations and Restrictions in Patients With Congenital Heart Disease

Lesion Type	Exercise: Restriction or Recommendation
ASD and PFO	Avoid scuba diving if persistent shunt
Corrected or unoperated with nl PAP (<30 mm Hg) and nl ventricular function (EF ≥50%)	No restrictions
With mild pulmonary HTN or other abnormal findings	See entry for CHD with mild pulmonary HTN... (next page)
VSD	
Closed or small unoperated with nl PAP and nl ventricular function	No restrictions
With mild pulmonary HTN or other abnormal findings	See entry for CHD with mild pulmonary HTN... (next page)
AVSD	No restrictions
PDA: Small untreated or closed with no evidence of pulmonary HTN or LV enlargement	No restrictions
Pulmonary stenosis	
Mild (PIG <40 mm Hg) or treated, no symptoms	No restrictions
Moderate (PIG >40 mm Hg): Treated + untreated, + severe PI with marked RV enlargement	Low to moderate dynamic/low static sports (IA and IB; see Table 8-12)
Aortic stenosis: Unoperated and operated	
Mild (PIG <40 mm Hg) with no abnormal findings	No restrictions
Moderate (PIG 40–70 mm Hg) with minimal abnormal findings (see text)	Low to moderate dynamic/low static sports (IA, IB, and IIA; see Table 8-12)
Severe (PIG >70 mm Hg)	No competitive athletics
Coarctation of the aorta: Mild untreated	No restrictions
Untreated with PIG arm/leg >20 mm Hg or exercise SBP >230 mm Hg	Low-intensity sports (IA; see Table 8-12)
Treated: Asymptomatic, PIG arm/leg <20 mm Hg, normal exercise SBP	No restrictions except no high-intensity static exercise (IIIA, IIIB, and IIIC; see Table 8-12) or sports with danger of bodily collision

Continued

TABLE 8-11: Exercise Recommendations and Restrictions in Patients With Congenital Heart Disease—Cont'd

Lesion Type	Exercise: Restriction or Recommendation
Coarctation of the aorta—Cont'd	
Treated with significant aortic root dilation, wall thinning, or aneurysm formation	Low-intensity sports (IA and IB; see Table 8-12)
Tetralogy of Fallot	
With excellent repair and minimal abnormal findings (see text)	No restrictions
With important residual abnormalities (see text)	Low dynamic and static sports (IA only; see Table 8-12)
TGA	
Arterial switch: Minimal abnormal findings	No restrictions
More than mild abnormalities + nl GXT	Low to high dynamic/low static and low dynamic/moderate static sports (IA, IB, IC, and IIA; see Table 8-12)
Atrial switch (Mustard or Senning operations) with minimal abnormal findings (see text)	Low dynamic/low to moderate static sports (IA and IIA; see Table 8-12)
Postoperative Fontan operation (e.g., HLHS)	Low dynamic/low static sports only (IA; see Table 8-12)
With nl ventricular function and O_2 saturation	Low-to-moderate dynamic/low static sports (IA and IB; see Table 8-12)
CHD with mild pulmonary HTN*	Low-intensity sports
With persistent, severe pulmonary HTN	No competitive sports
With PVOD, cyanosis + large R → L shunt	No competitive sports
CHD with symptomatic atrial or ventricular tachyarrhythmia	No competitive sports until adequate treatment and no recurrence for 2 to 4 wk, and then only IA sports (see Table 8-12) if status allows
CHD with moderate MR	Low to moderate dynamic/static sports (IA and IB, IIA and IIB; see Table 8-12)
With severe MR + LV enlargement, pulmonary HTN, or LV dysfunction at rest	No competitive sports
CHD with myocardial dysfunction[†]	
Mild (EF = 40%–50%)	Low-intensity static sports (IA, IB, and IC only; see Table 8-12)
Moderate to severe (EF <40%)	No competitive sports

Data from Bonow RO, Cheitlin MD, Crawford MH, et al. Task Force 3: Valvular heart disease. *J Am Coll Cardiol.* 2005;45:1334–1340; Graham TP Jr, Driscoll DJ, Gersony WM, et al. Task Force 2: Congenital heart disease. *J Am Coll Cardiol.* 2005;45:1326–1333; Hirth A, Reybrouck T, Bjarnason-Wehrens B, et al. Recommendations for participation and leisure sports in patients with congenital heart disease: A consensus document [position paper]. *Eur J Cardiovasc Prev Rehabil.* 2006;13:293–299; Pellica A, Fagard R, Bjørnstad HH, et al.: Recommendations for competitive sports participation in athletes with cardiovascular disease: A consensus document from the Study Group of Sports Cardiology of the Working Group of Cardiac Rehabilitation and Exercise Physiology and the Working Group of Myocardial and Pericardial Diseases of the European Society of Cardiology. *Eur Heart J.* 2005;26:1422–1445; Reybrouck T, Mertens L. Physical performance and physical activity in grown-up congenital heart disease. *Eur J Cardiovasc Prev Rehabil.* 2005;12:498–502; and Zipes DP, Ackerman MJ, Estes NAM, et al. Task Force 7: Arrhythmias. *J Am Coll Cardiol.* 2005;45:1354–1363.

arm/leg, Systolic arm-to-leg pressure gradient; ASD, atrial septal defect; AVSD, atrioventricular septal defect; CHD, congestive heart failure; EF, ejection fraction; GXT, graded exercise test; HLHS, hypoplastic left heart syndrome; HTN, hypertension; LV, left ventricular; MR, mitral regurgitation; nl, normal; PAP, pulmonary arterial pressure; PDA, patent ductus arteriosus; PFO, patent foramen ovale; PI, pulmonary insufficiency; PIG, peak instantaneous echo Doppler gradient; PVOD, pulmonary vascular obstructive disease; R → L, right to left; RV, right ventricular; SBP, systolic blood pressure; TGA, transposition of the great arteries; VSD, ventricular septal defect.

*Requires evaluation by echocardiography or and/or catheterization before engaging in competitive athletics.

[†]Requires periodic reassessment, because both unoperated and operated disease can deteriorate over time.

Patients with CHD are often treated with prophylactic antibiotics to prevent the development of infective endocarditis (IE). However, more recent guidelines from the American Heart Association have concluded that only an extremely small number of cases of IE might be prevented by antibiotic prophylaxis and therefore its use is reasonable only for patients with underlying cardiac conditions associated with the highest risk of adverse outcome from IE, which are listed in Box 8-2.[121] Good dental hygiene continues to play a critical role in preventing IE in all patients.

Beyond the scope of this chapter but worthy of mention is the emergence of a new cardiovascular subspecialty addressing the unique issues of the adult patient with CHD. Because of the advances made in detection and management, the number of patients with CHD who reach adulthood in the United States is estimated to be approximately 20,000 per year,[116] and most of these patients require continued surveillance because of risk of later complications (e.g., cardiac arrhythmia and ventricular dysfunction) and potential need for reoperation. This section provides information intended for use in the pediatric population but also serves as a resource for therapists working with adult patients with a history of congenital heart disease to better understand the lesions and their effects.

TABLE 8-12: Classification of Sports

	A. Low Dynamic (<40% $\dot{V}O_{2\,max}$)	B. Moderate Dynamic (40%–70% $\dot{V}O_{2\,max}$)	C. High Dynamic (>70% $\dot{V}O_{2\,max}$)
I. Low static (<20% MVC)	Billiards Bowling Cricket Curling Golf Riflery	Baseball/softball* Fencing Table tennis Tennis (doubles) Volleyball	Badminton Cross country skiing (classic technique) Field hockey* Orienteering Race walking Racquetball/squash* Running (long distance) Soccer* Tennis (singles)
II. Moderate static (20%–50% MVC)	Archery Auto racing*† Diving*† Equestrian*† Motorcycling*†	American football* Field events (jumping) Figure skating* Rodeoing*† Rugby* Running (sprint) Surfing*† Synchronized swimming†	Basketball* Cross-country skiing (skating technique) Ice hockey* Lacrosse* Running (middle distance) Swimming Team handball
III. High static (>50% MVC)	Bobsledding/luge*† Field events (throwing) Gymnastics*† Martial arts* Rock/sport climbing* Sailing Water skiing*† Weight lifting*† Windsurfing*†	Body building*† Downhill skiing*† Skateboarding*† Snowboarding*† Wrestling*	Boxing* Canoeing/kayaking Cycling*† Decathlon Rowing Speed skating*† Triathlon*†

Data from Mitchell JH, Haskell W, Snell P, et al. Task Force 8: Classification of sports. *J Am Coll Cardiol.* 2005; 45:1364–1367; and Pellica A, Fagard R, Bjørnstad HH, et al. Recommendations for competitive sports participation in athletes with cardiovascular disease: A consensus document from the Study Group of Sports Cardiology of the Working Group of Cardiac Rehabilitation and Exercise Physiology and the Working Group of Myocardial and Pericardial Diseases of the European Society of Cardiology. *Eur Heart J.* 2005;26:1422–1445.
MVC, Maximal voluntary contraction; $\dot{V}O_{2\,max}$, maximal oxygen uptake.
*Danger of bodily collision.
†Increased risk if syncope occurs.

Acyanotic Lesions

Acyanotic defects are usually associated with normal systemic arterial saturation as systemic output is frequently maintained. They may be divided into lesions with increased pulmonary blood flow due to left-to-right shunting through some communication between the two sides of the heart (e.g., atrial septal defect, ventricular septal defect, patent ductus arteriosus, arteriovenous malformation, endocardial cushion defect, and pulmonary hypertension due to any chronic left-to-right shunt) and lesions with normal blood pulmonary flow (e.g., coarctation of the aorta, mitral stenosis, pulmonary stenosis, aortic stenosis, endocardial fibroelastosis, and mitral regurgitation). The effect of the shunt depends on the size, location, and relative systemic and pulmonary vascular resistance (PVR) or, for atrial-level shunts, the relative compliance of the ventricles. The more common acyanotic defects are described in this section. On occasion, an acyanotic lesion may produce a shunt reversal (i.e., right-to-left shunting) in the presence of additional circumstances, as noted.

Atrial Septal Defect

An atrial septal defect (ASD) is a communication between the atria at the septal level, as shown in Figure 8-2. The atrial septum is composed of the septum primum and septum secundum. Ostium secundum ASD is a deficiency of the septum secundum in the region of the fossa ovalis and is the only true defect through the atrial septum proper.

BOX 8-2: Cardiac Conditions Associated With the Highest Risk of Adverse Outcome From Endocarditis for Which Prophylaxis With Dental Procedures Is Reasonable

Prosthetic cardiac valve or prosthetic material used for cardiac valve repair

Previous infective endocarditis

Congenital heart disease (CHD)*

- Unrepaired cyanotic CHD, including palliative shunts and conduits
- Completely repaired congenital heart defect with prosthetic material or device, whether placed by surgery or by catheter intervention, during the first 6 months after the procedure[†]
- Repaired CHD with residual defects at the site or adjacent to the site of a prosthetic patch or prosthetic device (which inhibit endothelialization)

Cardiac transplantation recipients who develop cardiac valvulopathy

Data from Wilson W, Taubert KA, Gewitz M, et al. Prevention of infective endocarditis: Guidelines from the American Heart Association. A guideline from the American Heart Association Rheumatic Fever, Endocarditis and Kawasaki Disease Committee, Council on Cardiovascular Disease in the Young, and the Council on Clinical Cardiology, Quality of Care and Outcomes Research Interdisciplinary Working Group. *Circulation* 2007;116:1736–1754.

*Except for the conditions listed above, antibiotic prophylaxis is no longer recommended for any other form of CHD.

[†]Prophylaxis is reasonable because endothelialization of prosthetic material occurs within 6 months of the procedure.

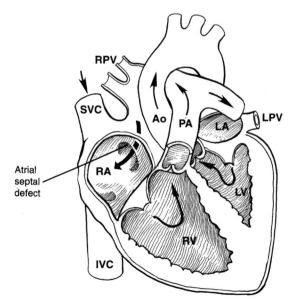

Figure 8-2: An atrial septal defect most commonly results in shunting of blood from the left atrium to the right atrium. Ao, Aorta; IVC, inferior vena cava; LA, left atrium; PA, pulmonary artery; LPV, left pulmonary vein; LV, left ventricle; PA, main pulmonary artery; RA, right atrium; RPV, right pulmonary vein; RV, right ventricle; SVC, superior vena cava.

- ASD occurring in isolation accounts for 5% to 10% of all CHD, with a 2:1 female-to-male preponderance; 50% to 70% are of the secundum type.[84] However, because the majority of individuals are asymptomatic until adulthood, it is likely that this prevalence is underestimated.
- ASD is present in one third to one half of all combination congenital heart defects.[85]
- *Patent foramen ovale (PFO)* is persistence of the normal fetal communication between the atria (see pages 342–343), which usually closes shortly after birth. In approximately one third of adults, the foramen ovale fails to achieve anatomic closure, which can lead to right-to-left shunting when RA pressure exceeds that in the LA or sometimes an acquired ASD when marked atrial dilation produces stretching of the atrial septum.[84]
- Infants born at high altitudes have a higher combined prevalence of ASD and PDA, most likely because of the relative hypoxemia at high elevations, which interferes with the normal mechanisms for closure (as opposed to true congenital malformations).[76]

Pathophysiology

- Left-to-right shunting usually occurs across an ASD, allowing blood that has arrived in the LA via the pulmonary veins to flow into the RA during both systole and diastole. The resultant volume overload on the RA, RV, and pulmonary circulation leads to dilatation of all of these structures, and pulmonary blood flow is increased compared with systemic blood flow.
- The degree of left-to-right shunt depends on the size of the ASD, the relative compliance of the ventricles during diastole, and the relative resistance in both the pulmonary and systemic circulations.
- With a large lesion, pulmonary hypertension frequently develops in adult life.
- In a small percentage of patients, increasing PVR results in a reduction of the left-to-right shunt. As RV and PA pressures increase and progressive pulmonary hypertension develops, shunt reversal may occur with subsequent cyanosis, heart failure, or pulmonary hemorrhage (see page 364 for further discussion of Eisenmenger's syndrome).

Clinical Manifestations and Natural History

- Despite substantial pulmonary blood flow, the majority of infants and children with ASD are asymptomatic, although the presence of the defect may exacerbate symptoms of bronchial or pulmonary disorders acquired through prematurity, infection, or asthma.
- Spontaneous closure of very small defects occurs during the first year of life in up to 85% of infants.[16,29,64]
- Older children and adults may experience palpitations, dyspnea, and decreased exercise tolerance over time.
- Pulmonary hypertension is uncommon during childhood but is more commonly encountered in the 20s and 30s, producing CHF if a large lesion has been left untreated. CHF is rarely seen in infancy.
- Adults over age 40 years with ASD may develop atrial flutter or fibrillation and right heart failure. However, the presence of symptoms at this age may also reflect the development of coronary artery disease (CAD) or systemic hypertension.

Management

- Surgical consideration is usually deferred during the first year of life given the high rate of spontaneous closure or narrowing of the lesion. Periodic follow-up with cardiology is recommended.
- Less common variants of ASD do not resolve spontaneously and require surgical closure, as do symptomatic ASDs and those with pulmonary-to-systemic flow ratios greater than 1.5, especially when the RA is dilated. Surgery is often performed in the pre-school years. If symptoms are present, elective repair at 1 year or earlier may reduce morbidity.[80] Closure options may include open repair with suture or patch, minithoracotomy, or transcatheter device closure (for secundum types).
- Full activity without restrictions should be encouraged in patients with unoperated or corrected ASD with normal PA pressures (peak systolic pressure ≤30 mm Hg), no significant arrhythmias (e.g., symptomatic atrial or ventricular tachyarrhythmias or second or third degree heart block), or ventricular dysfunction. Patients with pulmonary hypertension and other signs of dysfunction should restrict their participation in competitive athletics according to the recommendations listed in Table 8-11 on page 359.[40,49,77a,87]
    - ▸ Exercise tolerance tends to be normal or mildly impaired without surgical correction, with the limitation being related to the degree of pulmonary hypertension and not merely the size of the shunt.[70,91]
    - ▸ After surgical repair, exercise capacity may be normal or somewhat reduced. Some patients exhibit chronotropic incompetence and residual left or right ventricular dysfunction, which are more common when correction is performed in later childhood or adulthood.[70]
- Respiratory tract infections should be treated promptly.
- Antibiotic prophylaxis for infective endocarditis is unnecessary in isolated ASD.[121]

Ventricular Septal Defect

A ventricular septal defect (VSD) is an opening between the ventricles at the septal level (Figure 8-3), which occurs in or near the membranous or muscular portions of the septum. VSDs arise as isolated defects or in association with other major cardiac anomalies and are the most common form of CHD, representing 20% to 25% of all CHD not including those occurring as part of cyanotic CHD; 70% are the perimembranous type.[84] Diagnosis is often made within the first weeks of life after a systolic murmur is heard.

Pathophysiology

- As the PVR falls after birth, the developing pressure gradient between the LV and RV generates left-to-right shunting across the VSD, primarily during systole.
- The hemodynamic effects of a VSD depend on its size and the relative degree of PVR; the larger the defect and the lower the PVR, the greater the degree of left-to-right shunting.
    - ▸ Small defects are *restrictive,* producing a large resistance to flow and a small volume of shunt, so there is no elevation of RV or PA pressure.
    - ▸ In a moderately restrictive lesion, there is a moderate shunt that is proportional to the size of the lesion, producing LA

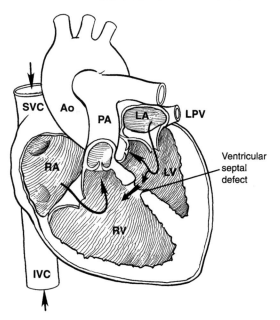

Figure 8-3: A ventricular septal defect usually allows blood to flow from the left ventricle into the right ventricle. Ao, Aorta; IVC, inferior vena cava; LA, left atrium; LPV, left pulmonary vein; LV, left ventricle; PA, main pulmonary artery; RA, right atrium; RV, right ventricle; SVC, superior vena cava.

and LV volume overload, but the pulmonary-to-aortic systolic pressure ratio is less than 0.66, so the right-sided chambers are rarely affected.
- ▸ A large *nonrestrictive* VSD produces little pressure difference between the left and right ventricles and is accompanied by a large shunt. The degree of shunting is dependent on the ratio of pulmonary to systemic vascular resistance:
  ⊙ If PVR is low, there is massive left-to-right shunting with increased pulmonary flow and PA pressures (PAPs), volume overload of the LA and LV, and heart failure.
  ⊙ As PAP rises over time, the degree of left-to-right shunting decreases.
  ⊙ When PVR approaches SVR, the left-to-right shunt is minimal or disappears, and the pathophysiological effects are those associated with pulmonary HTN and other coexistent anomalies.
- A perimembranous VSD located just below the aortic valve and doubly committed defects may be associated with progressive aortic regurgitation (AR).

Clinical Manifestations and Natural History

- Spontaneous closure of tiny, perimembranous VSDs occurs in 85% to 90% of infants by age 1 year.[50] Larger perimembranous defects may also resolve or become smaller over time; however, closure should be performed in adolescence if a significant left-to-right shunt is present.
- Because there is greater resistance to flow in the pulmonary vasculature at birth, left-to-right shunting may be minimal even in the presence of a larger VSD. Over the first few weeks of life, PVR naturally decreases, which reveals a progressive rise in shunting; in infants with a large VSD, CHF develops (usually between 3 and 12 wk of age).[29]

- Persistent VSDs may produce a range of clinical pictures:
  - Small VSDs (most common) typically are asymptomatic at birth and do not interfere with growth and development but do put the infant/child at relatively high risk for infective endocarditis. Classic signs include a holosystolic murmur (but no diastolic murmur) appearing in the first few days to weeks of life and a possible palpable thrill.
  - Moderate to large VSDs can result in delayed growth and development, recurrent pulmonary infections, decreased exercise tolerance, and CHF. Signs and symptoms occur between those described for small and large defects.
  - Large, unrestrictive VSDs often present later in the neonatal period (typically about 6 to 8 wk of age) because of equalization of pressures across the defect until decreased PVR allows significant left-to-right shunting. Then pulmonary hypertension and congestive heart failure develop (see Box 8-1, page 356) in the second or third month of life. Pulmonary vascular obstructive disease (PVOD) may arise, and up to 15% of patients develop Eisenmenger's syndrome (see the next entry) by age 20 years, leading to decreased exercise tolerance.
- *Eisenmenger's syndrome* refers to pulmonary vascular obstructive disease with right-to-left (or bidirectional) shunting that develops as a result of underlying CHD with a large left-to-right shunt (e.g., large VSD or patent ductus arteriosus and complex cyanotic defects; see pages 369–373). Chronic exposure to high pulmonary blood flow leads to increased PVR, pulmonary HTN, and irreversible damage to the pulmonary vessels (i.e., PVOD), often by the age of 2 years but more commonly in the teens or 20s.[117] When the PAP approaches that of the systemic circulation, Eisenmenger's syndrome is present and causes cyanosis.[96] Cardiac output may be inadequate at rest, and dyspnea, dizziness, and/or syncope with exertion are common symptoms. As RV dysfunction increases, RV failure develops. The right-to-left shunting also puts these patients at risk for brain abscess and systemic emboli.

Management

- Small shunts (pulmonary/systemic flow <1.5:1) require annual monitoring by a cardiologist for spontaneous closure or changes in symptoms.
- Shunts with greater than 2:1 ratios require surgical closure, often performed before 1 year of age.
- CHF is managed medically with the use of diuretics, angiotensin-converting enzyme (ACE) inhibitors, and digitalis. In addition to alleviating symptoms, this allows time for size reduction or spontaneous closure of the lesion as well as growth of the infant. Newborns with large VSDs may require supplemental nutrition with high-calorie formula or tube feedings.
- Surgical intervention is required for infants with CHF and failure to thrive who are unresponsive to medical management. Closure may be achieved via surgical suture or patch and more experimentally via transcatheter device closure for muscular and perimembranous VSDs.
  - Repair during the first year of life has been associated with better LV mechanics[18] and better weight gain in infants.[118]

- After surgical closure, residual, nonhemodynamically significant defects occur in 10% of cases.[84]
- Children with preoperative hypoxemia in infancy are at increased risk for neurodevelopmental impairments, including motor dysfunction.[52]
- Long-term follow-up is important because some patients develop late heart block or aortic regurgitation.
- Full activity without restrictions should be encouraged in patients with corrected or unoperated VSD with normal PA pressures, no significant arrhythmias, or ventricular dysfunction. Patients with pulmonary HTN and other signs of dysfunction should restrict their participation in competitive athletics according to the recommendations listed in Table 8-11 on page 359.[77a,87]
  - In unoperated patients, long-term follow-up has shown that exercise capacity is only mildly reduced, if at all, in selected patients with small VSDs (those with left-to-right shunt <50%; and no LV volume overload, elevation in PAP, VSD-related AR, or symptoms).[21a,32] A reduction in aerobic capacity has been correlated with a reduced level of physical activity.[91]
  - When surgical repair is made as an infant, exercise capacity is not significantly different from that of unaffected children at age 6 to 9 years.[52] At 12 to 17 years (after surgery in infancy or childhood), 84% of patients have normal values.[75] However, some patients may have difficulty tolerating the bursts of intensive activity that prevail in many types of sports.[35]
- Good dental hygiene practices are recommended for all patients and IE prophylaxis is required for appropriate patients (see Box 8-2, page 362).

Patent Ductus Arteriosus

Although the ductus arteriosus plays an important role in prenatal circulation, persistence of this communication between the PA and the proximal descending aorta past the first few weeks of life causes problematic shunting in the neonate. Patent ductus arteriosus (PDA) is illustrated in Figure 8-4.

PDA is an expected finding in premature infants. In term infants it represents 5% to 10% of all CHD and may occur alone or in combination with other cardiac anomalies.[84] As stated previously, the combined prevalence of PDA and ASD is increased in infants born at high altitudes, most likely because of interference with the normal mechanisms for closure caused by the relative hypoxemia at high elevations.[76]

Pathophysiology

PDA presents a unique situation because its existence as an isolated defect may cause a full spectrum of clinical presentations ranging from few, if any, problems to serious cardiac decompensation. It may also provide a life-sustaining conduit for systemic circulation when other cardiac anomalies are present (e.g., hypoplastic left heart syndrome, interrupted aortic arch, or severe aortic coarctation).

- Left-to-right shunting occurs in accordance with the size and length of the defect and the level of pulmonary versus systemic vascular resistance (as in VSD; see previous section).[29]
  - A small defect and shunt often has no hemodynamic significance but may increase the risk of infective endarteritis, especially when a murmur is heard.

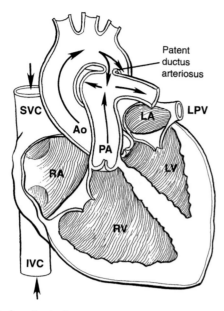

Figure 8-4: A patent ductus arteriosus (PDA) usually results in blood flow from the aorta back to the pulmonary arteries and lungs. Ao, Aorta; IVC, inferior vena cava; LA, left atrium; LPV, left pulmonary vein; LV, left ventricle; PA, main pulmonary artery; RA, right atrium; RV, right ventricle; SVC, superior vena cava.

▸ A moderate-sized duct and shunt create a volume load on the LA and LV with resultant dilation and dysfunction and possible eventual atrial fibrillation.

▸ A large PDA results in increased LA and LV volume overload and progressively rising PAPs, leading to pulmonary HTN and PVOD. The RV is thus subjected to an increased pressure load.

▸ Pulmonary congestion results from increased pulmonary blood flow and/or CHF due to LV dysfunction.

• If PAP exceeds aortic pressure, shunt reversal develops (Eisenmenger's syndrome) with preferential shunting of deoxygenated blood to the descending aorta, producing cyanosis of the lower part of the body and clubbing of the toes.

Clinical Manifestations and Natural History

• Prematurity interferes with the normal mechanisms for postnatal ductal closure (see page 343); almost all infants born weighing less than 1500 g have a PDA, as do approximately 20% of premature infants with birth weight under 1750 g. Small lesions are often asymptomatic, but large PDAs are associated with respiratory distress syndrome (see page 347) and CHF.

• Spontaneous closure is unlikely in full-term infants after the first days of life.

• Full-term infants with small PDAs are asymptomatic except for a grade 1 or 2 systolic to continuous murmur.

• Full-term infants with moderate to large defects have symptoms similar to those of VSD (see previous entry). They exhibit a louder, continuous or "machinery" murmur, widened pulse pressure, bounding peripheral pulses, and prominent suprasternal and carotid pulsations.

• Full-term infants with large PDAs and shunts often develop CHF and failure to thrive and are at high risk for recurrent pulmonary infections and pneumonia, PVOD, and possible premature death in late adolescence or young adulthood.

• Patients are at increased risk for infective endarteritis and endocarditis with age.

Management

• Primary prevention of premature birth.

• Asymptomatic premature infants with tiny left-to-right shunts require no intervention because of probable spontaneous closure with maturation.

• Premature infants with respiratory distress syndrome (RDS) are treated with indomethacin or possibly ibuprofen in addition to appropriate medical management of CHF (e.g., diuretics and fluid restriction). Indomethacin is ineffective in term infants.

• Surgical closure (ligation or division) is indicated for premature infants whose PDA fails to close after three doses of indomethacin or for term infants with a persistent PDA, especially those with CHF, failure to thrive, or pulmonary hypertension. Transcatheter device closure may be used for ducts smaller than 8 mm.

• Because infective endocarditis and heart failure are major causes of morbidity in older children, closure is recommended by 2 years of age in full-term children, even in the absence of symptoms.

• Patients with PDA should be encouraged to exercise on a regular basis unless pulmonary HTN is present. Asymptomatic patients with small PDAs and normal LV chamber size and those with corrected PDA without evidence of pulmonary HTN or LV enlargement can participate in competitive sports without restriction, as detailed in Table 8-11 on page 359.[40]

• Good dental hygiene practices are recommended for all patients and IE prophylaxis is required for appropriate patients (see Box 8-2, page 362).

Coarctation of the Aorta

A coarctation of the aorta (CoA) is a discrete narrowing of the distal segment of the aortic arch, most commonly in the vicinity of the former ductus arteriosus (Figure 8-5). The severity of the narrowing and the presence of associated lesions determine the effects of the obstruction. CoA is manifested in two different clinical presentations: One group exhibits symptoms in the first weeks of life and requires timely diagnosis and management, and the other remains essentially asymptomatic until hypertension is noted or other complications develop, usually in adolescence.

CoA accounts for 4%, to 8% to 10%, of all CHD, occurring two to five times more often in males than females.[30,84] Approximately 20% to 50% of infants born with CoA develop heart failure within the first 3 months of life, and about half of these have at least one other cardiac anomaly, including VSD, PDA, aortic or subaortic stenosis, mitral stenosis or regurgitation, and hypoplasia of the aortic arch.[30,84,117] A high percentage of patients with bicuspid aortic valve (up to 60%–85%) and gonadal dysgenesis (Turner's syndrome) also have CoA.

Pathophysiology

• During fetal life the descending aorta receives blood from the RV via the PDA and an amount of antegrade flow from the LV.

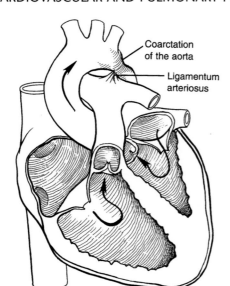

Figure 8-5: Coarctation of the aorta with narrowing in the juxtaductal location.

CoA creates an obstruction to aortic blood flow, which becomes more problematic after closure of the ductus arteriosus.

- Increased afterload caused by the obstruction provokes LV hypertrophy. The increase in LV pressures is reflected back to the left atrium and pulmonary vasculature, leading to CHF in symptomatic infants.
- Symptomatic infants with CoA tend to have a greater degree of obstruction and more limited flow through the aortic isthmus than asymptomatic infants. Because little aortic obstruction is present in utero, collateral vessels are poorly developed, and rapid constriction of the ductus arteriosus producing sudden severe aortic obstruction gives rise to rapidly increasing LV afterload, greater blood flow proximal to the defect, and significantly reduced flow with hypoperfusion distally.
- In asymptomatic infants and children, the LV afterload increases gradually, allowing the development of good collateral circulation, which provides adequate blood flow below the level of obstruction and preserves LV function. However, the severity of obstruction is almost always progressive, eventually producing signs and symptoms (see later).

Clinical Manifestations and Natural History

- Very severe obstruction results in critically ill, symptomatic infants who present with cyanosis (especially of the lower body) in the first few days to weeks of life as the result of right-to-left ductal shunting. If the ductus closes they may present with LV failure or shock.[54]
- Slightly less severe coarctation results in symptomatic infants who develop signs of CHF (see Box 8-1, page 356). Over time, significant narrowing of the aorta results in elevated systolic LV and aortic pressures proximal to the coarctation (i.e., to the brain and the upper extremities) and reduced systolic BP distal to the defect (i.e., to the kidneys and lower extremities).[54] Femoral pulses are weaker than brachial pulses.

- Asymptomatic infants with CoA are often discovered in adolescence on findings of systolic hypertension with BP differentials between upper and lower extremities. Presentation may also include symptoms of fatigue, complaints of leg pain/weakness after exercise or of headache or cold extremities, heart murmur, or endocarditis. Rib notching (scalloping of the undersides of the ribs) may be present because of increased size of the intercostal collateral vessels. If diagnosis is eluded until middle age, CoA may present with aortic rupture, intracranial hemorrhage, CHF often complicated by mitral or aortic valve disease, and atherosclerosis by age 40 years. The average life expectancy of untreated CoA is in the mid-30s.[54]
- CoA increases the risk of infective endocarditis.

Management

- The majority of infants with CHF respond well to medical management, including PGE_1 to maintain patency of the ductus arteriosus, inotropic agents, diuretics, and oxygen.
- Critically ill infants require immediate attention, with a short period of medical management to improve the infant's condition; ventilatory assistance may be required for infants with markedly increased work of breathing. Once the infant is stabilized, urgent surgery is usually performed.
- Primary surgical repair via end-to-end anastomosis, patch aortoplasty, or subclavian flap aortoplasty is recommended for all infants with other cardiac anomalies and those with isolated CoA who fail to respond to medical management.
  - The subclavian flap affords an autogenous patch with potential for growth, whereas end-to-end anastomosis carries a higher risk of restenosis if the area of repair does not grow with the child.
  - Primary surgical repair is recommended over balloon angioplasty (because of the higher incidence of recurrence and aneurysm formation with the latter); however, for high-risk surgical patients, balloon angioplasty may be a calculated option.[54]
  - Residual obstruction or recurrent coarctation occurs in 6% to 33% of all patients who undergo repair, with lower percentages after surgery than balloon angioplasty.[84] A small percentage of patients develop rapidly recurrent coarctation or moderate to severe mitral stenosis or regurgitation. For recurrent coarctation, balloon valvuloplasty or catheter angioplasty with or without stent placement is often performed.
- In infants whose obstruction is not clinically significant, monitoring occurs until the preschool or kindergarten years, when repair is performed (because of the decreased chance of reobstruction after this age).
- Older children and young adults will likely have chronic systemic HTN. After repair, β-blockers and ACE inhibitors are often prescribed. BP often improves with time, but these patients tend to have residual borderline HTN at rest and often have an exaggerated BP response to exercise.
- An adult with uncorrected CoA is usually asymptomatic although nonspecific symptoms such as headache, dyspnea with exertion, hypertension, and leg fatigue may develop. Diagnosis between 15 and 40 years of age often occurs at

the time of a severe medical emergency, such as cerebral hemorrhage, infective endocarditis, or aortic rupture.

- After surgery all individuals should receive at least an annual follow-up with a cardiologist to monitor for recoarctation.
- Exercise testing is helpful in identifying abnormal BP responses indicative of residual or recurrent coarctation and provides the best guidance regarding the need for exercise restriction.
  - ▸ The resting and exercise BPs will differ according to the type of CoA and the type of surgical repair.[94] Submaximal bicycle testing may be the best method for evaluating arm/leg BP gradients to distinguish patients with CoA from those without the defect.
  - ▸ Individuals with residual or recurrent CoA usually exhibit resting HTN with a BP differential between the arm and leg, which becomes more pronounced with exercise, as well as a hypertensive BP response to exercise.[91,94,97]
  - ▸ Patients who have had successful surgical repair or stent placement for CoA achieve normal values for exercise capacity and most have normal resting BP but may exhibit significantly higher BP than control subjects at all stages of exercise testing.[86,94,97] Persistent exercise HTN is more common in patients with later repair compared with those who undergo repair before the age of 1 year.
- Most patients should be encouraged to engage in regular physical exercise, although some should be restricted for participation in competitive athletics (see Table 8-11, page 359).[40,49,77a]
  - ▸ Patients with mild coarctation without large collateral vessels or significant aortic root dilation, a normal exercise test, a systolic arm/leg pressure gradient not exceeding 20 mm Hg, and a peak systolic blood pressure (SBP) not more than 230 mm Hg with exercise can engage in all competitive sports.
  - ▸ Patients with untreated CoA with a systolic arm/leg pressure gradient greater than 20 mm Hg or exercise-induced HTN with a SBP greater than 230 mm Hg should participate only in low-intensity competitive sports until treated.
  - ▸ Asymptomatic patients with treated CoA (surgery or balloon angioplasty) with an arm/leg pressure gradient of 20 mm Hg or less at rest and a normal peak SBP during exercise can engage in all competitive sports, except for high-intensity static exercise and sports that pose the danger of bodily collision, which should be avoided for one year after surgery.
  - ▸ Those with significant evidence of aortic root dilation, wall thinning, and aneurysm formation should be restricted to low-intensity competitive sports only.
- Good dental hygiene practices and SBE prophylaxis are required for all cases.[121]

Pulmonary Stenosis

Pulmonary stenosis (PS) may occur at the valvular, subvalvular, or supravalvular levels and creates an obstruction to RV outflow, with a pressure gradient between the RV and PA. Approximately 90% of cases are valvular, in which the valve is conical or dome-shaped with various degrees of fusion of the leaflets. A bicuspid valve is present in about 20% of cases; less commonly, the valve may be dysplastic ($\approx$15% of cases) as seen in Noonan's syndrome (phenotypically Turner's syndrome and genotypically normal [XX or XY]).

PS is one of the most common congenital heart defects, with isolated PS accounting for 5% to 12% of all CHD.[30,84] However, it usually occurs in combination with other cardiac anomalies, including VSD, tetralogy of Fallot, and single ventricle.

Pathophysiology

The pathophysiological and clinical manifestations of PS can be found in Chapter 4 on page 117.

- In general, when the effective valve area is reduced by about 60%, hemodynamically significant obstruction to flow occurs.
  - ▸ RV pressure increases in order to maintain flow across the stenotic site.
  - ▸ The pressure overload on the RV induces RV hypertrophy.
  - ▸ Poststenotic dilatation of the PA develops, likely as a result of the high-velocity jet across the stenotic valve.
- If normal RV output is not maintained, RV failure develops.
- Increasing RV pressures are reflected back to the RA, and increasing RA pressure may provoke right-to-left shunting in the presence of a PFO or ASD with systemic arterial desaturation and cyanosis.

Clinical Manifestations and Natural History

- The severity of stenosis is difficult to assess during the first days to week of life when PVR is normally higher and then falls rapidly. For the same reason, infants with mild to moderate symptoms initially may worsen over the first week of life.
- The effects of PS are related to the degree of obstruction. Stenosis is considered minimal if the pressure gradient is less than 35 to 40 mm Hg (the majority of patients) and severe when the gradient is greater than 70 mm Hg.[84]
  - ▸ Most infants and children with PS are asymptomatic and well developed, and the gradient does not increase with age. A systolic ejection murmur is present at the upper left sternal border when the stenosis occurs at the valvular level.
  - ▸ Moderately severe PS presents with mild fatigue and exertional dyspnea in some patients and may be progressive.
  - ▸ Severe PS may produce symptoms of CHF (see Box 8-1, page 356). Sudden death during strenuous activity has been reported in some patients.
  - ▸ Neonates with critical stenosis may exhibit difficulty feeding, tachypnea, and lethargy; cyanosis occurs if there is a PFO or ASD.
- Infective endocarditis occasionally occurs.

Management

- Balloon valvuloplasty is the treatment of choice for the valvular stenosis when RV systemic pressure exceeds 50% of systemic pressure, and is typically curative.[104,122]
- Infants with severe symptoms require immediate intervention regardless of valve gradient and may benefit from PGE$_1$ infusion to reopen the ductus arteriosus until balloon valvuloplasty can be performed.
- Surgical valvotomy is performed in patients with dysplastic pulmonary valves that do not respond to dilatation and the occasional patient in whom balloon valvuloplasty is not successful. Valve replacement is rarely performed in children.
- Some pediatric patients experience transient right ventricular outflow tract (RVOT) obstruction after relief of PS because of sudden decompression of the hypertrophied RV.[54]

- No activity restriction is necessary for asymptomatic patients with mild untreated or operated PS (peak systolic gradient <40 mm Hg) and normal RV function. Patients with untreated and operated PS with a persistent peak systolic gradient greater than 40 mm Hg and those with severe pulmonary incompetence with marked RV enlargement should be limited to low-intensity competitive sports, as described in Table 8-11 on page 359.[40,49,77a]
- Children and adults with mild valvular PS have nearly normal exercise tolerance, but it is reduced in those with moderate to severe stenosis as a result of their impaired ability to sustain adequate cardiac output.[21a,102,122]
  - ▸ During graded exercise the ability to increase cardiac output is diminished in accordance with the severity of the stenosis, and the transvalvular pressure gradient may increase.
  - ▸ In children who have undergone surgical valvotomy, exercise tolerance is slightly lower than age-predicted values, but it remains abnormal in adults who undergo corrective interventions.[91,102] Patients with fair or poor clinical status are most likely to have reduced exercise tolerance.
- Good dental hygiene practices are recommended for all patients. IE prophylaxis should be prescribed for appropriate patients (see Box 8-2).

Aortic Stenosis

Left ventricular outflow tract obstruction in the form of aortic stenosis (AS) may occur at the valvular (most common), subvalvular, or supravalvular level. Valvular AS is marked by thickening of the valvular tissue and various degrees of commissural fusion, which lead to subtotal obstruction of LV outflow. Bicuspid aortic valve is the most common cause of AS, or it may develop in a unicuspid or tricuspid valve. AS forms a continuum with hypoplastic left heart syndrome (HLHS), aortic atresia, and hypoplasia complexes.[117]

AS represents 5% to 10% of all CHD and occurs with a male-to-female predominance of 4:1.[84] It usually presents as an isolated defect, but it also occurs in combination with other cardiac anomalies, particularly PDA, CoA, and VSD.

Pathophysiology

- Few hemodynamic derangements occur until the valvular orifice is reduced to approximately one third its normal size, at which time AS produces a pressure and volume overload on the LV, as described on page 115.
- Specific considerations related to the pediatric population include the following:
  - ▸ The effects of congenital AS are reduced in the immediate postnatal period by the presence of a persistent PDA or stretched foramen ovale.
  - ▸ The aortic valve annulus may be relatively underdeveloped.
  - ▸ Endocardial fibrosis and papillary muscle necrosis may also occur.

Clinical Manifestations and Natural History

- Most infants and children with mild to moderate AS are asymptomatic, although occasionally there is exercise intolerance. They exhibit a harsh midsystolic murmur that is transmitted to the apex and carotid arteries; an ejection click may also be heard. Patients with bicuspid aortic valves may also

have a high-pitched, early diastolic decrescendo murmur due to aortic regurgitation.
- AS tends to progress with age, regardless of severity. Rapid progression is more likely before age 2 years or during puberty. Clinical symptoms do not always correlate with severity of AS.
- Infants with critical AS may present with symptoms ranging from mild CHF to shock, and signs of peripheral hypoperfusion may be present (see Box 8-1 on page 356).
- About half of infants born with severe AS require hospitalization for CHF during their first days to weeks of life.[84] Infants and children with a gradient greater than 65 to 70 mm Hg require intervention to prevent myocardial damage and eliminate the risk of sudden death.
- Rupture of the LV papillary muscles may occur with resultant acute mitral regurgitation, precipitating or intensifying CHF.
- Myocardial ischemia is often a significant problem in infants and children with severe AS despite normal coronary arteries. Syncope is also indicative of severe AS.

Management

- Critically ill infants are usually stabilized before surgery with PGE_1 to maintain patency of the ductus arteriosus, inotropic agents, diuretics, and oxygen; ventilatory assistance may be required for infants with markedly increased work of breathing.
- Percutaneous balloon valvuloplasty is the primary intervention for AS at many centers in the United States. Indications for its use in children and adolescents include the following[84]:
  - ▸ Symptomatic AS with a catheter pressure gradient (cath gradient) greater than 50 mm Hg
  - ▸ Asymptomatic AS with a cath gradient greater than 60 mm Hg
  - ▸ Asymptomatic patients who develop ST or T changes on ECG at rest or during exercise stress testing and who have a cath gradient greater than 50 mm Hg
  - ▸ Asymptomatic patients with a cath gradient greater than 50 mm Hg who want to play competitive sports
- Surgical valvotomy is performed if stenosis is not sufficiently reduced via valvuloplasty.
- Valve replacement is performed if significant aortic regurgitation (AR) develops. The Ross procedure (transfer of the pulmonary valve to the aortic position with placement of a pulmonary homograft) is the procedure of choice, especially for subvalvular aortic stenosis, because of its potential for growth with the child.
- Prosthetic valve replacement may be performed if there is significant valvular degeneration or calcification in adulthood.
- Exercise testing is indicated to define the appropriateness of individuals for sports participation and may reveal abnormalities even in the absence of moderate or severe AS. Radionuclide scans or stress echocardiography may provide additional information.
  - ▸ Children with mild unoperated AS have normal exercise capacity despite low peak HRs and sometimes blunted BP responses (the ability to increase systolic BP is inversely related to the degree of LV outflow obstruction in AS patients with moderate to severe aortic valve gradients).[21a,77]

Ventricular ectopy and ST-segment depression are common during exercise, but their significance in terms of risk is not clear.

▸ Children with operated AS usually achieve normal exercise capacity with significantly lower peak exercise HR, although some older studies report reduced exercise performance.[77]

- Activity restriction is recommended for patients with moderate to severe AS, both unoperated and operated, as listed in Table 8-11 on page 359, and even those with mild AS should be given activity guidelines and monitored for progression.[12a,40,77a]

  ▸ Patients with mild AS (<30 mm Hg peak-to-peak systolic gradient on catheterizations, <25 mm Hg mean echo Doppler gradient, or <40 mm Hg peak instantaneous echo Doppler gradient) can participate in all competitive sports if they have a normal ECG, normal exercise tolerance, and no history of exercise-related chest pain, syncope, or symptomatic atrial or ventricular tacyarrhythmias.[12a,40]

  ▸ Asymptomatic athletes with moderate AS (30- to 50-mm Hg peak-to-peak systolic gradient on catheterization, 25- to 40-mm Hg mean echo Doppler gradient, or 40- to 70-mm Hg peak instantaneous echo Doppler gradient) can engage in low to moderate dynamic and low to moderate static competitive sports if there is mild or no LV hypertrophy by echocardiography and no evidence of LV strain pattern on ECG, and exercise testing shows normal work capacity and BP responses without evidence of myocardial ischemia or atrial or ventricular tachyarrhythmias.[12a,40]

  ▸ Patients with severe AS (>50 mm Hg peak-to-peak systolic gradient on catheterization, >40 mm Hg mean echo Doppler gradient, or >70 mm Hg peak instantaneous echo Doppler gradient) should not participate in competitive athletics.[12a,40]

  ▸ The ability of patients with AS to reach or exceed normal exercise capacity makes activity restrictions difficult to impose and maintain. However, there is some evidence that the use of a personal HR monitor may enable the setting of and compliance with clear, precise, and observable limits on physical activity while also promoting self-control.[11]

- Patients with AS require annual follow-up with a cardiologist to monitor for progression of stenosis in nonoperated individuals or valvular insufficiency and ascending aortic aneurysmal dilatation in those who have had operative repair/replacement.

- Good dental hygiene practices are required for all patients and IE prophylaxis is recommended for patients with prosthetic aortic valves or previous history of infective endocarditis (see Box 8-2, page 362).[121]

Cyanotic Lesions

Cyanotic conditions are characterized by reduced systemic arterial saturation, which is usually due to shunting of systemic venous blood into the arterial circulation. The degree of desaturation is related to the severity of the lesion. These lesions can be divided into two main classifications:

- Defects with decreased pulmonary blood flow (e.g., severe pulmonary stenosis, pulmonary atresia without VSD, tetralogy of Fallot, tricuspid atresia with restrictive VSD, dextrotransposition of the great arteries with pulmonary stenosis, and Ebstein's anomaly)

- Defects with increased pulmonary blood flow (e.g., hypoplastic left heart syndrome, dextrotransposition of the great arteries, total and partial anomalous pulmonary venous connection, single ventricle without PS, tricuspid atresia with large VSD, and truncus arteriosus)

Because of persistent cyanosis or right-to-left shunts, these patients often have characteristic extracardiac complications, including polycythemia, relative anemia, central nervous system abscess, thromboembolic stroke, gum disease, gout, digital clubbing and hypoxic arthropathies, and increased incidences of infectious diseases. Several more commonly occurring cyanotic lesions are presented here.

Unoperated patients and those who have undergone palliative procedures can participate in low-intensity competitive sports only if they do not exhibit arterial oxygen desaturation to less than 80%, symptomatic tachyarrhythmias, or moderate/severe ventricular dysfunction.[40,49,87]

Tetralogy of Fallot

Tetralogy of Fallot (TOF), composed of four anatomic abnormalities including a large nonrestrictive VSD, overriding of the aorta over the VSD, severe RVOT obstruction, and RVH, is depicted in Figure 8-6. A right aortic arch occurs in 25% to 30% of patients.[84] If an ASD is also present, the combined lesion is termed *pentalogy of Fallot*. Coronary artery malformations may also exist.

TOF is the most common form of cyanotic CHD, accounting for 5% to 10% of all CHD.[84]

Pathophysiology

- In the absence of alternative sources of pulmonary blood flow, the degree of cyanosis reflects the severity of the RVOT obstruction and the level of SVR.[117]

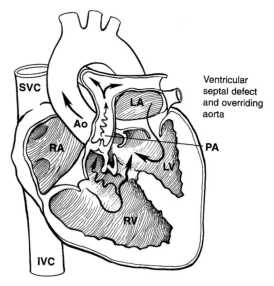

Figure 8-6: Classic tetralogy of Fallot: biventricular origin of the aorta, large ventricular septal defect, right ventricular hypertrophy, and obstruction to pulmonary flow. Ao, Aorta; IVC, inferior vena cava; LA, left atrium; LV, left ventricle; PA, main pulmonary artery; RA, right atrium; RV, right ventricle; SVC, superior vena cava.

- Because the VSD is nonrestrictive, systolic pressures are equal in the RV, LV, and aorta, making the degree of RVOT obstruction key in determining the type of shunting that occurs and the resultant clinical manifestations:
  - With mild PS and minimal obstruction to pulmonary blood flow, little to no right-to-left shunting occurs, and there may even be a left-to-right shunt. This is known as *acyanotic* or *pink* TOF. CHF may be provoked by large left-to-right shunts.
  - With severe PS (more common), a predominant right-to-left shunt exists, resulting in cyanosis and polycythemia.
  - Between the two extremes are relatively asymptomatic infants with mild hypoxemia (oxygen saturations, ≈90%) and "enough" PS to prevent overcirculation of the pulmonary arteries with resultant pulmonary hypertension.[99]

Clinical Manifestations and Natural History

- Most infants are symptomatic at birth or shortly thereafter with difficulty feeding and failure to thrive. RVOT obstruction may take time to develop and thus cyanosis may not occur immediately. An early systolic ejection murmur is heard, with the intensity and duration varying inversely with the severity of obstruction.
- Hypoxic, or hypercyanotic or "tet," spells occur most often in infants between 2 and 4 months of age, and are associated with irritability and prolonged, inconsolable crying, hyperpnea, marked cyanosis, and syncope.
  - They are triggered by an event that results in decreased SVR (including intense crying spells or defecation) or an increase in RVOT resistance causing an increase in right-to-left shunting.
  - A decrease in arterial Po_2 stimulates hyperpnea, which produces an increase in systemic venous return that, in the presence of RVOT obstruction, increases the right-to-left shunt, perpetuating the cycle.
  - A prolonged spell may result in loss of muscle tone or convulsions, and frequent spells may result in severe disability or death.
- Acyanotic TOF ultimately progresses to cyanotic TOF between ages 1 and 3 years.
- The prognosis is poorest in very young infants with cyanosis because of the severity of the obstruction, small size of the pulmonary arteries, and frequent hypoxic spells.
- Increasing cyanosis and polycythemia result in progressive obstruction to pulmonary blood flow, leading to hypoxic spells and possible syncope, especially in those under age 2 years. Digital clubbing develops. In addition, thrombi may develop in small pulmonary vessels, increasing the risk of cerebrovascular accidents (CVAs) and brain abscesses.
- The risk of infective endocarditis is markedly increased.
- Without surgery, one quarter of patients with TOF and severe PS die by age 1 year and three quarters by age 10 years.[56]

Management

- Medical management during a "Tet" spell aims at breaking the hypoxia–hyperpnea–increased venous return cycle and may include positioning to increase SVR (knee to chest), morphine sulfate (to suppress the respiratory center, abolish hyperpnea), sodium bicarbonate to treat acidosis, and agents to increase SVR. Oxygen may be used in an attempt to decrease cyanosis

but has limited value because the issue is reduced pulmonary blood flow, not impaired gas exchange.
- The use of oral propranolol may be considered to prevent hypoxic spells and delay corrective surgery.
- Monitoring should be done for anemia, which increases the risk of CVA.
- Palliative repair using a Blalock-Taussig shunt (subclavian artery to ipsilateral PA graft) is performed only if necessary for infants who are too small for standard repair or for those with limiting pulmonary arterial hypoplasia who may not be candidates for repair. More than 90% of infants have good results that persist for 1 year.[56]
- Complete surgical repair, usually performed between ages 6 months and 3 years depending on presentation, is a complex procedure given the many components of the defect.
- Exercise studies reveal mild to moderate reductions in exercise capacity after correction.[49,120] Patients who maintain an active lifestyle with regular aerobic training demonstrate better performance than those who are physically inactive.
- Participation in athletics for patients with postoperative TOF depends on whether there are residual defects (see Table 8-11, page 359)[40,77a]:
  - Individuals with an excellent repair can participate in all sports if they have normal or near-normal right heart pressures, no more than mild RV volume overload, and no evidence of significant residual shunt or atrial or ventricular tachyarrhythmias.
  - Those with marked pulmonary insufficiency and RV volume overload, residual RV hypertension (peak systolic RV pressure ≥50% of systemic pressure), or atrial or ventricular tachyarrhythmias should be restricted to low-intensity competitive sports only.
- Patients who have undergone corrective surgery require regular cardiology follow-up, as they may exhibit late complications, including residual peripheral pulmonary stenosis, occasional residual VSD, or rare AR. Long-term survivors sometimes develop atrial or, more commonly, ventricular arrhythmias and infective endocarditis.
- Meticulous dental hygiene and SBE prophylaxis are mandatory for all patients.[121]

Dextrotransposition of the Great Arteries

Complete transposition of the great arteries (D-TGA) is an anomaly in which the origin of the aorta arises anteriorly from the morphologic RV while the PA arises posteriorly from the morphologic LV (the aorta remains to the right, *dextro*, of the PA), resulting in separation of the systemic and pulmonary circuits into parallel rather than series circuits (Figure 8-7). Thus, deoxygenated blood circulates from the systemic veins through the RA and RV to the aorta without passing through the lungs, while oxygenated blood circulates from the lungs to the LA and LV and back to the lungs via the PA. The presence of other congenital lesions allowing exchange between the two systems is essential for survival (e.g. ASD, VSD, and PDA); about half of infants have only a PFO or a small PDA to provide intercirculatory mixing.

D-TGA accounts for 3% to 7% of all CHD.[30,84] Males are affected more often than females at a ratio of 2:1 to 3:1. VSD is present in 30% to 40% of infants, and 30% to 35% of these infants also have PS.

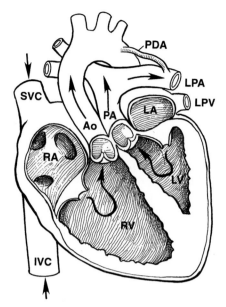

Figure 8-7: Complete transposition of the great arteries. When the interventricular septum is intact, there is usually a patent foramen ovale and enlarged bronchial arteries (Br. Art.). Otherwise, the ventricular septal defect allows connection of the systemic and pulmonary circulations. Ao, Aorta; IVC, inferior vena cava; LA, left atrium; LPA, left pulmonary artery; LPV, left pulmonary vein; LV, left ventricle; PA, main pulmonary artery; PDA, patent ductus arteriosus; RA, right atrium; RV, right ventricle; SVC, superior vena cava.

Pathophysiology

- The hemodynamics are dependent on the combination of defects present and particularly on the amount of mixing between the systemic and pulmonary circulations.
  - ▸ Bidirectional shunts must exist in order to deliver oxygenated blood to other organs and the periphery; intracardiac shunts include PFO, ASD, and VSD, and extracardiac shunts may include PDA or bronchopulmonary collateral circulation.
  - ▸ These shunts must also provide for equal net volume exchange between the systemic and pulmonary circulations over a given period of time in order to avoid volume depletion of one circuit at the expense of overloading the other.
- Without correction, patients are at high risk for the development of Eisenmenger's syndrome (see page 364) during the first year of life.[96]
- Often there is preferential blood flow to the right lung, causing greater PVOD on the right and more pulmonary thrombosis on the left.
- About one third of infants have abnormal coronary anatomy, including the left circumflex coronary arising from the right coronary artery (RCA), a single RCA, a single left CA, or inverted origin of the CAs.[30]

Clinical Manifestations and Natural History

- Clinical manifestations depend on the combination of defects each infant has, as well as the amount of mixing between the systemic and pulmonary circulations.

- ▸ Neonates with an intact ventricular septum present with severe progressive cyanosis within 1 hour of birth (>50% of cases) to a few days after birth. Persistent PDA in combination with PFO allows better oxygenation and on rare occasions permits survival for a few weeks.
- ▸ Infants with a sizable VSD usually exhibit minimal cyanosis initially (mostly during crying). However, as pulmonary blood flow increases, signs of severe CHF usually become evident over the first 3 to 6 weeks. These infants often develop moderate PVOD by 3 to 4 months of age.
- ▸ Infants with significant shunting via a persistent PDA present similar to those with large VSDs.
- ▸ Infants with a large VSD and severe PS present with cyanosis within a few days of birth; those with more moderate PS usually exhibit cyanosis and mild CHF within the first month. Infants with more moderate PS have longer survival without surgery because of protection of the pulmonary vascular bed and low incidence of pulmonary HTN. However, their surgical risk is higher.
- Without treatment, 30% of infants die in the first week of life, 50% within the first month, and 90% in the first 6 to 12 months as a result of progressive hypoxia, acidosis, and heart failure.[60,84]

Management

- Initial medical management consists of PGE₁ infusion to maintain patency of the ductus arteriosus for increased pulmonary blood flow and enhanced intercirculatory mixing. Oxygen should be administered for severe hypoxemia in an attempt to reduce PVR and thus increase pulmonary blood flow. If these do not improve arterial oxygen saturation, the foramen ovale or an ASD may be enlarged.
- Additional medical management includes treatment of symptoms of CHF and correction of metabolic acidosis.
- Palliative interventions designed to increase atrial mixing include balloon atrial septostomy to enlarge the foramen ovale and the Blalock-Hanlon procedure to create an ASD (see Table 8-9).
- Surgical correction is possible using procedures that switch right- and left-sided blood at three levels:
  - ▸ The arterial switch operation (Jatene procedure), which is the procedure of choice for D-TGA repair, involves anatomic correction of the great arteries with transplantation of the coronary arteries to the PA. It is usually performed at 2 to 4 weeks of age in D-TGA with intact ventricle septum and at about 2 months for D-TGA with VSD.
  - ▸ Atrial baffle operations, which reroute pulmonary and systemic venous return at the atrial level to create physiologic rather than anatomic correction, are performed only in rare situations (e.g., when coronary artery translocation is not possible) because of the high rate of complications.
  - ▸ The Mustard procedure uses a pericardial or prosthetic baffle.
  - ▸ The Senning operation uses the patient's own atrial septal flap and the RA free wall to redirect the venous return.
  - ▸ The Rastelli procedure is used in infants with D-TGA with VSD and severe PS to redirect blood at the ventricular level

(an intraventricular tunnel is created between the VSD and the aortic valve and a valved conduit or homograft is placed between the RV and PA). However, high surgical mortality rates (10%–29%), significant complications, poorer long-term survival rates, and the need to replace the conduit as the child grows limit the use of this procedure.

▸ When LV pressure is low, a PA band is placed for days to months to raise the LV pressure to more than 85% of the RV pressure before the switch operation is performed (a two-stage switch operation).

▸ Other staged operations using newer procedures are being used to repair D-TGA with VSD and severe PS.

⊙ The REV procedure (réparation à l'étage ventriculaire) involves infundibular resection to enlarge the VSD, placement of an intraventricular baffle to direct LV output to the aorta, aortic transection to bring the right PA anterior to the ascending aorta, and direct RV-to-PA reconstruction by means of an anterior patch. This procedure may require fewer reoperations than the Rastelli procedure.

⊙ The Nikaidoh procedure consists of aortic translocation without coronary transfer with biventricular outflow tract reconstruction.

⊙ The Damus-Kaye-Stansel procedure bypasses subaortic stenosis by connecting the proximal PA trunk, closes the VSD, and places a conduit between the RV and distal PA. It can also be used in patients with a single ventricle and other rare forms of TGA.

• Palliative interventions and subsequent corrective surgery produce excellent functional status and 30-year survival rates in more than 75% to 80% of patients.[30,84]

• Patients with successfully corrected TGA via arterial switch operation often have normal exercise capacity without ECG abnormalities, whereas those with intraatrial repair demonstrate moderately impaired exercise capacity.[49] Major limiting factors are RV dysfunction, tricuspid regurgitation, impaired chronotropic response, and atrial arrhythmias. All patients benefit from regular low- to moderate-intensity physical activity.

• Patients who have undergone procedures for repair of TGA may be able to participate in some competitive sports.[40,49,77a,87]

▸ Individuals who have had successful arterial switch operation with normal ventricular function and exercise test results and no atrial or ventricular tachyarrhythmias can participate in all sports. Those with more than mild hemodynamic abnormalities or ventricular dysfunction can participate in low-intensity exercise only (see Table 8-11, page 359).

▸ Selected asymptomatic patients who have had atrial switch (Mustard or Senning procedures) can participate in low dynamic/low to moderate static sports if they have no more than mild cardiac chamber enlargement, no evidence of atrial flutter, supraventricular or ventricular tachyarrhythmias, and a normal exercise test. Other patients require individualized exercise prescription based on diagnostic test results.

• Regular follow-up after surgical correction is important to detect possible complications, which occur at various frequencies depending on the operative procedure used.

• Good dental hygiene practices are recommended for all patients. SBE prophylaxis should be prescribed for appropriate patients (see Box 8-2 on page 362).

Hypoplastic Left Heart Syndrome

Hypoplastic left heart syndrome (HLHS) refers to a number of related anomalies that are associated with a markedly underdeveloped LV and ascending aorta, leading to compromised systemic circulation with resultant circulatory shock and metabolic acidosis. As shown in Figure 8-8, systemic circulation is dependent on patency of the ductus arteriosus, and the RV serves as a combined pump. Hypoplasia or atresia of the mitral valve, aortic valve, or both may also be present.

HLHS is found in 7% to 9% of all CHD diagnosed in the first year of life and is one of the most common causes of CHF during the first week of life.[30,84] Prenatal diagnosis is easily achieved by ultrasound.

Pathophysiology

• The LV is essentially nonfunctional, leaving the RV to pump blood to both the lungs (via the PAs) and the body (via the ductus arteriosus). This requires return from both systems to reach the RA, necessitating communication between the atria (via PFO or ASD) and left-to-right shunting.

• In the combined pump, systemic output is inversely related to pulmonary output and the pulmonary bed is exposed to systemic perfusion pressures.

• The RA and RV are markedly enlarged.

• Endocardial fibroelastosis is present in the LV.

Clinical Manifestations and Natural History

• With elevated PVR during fetal development, the dominant RV maintains perfusion pressure in the descending aorta through ductal right-to-left shunting. The proximal aorta and the cerebral and coronary arteries are perfused via retrograde aortic blood flow.

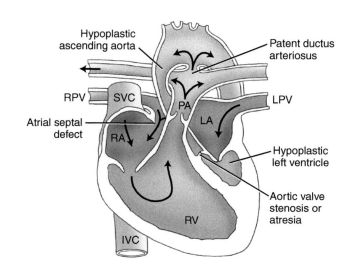

Figure 8-8: Hypoplastic left heart with mitral valve atresia or stenosis, hypoplastic left ventricle, aortic valve stenosis (or atresia), and hypoplastic ascending aorta. Systemic blood flow is provided via an atrial septal defect and patent ductus arteriosus. RA, Right atrium; RV, right ventricle; PA, pulmonary artery; PV, pulmonary vein.

- As the ductus arteriosus begins to close normally over the first 24 to 48 hours of life, signs of CHF and peripheral hypoperfusion rapidly develop (see Box 8-1 on page 356).
- Circulatory shock and progressive hypoxemia and acidosis result in death, usually within the first 2 weeks of life.

Management

- Early management includes PGE$_1$ to maintain ductal patency, supplemental tube feedings to decrease the work of breathing, and diuretics, inotropes, and/or afterload-reducing agents. Mechanical ventilation is not routinely used.
- Staged surgical intervention must be performed for long-term palliation and is essential for survival (see Table 8-10):
  ▸ Stage I, the Norwood procedure, is usually performed in the first weeks of life. It creates an unobstructed communication between the RV and the aorta by connecting the proximal pulmonary trunk to the ascending aorta, often with a patch extension around the augmented aortic arch. Pulmonary blood flow is established via an RV-to-PA conduit, the PDA is ligated, and a large interatrial communication is created.
  ▸ Stage II, which aims to unload the RV by partially separating the systemic and pulmonary circuits, is often performed at approximately 6 months of age, using the bidirectional Glenn procedure (an end-to-side superior vena cava-to-PA connection) or a hemi-Fontan procedure (incorporation of the roof of the atrium into the PA anastomosis) along with take-down of the previous systemic-to-pulmonary shunt placed in stage I.
  ▸ Stage III, the Fontan procedure, performed at 18 to 36 months of age, serves to complete the separation of the systemic and pulmonary circuits by funneling IVC and hepatic return into the PAs.
- Cardiac transplantation is a potential one-step surgical intervention for infants with HLHS. However, the shortage of transplant organs limits the availability of this option, and transplantation carries its own risks and burdens.
- Individuals who have had palliation of CHD by the Fontan procedure typically have markedly reduced exercise capacity and should be encouraged to perform regular physical activity to maximize performance level. They are usually restricted to low-intensity athletics at best, as listed in Table 8-11, page 359.
- Good dental hygiene practices are recommended for all patients. SBE prophylaxis should be administered to appropriate patients (see Box 8-2 on page 362).

OTHER CARDIAC DISORDERS SEEN IN CHILDHOOD

Cardiovascular disease in children may sometimes result from infection or inflammation of the cardiac structures, trauma, drug toxicity, cardiomyopathy, or involvement of the heart secondary to systemic diseases.

Myocarditis

Inflammation of the myocardium in children is most frequently the result of an infectious viral process, commonly coxsackievirus B or adenovirus. Much of the damage results from cell-mediated immunologic reactions. Because most cases are mild or subclinical in severity, only a small percentage of patients exhibit clinically significant symptoms. Of these, acute CHF is the most common presentation, which may require cardiac intensive care including ECMO. Other clinical features are similar to those found in adults (see pages 110 and 125). The majority of affected children recover completely, but up to one third of critically ill pediatric patients may die and one quarter of survivors suffer from persistent heart failure and chronic dilated cardiomyopathy, which can progress in severity to such an extent that heart transplantation must be considered.

Athletes with probable or definite evidence of myocarditis should be withdrawn from all competitive sports for 6 months after the onset of clinical manifestations.[67] They may resume training and competition after this period if LV function, wall motion, cardiac dimensions, serum markers of inflammation and heart failure, and 12-lead ECG (except for persistence of minor alterations, such as some ST–T changes) have returned to normal, and there are no clinically relevant arrhythmias (e.g., frequent or complex repetitive forms of ventricular or supraventricular arrhythmias).

Cardiomyopathies

Cardiomyopathy (CM) comprises a very small percentage of pediatric heart disease cases and the various types are presented in detail on pages 355 to 373.

- Dilated cardiomyopathy (DCM) is the most common type seen in the pediatric population and it is usually idiopathic in origin. Other causes include myocarditis, familial inheritance (e.g., Duchenne's and Becker's muscular dystrophies, Friedreich's ataxia), exposure to chemotherapeutic agents (mainly anthracyclines), recreational cocaine use by the child or adolescent, hypo- and hyperthyroidism, glycogen storage disease, and nutritional deficiencies of thiamine or selenium.
- Hypertrophic cardiomyopathy (HCM) is the leading cause of sudden death in children and young adults under 21 years of age.[101] Patients with probable or unequivocal clinical diagnosis of HCM should be restricted from participation in competitive athletics, with the possible exception of low-intensity sports (class IA in Table 8-12).[67] This recommendation includes patients with and without LV outflow obstruction and those who have had treatment with surgery, ablation, pacemaker, or implantable defibrillator.
- Arrhythmogenic right ventricular cardiomyopathy (ARVC) is a rare form of CM occurring in children that is characterized by the replacement of myocytes in the RV with fatty, fibrous tissue.
- Restrictive cardiomyopathy has a more malignant course in the pediatric population than in adults.[58]
- Cardiomyopathy resulting from etiologies other than myocarditis carries a poor prognosis in children. Treatment options that may be considered include automatic implantable cardioverter/defibrillators, ventricular assist devices (VADs), and heart transplantation.

There are preliminary data supporting the benefits of exercise rehabilitation for children with DCM, including increased cardiovascular fitness and strength, without deterioration of ventricular function.[95] Larger, prospective studies are warranted.

Infective Endocarditis

Infective endocarditis (IE) develops almost exclusively in children with a history of congenital or acquired heart disease who develop bacterial infection. If diagnosed in a child without known heart disease, an underlying bicuspid aortic valve is often revealed. With the exception of secundum ASD, all types of congenital heart defects predispose to IE when bacteremia (even transient, as occurs after dental procedures) is present, although it rarely occurs in infants except after open heart surgery. Diagnosis is made by pathologic evidence and fulfillment of certain clinical criteria.

- Initial symptoms are often noncardiac in nature and include fever, malaise, anorexia, arthralgia, and weakness.
- Cardiovascular symptoms include heart failure, hypotension, tachycardia, tachypnea, rales, and pulmonary edema.
- Infective endocarditis is suspected in any child presenting with a fever of unknown origin for several days along with any of the aforementioned symptoms or findings, especially in the presence of a congenital cardiac lesion.
- Although traditionally all patients with known heart disease have previously been treated with prophylactic antibiotics before dental and other procedures, data have revealed that only an extremely small number of cases of IE might be prevented, and therefore its use is currently recommended only for patients with underlying cardiac conditions associated with the highest risk of adverse outcome from IE, which are listed in Box 8-2 on page 362.[121]
- Good dental hygiene continues to play a critical role in preventing IE in all patients.

Rheumatic Fever

Acute rheumatic fever (ARF) is an inflammatory disease that occurs as a delayed sequela of group A β-hemolytic streptococcal (GABHS) pharyngitis. Most commonly presenting in children 5 to 15 years of age, it affects primarily the heart, joints, and central nervous system. The diagnosis of ARF is based on clinical and laboratory findings that occur as major and minor manifestations. Supporting evidence of previous group A streptococcal infection is a prerequisite.

- Typically, symptoms present 3 to 5 weeks after a sore throat or other presumed streptococcal infection and include migratory polyarthritis, carditis, chorea, erythema marginatum, and subcutaneous nodules.
- Carditis develops in at least 50% of patients with ARF and is usually mild or asymptomatic.[6,84,117] Clinical findings may include tachycardia, heart murmurs, pericarditis, cardiomegaly on chest x-ray, and signs of CHF, which usually results from LV volume overload associated with severe mitral regurgitation or occasionally aortic regurgitation. Most patients will develop some level of rheumatic heart disease (RHD). If carditis is not present, long-term effects are rare.
- Treatment for ARF may include antibiotics, antiinflammatory agents (most commonly aspirin), intravenous immunoglobulin (IVIG), and bed rest (progressing to restricted activity as clinical signs of carditis resolve). If chorea is present, haloperidol may be used to help control these involuntary movements.
- Both primary and secondary antibiotic prophylaxis is recommended to avoid initial occurrence of ARF (if GABHS infection present) and to avoid recurrence.

Pericarditis

In children, inflammation of the pericardium most commonly results from viral infections (in infancy), ARF (in less developed countries), or bacterial infections. It may also occur after heart surgery (postpericardiotomy syndrome), in the presence of collagen diseases, as a result of uremia, and as a complication of cancer or its therapy (chemo- and radiation therapy). It is discussed in more detail on page 127. Constrictive pericarditis is rare in children.

Athletes who develop pericarditis should not participate in competitive sports during the acute phase.[67] They can return to full activity when there is no evidence of active disease, including effusion by echocardiography, and when serum markers of inflammation have normalized. Chronic pericardial disease that results in constriction disqualifies the patient from all competitive athletics.

Lyme Disease

Lyme carditis occurs in about 10% of patients (including children) with Lyme disease, the leading tick-borne illness occurring in North America and Europe.[84] It often manifests 4 to 8 weeks (range, 4 d to 7 mo) after initial illness and appears primarily as various degrees of atrioventricular block. It is a growing cause of myocarditis in the school-aged population.[83] Symptoms of dizziness, syncope, chest pain, and easy fatigability generally occur only in the presence of complete heart block. Initial clinical manifestations of Lyme infection consist of erythema migrans and flulike symptoms, whereas secondary manifestations may include the reappearance of erythema migrans rash in multiple locations, asymmetrical oligoarthritis of the joints (particularly the larger ones), lymphocytic meningitis, and carditis. Treatment consists of antibiotic therapy.

Arrhythmias

Pediatric arrhythmias are not uncommon and range from benign to life-threatening. A child with arrhythmia is often asymptomatic, even when the abnormal rhythm is potentially life-threatening. Pediatric arrhythmias can result from intrinsic abnormalities of the myocardium or conduction system or extrinsic factors that alter the excitability of the heart, such as present or past infection, drug toxicity, structural lesions of the heart, and metabolic–endocrine disorders.

In infants who cannot verbally communicate symptoms, parents may report episodes of difficulty with feedings or increased irritability. In a young child, irregular heart beats may be sensed but difficult to articulate. Sudden death in the pediatric population is invariably linked with arrhythmias, although the underlying causes may be diverse. In teenagers and young adults, most arrhythmias are associated with previously operated CHD.[117]

- Supraventricular tachycardia (SVT) is the most commonly occurring arrhythmia in children.[62] Depending on the age of the patient and type of SVT, symptoms may include palpitations, chest pain, lack of energy, and dizziness.
- Atrial flutter is seen primarily in patients with CHD, and chronic atrial flutter is treated with digitalis in addition to procainamide, quinidine, or disopyramide.
- Atrial fibrillation is commonly seen after RHD affecting the mitral valve and in patients with poor LV function.

On occasion, idiopathic atrial fibrillation occurs in adolescents without CHD who, once converted, usually do not experience recurrence.

- Ventricular arrhythmias include premature ventricular contractions (PVCs), nonsustained or sustained ventricular tachycardia (VT), and ventricular fibrillation (VF). In pediatrics, PVCs are often benign but the significant difference in prognosis in children with normal versus abnormal hearts requires evaluation for underlying pathology. PVCs and VT resolve over time in one to two thirds of children without structural cardiac defects[115] but may evolve into more serious arrhythmias in children with underlying CHD.
- Pediatric cases of heart block (congenital, postoperative, or acquired), sinus node dysfunction (congenital or acquired), symptomatic hypervagal situations, and long Q–T syndromes (with severe bradycardia, uncontrolled ventricular arrhythmias, or both) may require pacemaker or occasionally automatic implantable cardioverter/defibrillator (AICD) placement.[41]

Some arrhythmias (e.g., ventricular tachyarrhythmias and atrial flutter or fibrillation with very rapid ventricular rates) are associated with increased risk of syncope and sudden death, particularly during exercise, and thus preclude participation in sports activities.[124] However, once the arrhythmia is brought under control through medication or other interventions (e.g., ablation, pacemaker, or AICD), many athletes are able to resume competitive athletics (see Table 8-11, page 359).

CLINICAL IMPLICATIONS FOR PHYSICAL THERAPY

- Infants and children with cardiovascular disease and the sequelae of its management are at risk for many of the same problems as adults, including the following:
  - Increased and/or retained secretions
  - Poor gas exchange; dyspnea
  - Pain or discomfort
  - Poor postural alignment
  - Decreased active range of motion
  - Impaired mobility
  - Reduced exercise tolerance
  - Diminished sense of wellness
  - Poor understanding of medical condition/medical status
- Postsurgical pediatric patients suffer depressed cardiorespiratory effects after general anesthesia similar to adults (see page 90). They are at higher risk for pulmonary dysfunction including atelectasis, infection, and airway obstruction, especially those who have preexisting lung disease. If sternal closure is delayed the child is usually sedated.
- In smaller, community-based hospitals where acute management of CHD is less common, the physical therapist (PT) may not have exposure to patients with these diagnoses acutely or subacutely. However, given the prevalence of CHD and its potential impact on cardiorespiratory function even after correction, it is good practice to inquire about any history of CHD in any older child or adolescent who is referred to PT.
- If working in an acute care, high-level subspecialty medical center, PTs are likely to encounter the majority of diagnoses

previously mentioned. In the intensive care units (ICUs), the role of PT depends on the acuteness of illness.

  - Initially, positioning, range of motion, sensorimotor stimulation, secretion clearance, breathing exercises, and patient and family education are often indicated for infants and small children.
  - For older children, immediate postoperative PT typically consists of breathing exercises, secretion clearance, range of motion, and bed mobility.
  - As the situation becomes less acute, PT interventions often progress to involve increased patient participation, including therapeutic exercise, therapeutic activities (using a play-based format, if appropriate), and more active airway clearance techniques.
  - Early mobilization, even if significant assistance is needed, is encouraged.
  - Ongoing monitoring of HR, RR, BP, oxygen saturation, and the overall clinical picture at rest and in response to activity is appropriate both in the ICUs and on inpatient floors.
- It is important to use appropriately sized equipment (BP cuff, stethoscope, and ECG electrodes) when assessing infants and children for findings to be valid.
- HR variability is common. Sinus bradycardia is present in infants and small children when the HR is less than 90 bpm. Normal decreases to 70 bpm may occur during bowel movements, eating, or hiccupping secondary to enhanced vagal tone; a HR less than 60 bpm is of concern.
- A wider range of normal ECG findings occurs in pediatric patients than in adults, with some predictable changes as the child ages:
  - Decrease in resting and maximal HRs
  - Increase in duration and intervals (P–R interval, QRS duration, and Q–T interval)
  - Increase in QRS voltage
  - Right ventricular dominant pattern converts to a left ventricular dominant pattern (reflective of age-related changes in the LV/RV weight ratio)
  - The most notable and rapid changes occur in the first month of life.
- Bradycardia can provoke a drop in cardiac output (because HR is the major determinant of cardiac output in infants and younger children as a result of increased cardiac compliance) and may be induced by hypoxemia.
- Some suggestions related to PT interventions for pediatric patients with cardiac disease are included here but are not intended to be inclusive. Refer to Section 8.6 for more information about pediatric PT treatment interventions.
  - Children are at additional risk for reduced active range of motion (AROM) at the sites of lines, tubes, drains, and/or incisions. Appropriate AROM of the extremities and the body should be encouraged through functional play, including functional respiration (e.g., reading aloud, singing, and bubble and other blowing activities). It is best to avoid drawing added attention to the site except for safety or patient/parent education.
  - Initial airway clearance interventions may include positioning, percussion, vibration, deep breathing activities (including

blowing bubbles and singing songs or facilitating laughter), movement play that incorporates thoracic expansion and arm movements (to avoid guarding), and instruction to splint incisions during coughing (e.g., by hugging a medium to large-sized stuffed animal to the site).

▸ In both neonatal and pediatric ICUs, developmental care practices are becoming more common and are designed to provide each infant with an environment conducive to sensorimotor development (e.g., dim lights, minimal noise, and supportive positioning).

▸ Infants with CHD are at risk to develop their gross and fine motor skills more slowly than healthy infants and may benefit from therapeutic developmental interventions, including supportive positioning, facilitation of flexor muscle activation patterns, and sensorimotor stimulation. Spending time with parents and caregivers to support infant/caregiver bonding is invaluable, especially when lines and tubes are daunting.

▸ Some infants with CHD may benefit from feeding interventions (which may be performed by physical therapists, occupational therapists, speech therapists, or nurses) to assist in facilitation of suck/swallow/breathing coordination.

▸ Regular physical exercise is important for all patients with CHD, as it optimizes physical performance and reduces the risk of early development of cardiovascular disease and other illnesses associated with physical inactivity. Many patients are able to participate in competitive athletics (see Table 8-11, page 359).

▸ Cardiac rehabilitation may be used in the pediatric population for children with severe congenital or acquired heart disease, cardiac transplantation, and high risk for developing atherosclerotic heart disease. Expected benefits are similar to those in adult patients (see page 309).

▸ The size and/or age of the child may limit the modes of exercise the child can perform, especially for exercise testing. Specially sized and programmed cardiovascular exercise equipment (e.g., treadmills, upright and recumbent bicycles, steppers, and elliptical trainers) is available and recommended.

8.4 SECONDARY CARDIOPULMONARY DYSFUNCTION IN PEDIATRIC DISEASES

This section focuses on secondary cardiopulmonary dysfunction associated with select neurological, neuromuscular, and musculoskeletal disorders occurring in the pediatric population. In these cases, cardiopulmonary problems are usually not the primary reason for PT referral, but it is important that physical therapists appreciate the interrelation between the cardiopulmonary system and all other systems, especially in a growing child and those with progressive conditions.

The gross cardiopulmonary impairments that can arise as secondary complications of other systemic processes include decreased ventilation (especially in the terminal airways), impaired airway clearance, impaired protective reflexes of the airway, increased work of breathing and potential respiratory failure, and decreased cardiovascular endurance. Chest wall deformities and spinal curvatures (especially kyphoscoliosis), whether congenital or acquired, negatively influence thoracic mobility as well as the mechanics of breathing. Cardiac manifestations of neuromuscular or musculoskeletal disease may range from incidental findings of changes on ECG to fully developed cardiomyopathies or serious arrhythmias. The presence of gastroesophageal reflux (GER), seizures, cognitive impairments, and limited mobility, as well as side effects of medications, may further complicate the clinical picture.

Several common pediatric disorders are presented including cerebral palsy, Down syndrome, Duchenne's and Becker's muscular dystrophies, spinal muscular atrophy, spina bifida with myelomeningocele, kyphoscoliosis, and obesity. Secondary impairments related to the cardiopulmonary system may also arise from neurological impairments due to infection, intracranial mass, CVA, or trauma. Other neuromuscular disorders with potential cardiopulmonary involvement that affect children include Guillain-Barré syndrome, multiple sclerosis, and spinal cord injury, which are presented in Chapter 4. Identification of those children at risk for secondary cardiopulmonary involvement and integration of interventions that aim to reduce potential complications are appropriate roles for the physical therapist.

CEREBRAL PALSY

Cerebral palsy (CP) refers to an acquired static encephalopathy resulting from insult during the perinatal period, which is associated with atypical tone, potential cognitive deficits, and impairments of motor control and function. Children with CP also may have vision, hearing, and other sensory deficits; learning disabilities; language impairments; and delay (or absence) of motor skill acquisition. Brain injury may result from anoxia, hypoperfusion, trauma, vascular events, or congenital anomalies. Spastic types of CP include diplegia, hemiplegia, and quadriplegia whereas hypotonic types include athetoid (predominant basal ganglia involvement) and ataxic (predominant cerebellar involvement). Cognitive and motor deficits range from very mild to severe. Cardiopulmonary complications may include abnormal mechanics of respiration, hypoventilation, difficulty in mobilizing and clearing secretions, increased work of breathing, and impaired phonation. Some of these children are also at risk for aspiration. Scoliosis may develop in some patients to further affect pulmonary function.

Children with CP have low physical activity and fitness levels and are therefore at increased risk for associated health problems.[28] Unfortunately, impairments such as muscle weakness, spasticity, contractures, and poor balance increase the energy demands of movement, particularly ambulation. Thus, they have limited cardiopulmonary reserves available for sustained physical activity. However, there is evidence that participation in generalized sports and exercise programs and formal exercise training can increase cardiorespiratory fitness in these children. Some physical therapists are becoming involved in establishing community- and school-based physical fitness programs for children with physical impairments.

DOWN SYNDROME

Down syndrome most often results from an extra copy of chromosome 21 (trisomy 21) and is the most common autosomal chromosomal abnormality in human live births. In addition to structural malformations associated with delays in development, one third to one half of infants diagnosed with Down syndrome have congenital heart defects, most frequently endocardial cushion defects, VSD, ASD, or TOF.

Clinical manifestations include various degrees of hypotonia, delay in motor skill acquisition, characteristic facies, bilateral hearing loss, cognitive impairments, and shorter stature than same-aged peers (see Table 8-8). Down syndrome has also been associated with increased incidence of leukemia and pulmonary hypertension. Cardiopulmonary manifestations include poor ability to clear secretions from both upper and lower airways, resulting in greater susceptibility to pulmonary infections, and postural abnormalities that may lead to restrictive lung dysfunction in older children. In addition, atlantoaxial instability and subluxation may result in compression of the medulla as the child ages, leading to respiratory compromise (see later section on spina bifida).

MUSCULAR DYSTROPHIES

Duchenne's muscular dystrophy and Becker's muscular dystrophy are hereditary, X-linked recessive myopathies related to abnormality of the dystrophin gene and characterized by progressive degeneration of the skeletal muscles, resulting in wasting and weakness (see page 140).

- Duchenne's muscular dystrophy (DMD) is most common. Classic clinical manifestations include waddling gait, increased lumbar lordosis, pseudohypertrophy of the calf muscles with eventual plantar flexion and inversion contractures, and transitions from floor to standing using the Gower's maneuver (using the arms to "climb up" the length of the legs to achieve an upright posture). Loss of functional ambulation often occurs by the end of adolescence.
  - ▶ Respiratory muscle weakness becomes a major problem by the teens, and most patients die of respiratory failure, usually related to pulmonary infection, if assisted ventilation is not instituted some time during the teens or 20s.[4] The degree of respiratory failure is related to the degree of skeletal muscle impairment and respiratory weakness. Before failure, dyspnea and tachypnea are common symptoms.
  - ▶ With increasing age, cardiac involvement becomes more prevalent and may include cardiomyopathy, arrhythmias, ECG abnormalities, and sudden death; however, the typical symptoms of reduced exercise tolerance are difficult to appreciate in nonambulatory patients. Instead, these patients may exhibit increased fatigue, difficulty sleeping, impaired concentration, and more subtle variants of poor performance.[21] Because of the associated musculoskeletal and respiratory impairments, cardiac transplant is not an option for these patients.
- Becker's muscular dystrophy occurs less frequently and noncardiac clinical manifestations are similar to but milder than in Duchenne's. The age of onset is later and musculoskeletal involvement progresses more slowly, so that there is preservation of ambulatory mobility into the fifth decade of life. Cardiac involvement occurs more frequently and with earlier onset (usually by age 30 yr) than in Duchenne's and its severity is out of proportion to the skeletal myopathy. Near-normal life expectancy is preserved with demise related to degree of heart failure present.

SPINAL MUSCULAR ATROPHY

Spinal muscular atrophy (SMA) that presents in infancy and childhood may be divided into three subtypes including type I (severe infantile SMA, Werdnig-Hoffman), type II (intermediate), and type III (mild, Kugelberg-Welander). Classification seeks to categorize type on the basis of age at onset/age of anticipated death, severity, and development (or lack of development) of functional motor skills including sitting, standing, and walking. In all types, the disease affects the motor neurons of the medulla and spinal cord, and SMA is characterized by hypotonia, weakness, and cranial nerve palsies (with sparing of the facial muscles). Research has yielded increased knowledge related to SMA, and the way it is classified has been reconsidered to more appropriately capture variability within types.[24]

Cardiopulmonary complications are associated with all types of SMA and range in severity on the basis of type and presentation. The most common consist of respiratory muscle weakness (leading to reduced thoracic compliance, diminished ventilatory volumes, and $\dot{V}/\dot{Q}$ mismatching) and impaired cough with retained secretions. For more involved cases, especially those with significant mobility impairments, respiratory support is often needed. Airway clearance techniques are often incorporated into daily management along with assisted cough techniques. Because intelligence is not affected, the severely involved infant or child who does not have the ability to perform functional movements is also at risk for social isolation and associated emotional issues.

SPINA BIFIDA

Spina bifida with myelomeningocele describes the herniation of meninges and spinal cord (exposed or within a sac) through a dorsal defect in the vertebral column at birth. It most commonly occurs in the lumbar region and results from failure of the neural folds to come together during the very early stages of fetal development. Folic acid supplementation before conception and during the first trimester of pregnancy has been associated with reduction in the incidence of neural tube defects.

The level of herniation is directly related to the degree of motor paresis. Other abnormalities that are often associated with myelomeningocele include Arnold-Chiari malformation (herniation of the inferior poles of the cerebellar hemispheres and medulla oblongata), progressive hydrocephalus, and some degree of scoliosis (existing from birth or developing over time). Cases of Arnold-Chiari malformation have also been associated with lower brainstem and cranial nerve dysfunction[37] that may have direct cardiopulmonary implications including apneic spells, impaired swallowing, and impaired cough generation of a central origin, which can lead to poor management of secretions and aspiration.

KYPHOSCOLIOSIS

Spinal deformities can exist at birth or develop as a result of neuromuscular disease or trauma. The more pronounced deformities may influence the mechanics of breathing, as described on page 88, because of reduced thoracic expansion and compression of the underlying structures. Kyphoscoliosis usually produces the most significant restriction of pulmonary function, resulting in a shallow, rapid breathing pattern, decreased total lung capacity and vital capacity, and increased dependence on the diaphragm and upper accessory muscles of breathing.[109]

OBESITY

Obesity has been defined by the Centers for Disease Control and Prevention as a body mass index (BMI) greater than or equal to the 95th percentile. The prevalence of childhood obesity has tripled between 1980 and 2002, such that 17.1% of children and adolescents in the United States are overweight or obese whereas another 16.5% are at risk of becoming overweight.[45] Overweight and obese children and adolescents have increased risk of cardiopulmonary morbidity.

- Pulmonary abnormalities that may be associated with childhood obesity include the following:
  ‣ Upper airway obstruction, sleep apnea
  ‣ Small airway disease; asthma
  ‣ Decreased functional residual capacity, diffusion impairment[59]
  ‣ Hypoventilation
  ‣ Pulmonary hypertension
- Similar to obese adults, overweight children often present with hypertension (HTN). The *Fourth Report on the Diagnosis, Evaluation, and Treatment of High Blood Pressure in Children and Adolescents* defines HTN in children as SBP and/or diastolic blood pressure that is, on greater than three measurements, at or above the 95th percentile.[112] This report presents tables to be used for identification of HTN in the pediatric population and that encompass age, height, and gender. These may be accessed at www.nhlbi.nih.gov/health/prof/heart/hbp/hbp_ped.pdf (accessed February 2009).
- Cardiovascular changes found in obese children and adolescents include the following:
  ‣ LV dilatation, increased wall stress, and compensatory LV hypertrophy[3]
  ‣ Increased left ventricular mass due to HTN[110]
  ‣ RV changes resulting from pulmonary complications[3]
  ‣ Deconditioning, reduced exercise tolerance
- Type 2 diabetes mellitus, once rare in children, is becoming more common in the pediatric population.[26]
- Overweight children are more likely to become obese adolescents and young adults. Increased body weight makes movement and exercise difficult and may also produce feelings of self-consciousness, which further inhibit the performance of physical activity. Conversely, longitudinal studies have shown that adaptation to a higher level of activity during childhood can result in reduced deposition of fat.[79]
- Obesity is more prevalent in children with several genetic syndromes and associated congenital heart defects including Down syndrome[15] and Prader-Willi syndrome.[51] Obesity is also common in children with neuromuscular diseases that limit mobility and activity, including cerebral palsy (especially spastic quadraparesis)[100] and spina bifida.[114]

- Studies examining the reversibility of cardiovascular changes in the pediatric population as the result of weight loss interventions yield mixed results.[53,113]
- Physical therapists are increasingly involved in programs aimed at both primary prevention and reversal of the current rise in childhood obesity and its effects.

CLINICAL IMPLICATIONS FOR PHYSICAL THERAPY

The clinical implications for physical therapy for infants and children with cardiopulmonary dysfunction associated with other chronic diseases are often similar to those for adults with similar diagnoses, which are presented in Chapter 4 (Cardiopulmonary Pathology; see pages 128 to 149). Clinical implications pertinent to the pediatric population are presented on pages 355 and 375; additional ones may apply to some of these patients:

- Physiological monitoring of responses to stimulation and activity/exercise is important.
- Besides the indications listed on page 355, positioning may also be used in appropriate patients to:
  ‣ Minimize scoliosis and its potential effects (often present and progressive in neurologically impaired children)
  ‣ Prevent upper airway obstruction during sleep
- Airway clearance techniques may be indicated to assist with the removal of secretions. Children with secondary cardiopulmonary dysfunction may also benefit from instruction in and reinforcement of coughing techniques, especially following activity. The mechanical insufflator–exsufflator (see page 326) can be used to stimulate coughing in those patients who are too weak or neurologically impaired to initiate it themselves.
- Manual stretching and mobilization of the rib cage are valuable for patients with reduced thoracic compliance resulting from muscle weakness, paralysis, or spasticity (see page 320).
- Diaphragmatic strengthening exercises using abdominal weights, inspiratory resistive devices, or incentive spirometry (see page 315) are beneficial for patients with neuromuscular disorders and can generally be performed by school-age children (or sometimes younger if they are part of a game or fun activity). Postural strengthening is also important.
- Activity level and ability to exercise vary a great deal according to the specific disorder and severity of involvement of each child.
  ‣ Neurodevelopmental interventions may be implemented to facilitate components of movement, muscle group activation (especially flexors), and/or acquisition of motor skills as appropriate.
  ‣ For nonambulatory patients, assistive technology, motorized wheelchairs, and other adaptive equipment may be appropriate and significantly improve quality of life, feelings of independence, and self-esteem.
  ‣ In addition, overall energy expenditure can be reduced by focusing on interventions to decrease spasticity, if present.
- Unless specifically contraindicated, regular physical activity is important for all children with secondary cardiopulmonary dysfunction to optimize functional capacity and prevent

complications associated with a sedentary lifestyle. In obese children, exercise is critical for weight loss and the prevention of type 2 diabetes (see page 128).

▸ Besides promoting cardiopulmonary fitness, aerobic exercise and recreational activities are crucial for achieving and maintaining weight loss and improving glucose metabolism.

▸ Strengthening exercises increase functional independence and also assist with weight loss and improved glucose metabolism.

▸ Stretching exercises maintain or improve flexibility to prevent injury and impairment of function caused by joint restrictions.

▸ Yoga and pilates techniques enhance postural strength and mobility, breath control and support, and focus and concentration.

8.5 ASSESSMENT OF THE PEDIATRIC PATIENT

Growth is an integral part of childhood and the cardiovascular system plays a key role in facilitating the development of all systems. Thus, all pediatric assessments should include, at minimum, a basic cardiopulmonary assessment. For those with known or suspected cardiopulmonary involvement, a more comprehensive examination is warranted. Biomechanical differences associated with congenital and acquired pediatric defects predispose the child to decreased cardiovascular efficiency and may interfere with typical development of motor function in young infants.

Assessment of ventilation in infants and children consists of observation, auscultation, palpation, and percussion with noted considerations. This section aims to identify modifications of cardiopulmonary PT assessment techniques (see Chapter 6) that are appropriate for the pediatric population. Other areas of assessment that are recommended in infants, children, and adolescents are also briefly described.

GENERAL CONSIDERATIONS

• Anatomic and physiologic differences in the pediatric population must be acknowledged and age-related differences in cognition and communication appreciated and respected.

• Incorporation of the parent or caregiver into the assessment process may be especially helpful with infants and younger children.

• Preservation of a comfortable, nonthreatening atmosphere will help ensure a more accurate physiological and behavioral baseline to serve for comparison with subsequent responses. Physiological parameters such as HR and BP may be falsely elevated if measurements are taken under duress.

▸ Initial interaction may rely more heavily on observational skills and less on hands-on assessment while the child gains a sense of trust and understanding of what the interaction is about. This is especially important when the child's cooperation may be affected by fear. Thus, observational skills are essential as are flexibility, creativity, and the ability to identify which components of the examination are necessary and which elements are supportive but not critical to the moment.

▸ Assessment components that may be perceived as scary or uncomfortable should be saved until the end of the examination.

• An age-appropriate explanation of procedures is warranted and, in particular, if the child is unable to directly communicate or comprehend what the assessment entails, a thorough explanation should be made to the parent or caregiver. In some situations explaining procedures to the parent or caregiver outside the range of the child's hearing is preferred.

MEDICAL CHART REVIEW

As with adults, a careful review of the medical record is extremely important. In the case of neonates, infants, and younger children, special attention is directed to the following items:

• Medical orders including medications prescribed, consultations requested, and diagnostic tests ordered

• History of prenatal course, labor and delivery, and relevant past medical history that may include the following:

▸ Apgar scores, reflective of the status of the newborn at noted intervals after birth, which are presented in Table 8-13

▸ New Ballard or Dubowitz gestational age scores, reflective of a compilation of both neurological and external characteristics present in premature infant[8,22,23]

• Calculation of chronological age and adjusted gestational age for infants with history of prematurity (commonly made until 24 mo chronological age)

• Clinical course from birth to the present including any cardiac or pulmonary diagnoses, previous surgeries or hospitalizations,

TABLE 8-13: Apgar Score for Newborn Infants*

Sign	Points		
	0	1	2
Heart rate	Absent	<100/min	>100/min
Respiration	Absent	Irregular, shallow, gasping, weak cry	Vigorous, crying
Skin color	Pale, blue	Pink body, blue extremities	Pink all over
Muscle tone/activity	Limp	Some flexion of extremities	Active movement
Reflex irritability (catheter in nostril)	None	Grimace, some motion	Active withdrawal

Data from Apgar V. Proposal for a new method of evaluation of the newborn infant. *Curr Res Anesth Analg.* 1953;32:260–267.

*The score is first taken 60 seconds after birth and may be repeated at 1- to 5-minute intervals until the total score reaches at least 8.

as well as current issues with any known intraoperative or postoperative complications

- Arterial blood gas history, other pertinent laboratory findings (e.g., presence of infection, and platelet counts), pulmonary function tests (commonly believed to be reliable in children greater than 6 yr old), and chest x-ray reports
- Mode and frequency of feedings; presence of reflux
- Prior level of function, including achievement of motor milestones when appropriate (autonomic, behavioral, and motor responses in the neonate) and history of therapeutic intervention including discipline, frequency, and location of service
- Social history including identification of the primary caregiver, support systems, and number of siblings

COMMUNICATION WITH THE NURSE, PHYSICIAN, AND PARENT/CAREGIVER

When dealing with infants and small children who are either not able to communicate verbally or who may be too young to communicate effectively with care providers, it is critical to check in with the primary caretakers before any intervention is initiated. Valuable information may be obtained from hospital personnel who have been taking care of the patient, especially if primary nursing is in practice. Never underestimate the value of information that may be obtained from the parent/caregiver. Although they may not have a professional medical background, most parents/caregivers have exceptional insight into their children, especially if the child has chronic needs. Specifically, they may be helpful in interpreting nonverbal or preverbal communication offered by the child or with key ways to motivate or console the child.

Important information to discuss and questions to ask may include the following:

- Up to the moment status of the infant or child (specifically, information that may not have been documented yet)
- Any evaluation or treatment procedures performed during the past few hours or planned for the next few hours
- Time and mode of the last feeding and the next planned feeding; course of feeding (e.g., typical vs. requiring increased time or effort)
- Response to handling (e.g., changes in HR, respiratory rate, and transcutaneous oxygen values, as well as state and behavioral changes) and time needed to recover after handling
- Method used to console the child and effectiveness of same
- Infant or child's activity level (current, past, and trends), including their ability to tolerate and participate in activities of daily living (e.g., feeding, dressing, sleeping, and play activities)
  - ▸ A parent may be able to use peers as a basis for comparison of activity level before admission.
  - ▸ Therapists may use standardized, norm-referenced developmental motor scales, developmental checklists, or clinical opinion in the acute setting to confirm or identify suspected delay in acquisition of motor skills.
  - ▸ Of note, the older child or teenager may be reluctant to expose limitations or disabilities, especially in front of others. Observational skills are critical when looking for signs and symptoms of potential limitations before actual assessment

begins or during functional activities (e.g., noting dyspnea during stair climbing).

- ▸ Heart failure will lead to decreased activity level and/or decreased exercise tolerance and dyspnea in infants and young children, but symptoms are difficult to identify in this population.
- Infant's sleep schedule
- Complaints of or observed signs of pain or discomfort; otherwise unexplainable irritability in an infant may be an expression of pain, while an older child may be better able to qualify and quantify pain similar to an adult. Pediatric pain scales using faces, body figures, or colors may be helpful in objectifying pain levels.
- Parent/caregiver perceptions as to the child's likes or dislikes, favorite types of toys, key motivators, and so on.

PHYSICAL ASSESSMENT

As with adults, the cardiopulmonary physical assessment of infants and children consists of observation, auscultation, palpation, and percussion. In addition, a functional assessment and evaluation of responses to exercise or therapeutic handling/positioning is performed. Observation is aided by removal of clothing and blankets but care must taken to preserve body temperature and state (i.e., neurobehavioral state: quiet awake, active awake, drowsy, crying, etc.) throughout the examination.

- Observation of the patient includes the following:
  - ▸ State and state control (all findings will be affected by the current neurobehavioral state of the infant and any changes that occur during the examination)
  - ▸ Observed signs of pain or discomfort (e.g., changes in facial expression, and withdrawal maneuvers)
  - ▸ Postural alignment (specifically to identify the presence of postural positions that suggest the baby is demonstrating a preference for positions that ease work of breathing including neck hyperextension, upper extremity elevation with scapular retraction, trunk extension with anterior pelvic tilt, and decreased lower extremity movements)
  - ▸ Rib cage shape, symmetry, alignment, and activation of oblique musculature, keeping in mind appropriateness for age (see page 345). Identification of congenital defects (e.g., pectus excavatum, pectus carinatum), acquired deformities (e.g., pectus excavatum, barrel-shaped chest), kyphosis, and scoliosis. Atypicalities in the rib cage may interfere with thoracic expansion and result in decreased lung volume or may reflect hyperinflation or air trapping within the lungs
  - ▸ Dysmorphic features (may reflect an underlying syndrome)
  - ▸ Skin inspection to include incisions, rash, scars, birth markings, color, and presence of lines, drains, and tubes.
    - ⊙ Skin integrity (preterm infants are especially prone to skin breakdown, especially in areas underlying adhesive monitoring pads, because of their extremely fragile, thin skin with little subcutaneous fat)
    - ⊙ Incisions (especially unilateral, which may produce asymmetry of movement)
    - ⊙ Scar mobility (presence of adhesions after adequate healing time, especially in a growing body)

⊙ Mottling, webbing, and color changes (indicating hypoxic stress)

⊙ Cyanosis (generalized, central, upper extremity vs. lower extremity; true arterial desaturation manifests in the lips, mucous membranes, and tongue)

⊙ Clubbing of digits (indicating prolonged tissue hypoxia)

⊙ Presence of indwelling lines (special care must be exercised during PT interventions to avoid dislodging lines in infants who have very fragile arteries and veins)

▸ Respiration/breathing pattern

⊙ Normal pattern (respiratory rate within normal limits [WNL] for age; short periods of apnea [<20 s] in neonates, ratio of inspiration to expiration of 1:2)

⊙ Head bobbing in synchrony with the respiratory cycle (indicates effort to use accessory muscles of inspiration in an infant with poor or immature head control)

⊙ Hypertrophy of accessory muscles of breathing suggesting chronic dyspnea

⊙ Signs of respiratory distress (see Table 8-7, page 348)

⊙ Bulging of the intercostal muscles caused by obstruction to expiration due to high expiratory pleural pressures in an infant whose chest wall compliance is increased (as expected at this age)

⊙ Sneezing (the primary means of airway clearance for the neonate and very young infant)

▸ Cough effectiveness (appropriate for older infants and children)

- Auscultation should be performed with a smaller, pediatric stethoscope. As appropriate to the child's age, the therapist may demonstrate its use before auscultation.

▸ Whenever possible, the infant's head should be placed in the midline position, because breath sounds will be decreased on the skull side. In addition, in the young or premature infant, muscle tone and movement patterns may also be influenced by head positioning out of midline.

▸ To improve the accuracy of findings, any water within the tubing used with ventilators or other systems delivering airway pressures (e.g., NCPAP and bilevel positive airway pressure [BiPAP]) should be emptied and auscultation of mechanically assisted breaths should be performed.

▸ In infants and younger children, the location of abnormal breath sounds does not necessarily correspond with the underlying lung segment because of the transmission of sounds through airways that are located in close proximity to a thin chest wall. Therefore, findings should be correlated with chest x-ray findings before providing treatment.

▸ Stridor on inspiration is often associated with upper airway obstruction in an infant. Expiratory grunting is often associated with airway collapse. Both may be audible without a stethoscope.

▸ Auscultation of the heart may reveal the murmurs of persistent fetal circulation (e.g., PDA or atrial septal defect, which can develop as a result of CHD or hypoxic vasoconstriction and pulmonary HTN due to neonatal lung disease).

- Chest palpation can be informative in pediatric patients.

▸ Palpation at the suprasternal notch may be performed to assess tracheal deviation (and thus mediastinal shift; see page 248).

▸ Because the chest walls of tiny infants move very little, the symmetry of their expansion is usually not palpated but asymmetry of retractions or movement surrounding surgical sites should be noted. Paradoxical chest motion can be palpated in the neonate.

▸ Symmetry of motion can be assessed in older infants and children.

▸ Peripheral edema is unusual in infants, even with congestive heart failure. If present it may be found in the scrotum or the eyelids.

▸ Palpation is also used to locate edema, subcutaneous emphysema, or fractured ribs.

- Percussion techniques are not commonly performed in neonates or younger infants. Mediate (indirect) percussion may be used in older infants and children to assess the density of underlying organs according to the techniques described on page 254.

ADDITIONAL CONSIDERATIONS FOR PEDIATRIC ASSESSMENT

- Vital signs vary with age, as depicted in Table 8-3 on page 344. Appropriately sized assessment tools including stethoscopes, BP cuffs, and oxygen saturation probes are required for accurate measurements.

▸ The pulse is taken at the brachial or femoral artery in infants and at the radial artery in older children.

▸ Palpation of pulses should be performed in both upper extremities and lower extremities. Patients with low cardiac output often have weak, thready pulses whereas those with systemic artery-to-pulmonary artery connections (e.g., PDA or arteriovenous malformation) may have bounding pulses. There is often a difference in force between upper and lower body pulses in patients with CoA.

▸ Vital signs are assessed in a variety of developmentally appropriate positions (e.g., supine, sitting, and standing).

▸ Physiologic signs of intolerance include excessive increases in HR and respiratory rate, oxygen desaturation, intercostal and other retractions, and skin color changes.

- Neurodevelopmental stress signs, such as arching and finger splaying, among others (for neonates) and observed signs of discomfort (for infants) must be noted and respected, as these signs communicate valuable information in patients who are unable to express themselves verbally.

- Gross screening for visual and auditory responsiveness is appropriate for young infants.

- Assessment of motor function and components of movement is required to fully assess the effectiveness of ventilation and respiration as well as the functional status of the child. Aerobic capacity in a neonate or infant may be assessed by looking at autonomic, behavioral, and motor responses. Exercise tolerance, strength, and flexibility can be measured in older children.

PHYSIOLOGICAL RESPONSE TO EXERCISE IN CHILDREN

Although pediatric cardiovascular responses to exercise are in many ways similar to those of adults, some important differences exist.[13] Factors that affect the normal child's physiological responses to exercise include the mode of exercise, body position, and protocol (running vs. walking).

- Resting HR decreases progressively throughout childhood, falling 10 to 20 bpm from age 5 to 15 years, which appears to parallel the decrease in basal metabolic rate that occurs at the same ages.
- Submaximal HRs at any given workload are usually higher in girls than boys (by as much as 10–20 bpm), which probably reflects lower SVs in females and sex-related differences in autonomic cardiac regulation.
- Maximal heart rate (HR$_{max}$), which is dependent on the mode of exercise, exercise position, and level of motivation, is fairly stable throughout childhood until late adolescence, when it begins to decrease throughout adult life. The standard formula for maximal predicted HR (220 − age in years) holds true, given a ±10 bpm range.[81]
  ▸ Running protocols produce greater HR$_{max}$ values than walking protocols.
  ▸ Treadmill exercise produces higher HR$_{max}$, maximal cardiac output ($CO_{2\ max}$), and $\dot{V}O_{2\ max}$ compared with cycle ergometry.
  ▸ Supine cycle exercise provokes a 25% higher resting SV and thus lower HR values at rest and at maximal exercise. Therefore, upright cycling produces higher $\dot{V}O_{2\ max}$ values and more marked changes in maximal cardiac output.
- The maximal SV response to exercise is lower in children than in adults and increases with increasing age and height.
- Maximal systolic BP, diastolic BP, and mean arterial pressure increase with age, most likely as a result of increasing body size.
- Resting and maximal arteriovenous oxygen differences are independent of age, and maximal values range from 10.3 to 15 mL/100 mL of blood.
- $\dot{V}O_{2\ max}$ increases with age with little difference between the genders until puberty, when it levels off for girls and accelerates for boys throughout adolescence (due to increasing lean body mass and hemoglobin)
- Higher pediatric resting metabolic rates inherently require greater oxygen consumption and the heightened demands placed on their systems may produce hypoxia more quickly. In infants, hypoxia leads to bradycardia, not tachycardia as in adults.
- Close clinical monitoring of infants and children with possible cardiopulmonary dysfunction is recommended because of their decreased tolerance for hemodynamic changes, age-related differences in ability to communicate, and sometimes unpredictable behavior.

Before puberty the effects of training on the cardiovascular responses to exercise are somewhat depressed in children as compared with adults, with most studies demonstrating training-induced increases in $\dot{V}O_{2\ max}$ not exceeding 11%.[13] Postpuberty responses are similar to those found in adults (see page 309).

8.6 PEDIATRIC CARDIOVASCULAR AND PULMONARY PHYSICAL THERAPY TREATMENT

The underlying principles of intervention for infants, children, and adolescents with primary and secondary cardiopulmonary dysfunction are similar to those for adults. Many of the techniques used in the adult population (see Chapter 7) are appropriate for use in pediatrics, with some obvious adjustments required because of differences in physical size and cognitive level. Modifications may also be necessary to account for physiological and motivational differences that exist across age groups.

This section aims to complement the problem-based format used in Chapter 7 and to identify known and suspected differences that exist in the pediatric population. It is intended to serve as a resource for methods of adapting techniques the clinician is already familiar with and to highlight additional considerations. Specific precautions and contraindications are presented when unique to the population. Please refer to the sections, entitled Clinical Implications for Physical Therapy, that appear throughout the chapter for additional ideas and recommendations related to specific pathologies.

Careful assessment and decision-making regarding the potential risks and benefits of each intervention are especially critical in the neonatal population given their sensitivity to stimulation, including routine care. Specialized, advanced-level training is recommended for clinicians who provide PT interventions of any kind to neonates, as well as to patients with ventricular assist devices (e.g., left or biventricular assist devices) and those who have undergone heart, lung, or heart–lung transplantation.

GENERAL CONSIDERATIONS

- Interventions specifically designed for the pediatric population with known or suspected atypicalities in motor development (particularly upright postural control issues) should address goals related to the respiratory system, because these patients have an inherent risk for cardiopulmonary dysfunction.
- The needs, realities, and goals of the family or caregiver (as well as the child, if able to participate) must be considered when developing a plan of care for pediatric patients, especially those requiring significant amounts of assistance or guidance to participate in PT interventions. Including the parent, caregiver, and/or sibling(s) throughout the process of creating, executing, or modifying the plan of care will help to facilitate follow-through of a realistic, individualized home program and therefore help maximize success. Therapeutic interventions provide the family or caregiver with a unique opportunity to directly participate in the child's medical care and thus can facilitate feelings of usefulness and purpose, especially during hospitalization. However, it may also inadvertently foster feelings of guilt if other needs and priorities for the family (including care for siblings) must compete with the therapeutic plan because of time constraints.
- Creativity, patience, and flexibility are invaluable tools when working with the pediatric population. Pediatric therapists are challenged to find activities that the child enjoys and identify appropriate methods of motivation to facilitate their participation.
- When working with teenagers, establishing adequate motivation to perform interventions that are within their physical and cognitive capabilities is especially challenging. Taking the time to educate the older adolescent as well as to attempt to identify their priorities is often helpful in designing a program that will both address impairments and promote compliance. It is important to recognize that participation in a program that ameliorates some but not all of the teenager's impairments is

more productive than designing a plan that is all encompassing but is not adhered to with regularity.

- It is also helpful to be aware of the parents' or primary caregiver's concerns about allowing their older adolescent to participate in decision-making when designing and implementing strategies for intervention.

ELEVATED CARDIOVASCULAR RISK IN CHILDREN

Because the atherosclerotic disease process begins in childhood, it is important to identify the presence of coronary risk factors in the pediatric population (see Table 4-7 on page 103). Evidence suggests that known risk factors for adult cardiovascular disease (CVD) might influence the rate of progression of atherosclerosis in children and young adults. It is also suspected that prevention may be more successful if started earlier in life.[44,71-74]

- Findings from the Cardiovascular Risk in Young Finns Study suggest that exposure to risk factors in childhood may increase vulnerability of the vascular wall to atherosclerosis.[89] They have also shown that lifestyle habits adopted in childhood are clearly predictive of diet and physical activity in adulthood.
- The prevalence of primary HTN in children and adolescents is relatively low (1%–3%) compared with adults, but is increasing (largely related to the increasing prevalence of obesity in this population). There are data suggesting that elevated BP during adolescence influences brachial artery endothelial function later in adulthood.[89]
- In the pediatric population, the efficacy of lower fat diets[82] and drug therapy[39] has been examined in short-term studies, but no long-term drug therapy studies exist.
- Weight loss has been associated with improvements in CVD risk factors in children.[25]
- The U.S. Department of Health and Human Services estimates that less than one third of American adolescents engage in more than 30 minutes of moderate-intensity activity on most days of the week (as recommended for this population). Approximately 65% of high school students meet the recommendation for vigorous activity on three or more days per week for greater than 20 minutes (self-reported measures).[111] Of note, the number of youths participating in these activities decreases with each year of high school.
- There has been a dramatic increase in the prevalence of type 2 diabetes in children and adolescents.[26]
- More than 2000 children under the age of 18 years became regular smokers each day during 2002.[106]

Therefore, physical therapists should assess cardiovascular risk factors in the children and adolescents referred for treatment. The participation of children and adolescents in regular physical activity and sports should be encouraged. It has been demonstrated that a high level of physical activity at ages 9 to 24 years is associated with high levels of high-density lipoprotein (HDL)–cholesterol and low levels of triglycerides, apolipoprotein B, and insulin in males.[89] More specific education regarding risk factor reduction may be indicated in youths at higher risk for the development of cardiovascular disease (e.g., those with hypertension, obesity, diabetes, and renal disease).

IMPAIRED EXERCISE TOLERANCE

Older children with cardiovascular and pulmonary disease, as well as other chronic diseases, commonly experience decreased exercise tolerance compared with their healthy peers. The same downward cycle that often presents with adult patients (decreased activity over time resulting in increased symptomatology during attempted exertion, and future reluctance to attempt activity because of the anticipated discomfort and fatigue, as shown in Figure 7-1 on page 300) may be found in the pediatric population. This is sometimes compounded by feelings of self-consciousness in situations in which peer comparisons are inevitable.

Infants with underlying primary cardiopulmonary impairments are also more likely to demonstrate impaired exercise tolerance reflected by slowed or absent development of motor skills. PT intervention must focus on providing the infant with movement and sensory experiences that facilitate the development of components of movement while also providing adequate ventilation.

- For infants whose cardiopulmonary impairments are secondary, equal attention should be focused on facilitation of ventilation and movement patterns. Provision of such items as abdominal binders or rigid body jackets may be supportive of both respiratory and developmental goals.
- It is imperative that neck, trunk, and proximal extremity range of motion be assessed and ventilation supported during handling techniques focused on facilitation of developmental motor patterns. Techniques that provide passive elongation followed by functional muscle activation are commonly used.
- Manual stabilization and realignment of the rib cage (toward a lower and more medial position) and shoulder girdles (toward external rotation, adduction, and/or depression), and facilitation of activation of the abdominal obliques are commonly needed interventions.
- In general, attempts should be made to couple extension movement patterns with inspiration and flexor movement patterns with expiration.
- Passive positioning interventions at the pelvis or upper thorax may also be used to facilitate ventilation (see next page).

Exercise studies involving prepubescent children are limited, but there is ample evidence supporting the importance of regular physical activity in enhancing physical and psychosocial development and establishing good health habits at an early age.

- All children should be encouraged to be as physically active as possible, through play, games, sports, transportation, chores, recreation, physical education, and planned exercise. Before adolescence (with its associated developmental and social influences), children with cardiopulmonary dysfunction are reliable at self-limiting exercise according to tolerance and therefore do not need to be told to restrict their activity. The main problems occur when overzealous coaches or parents don't allow children to act according to their instincts.
- The vast majority of children's spontaneous physical activity is characterized by intermittent rather than continuous activity, with only 5% of their high-intensity activities lasting more than 15 seconds.[90] By purposefully incorporating these repeated bouts of high-intensity activity in physical activity programs for

children, including those with cardiopulmonary dysfunction, both aerobic and anaerobic fitness may be enhanced.[9,90]

- For aerobic training, it appears that exercise intensity greater than 80% of HR_{max} is required to obtain significant improvements in peak $\dot{V}O_{2\ max}$.[9] However, because children are characterized by large interindividual variability in HR_{max}, exercise intensity calculated using absolute HR relative to predicted HR_{max} may be associated with significant error, particularly in children with congenital heart disease who may demonstrate chronotropic incompetence.
- Muscular strength training is beneficial for children and should be included as part of a well-balanced fitness program. Besides increasing muscular strength, properly designed strength training programs have been shown to increase bone mineral density, improve body composition, augment motor performance skills, enhance sports performance, and reduce injuries.[27,42]
  - ▸ Strength training is advantageous for children as young as 6 years of age, as long as they have the emotional maturity to accept and follow directions and can appreciate the risks and benefits associated with training.
  - ▸ A 10-minute warm-up period of light aerobic and stretching exercises should precede resistance training.
  - ▸ Modes of training that are successful with children include body weight exercises, rubber tubing, medicine balls, free weights, and appropriately sized weight machines.
  - ▸ Training should begin at a level commensurate with each child's physical abilities and emphasize high repetition–moderate load training (13- to 15-repetition maximal [RM] load) rather than low repetition–heavy load training.
  - ▸ Once the child can demonstrate proper exercise technique and safe training procedures, resistance can be increased gradually as strength improves (e.g., approximately 5%–10%).
  - ▸ The strength training program should be systematically varied over time to optimize training adaptations and prevent boredom.

The principles of exercise training and basic components of an exercise training session for adolescents are similar to those for adults, and many individuals with cardiopulmonary dysfunction can participate in and achieve the same benefits of training as their healthy peers.

- All individuals, even those with significant cardiopulmonary dysfunction, should be encouraged to perform regular physical activity within the limits of their abilities. Aerobic exercise optimizes physical performance and reduces the risk of early development of cardiovascular disease and other illnesses associated with a sedentary lifestyle. Refer to pages 301 to 308 for detailed information on aerobic exercise training.
- The ability for adolescents to benefit from resistance training is well documented. With careful instruction and proper supervision, adolescents can achieve significant gains in muscle strength and endurance without increased risk of injury following similar guidelines as those for adults (see page 309), keeping in mind the preceding recommendations for children.

IMPAIRED ABILITY TO MEET DEMANDS OF ACTIVITIES OF DAILY LIVING

Youths with severe cardiopulmonary dysfunction may have difficulty performing activities of daily living (ADLs) and may benefit from interventions described in Chapter 7 (see pages 310 to 311).

- For younger infants and children, the primary caregiver is often responsible for performing or assisting with ADLs and therefore must be considered when completing the assessment and formulating a treatment plan.
- In the presence of cardiopulmonary impairments, increased time and/or effort may be required for the child to be able to perform basic ADL tasks with or without assistance. Children with more significant functional impairments may be dependent on the caregiver for all aspects of ADLs.
- For children with impairments in upright control, appropriate positioning devices and supports are important, and strategies that address ease in performing ADLs are truly appreciated by caregivers.

IMPAIRED VENTILATION AND GAS EXCHANGE

The causes of impaired ventilation and gas exchange are detailed in Section 7.5. In the pediatric population, more commonly utilized techniques to address these impairments include positioning, functional mobility training, proprioceptive neuromuscular facilitation (PNF) techniques, incentive spirometry (IS), diaphragmatic strengthening exercises, and thoracic mobilization techniques (active and facilitated), which are described in Chapter 7 (see pages 311 to 318).

- Frequent position changes are important for infants, as they not only improve ventilation–perfusion relationships, but they also provide skin and skull pressure relief and stimulate circulation.
  - ▸ In general, positioning into a more posterior pelvic tilt will encourage diaphragmatic function and a more anterior pelvic tilt will encourage a more open position of the upper thorax and more of an upper airway or accessory muscle breathing pattern.
  - ▸ Placing the arms overhead when supine elicits greater upper chest expansion.
  - ▸ Prone positioning is especially beneficial for improving ventilation, especially of the posterior lung segments, but may require additional support for infants with low muscle tone and to accommodate those with umbilical arterial catheters, anterior chest tubes, or abdominal distension.
  - ▸ Semierect positions may also promote better oxygenation than flat positions, especially in infants with abdominal wall defects or distension.
- Techniques that require sequenced breathing patterns or the following of complex directions are likely not appropriate for younger children.
- The majority of other techniques may be used with children and adolescents as long as the physical therapist is skilled and creative enough to keep activities interesting, nonthreatening, and purposeful.

IMPAIRED CLEARANCE OF SECRETIONS

- Impaired secretion clearance in infants, children and adolescents can be addressed using the airway clearance techniques presented in Section 7.6 (see pages 328 to 336). Increased patience and creativity are frequently required to find adequate motivation for effective participation and compliance with many children, especially if the technique is challenging for them.
- Frequently used techniques with infants and small children include bronchial, or postural, drainage positioning, chest percussion, vibration, cough stimulation, and airway suctioning.

▸ Because the bronchial tree (exclusive of the alveoli) is fully developed before birth, the same 12 bronchial drainage positions used for adults are used for infants and children.

⊙ Positioning the infant or toddler over the caregiver's lap, as shown in Figure 8-9, makes transition between positions less troublesome for the caregiver. Use of a thin pillow on the caregiver's lap may reduce irritation and increase comfort for the infant.

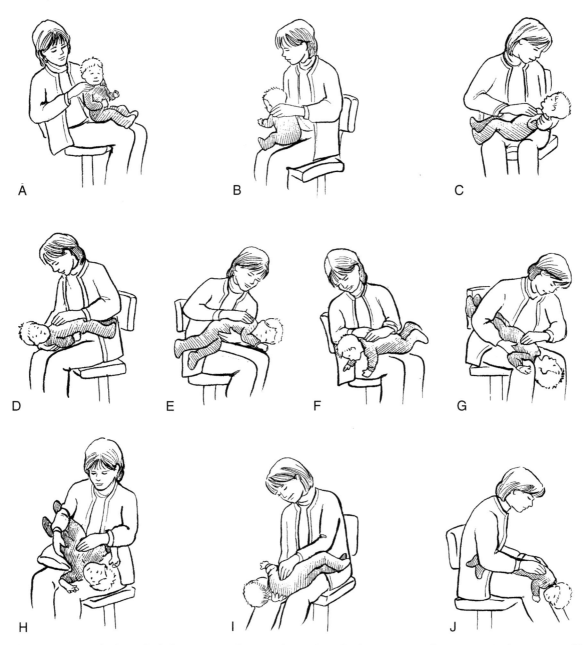

Figure 8-9: The 12 positions for bronchial drainage in infants performed on the lap or using pillows. **A,** Apical segments of both upper lobes (BUL). **B,** Posterior segment of left upper lobe (LUL). **C,** Anterior segment of LUL. **D,** Anterior segment of right upper lobe (RUL). **E,** Posterior segment of RUL. **F,** Superior, or apical, segments of both lower lobes (BLL). **G,** Anterior segments of BLL. **H,** Right middle lobe (also done on other side for lingular segment of LUL). **I,** Lateral segment of right lower lobe (RLL) (also done on other side for lateral segment of left lower lobe). **J,** Posterior segments of BLL.

⊙ Once the child is too large for the caregiver's lap, positioning is the same as for adults. Some children use very large stuffed animals or large floor pillows to assist with positioning.

⊙ Precautions and contraindications for bronchial drainage in the neonate are presented in Table 8-14. Controversy exists over the use of the Trendelenburg position in the younger population with known or suspected gastroesophageal reflux, especially when feedings are frequent.

⊙ Essential points for performing bronchial drainage in infants are listed in Box 8-3.

▸ Manual chest percussion and vibration, which are used in conjunction with bronchial drainage to assist in the removal of secretions, are often modified to conform to the size of the infant or child.

⊙ Precautions and contraindications for the use of chest percussion and vibration in the neonate are listed in Boxes 8-4 and 8-5.

⊙ When chest percussion is employed to treat small infants, a commercially available or adapted percussion device can be used, as shown in Figure 8-10, or the hand position can be modified to use three fingers in a tented position (see Figures 8-11 and 8-12).

⊙ Vibration is performed with one hand (or sometimes only several fingers) for premature and small infants, as demonstrated in Figure 8-13.

⊙ Essential points for performing chest percussion and vibration in small infants are listed in Box 8-6. Higher respiratory rates make it more challenging to provide vibration during exhalation.

BOX 8-3: Essential Points in Performing Bronchial Drainage in Infants

- Care should be taken to coordinate any change in the infant's position with other nursing procedures to avoid unnecessary stimulation.
- Infants should never be left unattended when in a head-down position.
- Vital signs should be monitored closely by respiration and heart rate monitors. The alarms should be turned on.
- The infant's chest should be auscultated for adventitious breath sounds after positioning.
- While the infant is in a drainage position, secretions will be more easily mobilized. The infant's trachea or endotracheal tube should be suctioned as needed.
- Avoid placing the infant in a head-down position for approximately 1 hour after eating to avoid aspiration of regurgitated food.
- Any change in the infant's position should be done slowly to minimize stress on the cardiovascular system.
- Infants with umbilical arterial lines can be placed on their abdomens; however, one should always check that the line has not been kinked.
- Some infants might require modified drainage positions. Infants with severe cardiovascular instability or suspected intracranial bleeding should not be placed in a head-down position.

From Moerchen VA, Crane LD. The neonatal and pediatric patient. In Frownfelter D, Dean E. *Cardiovascular and Pulmonary Physical Therapy: Evidence and Practice*, 4th ed. St. Louis: Mosby; 2006.

TABLE 8-14: **Precautions and Contraindications for Postural Drainage in Neonates**

Position	Precaution	Contraindication
Prone	Umbilical arterial catheter	Untreated tension pneumothorax
	Continuous positive airway pressure in nose	
	Excessive abdominal distension	
	Abdominal incision	
	Anterior chest tube	
Trendelenburg position (head-down)	Distended abdomen	Untreated tension pneumothorax
	SEH/IVH (grades I and II)	Recent tracheoesophageal fistula repair
	Chronic congestive heart failure or cor pulmonale	Recent eye or intracranial surgery
	Persistent fetal circulation	Intraventricular hemorrhage (grades III and IV)
	Cardiac dysrhythmias	Acute congestive heart failure or cor pulmonale
	Apnea and bradycardia	
	Infant exhibiting signs of acute respiratory distress	
	Hydrocephalus	
	Gestational age of less than 28 wk	

From Crane LD, Physical therapy for the neonate with respiratory diease. In Irwin S, Tecklin JS, editors. *Cardiopulmonary physical Therapy*. 3rd ed. St. Louis: Mosby; 1995.
SHE/IVH, Subependymal hemorrhage/intraventricular hemorrhage.

BOX 8-4: Precautions and Contraindications for Chest Percussion in Neonates

Precautions

- Poor condition of skin
- Coagulopathy
- Presence of a chest tube
- Healing thoracic incision
- Osteoporosis and rickets
- Persistent fetal circulation
- Cardiac arrhythmias
- Apnea and bradycardia
- Signs of acute respiratory distress
- Increased irritability during treatment
- Subcutaneous emphysema
- Bronchospasm, wheezing, rhonchi
- Subependymal hemorrhage/intraventricular hemorrhage (SEH/IVH)
- Prematurity (gestational age of less than 28 wk)

Contraindications

- Intolerance to treatment as indicated by low transcutaneous oxygen values
- Rib fracture
- Hemoptysis

From Crane LD. Physical therapy for the neonate with respiratory disease. In Irwin S, Tecklin JS, editors. *Cardiopulmonary Physical Therapy*, 3rd ed. St. Louis: Mosby; 1995.

BOX 8-5: Precautions and Contraindications for Vibration in Neonates

Precautions

- Increased irritability/crying during treatment
- Persistent fetal circulation
- Apnea and bradycardia

Contraindications

- Untreated tension pneumothorax
- Intolerance to treatment as indicated by low transcutaneous oxygen values
- Hemoptysis

From Crane LD. Physical therapy for the neonate with respiratory disease. In Irwin S, Tecklin JS, editors. *Cardiopulmonary Physical Therapy* 3rd ed. St. Louis: Mosby; 1995.

▶ After bronchial drainage with or without chest percussion and vibration, infants may require assistance in clearing the loosened secretions, especially if cough production is impaired (recall that neonates and young infants use sneezing to assist with airway clearance).

⊙ If the infant demonstrates adequate means to clear the airways, suctioning should be deferred. If required, nasal or oropharyngeal suctioning may be performed. The catheter may help to stimulate a cough. Lubricating agents are never used in infants and smaller diameter catheters are used to accommodate smaller nasal passageways.

⊙ The suggested procedure for performing suctioning is described in Table 8-15.

⊙ Hypoxemia and hyperoxemia can be minimized during suctioning if transcutaneous oxygen levels are monitored.

⊙ Children capable of cough production should be encouraged to both cough and huff to clear secretions. Both laughing and crying often lead to cough stimulation. Singing, blowing bubbles, playing musical toys that require breath production (e.g., whistles, horns, harmonicas), playing other games (including those made up by the child or therapist) that require breath production (e.g., blowing miniature hockey "pucks" across a goal line) may also be used.

- For older children, specifically those taking more responsibility for their own airway clearance, frequently used methods include oscillatory positive expiratory pressure (e.g., the Acapella and the Flutter) and high-frequency chest wall compression (HFCWC) systems including The Vest, The InCourage System, and Smart Vest (see pages 334–335).

IMPAIRED ABILITY TO PROTECT AIRWAY

Pediatric patients at risk for aspiration are frequently treated with prophylactic airway clearance techniques. It is not uncommon for physical therapists, occupational therapists, and speech therapists to all be involved with pediatric patients who have an impaired ability to protect their airway.

INCREASED WORK OF BREATHING

Pediatric patients with cardiopulmonary dysfunction often experience increased work of breathing, which may be alleviated by treating the underlying problem(s) and using some of the treatment techniques described in Chapter 7 (see page 337), according to age-appropriateness.

- Infants and children of all ages can benefit from positioning to relieve dyspnea. Positioning will be passive in infants and sometimes very small children, but older children and adolescents can be instructed in active positioning.
  ▶ Positions that facilitate ventilation–perfusion relationships have already been described (see page 384).
  ▶ Often children spontaneously assume positions that relieve their dyspnea. Infants and toddlers may play actively for a few minutes and then sit or lie down. Older children typically catch their breath by leaning forward with their hands on their knees or thighs. Those with cyanotic heart disease typically assume a squatting position to reduce venous return and dyspnea associated with exertion.
  ▶ Children with asthma and other pulmonary disorders can be taught to use positioning to relieve their dyspnea, as described on page 338.

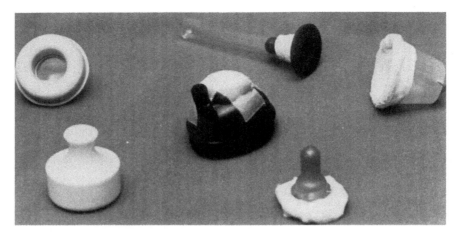

Figure 8-10: Commercially available (two devices on the left) and adapted devices for chest percussion on small infants. (From Irwin S, Tecklin JS. *Cardiopulmonary Physical Therapy: A Guide to Practice.* 4th ed. St. Louis: Mosby; 2004.)

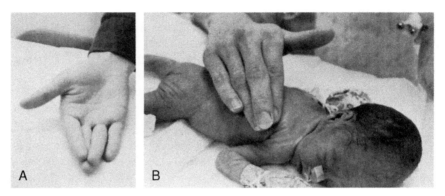

Figure 8-11: "Tenting" of the fingers for performing manual chest percussion on premature or small infants. (From Moerchen VA, Crane LD. The neonatal and pediatric patient. In Frownfelter D, Dean E, editors. *Cardiovascular and Pulmonary Physical Therapy: Evidence and Practice.* 4th ed. St. Louis: Mosby; 2006.)

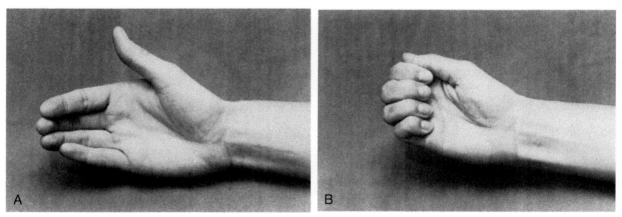

Figure 8-12: Hand modifications with fully cupped hand **(A)** and four fingers cupped **(B)** for performing manual chest percussion on infants and small toddlers. (From Irwin S, Tecklin JS. *Cardiopulmonary Physical Therapy: A Guide to Practice.* 4th ed. St. Louis: Mosby; 2004.)

- Youths who can follow directions can be instructed in specific breathing strategies, such as diaphragmatic breathing, pursed-lip breathing, and coordination of breathing with exertion, to gain control over their dyspnea.

- Yoga and pilates techniques are valuable forms of exercise for improving breath control and support and increasing focus and concentration and thus can lead to reduced work of breathing.

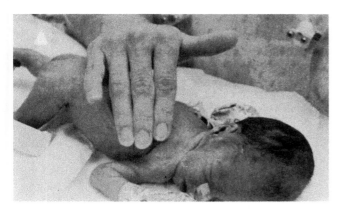

Figure 8-13: Manual chest wall vibration of a premature infant. (From Moerchen VA, Crane LD. The neonatal and pediatric patient. In Frownfelter D, Dean E. *Cardiovascular and Pulmonary Physical Therapy: Evidence and Practice.* 4th ed. St. Louis: Mosby; 2006.)

BOX 8-6: **Essential Points for Performing Chest Percussion and Vibration in Small Infants**

- Chest percussion can be administered manually or with one of a variety of percussion devices; the choice is personal and depends on the size of the therapist's hand, the infant, and the shape of the area to be treated. Regardless of the method used, a cupping effect should be maintained.
- Although most percussion techniques cover a larger area than the specific lung segment being treated, it is important to avoid percussing over the liver, spleen, and kidneys by paying close attention to the borders of the lungs and surface anatomy.
- In most cases a thin sheet or article of clothing can be used to cover the area being treated. The exception is when careful observation of anatomic landmarks and signs of respiratory distress is important.
- The infant's chest should be supported firmly during percussion.
- Vibration can be applied manually or using a mechanical vibrator or an electric toothbrush with foam padding of the bristle portion.
- The time necessary for effective drainage is considered to be a minimum of 3 to 5 minutes per position, but sometimes must be shortened if a position is not tolerated well.
- Because bronchial drainage is often fatiguing, the areas of greatest involvement should be treated first, followed by the less involved areas.
- Careful attention to the infant's responses to treatment is important, particularly in sick neonates; heart rate, respiratory rate, and transcutaneous oxygen values should be monitored, if available.

- Relaxation techniques may be particularly valuable for pediatric patients with chronic illnesses and their families. Guided imagery, yoga, and guided breathing control exercises may be appropriate, with appropriate adjustments according to age.

TABLE 8-15: Procedure for Suctioning Infants

Step	Procedures
Preparation	1. Place the infant in the supine position, preferably with the head in the midline position
	2. Check that the suction apparatus is functioning properly and is connected, the suction is turned on, and the vacuum level is set between −50 and −80 cm H_2O
	3. Make sure the oxygen flow is turned on and attached to the self-inflating breathing bag and the pressure manometer is connected
	4. Check to see what pressures the ventilator is delivering or what pressure is required to properly ventilate the infant
Hyperoxygenation	1. Hyperoxygenate the infant using an oxygen concentration 10%–20% higher than the level set on the ventilator; if the FIO_2 is 0.5 or higher, use 100% oxygen
	2. Hyperoxygenation should precede and follow each pass with the suction catheter
Lavage (optional)	Instill 0.5–1.0 mL, or 2–3 drops, of sterile normal saline solution (NaCl) directly into the endotracheal or tracheostomy tube
Suction	Using sterile technique:
	1. Wet the catheter in the sterile solution
	2. Insert the catheter (with no suction applied) into the airway until resistance is met. To avoid mucosal damage, premeasure the length of catheter against the endotracheal tube length allowing no more than a 0.5-cm length greater than the tube
	3. Pull the catheter back slightly and then withdraw the catheter while applying intermittent suction and turning the catheter (should not last longer than 5 s)
	4. Repeat if necessary until there are no more secretions
	5. Suction the nasal and oral pharynges

FIO_2, Fraction of inspired oxygen.

WELLNESS AND PREVENTION IN THE PEDIATRIC POPULATION

Pediatric physical therapists routinely work toward the prevention, abatement, or reversal of impairments and functional limitations resulting from disease processes. Goals and intervention related to wellness and fitness also fall within the scope of PT practice, and an increasing number of physical therapists are creating or participating in such programs.

Primary prevention programs target many issues that affect children and their families and are appearing at both the community-based and school-based levels. Programs relevant to optimal cardiopulmonary function focus on identifying and ameliorating coronary risk factors, (see Table 7-1, page 299), and addressing and preventing obesity and diabetes in children. In general, these programs provide education related to healthy eating, risk factor reduction, and increasing physical activity for children and their families.

Physical therapists have the opportunity (especially in states with direct access) to intervene at the individual level with each patient assessment and through each plan of care they develop, regardless of the referral diagnosis. Physical therapists are uniquely qualified to assist in fighting the growing national health crisis related to these problems and are stepping in to contribute their expertise in increasing numbers. Research is needed to determine which types of interventions (both PT and nonPT related) are the most effective across different age, gender, and ethnic groups.

REFERENCES

1. Ahanya SN, Lakshmanan J, Morgan BLG, et al. Meconium passage in utero: mechanisms, consequences, and management. *Obstet Gynecol Surv.* 2005;60:45-56.
2. Ainsworth SB. Pathophysiology of neonatal respiratory distress syndrome: implications for early treatment strategies. *Treat Respir Med.* 2005;4: 423-437.
3. Alpert MA. Obesity cardiomyopathy: pathophysiology and evolution of the clinical syndrome. *Am J Med Sci.* 2001;321(4):225-236.
4. American Academy of Pediatrics. American Academy of Pediatrics Clinical Report: cardiovascular health supervision for individuals affected by Duchenne or Becker muscular dystrophy. *Pediatrics.* 2005;116: 1569-1573.
5. American Academy of Pediatrics Task Force on Prolonged Apnea. Prolonged apnea. *Pediatrics.* 1978;61:651-652.
6. Anderson JL, Sande MA, Kartalija M, et al. Infective endocarditis. In: Fuster V, Alexander RW, O'Rourke RA, eds. *Hurst's The Heart.* 11th ed. New York: McGraw-Hill; 2004.
7. Baldwin HS, Grindley JC. Molecular determinants of embryonic vascular development. In: Polin RA, Fox WW, Abman SH, eds. *Fetal and Neonatal Physiology.* 3rd ed. Philadelphia: W.B. Saunders; 2004.
8. Ballard JL, Khoury JC, Wedig K, et al. New Ballard score, expanded to include extremely premature infants. *J Pediatr.* 1991;119:417-423.
9. Baquet G, Van Praagh E, Berhoin S. Endurance training and aerobic fitness in young people. *Sports Med.* 2003;33:1127-1143.
10. Baraldi E, Filippone M. Chronic lung disease after premature birth. *N Engl J Med.* 2007;357:1946-1955.
11. Bar-Mor G, Zeevi B, Yaaron M, et al. Use of the heart rate monitor to modulate physical activity in adolescents with congenital aortic stenosis: an innovative approach. *J Pediatr Nurs.* 1999;14:273-277.
12. Bloom B, Dey AN. Summary Health Statistics for U.S. Children: National Health Interview Survey, 2004. National Center for Health Statistics. *Vital Health Stat.* 2006;10(227):1-85.
12a.Bonow RO, Cheitlin MD, Crawford MH, et al. Task Force 3: valvular heart disease. *J Am Coll Cardiol.* 2005;45:1334-1340.
13. Braden DS, Carrol JF. Normative cardiovascular responses to exercise in children. *Pediatr Cardiol.* 1999;20:4-10.
14. Bush A, Chodhari R, Collins N, et al. Primary ciliary dyskinesia: current state of the art. *Arch Dis Child.* 2007;92:1136-1140.
15. Chumlea WC, Cronk CE. Overweight among children with trisomy 21. *J Ment Defic Res.* 1981;25:275-280.
16. Cockerham JT, Martin TC, Guitierrez FR, et al. Spontaneous closure of secundum atrial septal defect in infants and young children. *Am J Cardiol.* 1983;52:1267-1271.
17. Committee on Obstetric Practice. American College of Obstetricians and Gynecologists: ACOG Committee opinion No. 379: management of delivery of a newborn with meconium-stained amniotic fluid. *Obstet Gynecol.* 2007;100:739.
18. Cordell D, Graham TP, Atwood GF, et al. Left heart volume characteristics following ventricular septal defect closure in infancy. *Circulation.* 1976;54:294-298.
19. Cotes JE, Chinn DJ, Miller MR. *Lung Function: Physiology, Measurement and Application in Medicine.* Boston: Blackwell; 2006.
20. Cystic Fibrosis Foundation. *Patient Registry 2006 Annual Report.* Bethesda, MD: Cystic Fibrosis Foundation; 2006.
20a.de Benedictis D, Bush A. The challenge of asthma in adolescence. *Pediatr Pulmonol.* 2007;42:683-692.
21. Dellefave LM, McNally EM. Cardiomyopathy in neuromuscular disorders. *Prog Pediatr Cardiol.* 2007;24:35-46.
21a.Driscoll DJ, Wolfe RR, Gersony WM, et al. Cardiorespiratory responses to exercise of patients with aortic stenosis, pulmonary stenosis, and ventricular septal defect. *Circulation.* 1993;87(suppl 2):1102-1113.
22. Dubowitz L, Mercuri E, Dubowitz V. An optimality score for the neurologic examination of the term newborn. *J Pediatr.* 1998;133:406-415.
23. Dubowitz LMS, Dubowitz V, Goldberg C. Clinical assessment of gestational age in the newborn infant. *J Pediatr.* 1970;77(1):1-10.
24. Dubowitz V. Chaos in the classification of SMA: a possible resolution. *Neuromusc Disord.* 1995;5(1):3-5.
25. Epstein LH, Kuller LH, Wing RR, et al. The effect of weight control on lipid changes in obese children. *Am J Dis Child.* 1989;143:454-457.
26. Fagot-Campagna A, Pettit DJ, Engelgau MM, et al. Type 2 diabetes among North American children and adolescents: an epidemiologic review and a public health perspective. *J Pediatr.* 2000;136:664-672.
27. Faigenbaum AD. Strength training for children and adolescents. *Clin Sports Med.* 2000;19:593-619.
28. Fowler EG, Kolobe THA, Damiano DL, et al. Promotion of physical fitness and prevention of secondary conditions for children with cerebral palsy: Section on Pediatric Research Summit Proceedings. *Phys Ther.* 2007; 87:1495-1510.
29. Deleted in pages.
30. Fulton DR, Freed MD. The pathology, pathophysiology, recognition, and treatment of congenital heart disease. In: Fuster V, Alexander RW, O'Rourke RA, eds. *Hurst's The Heart.* 11th ed. New York: McGraw-Hill; 2004.
31. Fyler DC, Buckley LP, Hellenbrand WE, et al. Report of the New England Regional Infant Cardiac Program. *Pediatrics.* 1980;65(suppl):376-460.
32. Gabriel HM, Heger M, Innerhofer P, et al. Long-term outcome of patients with ventricular septal defect considered not to require surgical closure during childhood. *J Am Coll Cardiol.* 2002;39:1066-1071.
33. Gauderman WJ, Vora E, McConnell R, et al. Effect of exposure to traffic on lung development from 10-18 years of age: a cohort study. *Lancet.* 2007;369:571-577.
34. Gerdes JS. Bronchopulmonary dysplasia. In: Polin RA, Yoder MC, Burg FD, eds. *Workbook in Practical Neonatology.* 3rd ed. Philadelphia: W.B. Saunders; 2001.
35. Gildein P, Mocellin R, Kaufmehl K. Oxygen uptake transient kinetics during constant-load exercise in children after operations of ventricular septal defect, tetralogy of Fallot, transposition of the great arteries, or tricuspid valve atresia. *Am J Cardiol.* 1994;74:166-169.
36. Gittenberger-de Groot AC, DeRuiter MC, Bartelings MM, et al. Embryology of congenital heart disease. In: Crawford MH, DeMarco JP, Paulus WJ eds. *Cardiology.* 2nd ed. Spain: C.V. Mosby; 2004.
37. Golden JA, Bönnemann CG. Developmental structural disorders. In: Goetz CG, ed. *Textbook of Clinical Neurology.* 2nd ed. Philadelphia: W.B. Saunders; 2003.
38. Gomella TL. *Neonatology: Management, Procedures, On-Call Problems, Diseases, and Drugs.* 5th ed. New York: McGraw-Hill; 2004.
39. Gotto Jr AM. Targeting high-risk young patients for statin therapy. *JAMA.* 2004;292:377-378.
40. Graham Jr TP, Driscoll DJ, Gersony WM, et al. Task Force 2: congenital heart disease. *J Am Coll Cardiol.* 2005;45:1326-1333.
41. Gregoratos G, Abrams J, Epstein AE, et al. ACC/AHA 2002 guideline update for implantation of cardiac pacemakers and antiarrhythmia

devices: a report of the American College of Cardiology/American Heart Association Task Force on Practice Guidelines (ACC/AHA/NASPE Committee on Pacemaker Implantation). *Circulation.* 2002;106:2145-2161.

42. Guy JA, Micheli LJ. Strength training for children and adolescents. *J Am Acad Orthop Surg.* 2001;9:29-36.

43. Halliday HL. Respiratory distress syndrome. In: Greenough A, Milner AD, eds. *Neonatal Respiratory Disorders.* London: Arnold; 2003.

44. Haust MD. The genesis of atherosclerosis in the pediatric age-group. *Pediatr Pathol.* 1990;10:253-271.

45. Hedley AA, Ogden CL, Johnson CL, et al. Prevalence of overweight and obesity among U.S. children, adolescents, and adults. *JAMA.* 2004;291 (23):2847-2850.

46. Hermansen CL, Lorah KN. Respiratory distress in the newborn. *Am Fam Physician.* 2007;76:987-994.

47. Hibbert M, Lannigan A, Raven J, et al. Gender differences in lung growth. *Pediatr Pulmonol.* 1995;19:129-134.

48. Hilsop AA. Fetal and postnatal anatomical lung development. In: Greenough A, Milner AD, eds. *Neonatal Respiratory Disorders.* London: Arnold; 2003.

49. Hirth A, Reybrouck T, Bjarnason-Wehrens B, et al. Recommendations for participation and leisure sports in patients with congenital heart disease: a consensus document. Position paper. *Eur J Cardiovasc Prev Rehabil.* 2006;13:293-299.

50. Hoffman JIE, Kaplan S. The incidence of congenital heart disease. *J Am Coll Cardiol.* 2002;39:1890-1900.

51. Holm VA, Cassidy SB, Butler MG, et al. Prader-Willi syndrome: consensus diagnostic criteria. *Pediatrics.* 1991;91(2):398-402.

52. Hövels-Gürich HH, Konrad J, Skorzenski D, et al. Long-term neurodevelopmental outcome and exercise capacity after corrective surgery for tetralogy of Fallot or ventricular septal defect in infancy. *Ann Thorac Surg.* 2006;81:958-966.

53. Humphries MC, Gutin B, Barbeau P, et al. Relations of adiposity and effects on training on the left ventricle in obese youths. *Med Sci Sports Exer.* 2002;34(9):1428-1435.

54. Joshi VM, Sekhavat S. Acyanotic congenital heart defects. In: Vetter VL, ed. *Pediatric Cardiology: The Requisites in Pediatrics.* Philadelphia: C.V. Mosby; 2006.

55. Kennaird DL. Oxygen consumption and evaporative water loss in infants with congenital heart disease. *Arch Dis Child.* 1976;51:34-41.

56. Kirklin JW, Barratt-Boyes BG. *Cardiac Surgery.* 2nd ed. New York: Churchill Livingstone; 1993.

57. Lamour JM, Addonizio LJ, Galantowicz ME, et al. Outcome after orthotopic cardiac transplantation in adults with congenital heart disease. *Circulation.* 1999;100(suppl.):II200-II205.

58. Lewis AB. The failing myocardium. In: Chang AC, Hanley FL, Wernovsky G et al, eds. *Pediatric Cardiac Intensive Care.* Baltimore: Lippincott Williams & Wilkins; 1998.

59. Li AM, Chan D, Wong E, et al. The effects of obesity on pulmonary function. *Arch Dis Child.* 2003;88(4):361-363.

60. Liebman J, Cullum L, Belloc NB. Natural history of transposition of the great arteries—anatomy and birth and death characteristics. *Circulation.* 1969;40:237-262.

61. Lopes J, Muller NL, Bryan MH, et al. Importance of inspiratory muscle tone in maintenance of FRC in the newborn. *J Appl Physiol.* 1981;51:830-834.

62. Ludomirsky A, Garson Jr A. Supraventricular tachycardia. In: Garson A Jr Gillette PC, eds. *Pediatric Arrhythmias: Electrophysiology and Pacing.* Philadelphia, W.B. Saunders; 1990.

63. Magee CL. Physical therapy for the child with asthma. *Pediatr Phys Ther.* 1991;3:23-28.

64. Mahoney LT, Truesdell SC, Krzmarzick TR, et al. Atrial septal defects that present in infancy. *Am J Dis Child.* 1986;140:1115-1118.

65. Majnemer A, Riley P, Shevell M, et al. Severe bronchopulmonary dysplasia increases risk for later neurological and motor sequelae in preterm survivors. *Dev Med Child Neurol.* 2000;42:53-60.

66. Mansell AL, Bryan AC, Levison H. Relationship of lung recoil to lung volume and maximum expiratory flow in normal children. *J Appl Physiol.* 1977;42:813-823.

67. Maron BJ, Acherman MJ, Nishimura RA, et al. Task Force 4: HCM and other cardiomyopathies, mitral valve prolapse, myocarditis, and Marfan syndrome. *J Am Coll Cardiol.* 2005;45:1340-1345.

68. Massery M. Chest development as a component of normal motor development: implications for pediatric physical therapists. *Pediatr Phys Ther.* 1991;3(1):3-8.

69. Massery M. Multisystem consequences of impaired breathing mechanics and/or postural control. In: Frownfelter D, Dean E, eds. *Cardiovascular and Pulmonary Physical Therapy: Evidence and Practice.* 4th ed. St. Louis: C.V. Mosby; 2006.

70. Matthys D. Pre-and postoperative exercise testing of the child with atrial septal defect. *Pediatr Cardiol.* 1999;20:22-25.

71. McGill Jr HC, McMahan CA, Zieske AW, et al. Associations of coronary heart disease risk factors with the intermediate lesion of atherosclerosis in youth. *Arterioscler Thromb Vasc Biol.* 2000;20:1998-2004.

72. McGill Jr HC, McMahan CA, Zieske AW, et al. Association of coronary heart disease risk factors with microscopic qualities of coronary atherosclerosis in youth. *Circulation.* 2000;102:374-379.

73. McGill Jr HC, McMahan CA, Zieske AW, et al. Effects of non-lipid risk factors on atherosclerosis in youth with a favorable lipoprotein profile. *Circulation.* 2001;103:1546-1550.

74. McGill Jr HC, McMahan CA, Zieske AW, et al. Effects of serum lipoproteins and smoking on atherosclerosis in young men and women. *Arterioscler Thromb Vasc Biol.* 1997;17:95-106.

75. Meijboom F, Szatmari A, Utens E, et al. Long-term follow-up after surgical closure of ventricular septal defect in infancy in childhood. *J Am Coll Cardiol.* 1994;24:1358-1364.

76. Miao C, Zuberbuhler JA, Zuberbuhler JR. Prevalence of congenital cardiac anomalies at high altitude. *J Am Coll Cardiol.* 1988;12:224-228.

76a.Milner AD, Boon AW, Saunders RA, et al. Upper airways obstruction and apnoea in preterm babies. *Arch Dis Child.* 1980;55:2-25.

77. Mitchell BM, Strasburger JF, Hubbard JE, et al. Serial exercise performance in children with surgically corrected congenital aortic stenosis. *Pediatr Cardiol.* 2003;24:319-324.

77a.Mitchell JH, Haskell W, Snell P, et al. Task Force 8: classification of sports. *J Am Coll Cardiol.* 2005;45:1364-1367.

78. Mitchell SC, Korones SB, Berendes HW. Congenital heart disease in 56,109 live births: incidence and natural history. *Circulation.* 1971;43:323-332.

79. Moore LL, DiGao M, Loring Bradlee L, et al. Does early physical activity predict body fat change throughout childhood? *Prev Med.* 2003; 37(1):10-17.

80. Murphy JG, Gersh BJ, McGood MD, et al. Long-term outcome after surgical repair of isolated atrial septal defect. *N Engl J Med.* 1990;323:1645-1650.

81. Nixon PA, Orenstein DM. Exercise testing in children. *Pediatr Pulmonol.* 1988;5:107-122.

82. Ornish D, Brown SE, Scherwitz LW, et al. Can lifestyle changes reverse coronary heart disease? The Lifestyle Heart Trial. *Lancet.* 1990;336:129-133.

83. Paridon S. Acquired heart disease. In: Vetter VL, ed. *Pediatric Cardiology: The Requisites in Pediatrics.* Philadelphia: C.V. Mosby; 2006.

84. Park MK. *Pediatric Cardiology for Practitioners.* 5th ed. Philadelphia: C.V. Mosby; 2008.

85. Park MK. *The Pediatric Cardiology Handbook.* 3rd ed. Philadelphia: C.V. Mosby; 2003.

86. Peirone AR, Lee KJ, Golding IF, et al. Exercise performance and blood pressure responses in children after stenting of aortic coarctation. *Prog Pediatr Cardiol.* 2006;22:161-164.

87. Pellica A, Fagard R, Bjørnstad HH, et al. Recommendations for comptetitive sports participation in athletes with cardiovascular disease. A consensus document from the Study Group of Sports Cardiology of the Working Group of Cardiac Rehabilitation and Exercise Physiology and the Working Group of Myocardial and Pericardial Diseases of the European Society of Cardiology. *Eur Heart J.* 2005;26:1422-1445.

88. Pierce MR, Bancalari E. The role of inflammation in the pathogenesis of bronchopulmonary dysplasia. *Pediatr Pulmonol.* 1995;19:371-378.

89. Raitakari OT, Juonala M, Rönnemaa T, et al. Cohort profile: The Cardiovascular Risk in Young Finns Study. *Int J Epidemiol.* 2008;37(6):1220-1226.

90. Ratel S, LAzaar N, Dore E, et al. High-intensity intermittent activities at school: controversies and facts. *J Sports Med Phys Fitness.* 2004;44:272-280.

91. Reybrouck T, Mertens L. Physical performance and physical activity in grown-up congenital heart disease. *Eur J Cardiovasc Prev Rehabil.* 2005;12:498-502.

91a. Rigatto H, Brady JP. Periodic breathing and apnea in preterm infants. I. Evidence for hypoventilation possibly due to central respiratory depression. *Pediatrics*. 1972;50:202-218.

92. Rosenstein BJ, Cutting GR. Cystic Fibrosis Foundation Consensus Panel: the diagnosis of cystic fibrosis: a consensus statement. *J Pediatr*. 1998; 132(4):589-595.

93. Rudolph AM. *Congenital Diseases of the Heart: Clinical-Physiological Considerations*. 2nd ed. Armonk: Futura; 2001.

94. Ruttenberg HD. Pre- and postoperative exercise teating of the child with coarctation of the aorta. *Pediatr Cardiol*. 1999;20:33-37.

95. Somarriba G, Extein J, Miller TL. Exercise rehabilitation in pediatric cardiomyopathy. *Prog Pediatr Cardiol*. 2008;25(1):91-102.

96. Schultz AH, Kreutzer J. Cyanotic heart disease. In: Vetter VL, ed. *Pediatric Cardiology: The Requisites in Pediatrics*. Philadelphia: C.V. Mosby; 2006.

97. Sigurðardóttir LÝ, Helgason H. Exercise-induced hypertension after corrective surgery for coarctation of the aorta. *Pediatr Cardiol*. 1996; 17:301-307.

98. Splitt MP, Burn J, Goodship J. Defects in the determination of left–right asymmetry. *J Med Genet*. 1996;33:498-503.

99. Spray TL, Wernovsky G. Right ventricular outflow tract obstruction: Tetralogy of Fallot. In: Chang AC, Hanley FL, Wernovsky G, Wessel DL, eds. *Pediatric Cardiac Intensive Care* Baltimore: Lippincott Williams & Wilkins; 1998.

100. Stallings VA, Zemel BS, Davies JC, et al. Energy expenditure of children and adolescents with severe disabilities: a cerebral palsy model. *Am J Clin Nutr*. 1996;64:627-634.

101. Stefanelli CB. Sudden cardiac death in the young. In: Dick MII, ed. *Clinical Cardiac Electrophysiology in the Young*. New York: Springer; 2006.

102. Steinberger J, Moller JH. Exercise testing in children with pulmonary valvar stenosis. *Pediatr Cardiol*. 1999;20:27-31.

103. Storms WW. Asthma associated with exercise. *Immunol Allergy Clin North Am*. 2005;25:31-43.

104. Stranger P, Cassidy SC, Girod DA, et al. Balloon pulmonary valvuloplasty: Results of the Valvuloplasty and Angioplasty of Congenital Anomalies Registry. *Am J Cardiol*. 1990;65:775-783.

105. Strunk RC, Bacharier LB, Bloomberg GR. Asthma in adolescence. In: Szefler SJ, Pederson S, eds. *Childhood Asthma*. New York: Taylor & Francis; 2006.

106. Substance Abuse and Mental Health Services Administration. *Results from the 2002 National Survey on Drug Use and Health: National Findings* (NHSDA Series H-22, DHHS Publication No. SMA 03-3836). Rockville, MD: Department of Health and Human Services; 2003. Available at http://www.oas.samhsa.gov/nhsda/2k2nsduh/results/2k2Results.htm (accessed February 2009).

107. Sweeney JK, Heriza CB, Reilly MA, et al. Practice guidelines for the physical therapist in the neonatal intensive care unit (NICU). *Pediatr Phys Ther*. 1999;11:119-132.

108. Thach BT, Stark AR. Spontaneous neck flexion and airway obstruction during apneic spells in preterm infants. *J Pediatr*. 1979;94:275-279.

109. Tzelepis GE, McCool FD. The lungs and chest wall disease. In: Mason RJ, Broaddus VC, Murray JF, Nadel JA, eds. *Murray and Nadel's Textbook of Respiratory Medicine*. 4th ed. Philadelphia: W.B. Saunders; 2005.

110. Urbina EM, Gidding SS, Bao W, et al. Effect of body size, ponderosity, and blood pressure on left ventricular growth in children in young adults in the Bogalusa Heart Study. *Circulation*. 1995;91(9):2400-2406.

111. U.S. Department of Health and Human Services. *Healthy People 2010* (017-001-00547-9), Washington, DC; 2000. Available at:www.healthy-people.gov/ (accessed February 2009).

112. U.S. Department of Health and Human Services, National Institutes of Health. *The Fourth Report on the Diagnosis, Evaluation, and Treatment of High Blood Pressure in Children and Adolescents*. Bethesda, MD; 2005.

113. Uwaifo GI, Fallon EM, Calis KA, et al. Improvement in hypertrophic cardiomyopathy after significant weight loss: case report. *South Med J*. 2003;96(6):626-631.

114. van den Berg Emons HJ, Jentrika J, Bussman B, et al. Everyday physical activity in adolescents and young adults with meningomyelocele as measured with a novel activity monitor. *J Pediatr*. 2001;139:880-886.

115. Vetter VL, Rhodes LA. Evaluation and management of arrhythmias in a pediatric population. In: Saksena S, Camm AJ, eds. *Electrophysiological Disorders of the Heart* Philadelphia: Churchill Livingstone; 2005.

115a. Walsh MC, Fanaroff JM. Meconium stained fluid: approach to the mother and the baby. *Clin Perinatol*. 2007;34:653-665.

116. Warnes CA, Liberthson R. Danielson Jr GK, et al.: 32nd Bethesda Conference: care of the adult with congenital heart disease. Task Force 1: the changing profile of congenital heart disease in adult life. *J Am Coll Cardiol*. 2001;37:1170-1175.

117. Webb GD, Smallhorn JF, Therien J, et al. Congenital heart disease. In: Zipes DP, Libby P, Bonow RO, Braunwald E, eds. *Braunwald's Heart Disease: A Textbook of Cardiovascular Medicine*. 7th ed. Philadelphia: W.B. Saunders; 2005.

118. Weintraub RG, Menahem S. Early surgical closure of a large ventricular septal defect: influence on long term growth. *J Am Coll Cardiol*. 1991;18:552-558.

119. Welsh L, Kemp JG, Roberts RGD. Effects of physical conditioning on children and adolescents with asthma. *Sports Med*. 2005;35:127-141.

120. Wessel HU, Paul MH. Exercise studies in tetralogy of Fallot: a review. *Pediatr Cardiol*. 1999;20:39-47.

121. Wilson W, Taubert KA, Gewitz M, et al. Prevention of infective endocarditis: guidelines from the American Heart Association. A guideline from the American Heart Association Rheumatic Fever, Endocarditis and Kawasaki Disease Committee, Council on Cardiovascular Disease in the Young, and the Council on Clinical Cardiology, Quality of Care and Outcomes Research Interdisciplinary Working Group. *Circulation*. 2007;116: 1736-1754.

122. Witsenburg M, Talsma M, Rohmer J, et al. Balloon valvuloplasty for valvular pulmonary stenosis in children over 6 months of age: initial results and long-term follow-up. *Eur Heart J*. 1993;14:1657-1660.

123. Zeltser I, Tabbutt S. Critical heart disease in the newborn. In: Vetter VL, ed. *Pediatric Cardiology: The Requisites in Pediatrics*. Philadelphia: C.V. Mosby; 2006.

124. Zipes DP, Ackerman MJ, Estes NAM, et al. Task Force 7: Arrhythmias. *J Am Coll Cardiol*. 2005;45:1354-1363.

ADDITIONAL REFERENCES

Behrman RE, Kliegman RM, Jensen HB. eds. *Nelson Textbook of Pediatrics*. 17th ed. Philadelphia: W.B. Saunders; 2004.

Berg BO. Chromosomal abnormalities and neurocutaneous disorders. In: Goetz CG, ed. *Textbook of Clinical Neurology*. 2nd ed. Philadelphia: W.B. Saunders; 2003.

Chang AC, Hanley FL, Wernovsky G, Wessel DL (editors-in-chief). *Pediatric Cardiac Intensive Care*. Baltimore: Lippincott Williams & Wilkins; 1998.

Marino BS, Wernovsky G. General principles: preoperative care. In: Chang AC, Hanley FL, Wernovsky G, Wessel DL, eds. *Pediatric Cardiac Intensive Care*. Baltimore: Lippincott Williams & Wilkins; 1998.

Pyeritz RE. Genetics and cardiovascular disease. In: Zipes DP, Libby P, Bonow RO, Braunwald E, eds. *Braunwald's Heart Disease: A Textbook of Cardiovascular Medicine*. 7th ed. Philadelphia: Elsevier/Saunders; 2005.

CHAPTER 9

Laboratory Medicine

Joel D. Hubbard, PhD, MT (ASCP) and Joanne Watchie, PT, CCS

This chapter presents common laboratory investigations, normal reference intervals, and the more notable causes of abnormal values, as well as a some common diagnostic profiles. This information is valuable to physical therapists as it aids in differential diagnosis of a variety of signs and symptoms that patients present and adds to the appreciation of the impact of cardiopulmonary dysfunction on other bodily systems. Furthermore, some data may have a direct impact on choice of treatment, both in terms of appropriate interventions and those that might be contraindicated.

The normal reference intervals presented in this chapter are for adults and some vary significantly with gender and age, as noted, in which case one of the reference sources should be consulted for more specific information. These reference intervals should be used only as a general guide, as they vary somewhat between laboratories. Thus, each patient's test results should be evaluated according to the reference values established by the laboratory that ran the tests. Most laboratory values are given in conventional units as well as Système International (SI) units to accommodate the various presentations in different parts of the nation and in the world.

9.1 SERUM CHEMISTRY

Analysis of blood chemistry is typically performed as an adjunct to physical examination to determine the presence of medical problems, clarify a diagnosis, and monitor the progression of disease. Typically, several blood chemicals must be measured to establish a pattern of abnormalities, and therefore laboratories perform standardized "profile" or "panel" tests from a single blood sample.

- Profiles are a group of select tests that are used to screen for certain conditions. Common screening profiles include the following:
  - Lipid profile (coronary risk): Cholesterol, triglycerides, lipoprotein electrophoresis (high-density lipoprotein, low-density lipoprotein, and very low-density lipoprotein; HDL, LDL, and VLDL, respectively)
  - Cardiac markers: Chemical panels, cardiac troponin, creatine kinase (CK), myocardial bands (MB), and homocysteine
  - Thyroid function: total triiodothyronine (T_3) uptake, total thyroxine, T_4, free T_3, free T_4, free thyroxine index (FTI or FT_4I), T_4 by radioimmunoassay (T_4 by RIA, also called T_7), thyroid-stimulating hormone (TSH)
  - Metabolic syndrome: Blood lipids, glucose, insulin
- Two of the most commonly performed panels are as follows:
  - The basic metabolic panel (BMP), which includes chloride, sodium, potassium, carbon dioxide (CO_2), creatinine, blood urea nitrogen (BUN), glucose, and calcium
  - The comprehensive metabolic panel (CMP), which includes the tests from the BMP along with total protein, albumin, alanine aminotransferase (ALT), aspartate transaminase (AST), alkaline phosphatase, and total bilirubin
- Among other standardized panels are the following:
  - Electrolyte panel: Sodium, potassium, chloride, CO_2, and pH
  - Hepatic function panel: ALT, albumin, alkaline phosphatase, AST, direct bilirubin, total bilirubin, and total protein
  - Renal function panel: Albumin, calcium, CO_2, chloride, BUN, creatinine, glucose, phosphorus (inorganic), potassium, sodium, and BUN-to-creatinine ratio as a calculated value
  - Arthritis panel: Uric acid, erythrocyte sedimentation rate (ESR), anti-nuclear antibody (ANA) screen, rheumatoid factor
  - Shorthand notation is often used for recording laboratory results, as illustrated in Figure 9-1.
- Normal reference intervals for serum chemistry analytes are available in a number of clinical laboratory science references. Table 9-1 lists normal reference intervals for adults, along with common causes of abnormally high or low values.[1,3-5,7-9]

9.2 HEMATOLOGY

Analysis of the blood cells themselves is achieved through the complete blood cell count, which indicates the number of red and white blood cells in a cubic millimeter of blood; the erythrocyte indices; hematocrit; and differential percentages and absolute values of the various types of white blood cells in circulation.

- Table 9-2 lists normal reference intervals for the complete blood cell count and some common causes of abnormally high and low values.[5,6,8]
- Other hematologic analytes, that is, the erythrocyte sedimentation rate and the reticulocyte count, are presented with some common causes of excessively high and low values in Table 9-3.[5,6]
- Common terminology for various hematologic abnormalities and their clinical definitions are included in Table 9-4.[5,6,8]

9.3 COAGULATION STUDIES

Another important function that can be monitored via blood tests is the status of blood coagulation, testing for risks of excessive bleeding or clot formation.

Normal reference values for coagulation studies and some common causes of abnormalities are listed in Table 9-5.[5-8]

9.4 SELECTED IMMUNOLOGIC STUDIES

Immunologic testing monitors the function of the immune system for the presence of antigen–antibody reactions and related changes within the blood in order to diagnose infectious disease, autoimmune disorders, immune allergies, and neoplastic disease.

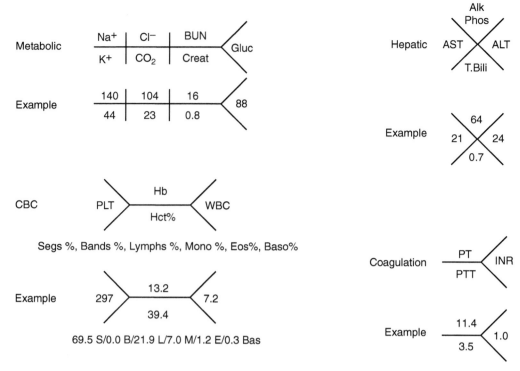

Figure 9-1: Shorthand notation for recording laboratory values. (Adapted from Wiese JG. *The Answer Book: Saint Francis Guide to the Clinical Clerkships.* 7th ed. Philadelphia: Lippincott Williams & Wilkins; 2005.)

Table 9-6 enumerates selected immunologic analytes, their normal reference intervals, and common causes of abnormalities.[5,6,8]

 9.5 OTHER LABORATORY DISCIPLINES

URINALYSIS

The routine analysis is important to monitor renal and liver diseases. A urinalysis consists of a report of physical characteristics (e.g., color and clarity), a chemical screen, and a microscopic analysis of the sediment. The chemical screen consists of protein, blood, pH, glucose, ketones, bilirubin, urobilinogen, specific gravity, nitrite, and leukocyte esterase.

IMMUNOHEMATOLOGY

Immunohematology is commonly referred to in the clinical laboratory as the blood bank, and it is here that blood is processed and cross-matched for use in surgery or for patients with significant anemia. Units of donated blood are screened for the matching blood type and for possible antibodies that may interfere with compatibility of the transfusion. The majority of hospital immunohematology departments do not serve as a blood collection site for donors.

MICROBIOLOGY

Microbiology, in laboratory medicine, is devoted to the identification of pathogenic bacteria isolated from clinical specimens. Specimen sources include urine, feces, sputum, wounds, surgical biopsies, blood, and body fluids such as cerebral spinal fluid, pleural or pericardial effusions, and ascites. Cultures are assessed for the presence of normal bacterial flora and potential pathogens. Pathogenic isolates are identified and antibiotic susceptibility testing is preformed to aid in the determination of appropriate antimicrobial therapy. Routine bacterial cultures take 24 to 72 hours to complete and report. Some microbiology departments include testing for mycobacteria, parasites, viruses, and fungal pathogens. These types of cultures may take up to 4 to 6 weeks for positive identification.

9.6 ABNORMALITIES SEEN IN SPECIFIC DISEASE STATES

Frequently, disease states produce specific abnormalities in a number of laboratory blood tests. Some of these of particular importance in patients with cardiopulmonary dysfunction are described here.

- Disorders of lipid metabolism play a major role in the development of atherosclerosis and coronary artery disease. The various types of hyperlipidemias are shown in Table 9-7[2,7,8]
- Other substances that have been associated with arterial damage, especially coronary artery disease (CAD), are used to assess cardiovascular risk, including homocysteine, C-reactive protein (CRP), and fibrinogen.
- Tests for the measurement of cardiac markers (proteins that are released into the circulation from damaged heart muscle) are important for diagnosing acute coronary syndrome (see page 105). These cardiac markers are listed in Table 9-8.[4,5,8,9] In addition, changes in their levels as a function of time are illustrated in Figure 9-2.

TABLE 9-1: Normal Reference Intervals in Adults for Serum Analytes

Analyte	Reference Intervals		Some Causes of Abnormal Results
	Standard	SI*	
Alanine aminotransferase (ALT, SGPT)	6–37 U/L†	1.0–6.2 × 10⁻⁷ kat/L	Increased: Liver disease (hepatitis, cirrhosis, biliary disease), muscle trauma, rhabdomyolysis, acute pancreatitis, myositis, drugs (e.g., heparin, salicylates), obesity, anorexia nervosa, severe preeclampsia, acute MI
			Decreased: GI tract infection, malnutrition, malignancy
Albumin	3.5–5.5 g/dL	35–55 g/L	Increased: Dehydration, IV albumin infusions
			Decreased: Inadequate intake (malnutrition), malabsorption syndromes, ↑ need (hyperthyroidism, pregnancy), impaired synthesis (liver disease, chronic infection, hereditary analbuminemia), ↑ breakdown (neoplasms, infection, trauma), ↑ loss (edema, ascites, burns, hemorrhage, nephrotic syndrome, protein-losing enteropathy), dilutional states (IV fluids, SIADH, water intoxication)
Aldolase	2.5–10 U/L	0.04–0.13 μKat/L	Increased: Cell destruction (acute MI, burns, hemolytic anemia, acute hepatitis, acute pancreatitis, muscular dystrophies, myopathies, polymyositis, prostate cancer, gangrene, rhabdomyolysis)
Alkaline phosphatase: Bowers and McComb method	30–100 U/L	0.51–1.70 μKat/L	Increased: ↑ Deposition of calcium in bone (hyperparathyroidism, Paget's disease, osteoblastic bone tumors, osteogenesis imperfecta, osteomalacia, rickets, late pregnancy), liver disease with obstruction of the biliary system (stone, carcinoma, metastatic tumor, abscess, cyst, TB, amyloid, sarcoid, leukemia), drugs (phenobarbital, phenytoin); normal children <12 yr of age
			Decreased: Excess vitamin D, milk-alkali syndrome, hypothyroidism, celiac disease, malnutrition, scurvy
Ammonia (plasma)	19–60 μg/dL	11–35 mmol/L	Increased: Severe liver disease, GU tract infection with distension and stasis, Reye's syndrome, severe CHF, severe GI bleeding, drugs (e.g., alcohol, barbiturates, diuretics, valproic acid, narcotics)
			Decreased: HTN, drugs (e.g., neomycin, tetracycline, lactulose, MAO inhibitors)
Amylase	24–125 U/L‡	0.41–2.13 μKat/L	Increased: Acute pancreatitis, pancreatic duct obstruction (stones, stricture, tumor, sphincter spasm due to drugs), mumps, renal disease, peptic ulcers, cholecystitis, diabetic ketoacidosis, parotiditis, intestinal obstruction
			Decreased: Advanced chronic pancreatitis, cystic fibrosis, hepatic necrosis
Angiotensin-converting enzyme (ACE)	10–50 U/L	0.15–1.14 μKat/L	Increased: Sarcoidosis, primary biliary cirrhosis, alcoholic cirrhosis, hyperthyroidism, hyperparathyroidism, DM, amyloidosis, multiple myeloma, lung disease (asbestosis, berylliosis, silicosis, allergic alveolitis, coccidioidomycosis), Gaucher's disease, leprosy
			Decreased: Azotemia, chronic renal dialysis; factitiously in diabetic ketoacidosis, beriberi, severe liver disease
Aspartate aminotransferase (AST, SGOT)	5–30 U/L	8.3–50 × 10⁻⁸ kat/L	Increased: Acute MI, liver disease, musculoskeletal diseases (including trauma, surgery, IM injections), acute pancreatitis, other organ infections, local radiation therapy, burns, heat exhaustion
Bicarbonate (HCO₃⁻)	22–26 mEq/L†	22–26 mmol/L	Increased: Respiratory acidosis (emphysema, respiratory failure), compensated metabolic alkalosis (severe vomiting, NG suction), primary aldosteronism, Barter's syndrome
			Decreased: Respiratory alkalosis (hyperventilation, severe CNS damage), compensated metabolic acidosis (ketoacidosis, lactic acidosis), renal failure, toxins, adrenal insufficiency, drugs (e.g., salicylates, acetazolamide)

Continued

TABLE 9-1: Normal Reference Intervals in Adults for Serum Analytes—Cont'd

	Reference Intervals		
Analyte	**Standard**	**SI***	**Some Causes of Abnormal Results**
Bilirubin			Increased: Hepatic cellular damage, biliary obstruction, hemolytic diseases, prolonged fasting
Total	0.2–1.0 mg/dL	3–17 μmol/L	
Direct	<0.2 mg/dL	0–3 μmol/L	Decreased: Drugs (barbiturates)
Blood urea nitrogen (BUN)	7–18 mg/dL	2.5–6.4 mmol/L	Increased: Renal failure, prerenal azotemia (CHF, salt and water depletion, shock), postrenal azotemia, GI bleed, acute MI, stress, drugs (e.g., aminoglycosides)
			Decreased: Diuresis, severe liver damage (drugs, poisoning, hepatitis, cirrhosis), ↑ use of protein for synthesis (late pregnancy, infancy, acromegaly, malnutrition, anabolic steroids), diet (low protein and high carbohydrate, IV feedings only, impaired absorption [celiac disease], malnutrition), nephrotic syndrome (some patients), SIADH
B-type natriuretic peptide (BNP)	<100 pg/mL	<100 ng/L	Increased: CHF (levels are proportional to severity of failure), LV dysfunction, MI, ventricular hypertrophy, cardiomyopathy, tuberculosis, lung cancer, pulmonary embolism, renal failure, chronic obstructive pulmonary disease
Calcium (Ca^{2+})			Increased: Hyperparathyroidism, malignant tumors, vitamin D intoxication, milk-alkali syndrome, acute osteoporosis (immobilization of young patients, Paget's disease), granulomatous diseases (sarcoidosis, TB, mycoses, berylliosis), some patients with hyperthyroidism or hypothyroidism, following renal transplantation, polyuric phase of renal failure, multiple myeloma, drugs (e.g., diuretics, thyroid hormone, estrogens, androgens, progestins, tamoxifen, lithium)
Total	8.5–10.5 mg/dL	2.15–2.50 mmol/L	
Ionized (plasma)	1.6–5.3 mg/dL	1.16–1.32 mmol/L	
			Decreased: Hypoparathyroidism, malabsorption of Ca^{2+} and vitamin D, obstructive jaundice, hypoalbuminemia, acute pancreatitis, chronic renal disease, osteomalacia, rickets, starvation, late pregnancy, drugs (e.g., citrated banked blood, mithramycin, fluoride intoxication, gentamicin, phenobarbital, phenytoin, cisplatin, loop diuretics, calcitonin), respiratory distress, asphyxia, cerebral injuries, neonates with high bilirubinemia
Carcinoembryonic antigen (CEA)	0–3.0 ng/mL	<3 μg/L	Increased: Carcinoma (colon, pancreas, lung, stomach), smokers, nonneoplastic liver disease, Crohn's disease, ulcerative colitis
Chloride (Cl^-)	100–108 mEq/L	100–108 mmol/L	Increased: Metabolic acidosis due to prolonged diarrhea or renal disease, respiratory alkalosis (hyperventilation, severe CNS damage), diabetes insipidus, intestinal fistulas, dehydration, ureterosigmoidostomy, certain drug excesses (e.g., ammonium chloride, IV saline, steroids, salicylates, acetazolamide)
			Decreased: Prolonged vomiting or NG suction, metabolic acidosis with accumulation of organic anions, chronic respiratory acidosis, salt-losing renal diseases, water intoxication, adrenocortical insufficiency, SIADH, primary aldosteronism, hyponatremia, CHF, burns
Cholesterol, total desirable	140–200 mg/dL[†‡]	3.6–5.2 mmol/L	Increased: Hyperlipoproteinemia, idiopathic hypercholesterolemia, biliary obstruction, nephrosis, hypothyroidism, DM, pregnancy, MI, drugs (e.g., steroids, phenothiazines, oral contraceptives)
			Decreased: Starvation, malabsorption, sideroblastic anemia, thalassemia, hyperthyroidism, hypolipoproteinemias, liver failure, Cushing's syndrome, multiple myeloma, CML, myeloid metaplasia, myelofibrosis

Continued

TABLE 9-1: Normal Reference Intervals in Adults for Serum Analytes—Cont'd

Analyte	Reference Intervals Standard	SI*	Some Causes of Abnormal Results
C-reactive protein (CRP)	<0.5 mg/dL	<5 mg/L	Increased: Acute inflammation or infection, connective tissue disease, inflammatory bowel disease, lymphoma, rheumatic fever, tuberculosis, and many more; late pregnancy.
High-sensitivity (hs-CRP)	<9 mg/L	<9 mg/L	↑ hs-CRP, especially >3 mg/L, indicates ↑ risk of CVD
Creatine kinase (CK, CPK)	F: 15–130 U/L M: 15–160 U/L	F: $0.25-2.17 \times 10^{-6}$ kat/L M: $0.25-2.67 \times 10^{-6}$ kat/L	Increased: Muscle damage (acute MI, myocarditis, muscular dystrophy, trauma, IM injections, after surgery, status epilepticus, thermal and electrical burns), brain infarction, rhabdomyolysis, myositis, hypothyroidism, acromegaly, malignant hyperthermia, late pregnancy and parturition, vigorous exercise
CK myocardial band (MB) fraction	<3.9 total CK	<0.039 fractional	Increased: Necrosis of myocardial cells (acute MI, contusion, PTCA, cardioversion, surgery, pericarditis, prolonged SVT), skeletal muscle disease or trauma, alcoholism, Reye's syndrome, acute cholecystitis, carcinomas, hypothyroidism, drugs (e.g., aspirin, tranquilizers)
Creatinine	F: 0.5–1.1 mg/dL‡ M: 0.6–1.2 mg/dL‡	F: 44–97 mmol/L M: 53–106 mmol/L	Increased: Ingestion of raw meat, acromegaly, gigantism, azotemia, impaired renal function Decreased: Not clinically significant
Ferritin	F: 10–106 ng/mL M: 15–400 ng/mL	F: 10–106 μg/L M: 15–400 μg/L	Increased: Hyperthyroidism, inflammatory diseases, liver disease, neoplasms, iron replacement therapy, hemochromatosis, chronic renal disease Decreased: Iron deficiency anemia

Folate (folic acid)
  Serum
  RBC
	
	2.0–10.0 ng/mL†
	>120 ng/mL†
		
		4.5–22.7 nmol/L
		>270 nmol/L
			Decreased: Folic acid deficiency (inadequate intake, malabsorption, alcoholism), drugs (e.g., methotrexate, trimethoprim, phenytoin, oral contraceptives, aminopterin, azulfadine), vitamin B_{12} deficiency, hemolytic anemia

γ-Glutamyl transpeptidase (GGT) (plasma)	F: 5–30 U/L M: 6–45 U/L	F: $8-50 \times 10^{-6}$ kat/L M: $10-75 \times 10^{-6}$ kat/L	Increased: Liver disease, pancreatitis, acetaminophen toxicity, acute MI, alcoholism, drugs (barbiturates, phenytoin), neoplasms, CHF
Gamma Immunoglobulins			
IgG	600–1600 mg/dL	6–16 g/L	Increased: Infections of all types, severe malnutrition, RA, myeloma, hyperimmunization, liver disease Decreased: Hereditary or acquired deficiency, CLL, protein-losing syndromes, pregnancy, IgA myeloma
IgA	70–312 mg/dL‡	0.7–3.12 g/L	Increased: Cirrhosis, hepatitis, gamma A myeloma, subacute and chronic infections, RA, SLE, CML, exercise Decreased: Hereditary deficiency, lymphocytic leukemias, ataxia telangiectasia, acquired immunodeficiency states, chronic sinopulmonary disease, protein-losing enteropathy, late pregnancy
IgM	50–280 mg/dL‡	5–2.8 g/L	Increased: Liver disease, chronic infections, primary biliary cirrhosis, Waldenström's macroglobulinemia, RA, SLE. Decreased: Hereditary deficiency, CLL, protein-losing syndromes, IgG and IgA myelomas, hepatoma, lymphoid aplasia, infancy and early childhood
IgE	0.01–0.06 mg/dL‡	0.1–0.6 mg/L	Increased: Atopic diseases (exogenous asthma, allergic eczema, hay fever), parasitic diseases, IgE myeloma Decreased: Hereditary deficiency, acquired immunodeficiency, ataxia telangiectasia, non-IgE myelomas

Continued

TABLE 9-1: Normal Reference Intervals in Adults for Serum Analytes—Cont'd

	Reference Intervals		
Analyte	**Standard**	**SI***	**Some Causes of Abnormal Results**
Glucose (fasting) (plasma)	70–99 mg/dL‡	3.9–5.5 mmol/L	Increased: Diabetes mellitus
			Decreased: Pancreatic disorders, neoplasms (adrenal gland, stomach, fibrosarcoma, others), hepatic disease (diffuse or severe), endocrine disorders (Addison's disease, hypopituitarism, hypothyroidism, early DM), functional disturbances (following gastrectomy or gastroenterostomy, ANS disorders), malnutrition, alcoholism, some pediatric anomalies and enzyme diseases
Glycosylated hemoglobin (HbA$_{1c}$)	2.5%–6.0%	0.040–0.060 of Hb fraction	Increased: DM with poor blood sugar control, glycosuria, hyperglycemia, polycystic ovary syndrome
High-density lipoprotein (HDL) cholesterol	F: 38–75 mg/dL‡ M: 29–60 mg/dL‡	F: 1.00–1.94 mmol/L M: 0.75–1.60 mmol/L	Decreased: Uremia, diabetes, liver disease, ↓ apoproteins, Tangier's disease
			Note: Guidelines from the National Cholesterol Education Program state that values <40 are low and >60 are high
Homocysteine	Folate sufficient Folate deficient	<16 μmol/L <20 μmol/L	Increased: Deficiency of vitamins B$_6$, B$_{12}$, and folate, renal failure, drugs (e.g., carbamazepine, methotrexate, and phenytoin); associated with ↑ risk of atherosclerotic CVD
Iron	F: 50–170 μg/dL M: 65–170 μg/dL	F: 8.9–30.3 μmol/L M: 11.7–30.3 μmol/L	Increased: Hereditary hemochromatosis, sideroblastic anemia, aplastic anemia from treatment, hemoglobinopathies, thalassemias
			Decreased: Iron deficiency anemia, polycythemia vera from treatment, chronic blood loss, anemia of chronic disorders
Iron-binding capacity	250–435 μg iron/dL plasma	44.75–80.55 μmol/L	Increased; Iron deficiency anemia, pregnancy
			Decreased: Anemia of chronic disorders, thalassemia, hemochromatosis, sideroblastic anemia
Lactate dehydrogenase (LDH)	(L → P) 100–225 U/L (P → L) 80–280 U/L	1.7–3.7 μKat/L 1.4–6.1 μKat/L	Increased: Acute MI, cardiac surgery, prosthetic heart valve, hepatitis, malignant tumors, pulmonary embolus and infarction, myelogenous leukemia, diseases of muscle, burns, trauma, renal diseases (nephrotic syndrome, nephritis), hemolytic anemia, pernicious anemia, various infections and parasitic diseases, hypothyroidism, collagen vascular diseases, acute pancreatitis, intestinal obstruction, sarcoidosis
			Decreased: x-ray irradiation
LDH isoenzymes	LDH$_1$, 17%–27% LDH$_2$, 28%–38% LDH$_3$, 18%–28% LDH$_4$, 5%–15% LDH$_5$, 5%–15%		If LDH$_1$/LDH$_2$ >1.0: Recent MI (level starts to rise at 12–48 h) If LDH$_5$ >LDH$_4$: Liver disease
Lactic acid (plasma)	5–22 mg/dL	0.5–2.2 mmol/L	Increased lactic acidosis due to hypoxia, hemorrhage, shock, sepsis, cirrhosis, exercise
Lipase	4–24 U/dL	0.1–0.4 μKat/L	Increased: Acute pancreatitis, pancreatic duct obstruction, fat embolus syndrome, perforated peptic ulcer
Low-density lipoprotein (LDL) cholesterol	Desirable: ≤100 mg/dL Borderline: 130–159 mg/dL High risk: ≥160 mg/dL	<2.59 mmol/L	Increased: Excess dietary saturated fats, acute MI, DM, primary hyperlipoproteinemia, primary biliary cirrhosis, nephrosis, hypothyroidism

Continued

TABLE 9-1: Normal Reference Intervals in Adults for Serum Analytes—Cont'd

Analyte	Reference Intervals		Some Causes of Abnormal Results
	Standard	**SI***	
Magnesium (Mg^+)	1.2–2.1 mEq/L	0.60–1.05 mmol/L	Increased: Renal failure, hypothyroidism, Mg^+-containing antacids, Addison's disease, diabetic coma, severe dehydration, lithium intoxication
Myoglobin	≤90 ng/mL		Increased: Acute MI; skeletal muscle inflammation (myositis), ischemia, or trauma; muscular dystrophy, rhabdomyolysis, surgery, seizures
Osmolality			Increased: Hyperglycemia, alcohol ingestion, ↑ sodium with dehydration (diarrhea, vomiting, fever, ↓ water intake, hyperventilation, diabetes insipidus, osmotic diuresis), ↑ sodium with normal hydration (hypothalamic disorders), ↑ sodium with overhydration ($NaHCO_3$ for respiratory distress or cardiac arrest, infants given feedings with high Na^+ content)
Serum	280–296 mOs/kg	280–296 mmol/kg	
Urine	300–900 mOs/kg	300–900 mmol/kg	
			Decreased: Hyponatremia with hypovolemia (adrenal insufficiency, renal losses, GI tract loss [diarrhea, vomiting], burns, peritonitis, pancreatitis), hyponatremia with normal or ↑ hydration (CHF, cirrhosis, nephrotic syndrome, SIADH)
Phosphorus (inorganic)	2.7–4.5 mg/dL	0.87–1.45 mmol/L	Increased: ↑ Phosphate load (↑ vitamin D intake, massive transfusions, phosphate enemas, laxatives or infusion), excess tissue turnover (neoplasms, trauma, rhabdomyolysis, chemotherapy), acromegaly, hypoparathyroidism with ↓ Ca^{2+}, high intestinal obstruction, ↓ Mg^+, sarcoidosis
Females >60 yr	2.8–4.1 mg/dL	0.90–1.30 mmol/L	
Males >60 yr	2.3–3.7 mg/dL	0.74–1.20 mmol/L	
			Decreased: Renal or intestinal loss (diuretics, renal tubular defects, hyperthyroidism, hyperparathyroidism, ↓ K^+, ↓ Mg^+, others), ↓ intestinal absorption (malabsorption, malnutrition, ↓ vitamin D, osteomalacia, diarrhea, vomiting, phosphate-binding antacids), alcoholism, DM, hyperalimentation, nutritional recovery syndrome, alkalosis, drugs (e.g., salicylate poisoning, anabolic steroids, epinephrine, glucagon, insulin, IV glucose)
Potassium (K^+)	3.5–5.0 mEq/L	3.5–5.0 mmol/L	Increased: Impaired excretion (renal failure, oliguria, severe dehydration, ↓ blood volume, ↓ mineralocorticoids, Addison's disease), K^+ redistribution (acute acidosis, insulin, intravascular hemolysis, drugs [e.g., succinylcholine, digitalis toxicity, β-adrenergic blockade, arginine infusion]), release of extracellular K^+ (burns, crush injury, severe infections, rhabdomyolysis), ↑ supply of K^+ (factitiously if thrombocytosis or leukocytosis, hemolysis of sample, incomplete separation of serum and clot, prolonged use of tourniquet or hand exercise when drawing blood)
			Decreased: Hyperglycemia, nephropathies, mineralocorticoid excess, drugs (e.g., diuretics, insulin, adrenergics, antibiotics [amphotericin B, gentamicin, carbenicillin, ticarcillin]), GI loss (vomiting, diarrhea, NG suction, bowel obstruction, small bowel or biliary fistula, laxative abuse, neoplasms), skin loss (excess sweating, cystic fibrosis, severe burns, draining wounds), alkalosis, severe eating disorders, dietary deficiency, licorice abuse
Protein, total (serum)	6.5–8.3 g/dL	65–83 g/L	Increased: Hypergammaglobulinemias, hypovolemic states, dehydration, multiple myeloma, Waldenström's macroglobulinemia, sarcoidosis, collagen vascular diseases
			Decreased: Nutritional deficiency, ↓ or ineffective protein synthesis (severe liver disease, agammaglobulinemia), ↑ loss (renal [nephrotic syndrome], GI [protein-losing enteropathies or surgical resection], severe skin disease, burns), ↑ catabolism (fever, inflammation, hyperthyroidism, malignancy, chronic diseases), dilutional (IV fluids, SIADH, water intoxication)

Continued

TABLE 9-1: Normal Reference Intervals in Adults for Serum Analytes—Cont'd

Analyte	Reference Intervals Standard	SI*	Some Causes of Abnormal Results
Sodium (Na$^+$)	135–145 mEq/L	135–145 mmol/L	Increased: Osmotic diuresis (glycosuria, mannitol, urea), excess sweating, diabetes insipidus, respiratory loss (hyperpnea), administration of hypertonic NaHCO$_3$ or dialysis, salt tablets
			Decreased: Nephrotic syndrome, CHF, cirrhosis, renal failure, SIADH, hypothyroidism, adrenal insufficiency, urea, ↓ mineralocorticoids, GI or skin loss (vomiting, diarrhea, burns, pancreatitis, peritonitis), renal loss (diuresis, ketonuria, metabolic alkalosis, salt-losing nephritis, renal tubular acidosis), drugs that stimulate ADH release (chlorpropamide, tolbutamide, clofibrate, morphine, barbiturates, carbamazepine, acetaminophen, isoproterenol, indomethacin)
Triglycerides	67–157 mg/dL	0.11–2.15 mmol/L	Increased: Hyperlipoproteinemias,[§] hypothyroidism, liver diseases, alcoholism, pancreatitis, acute MI, nephrotic syndrome, DM, pregnancy, estrogens, glycogen storage disease
			Decreased: Malnutrition, congenital abetalipoproteinemia, drugs (e.g., clofibrate)
Troponins			Increased: Acute MI, angina, coronary syndromes, cardiac surgery or trauma, electrical countershock, myocarditis, heart failure, cardiomyopathy, percutaneous coronary interventions, renal failure, pulmonary HTN, PE, sepsis, stroke, high-dose chemotherapy, critically ill patients
Troponin I	<0.1 ng/mL	<0.1 µg/L	
Troponin T	<0.01 ng/mL	<0.01 µg/L	
Uric acid	F: 2.6–6.0 mg/dL M: 3.5–7.2 mg/dL	F: 155–357 µmol/L M: 208–428 µmol/L	Increased: Gout, renal failure, asymptomatic hyperuricemia, ↑ destruction of nucleoproteins (leukemia, multiple myeloma, polycythemia, lymphoma [especially after radiation therapy], other disseminated neoplasms, cancer chemotherapy, hemolytic anemia, sickle cell anemia, resolving pneumonia, toxemia of pregnancy), diet (high-protein weight loss, excess nucleoproteins [sweetbreads, liver]), lead poisoning, polycystic kidneys, sarcoidosis, hypoparathyroidism, hypothyroidism, metabolic acidosis, drugs (e.g., diuretics, small doses of salicylates).
			Decreased: ACTH therapy, drugs (probenecid, cortisone, allopurinol, coumarins, high doses of salicylates, glycerol guaiacolate), x-ray contrast agents, Wilson's disease, Fanconi's syndrome
Very low-density lipoprotein (VLDL) cholesterol	5–40 mg/Dl (Standard)		Increased: Genetic lipid disorders, DM, bile duct obstruction, nephrotic syndrome, hypothyroidism
Vitamin B$_{12}$	200–850 pg/mL	151–497 pmol/L	Increased: Chronic granulocytic leukemia, myelodysplastic disorders
			Decreased: Nutritional deficiency, pernicious anemia, malabsorption diseases, intestinal blind loop syndrome, megaloblastic anemia

↓, Decreased; ↑, increased; ACTH, adrenocorticotropic hormone; ADH, antidiuretic hormone; ANS, autonomic nervous system; CHF, congestive heart failure; CLL, chronic lymphocytic leukemia; CML, chronic myelogenous leukemia; CNS, central nervous system; CVD, cardiovascular disease; DM, diabetes mellitus; F, female; GI, gastrointestinal; GU, genitourinary; HTN, hypertension; IM, intramuscular; IV, intravenous; L → P, liver → pancreas; LV, left ventricular; M, male; MAO, monoamine oxidase; MI, myocardial infarction; P → L, pancreas → liver; NG, nasogastric; PE, pulmonary embolism; PTCA, percutaneous translumenal coronary angioplasty; RA, rheumatoid arthritis; RBC, red blood cell; SIADH, syndrome of inappropriate secretion of antidiuretic hormone; SLE, systemic lupus erythematosus; SVT, supraventricular tachycardia; TB, tuberculosis.
*SI, Systéme International units.
[†]Varies with gender.
[‡]Varies with age.
[§]See Table 9-7.

TABLE 9-2: Normal Adult Reference Intervals for a Complete Blood Cell Count and Some Common Causes of Abnormalities

Analyte	Reference Intervals		Some Causes of Abnormal Results
	Standard	**SI***	
White blood cell count (WBC)	$4.0\text{--}11.0 \times 10^3/mm^3$	$4.3\text{--}10.8 \times 10^5/L$	Increased: Most commonly related to ↑ numbers of neutrophils, lymphocytes, eosinophils, or monocytes (see entry for Differential count)
			Decreased: Viral infections, hypersplenism, bone marrow suppression due to drugs (e.g., antimetabolites, barbiturates, antibiotics, antihistamines, anticonvulsants, antithyroid medications, arsenicals, cancer chemotherapy, cardiovascular drugs/analgesics, antiinflammatory drugs), primary bone marrow disorders (leukemia, myeloma, aplastic anemia, congenital disorders, myelodysplastic syndromes), immune-associated neutropenia, marrow-occupying diseases (fungal infection, metastatic tumor)
Red blood cell count (RBC)	F: $4.00\text{--}5.40 \times 10^6/mm^3$ M: $4.60\text{--}6.00 \times 10^6/mm^3$	F: $4.00\text{--}5.40 \times 10^{12}/L$ M: $4.60\text{--}6.00 \times 10^{12}/L$	Increased: Hemoconcentration, dehydration, COPD, CHF, high altitude, polycythemia vera, smokers, cardiovascular disease, congenital heart disease, chronic lung disease, renal cell carcinoma, other erythropoietin-producing neoplasms, stress, hemoconcentration/dehydration
			Decreased: Anemias, hemolysis, chronic renal failure, hemorrhage, marrow failure, Hodgkin's disease, lymphoma, multiple myeloma, leukemia, SLE, Addison's disease, rheumatic fever, SBE, hyperthyroidism, cirrhosis
Hemoglobin (Hb)	F: 12–16 g/dL M: 13–18 g/dL	F: 7.45–9.93 mmol/L M: 8.06–11.17 mmol/L	Note: Causes of abnormal results same as for RBC
Hematocrit (Hct)	F: 37%–48% M: 42%–52%	F: 0.37–0.48 L/L M: 0.42–0.52 L/L	Note: Causes of abnormal results same as for RBC
Mean corpuscular hemoglobin (MCH)	28–33 pg/cell	1.73–2.05 fmol	Increased: Macrocytic anemias Decreased: Microcytic anemias
Mean corpuscular hemoglobin concentration (MCHC)	32%–36%	19.2–23.58 mmol/L	Increased: High-titer cold agglutinins, severe plasma lipemia Decreased: Hypochromatic anemia, iron deficiency, macrocytic anemias, anemia of chronic disease
Mean corpuscular volume (MCV)	80–98 μm^3	80–98 fL	Increased: ↓ Vitamin B, ↓ folic acid, chronic liver disease, alcoholism, reticulocytosis, myelodysplastic syndromes, myelofibrosis, hypothyroidism, cytotoxic chemotherapy Decreased: Chronic ↓ iron, thalessemia, other hemo-globinopathies, anemia of chronic disease, CRF
Red cell distribution width (RDW)	11.5%–14.5%		Related to MCV level: • *If normal RDW and ↑ MCV:* Aplastic anemia, preleukemia • *If normal RDW and normal MCF:* Normal, anemia of chronic disease, acute blood loss or hemolysis, CLL, CML, others • *If normal RDW and ↓ MCV:* Anemia of chronic disease, heterozygous thalassemia

Continued

TABLE 9-2: Normal Adult Reference Intervals for a Complete Blood Cell Count and Some Common Causes of Abnormalities—Cont'd

	Reference Intervals		
Analyte	**Standard**	**SI***	**Some Causes of Abnormal Results**
			• *If ↑ RDW and ↑ MCV:* ↓ Vitamin B, ↓ folate, autoimmune hemolytic anemia, cold agglutinins, CLL with high count, neonates
			• *If ↑ RDW and normal MCV:* Early iron deficiency, early ↓ vitamin B, early ↓ folate, sickle cell diseases, myelofibrosis, sideroblastic anemia
			• *If ↑ RDW and ↓ MCV:* Iron deficiency, RBC fragmentation, thalassemia intermedia
Platelets	$150-450 \times 10^3/mm^3$	$150-450 \times 10^9/L$	Increased: Malignancy (especially disseminated or advanced), myeloproliferative diseases, after splenectomy, collagen disorders, iron deficiency anemia, pseudothrombocytosis, acute infections, chronic pancreatitis, cirrhosis, cardiac disease
			Decreased: Thrombocytopenia (acquired and hereditary)
Differential count (leukocytes)			
Neutrophils, segmented (segs, polys)	Relative: 40%–80% Absolute: 2000–6800/mm³	$2.0-6.8 \times 10^9/L$	Increased: Acute infections, tissue breakdown (trauma, burns, tumors, gangrene, acute MI, acute stress), rheumatic and autoimmune disorders (e.g., RA, RF, inflammatory bowel disease, gout), hemolytic anemia, neoplastic disorders, myelogenous leukemia, metabolic disorders (e.g., ketoacidosis, lactic acidosis), pregnancy, drugs
Bands (stabs, early mature neutrophils)	Relative: 0%–4% Absolute: 0–600/mm³	$0-0.5 \times 10^9/L$	Decreased: Aplastic anemia, nutritional deficiencies (e.g., vitamin B_{12}, folate), overwhelming bacterial infection, viral infections (e.g., hepatitis, influenza, measles), cytotoxic and many other drugs, XRT
Lymphocytes (lymphs)	Relative: 20%–35% Absolute: 1250–3400/mm³	$1.0-4.0 \times 10^9/L$	Increased: Chronic bacterial infection, viral infection (e.g., mumps, rubella, mononucleosis, CMV, hepatitis), lymphocytic leukemias, multiple myeloma, Hodgkin's disease, XRT
			Decreased: Stress situations (burns, trauma, acute infections, sepsis) and corticosteroids, leukemia, immunodeficiency diseases (e.g., HIV, SLE), drug therapy (e.g., chemotherapy, immunosuppressants), XRT
Monocytes (monos)	Relative: 2%–10% Absolute: 150–1100/mm³	$0.2-1.0 \times 10^9/L$	Increased: Chronic inflammatory disorders, viral infections, recovery phase of acute infection, TB, collagen disorders (RA, SLE), neoplastic diseases (Hodgkin's disease, carcinoma, myelomonocytic leukemias, myelodysplasias), GI disorders
			Decreased: Aplastic anemia, hairy cell leukemia, lymphocytic leukemias, prednisone
Eosinophils (eos)	Relative: 1%–5% Absolute: 43–432/mm³	$0-0.5 \times 10^9/L$	Increased: Allergic reactions, eczema, parasitic infections, leukemia, autoimmune diseases, PIE, reaction to certain drugs (e.g., iodides, sulfa drugs, chlorpromazine), chronic granulomatous diseases

Continued

TABLE 9-2: Normal Adult Reference Intervals for a Complete Blood Cell Count and Some Common Causes of Abnormalities—Cont'd

	Reference Intervals		
Analyte	**Standard**	**SI***	**Some Causes of Abnormal Results**
Basophils (basos)	Relative: 0%–2% Absolute: 0–216/mm³	0–0.2 × 10⁹/L	Decreased: Stress situations resulting in adrenal corticoid or epinephrine production (burns, post surgery, SLE, CHF), acute infections, sepsis, certain drugs
			Increased: Myeloproliferative disease, leukemia, inflammatory processes, polycythemia vera, Hodgkin's disease after splenectomy or XRT, chronic sinusitis
			Decreased: Stress reactions (acute MI, bleeding ulcer), hypersensitivity reactions, hyperthyroidism, certain drugs (e.g., corticosteroids, chemotherapy)

↓, Decreased; ↑, increased; AML, Acute myelogenous leukemia; CHF, congestive heart failure; CML, chronic myelogenous leukemia; CMV, cytomegalovirus; COPD, chronic obstructive pulmonary disease; GI, gastrointestinal; HIV, human immunodeficiency virus; MI, myocardial infarction; MS, multiple sclerosis; PIE, pulmonary infiltrates with eosinophilia; RA, rheumatoid arthritis; RF, rheumatic fever; SBE, subacute bacterial endocarditis; SLE, systemic lupus erythematosus; TB, tuberculosis; XRT, radiation therapy.
*SI, Systéme International units.

TABLE 9-3: Other Hematologic Analytes

Analyte	**Reference Interval**	**Some Causes of Abnormal Results**
Erythrocyte sedimentation rate (ESR, sed rate)	F: 0–20 mm/h M: 0–10 mm/h (Westergren scale)	Increased: Severe anemia, macrocytosis, collagen diseases, hypercholesterolemia, infections, acute rheumatic fever, carcinoma, acute MI, nephrosis, pregnancy, chronic inflammatory diseases, ↑ fibrinogen, gamma or beta globulins, toxemia
		Decreased: Polycythemia, abnormal RBCs (especially sickle cell disease), microcytosis, ↓ fibrinogen, cachexia, ↑ WBC, overanticoagulation, CHF
Reticulocyte count	Relative: 0.5%–2.5% Absolute: Standard units: 18000–158000/mm³ SI units: 18–158 × 10⁹/L	Increased: Hemolytic anemias, hemorrhage, sickle cell crisis, thalassemia, autoimmune hemolysis, postanemia therapy (folic acid, ferrous sulfate, vitamin B₁₂)

↓, Decreased; ↑, increased; CHF, congestive heart failure; F, female; M, male; MI, myocardial infarction; RBC, red blood cell; WBC, white blood cell.

- B-type natriuretic protein (BNP), which is secreted by the ventricles in response to wall-stretch stimuli, is a marker of the presence and severity of heart failure.[1a]
- The digitalis glycosides, which are used to treat systolic dysfunction in heart failure, have a very narrow therapeutic range, below which they lose their effect and above which they become toxic. Digoxin is the most commonly used digitalis preparation in the United States, and its therapeutic trough range is 0.5 to 2.0 ng/mL.[2] Toxicity occurs at levels above 2.0 ng/mL and sometimes even lower, especially in the elderly and in the presence of hypokalemia or hypomagnesemia, and is manifested as cardiac arrhythmias, gastrointestinal symptoms (e.g., anorexia, nausea, and vomiting), and neurological complaints (e.g., visual disturbances, disorientation, and confusion). Digitalis toxicity is more common in individuals with renal or liver dysfunction and can be provoked by a great number of medications, including amiodarone, antacids, captopril, cholestyramine, clarithromycin, erythromycin, flecainide, fluoxetine, heparin, ibuprofen, itraconazole, kaolin-pectin, midazolam, neomycin, nitrendipine, phenobarbital, phenytoin, propafenone, quinidine, rifampin, spironolactone, and verapamil. In addition, some herbal supplements are known to

TABLE 9-4: Some Hematologic Abnormalities

Term/Abnormality	Definition
Leukocytosis	Total WBC count >10,000–15,000/mm^3
Leukopenia	Total WBC count <4000/mm^3
Neutrophilia	Absolute neutrophil count >8000/mm^3
Neutropenia	Absolute neutrophil count <1500–2000/mm^3, <1000–1500/mm^3 in black population
Lymphocytosis	Lymphocyte count >4000/mm^3 in adults, >7200 in adolescents, >9000 in young children and infants
Lymphocytopenia	Lymphocyte count <1500/mm^3 in adults, <3000/mm^3 in children
Monocytosis	Monocyte count >10% in differential count, or absolute count >500/mm^3
Eosinophilia	Eosinophil count >500/mm^3, or >10% in differential count
Basophilia	Basophil count >150/mm^3, or >3% in differential count
Granulocytosis	Abnormally high count of PMNs (includes neutrophils, eosinophils, and basophils)
Granulocytopenia	Abnormally low count of PMNs
Agranulocytosis	Extremely low count of PMNs (<500/mm^3)
Thrombocytosis	Platelet count >500,000/mm^3
Thrombocytopenia	Platelet count <100–150 × 10^3/mm^3
Pancytopenia	Abnormally low counts of RBCs, all WBC types, and platelets
Polycythemia	RBC count >5.1–5.5 × 10^6/mm^3
Reticulocytosis	Reticulocyte (young RBCs) count >2.5%–4% of RBCs
Anemia	Any condition in which the RBC count, the Hb level, or the Hct are less than normal:
Aplastic	Failure of bone marrow with pancytopenia
Fanconi's	Congenital aplastic anemia
Hemolytic	Hemolysis of RBCs caused by RBC injury
Iron deficiency	↓ Iron for RBC production, resulting in ↓ Hb levels
Megaloblastic	↑ Megaloblasts due to ↓ vitamin B$_{12}$ or folate
Macrocytic	With ↑ size of RBCs (↑ MCV)
Microcytic	With ↓ size of RBCs (↓ MCV)
Normocytic	With normal-sized RBCs (normal MCV)
Pernicious	Chronic anemia caused by malabsorption of B$_{12}$
Hemoglobinopathy	Any disorder affecting the structure, function, or production of Hb (e.g., sickle cell syndromes, thalassemia)
Myeloproliferative disorders	Acquired clonal abnormalities of hematopoietic stem cells resulting in changes in myeloid, erythroid, and platelet cells (e.g., polycythemia vera, primary thrombocytopenia)
Myelodysplastic syndromes	A group of disorders characterized by cytopenias of one to three cell lines and abnormal cellular morphology in the bone marrow and peripheral blood (e.g., refractory anemia)
Leukemia	Uncontrolled proliferation of a malignant clone of hematopoietic stem cells, resulting in marked increase in functionless cells and decreased normal cells
Acute	Characterized by anemia, thrombocytopenia, and granulocytopenia:
ALL	Acute lymphocytic leukemia (↑ number of lymphoid cells)
AML	Acute myelogenous leukemia (↑ number of granulocytes)
ANLL	Acute nonlymphocytic leukemias—all others (myeloid, promyeloid, monocytic, myelomonocytic, erythroleukemia)
Chronic	Proliferative disorders derived from myeloid or lymphoid precursor cells that retain some capacity for differentiation to recognizable mature elements:
CLL	Chronic lymphocytic leukemias (B cell is more common, T cell more aggressive)
CML	Chronic myelocytic/myelogenous leukemia
HCL	Hairy cell leukemia
Leukemoid reaction	A nonleukemic WBC count >50,000/mm^3 or differential with >5% metamyelocytes or earlier cell
Lymphoma	Can be Hodgkins or non-Hodgkins. A variety of lymphocytic malignancies that originate in the lymph nodes and spread systematically via the lymphatic system. Often presents with a normal CBC. Most commonly diagnosed with a lymph node biopsy

↓, Decreased; ↑, increased; CBC, complete blood count; Hct, hematocrit; Hb, hemoglobin; MCV, mean corpuscular volume; PMN, polymorphonuclear leukocyte; RBC, red blood cell; WBC, white blood cell.

TABLE 9-5: Normal Reference Intervals for Coagulation Studies and Common Causes of Abnormalities

Analyte	Reference Intervals	Common Causes of Abnormal Results
Antithrombin III	Activity: 80%–120%	Increased: Warfarin, post-MI
	Antigen: 22–39 mg/dL	Decreased: Hereditary deficiency, DIC, PE, thrombolytic therapy, cirrhosis, chronic liver failure, postsurgery, late pregnancy, oral contraceptives, sepsis, nephrotic syndrome, IV heparin >3 d
Bleeding time	2–8 min	Increased: Thrombocytopenia, capillary wall abnormalities, platelet abnormalities, drugs (e.g., aspirin, warfarin, antiinflammatory drugs, streptokinase, urokinase, dextran, β-lactam antibiotics, moxalactin)
Coagulation factors		
I (fibrinogen)	0.15–0.35 g/dL	Increased: Acute inflammatory reactions, trauma, CAD, smoking, oral contraceptives, pregnancy
		Decreased: DIC, hereditary afibrinogenemia, liver disease, fibrinolysis, abnormal fibrinogen or abnormal prothrombin
II (prothrombin)	60%–140%	Decreased: Vitamin K deficiency, liver disease, congenital deficiency, warfarin
V (proaccelerin, labile factor)	60%–140%	Decreased: Factor V Leiden, liver disease, DIC, fibrinolysis
VII (proconvertin, stable factor)	60%–140%; 60–140 AU	Decreased: Congenital deficiency, ↓ vitamin K, liver disease, warfarin
VIII (antihemophilic factor + von Willebrand factor)	50%–150%; 50–150 AU	Increased: Acute inflammatory reactions, trauma, stress, late normal pregnancy, thromboembolic conditions, liver disease, normal newborns
		Decreased: Hemophilia A, von Willebrand's disease, DIC, factor VIII inhibitor (e.g., from childbirth, multiple myeloma, penicillin allergy, RA, SLE, surgery), fibrinolysis
IX (Christmas factor)	60%–140%; 60–140 AU	Decreased: Hemophilia B (Christmas disease), liver disease, nephrotic syndrome, warfarin, DIC, ↓ vitamin K
X (Stuart-Prower factor)	60%–140%; 60–140 AU	Decreased: Congenital deficiency, liver disease, warfarin, ↓ vitamin K
XI (prekallikrein)	60%–140%; 60–140 AU	Decreased: Congenital heart disease, congenital deficiency, liver disease, pregnancy, ↓ vitamin K, drugs
XII (Hageman factor)	50%–150%; 50–150 AU	Decreased: Congenital deficiency, ↓ vitamin K, liver disease, nephrotic syndrome, warfarin, DIC
XIII (fibrin-stabilizing factor)	Negative screen	
Partial thromboplastin time (PTT)	24–37 s	Prolonged: Anticoagulation therapy, coagulation factor deficiencies (hemophilia, ↓ fibrinogen, etc.), liver disease, ↓ vitamin K, DIC, prolonged use of tourniquet before drawing blood sample
		Decreased: Extensive cancer without liver involvement, immediately after acute hemorrhage, early DIC
Platelet count	150–450 × 10³/mm³	See Table 9-2
Prothrombin time (PT)	8.8–11.6 s	Prolonged PT or ↑ INR or P/C ratio: anticoagulation therapy, DIC, liver disease, ↓ vitamin K, coagulation factor deficiencies, drugs (e.g., salicylates, chloral hydrate, diphenylhydantoin, estrogens, antacids, phenylbutazone, quinidine, antibiotics, allopurinol, anabolic steroids), biliary obstruction, prolonged use of tourniquet before drawing blood sample
International normalized ratio (INR)	<1.5	
		Decreased: Vitamin K supplementation, thrombophlebitis, drugs (e.g., gluthetimide, estrogens, griseofulvin, diphenhydramine)
Thrombin time	±5 s of control	Prolonged: Heparin therapy, DIC, fibrinogen, streptokinase, urokinase

↓, Decreased; ↑, increased; AU, Arbitrary Units; DIC, disseminated intravascular coagulation; IV, intravenous; MI, myocardial infarction; P/C ratio, ratio of patient PT value to control PT value; PE, pulmonary embolism; RA, rheumatoid arthritis; SLE, systemic lupus erythematosus.

TABLE 9-6: Normal Reference Values for Selected Immunologic Analytes and Common Causes of Abnormalities

Analyte	Reference Value	Common Causes of Abnormal Values
Autoantibodies		
Anti-nuclear (ANA)	Negative at 1:8 dilution	Positive: Mixed connective tissue diseases (SLE, RA, scleroderma, dermatomyositis, polyarteritis), drug-induced lupus-like syndromes, chronic active lupoid hepatitis, pulmonary interstitial fibrosis, TB, necrotizing vasculitis, Sjögren's syndrome, idiopathic
Mitochondrial	Negative at 1:20 dilution	Positive primary biliary cirrhosis, long-standing hepatic obstruction, chronic hepatitis, cryptogenic cirrhosis
Smooth muscle	Negative at 1:20 dilution	Positive: Chronic active hepatitis, lupoid hepatitis, intrinsic asthma, acute viral hepatitis, biliary cirrhosis
Cold agglutinins	<1:32	Increased: Mycoplasma pneumonia, CMV infections, infectious mononucleosis, cirrhosis, acquired hemolytic anemia, frostbite, malaria
Complement		
C3	83–177 mg/dL	Increased: Inflammatory states as acute-phase response (RA, rheumatic fever, early SLE), neoplasms
		Decreased: Active SLE, glomerulonephritis, chronic active hepatitis, DIC, hereditary C3 deficiency, celiac disease, anorexia nervosa, SBE, chronic liver disease, gram-negative sepsis, fungemia, cryoglobulinemia, immune complex disease
C4	15–45 mg/dL	Increased: Neoplasms, juvenile RA, ankylosing spondylitis
		Decreased: Acute early SLE, early glomerulonephritis, hereditary angioneurotic edema, hereditary C4 deficiency, cryoglobulinemia, immune complex disease
Rheumatoid factor (fasting)	<30 U/mL	Increased: RA, SLE, syphilis, chronic inflammation, SBE, cancer, some lung diseases (i.e., TB), sarcoidosis, viral infections

CMV, Cytomegalovirus; DIC, disseminated intravascular coagulation; RA, rheumatoid arthritis; SBE, subacute bacterial endocarditis; SLE, systemic lupus erythematosus; TB, tuberculosis.

TABLE 9-7: Hyperlipidemias

		Plasma Lipids			
Type	Lipoprotein Abnormality	Cholesterol	Triglycerides	CAD Risk	Prevalence
I	↑↑↑ Chylomicrons	nl–↑	↑↑↑	Low	Rare
IIa	↑↑↑ LDL cholesterol	↑↑↑	nl	Very high	Common
IIb	↑↑ LDL, ↑ VLDL	↑↑	↑	Very high	Probably common
III	Broad band B-lipoprotein	↑↑	↑↑	Very high	Rare
IV	↑ VLDL	nl–↑	↑↑	High	Most common
V	↑↑ VLDL, ↑↑ chylomicrons	↑	↑↑	Low	Rare

↑, Somewhat increased; ↑↑, moderately increased; ↑↑↑, markedly increased; CAD, coronary artery disease; LDL, low-density lipoprotein; nl, normal; VLDL, very low-density lipoprotein.

TABLE 9-8: Serum Cardiac Markers After Acute Myocardial Infarction

Analyte and Normal Value	Begins to Rise at:	Reaches Peak at:	Returns to Normal at:
Myoglobin			
≤90 ng/mL	1–3 h	6–12 h	24–36 h
Troponin I (cTnI)			
<0.10 ng/mL	3–4 h	8–24 h	4–12 d
Troponin T (cTnT)			
<0.01 ng/mL	3–4 h	12–16 h	6–14 d
Creatine kinase (CPK)			
F: 15–130 U/L	2–12 h	12–40 h	2–6 d
M: 15–160 U/L			
Myocardial bands (MB)			
<6% total CK	2–12 h	12–24 h	1.5–3 d
Aspartate aminotransferase (AST)			
5–30 U/L	6–24 h	24–48 h	3–6 d
Lactate dehydrogenase (LDH)			
(L → P) 100–225 U/L	12–48 h	2–6 d	7–14 d
(P → L) 80–280 U/L			
LDH-1 isoenzyme			
17%–27%	12–48 h	2–6 d	7–14 d
LDH-1 <LDH-2			

F, Female; L→ P, liver → pancreas; M, male; P → L, pancreas → liver.

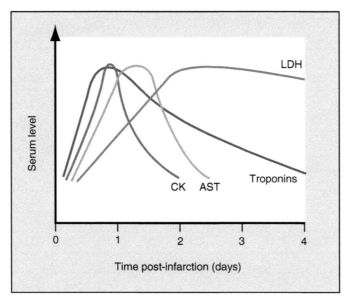

Figure 9-2: Changes in serum cardiac markers after acute myocardial infarction (MI). The troponins are detectable within 2 to 4 hours of MI and are very specific for cardiac injury. Creatine kinase (CK), which is muscle specific, also rises rapidly and earlier than detectable changes in aspartate transaminase (AST) or lactate dehydrogenase (LDH). Another cardiac marker, myoglobin, is not illustrated. (From Forbes CD, Jackson WF. *Color Atlas and Text of Clinical Medicine.* 3rd ed. St. Louis: Mosby; 2003.)

TABLE 9-9: Normal Adult Reference Values of Endocrine Function

	Reference Intervals		
Test	**Standard**	**SI Units***	**Common Causes of Abnormal Results**
Thyroid Function			
Total thyroxine (T$_4$)	5–12 µg/dL	65–155 nmol/	Increased: Graves' disease, toxic goiter
			Decreased: Primary hypothyroidism, secondary hypothyroidism
Total triiodothyronine (T$_3$)	100–200 ng/dL	1.62–4.14 nmol/L	Same as T$_4$
Adrenal Function			
Epinephrine (24-h urine)	0–20 µg/day	0–109 nmol/day	Increased: Stress, hypothyroidism, chronic low blood pressure, congestive heart failure, pheochromocytoma and other catecholamine-secreting tumors
			Decreased: Idiopathic postural hypotension, anorexia nervosa, familial dystonia
Norepinephrine (24-h urine)	15–80 µg/day	80–473 nmol/day	Increased: Stress, hypothyroidism, chronic low blood pressure, congestive heart failure, pheochromocytoma and other catecholamine-secreting tumors
			Decreased: Idiopathic postural hypotension, anorexia nervosa, familial dystonia
Cortisol: Morning – evening	10–100 µg/day	27.6–276 nmol/day	Increased: Cushing's syndrome
			Decreased: Addison's disease
Pancreatic Function			
Glucose tolerance test			Increased: DM if fasting value >125 mg/dL or 2-h value ≥200 mg/dL; Impaired fasting glucose (IFG) if fasting values of 100–125 mg/dL; Impaired glucose tolerance (IGT) if 2-h values of 121–199 mg/dL. Many drugs (e.g., steroids, diuretics, oral contraceptives, phenytoin, cimetidine, levodopa)
Fasting	70–99 mg/dL	3.9–5.5 nmol/L	
30 min	110–170 mg/dL	6.1–9.4 nmol/L	
60 min	120–170 mg/dL	6.7–9.4 nmol/L	
90 min	100–140 mg/dL	5.6–7.8 nmol/L	
2h	70–120 mg/dL	3.9–6.7 nmol/L	Decreased: Hypoglycemia, celiac disease, hepatic disease, various drugs (e.g., β-blockers, ethanol, oral hypoglycemic agents, clofibrate)
Insulin: 12-h fasting	2–25 µU/mL	13–174 pmol/L	Increased: Insulin resistance (as in type 2 DM and metabolic syndrome), obesity, insulinoma, various drugs (e.g., corticosteroids, levodopa, oral contraceptives)
			Decreased: DM, hypopituitarism, chronic pancreatis (including cystic fibrosis), various drugs (e.g., β-blockers, calcitonin, cimetidine, thiazide diuretics, furosemide)
Amylase (serum)	See Table 9-1 for normal ranges		See Table 9-1

DM, Diabetes mellitus.
*SI, Systéme International units.

increase digoxin levels: ephedra (*ma huang,* ephedrine), pleurisy root, and sarsaparilla root.

- Metabolic syndrome is characterized by impaired glucose tolerance (Table 9-9, and see page 130) and dyslipidemia (as well as obesity and hypertension).[5,6]
- Abnormalities of endocrine function have a direct effect on metabolism and the physiological responses to increasing metabolic demands, as in exercise or the stress of illness or trauma. Normal endocrine function provides for the augmentation of blood flow and pressure and reduction in peripheral resistance

that are required when demand is increased. Some common tests of endocrine function are listed in Table 9-9, along with their normal reference intervals and some common causes of abnormalities.

- Diabetes mellitus (DM) is diagnosed by fasting glucose levels greater than 125 mg/dL (see Table 9-9). In type 1 DM, insulin levels are reduced, whereas in type 2 DM, insulin levels are increased. Glycosylated hemoglobin (HbA$_{1c}$) levels are elevated in patients with poor blood sugar control over the previous 8 to 12 weeks. In nondiabetics HbA$_{1c}$ levels are typically 4% to 6%; individuals with DM rarely achieve levels less than 7%, and HbA$_{1c}$ levels greater than 9% indicate poor control and greater than 12% signify very poor control.

- α_1-Protease inhibitor (API), or α_1-antitrypsin, deficiency results in the inhibition of the activities of a number of enzymes in the body, leading to the premature development of severe emphysema, as well as chronic bronchitis and bronchiectasis, and liver disease. Normal API levels are 80 to 260 mg/dL (0.8–2.6 g/L, SI units). Decreased levels are also seen in congenital deficiency, premature infants (usually transient), severe liver disease, malnutrition, renal losses (e.g., nephrosis), gastrointestinal (GI) losses (e.g., pancreatitis and protein-losing diseases), and exudative dermopathies. Increased levels occur in acute and chronic infections, cancer (especially cervical cancer and lymphoma), pregnancy, chronic liver disease, systemic lupus erythematosus (SLE), and ulcerative colitis, and with the use of birth control pills, estrogens, and steroids.

- Polycythemia (increased red blood cell [RBC] mass, also known as erythrocytosis) usually results from stimulation of normal hematopoietic progenitors by extrinsic factors, such as tissue hypoxia (e.g., chronic high-altitude exposure, severe lung disease, cyanotic congenital heart disease, and severe congestive heart failure [CHF]) or increased production of erythropoietin (EPO, due to cerebellar hemangioblastoma, hepatocellular carcinoma and other tumors, renal disease, and uterine fibromyoma), although it may also occur as a primary disorder (polycythemia vera).

- Cystic fibrosis (CF) is diagnosed by a sweat chloride test performed in infants who are at least 3 months old. Normally, sweat chloride values are 10 to 35 mEq/L; a value greater than 60 mEq/L is diagnostic of CF.

- Renal insufficiency and failure result in the accumulation of water, crystalloid solids, and waste products, which leads to altered electrolyte and acid–base balances, hypertension, gastrointestinal dysfunction, severe anemia, and multiple other abnormalities involving all body organs. The typical progression of nonspecific symptoms and signs of chronic renal failure is depicted in Figure 9-3. Characteristic patterns of renal impairment and failure are found in Table 9-10.[7–9]

- The liver plays important roles in carbohydrate, fat, and protein metabolism; aids in digestion through the production of bile; serves as a storage site for many vitamins and iron (as ferritin); forms a number of substances used in the coagulation process; and is responsible for detoxifying the blood and excreting into bile many drugs, hormones, and other substances. Some possible patterns of abnormalities seen in liver disease are presented in Table 9-11.[7–9]

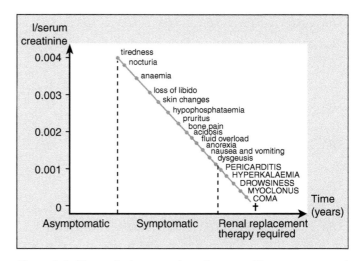

Figure 9-3: The typical progression of nonspecific symptoms and signs of chronic renal failure as related to creatinine levels. (From Forbes CD, Jackson WF. *Color Atlas and Text of Clinical Medicine.* 3rd ed. St. Louis: Mosby; 2003.)

TABLE 9-10: **Characteristic Patterns of Renal Impairment and Failure**

Analyte (Normal Value)	Prerenal Azotemia	Acute Tubular Injury	Chronic Renal Failure
Urine osmolality (500–1200 mOsm/L)	>500	<350	<50
Urine/serum urea	>10	<10	>10
Urine/serum creatinine	>40	<20	<20
Urine Na$^+$ (40–240 mEq/24 h)	<10–20	>40	May be ↑ or may be ↓
Other	No casts in UA, ↑ BUN >↑ creatinine	Clinical evidence of acute onset, positive casts or cells in UA, ↑ serum WBC, slight ↑ BUN, ↑ serum creatinine, metabolic acidosis; may be ↓ Ca^{2+}, ↑ K$^+$, normal–↓ serum Na$^+$	Proteinuria, ↑ BUN, ↑ serum creatinine, ↓ serum Na$^+$, ↑ serum K$^+$, metabolic acidosis, ↑ serum Ca^{2+}, ↑ triglycerides, ↑ cholesterol, ↑ VLDL, ↓ Hct (anemia), ↓ serum albumin, ↓ total protein, ↑ phosphate

↓, Decreased; ↑, increased; BUN, blood urea nitrogen; Hct, hematocrit; UA, urinalysis; VLDL, very low-density lipoprotein; WBC, white blood cell.

TABLE 9-11: Characteristic Patterns of Liver Function Tests

Disorder	Bilirubin	Alkaline Phosphatase	AST (SGOT)	ALT (SGPT)	PTT	Other
Hepatocellular jaundice	↑	↑–↑↑	↑ AST <ALT	↑	nl–↑ (poor response to vitamin K)	↓ Serum albumin ↓↓ Cholesterol (total and esters)
Uncomplicated obstructive jaundice	↑–↑↑↑	↑↑↑	nl–↑ AST >ALT	nl–↑	nl–↑↑ (responds to vitamin K)	↑ Total cholesterol (normal esters) nl–↓ albumin ↑ GGT
Acute viral or toxic hepatitis	↑–↑↑↑	↑–↑↑	↑↑↑	↑↑↑	nl–↑↑↑	↑ IgM if hepatitis B
Chronic active (non-A, non-B) hepatitis	nl–↑	nl–↑	↑–↑↑	↑–↑↑	nl–↑↑ (no response to vitamin K)	nl–↑ serum albumin ↑ IgG, IgM
Alcoholic hepatitis	nl–↑↑	nl–↑↑	nl–↑↑↑	nl–↑↑	nl–↑↑	nl–↓ serum albumin ↑ Gamma globulin ↑ GGT ↑ MCV Possible anemia
Cirrhosis	nl–↑	nl–↑	nl–↑↑	nl–↑	nl–↑↑	Anemia is common ↑ Gamma globulin, especially IgM ↓ Serum albumin Positive mitochondrial antibody

↓, Decreased; ↑, somewhat increased; ↑↑, moderately increased; ↑↑↑, markedly increased; ALT (SGPT), alanine aminotransferase (serum glutamic pyruvic transaminase); AST (SGOT), aspartate aminotransferase (serum glutamic oxaloacetic transaminase); GGT, γ-glutamyl transpeptidase; Ig, immunoglobulin; MCV, mean corpuscular volume; nl, normal; PTT, prothrombin time.

REFERENCES

1. Burtis CA, Ashwood ER, Bruns DE. *Tietz Fundamentals of Clinical Chemistry.* 6th ed. Philadelphia: W.B. Saunders; 2008.

1a. Carderelli R, Lumicao TG. B-type natriuretic peptide: a review of its diagnostic, prognostic, and therapeutic monitoring value in heart failure for primary care physicians. *J Am Board Fam Pract.* 2003;16:327-333.

2. Chernecky CC, Berger BJ. *Laboratory Tests and Diagnostic Procedures.* 4th ed. Philadelphia: W.B. Saunders; 2004.

3. Fischbach F. *A Manual of Laboratory & Diagnostic Tests.* 7th ed. Philadelphia: Lippincott Williams & Wilkins; 2004.

4. Holmes HN, ed. *Clinical Laboratory Tests, Values and Implications.* 3rd ed. Philadelpia: Springhouse Publishing.; 2001.

5. Mahon CR, Fowler DG. *Diagnostic Skills in Clinical Laboratory Science.* New York: McGraw-Hill; 2004.

6. McKenzie SB. *Clinical Laboratory Hematology.* 2nd ed. Prentice Hall; 2003.

7. McPherson RA, Pincus MR, eds. *Henry's Clinical Diagnosis and Management by Laboratory Methods.* 21st ed. Philadelphia: W.B. Saunders; 2006.

8. Pagana KD, Pagana TJ. *Mosby's Diagnostic and Laboratory Test Reference.* 7th ed. St. Louis: C.V. Mosby.; 2004.

9. Wallach J. *Interpretation of Diagnostic Tests.* 7th ed. Philadelphia: Lippincott Williams & Wilkins; 2000.

Abbreviations

6MWT 6-Minute walk test

α_1 PI Alpha$_1$-proteinase inhibitor

AAA Abdominal aortic aneurysm

A–a gradient Alveolar-to-arterial gradient

AAI Ankle-arm index (BP measure) (= ABI)

A & B Apnea and bradycardia

ABE Acute bacterial endocarditis

ABGs Arterial blood gases

ABI Ankle-brachial index (BP measure) (= AAI)

A/C Assist control (mode on ventilator)

ACB Aortocoronary bypass, active cycles of breathing

ACBT Active cycles of breathing technique

ACE Angiotensin-converting enzyme

ACEIs ACE inhibitors

ACLS Advanced cardiac life support

ACS Acute coronary syndrome

AD Autogenic drainage

AF Aortofemoral, atrial fibrillation or flutter

A-fib Atrial fibrillation

AI Aortic insufficiency

AICD Automatic implantable cardiac defibrillator

AIDS Acquired immune deficiency syndrome

ALT Serum alanine aminotransferase (= SGPT)

ALS Amyotrophic lateral sclerosis (Lou Gehrig's Disease)

AMI Acute myocardial infarction

AML Anterior mitral leaflet, acute myelogenous leukemia

AMV Augmented minute ventilation

Ao Aorta

AoV Aortic valve

AP Anteroposterior, aortopulmonary

APB Atrial premature beat (= PAC)

APC Atrial premature complex/contraction (= PAC)

APRV Airway pressur-release ventilation (added to CPAP)

ARBs Angiotensin II receptor blockers

ARD Autoimmune rheumatic disease

ARDS Acute respiratory distress syndrome

ARF Acute renal failure, acute rheumatic fever

AS Aortic stenosis

ASCAD Atherosclerotic coronary artery disease

ASCVD Atherosclerotic cardiovascular or cerebrovascular disease

ASD Atrial septal defect

ASHD Atherosclerotic heart disease

AST Serum aspartate aminotransferase (= SGOT)

AT Anaerobic threshold

AV Atrioventricular, aortic valve

AVB Atrioventricular node block

(a–v)o$_2$ Arteriovenous oxygen difference

AVR Aortic valve replacement

BBB Bundle branch block

BCLS Basic cardiac life support

BE Base excess/deficit

BG Blood glucose

BIA Bioelectrical impedance analysis

bi-PAP Bilevel positive airway pressure

biVAD Biventricular assist device

BMI Body mass index

BMT Bone marrow transplant

BNP B-type natruiretic peptide

BO(S) Bronchiolitis obliterans (syndrome)

BOOP Bronchiolitis obliterans with organizing pneumonia

BP Blood pressure

BPD Bronchopulmonary dysplasia

bpm Beats per minute, breaths per minute

BR Breathing reserve

BS Breath sounds, bowel sounds

BSA Body surface area

BUN Blood urea nitrogen

C & S Culture and sensitivity

CABG Coronary artery bypass graft (surgery)

CAD Coronary artery disease

CAN Cardiovascular autonomic neuropathy

Cath Catheterization

CBD Chronic berrylium disease (berrylliosis)

CBF Coronary blood flow

CCBs Calcium channel blockers

CCU Coronary care unit

CDH Congenital diaphragmatic hernia

CF Cystic fibrosis

CHD Coronary heart disease, congenital heart disease

CHF Congestive or chronic heart failure

CI Cardiac index

circ Circumflex (coronary artery) (= Cx)

CK Creatine kinase (= CPK)

CKD Chronic kidney disease

CMC Closed mitral commissurotomy

CMR Cardiac magnetic resonance (imaging)

CMV Cytomegalovirus

CNS Central nervous system

CO Cardiac output, carbon monoxide

CO$_2$ Carbon dioxide

CoA Coarctation of the aorta

COAD Chronic obstructive airway disease

COLD Chronic obstructive lung disease

COP Cryptogenic organizing pneumonia (= BOOP)

COPD Chronic obstructive pulmonary disease

cp Chest pain

CPA Cardiophrenic angle (on CXR examination)

CPAP Continuous positive airway pressure

CPB Cardiopulmonary bypass

CPET Cardiopulmonary exercise test (= CPX)

CPK Creatine phosphokinase (= CK)

CPR Cardiopulmonary resuscitation

CPT Chest physical therapy

CPX Cardiopulmonary exercise test (= CPET)

CR(P) Cardiac rehabilitation (program)

CRF Chronic renal failure

CRP C-reactive protein

CRT Cardiac resynchronization therapy

CSII Continuous subcutaneous insulin infusion

CT Computed tomography

CTD Connective tissue disease

CV Cardiovascular

CVA Cerebrovascular accidet

CVD Cardiovascular disease

CVP Central venous pressure

CVS Cardiovascular system

CWE Chest wall excursion

Cx Circumflex (coronary artery)

CXR Chest x-ray

DB Diaphragmatic breathing, deep breathing

DBP Diastolic blood pressure

DCM Dilated cardiomyopathy

dig Digitalis

DKA Diabetic ketoacidosis

Dl$_{CO}$ Diffusion capacity for carbon monoxide

DLD Diffuse lung disease

DM Diabetes mellitus

DOE Dyspnea on exertion

DPI Dry-powder inhaler

D-TGA Dextrotransposition of the great arteries

DTIs Direct thrombin inhibitors

DVT Deep venous thrombosis

EBCT Electron beam computed tomography

ECG Electrocardiogram

Echo Echocardiogram

ECMO Extracorporeal membrane oxygenation

EDP End-diastolic pressure

EDV End-diastolic volume

EECP Enhanced extracorporeal counterpulsation

EF Ejection fraction

EIA Exercise-induced asthma (= EIB)

EIB Exercise-induced bronchoconstriction (= EIA)

EPS Electrophysiological studies

ESRD End-stage renal disease

EST Exercise stress test

ESV End-systolic volume

ET Endotracheal

ETT Exercise tolerance test, endotracheal tube

f Respiratory rate

FEF$_{25\%-75\%}$ Forced expiratory flow during mid-half of forced vital capacity (formerly NMFR)

FET Forced expiratory technique

FEV$_1$ Forced expiratory volume in 1 second

FEV$_1$/FVC FEV$_1$ expressed as a percentage of forced vital capacity

FH Family history

F$_{IO_2}$ Fraction of inspired oxygen

FRC Functional residual capacity

FVC Forced vital capacity

FWC Functional work capacity

GA General anesthesia

GBPS Gated blood pool study (= MUGA, RNA)

GBS Guillian-Barré syndrome

GDM Gestational diabetes (mellitus)

GPB Glossopharyngeal breathing

GTT Glucose tolerance test

GXT Graded exercise test

HAART Highly-active antiretroviral therapy (for HIV)

Hb Hemoglobin

HbA$_{1c}$ Glycosylated hemoglobin

HBP High blood pressure

HCM Hypertrophic cardiomyopathy

HCO$_3^-$ Bicarbonate

Hct Hematocrit

HCTZ Hydrochlorothiazide

HCVD Hypertensive cardiovascular disease

HDL High-density lipoproteins

HFCWC High-frequency chest wall compression

HFCWO High-frequency chest wall oscillation

HFNEF Heart failure with normal ejection fraction

HIV Human immunodeficiency virus

HJR Hepatojugular reflex

HLHS Hypoplastic left heart syndrome

HOCM Hypertrophic obstructive cardiomyopathy

HoTN Hypotension

HR Heart rate

HRCT High-resolution computed tomography

HR$_{max}$ Maximal heart rate (= MHR)

HRR Heart rate reserve

hs-CRP High-sensitivity C-reactive protein

HSCT Hematopoietic stem cell transplant

HTN Hypertension

I & O Intake and output

IABP Intraaortic balloon pump

IC Inspiratory capacity

ICP Intracranial pressure

ICS Intercostal space, inhaled corticosteroid

IE Infective endocarditis

I:E Inspiratory-to-expiratory ratio

IFG Impaired fasting glucose

IGT Impaired glucose tolerance

IHSS Idiopathic hypertrophic subaortic stenosis (now termed HOCM)

ILD Interstitial lung disease

IMV Intermittent mandatory ventilation

INR International normalized ratio (prothrombin time)

IPF Idiopathic pulmonary fibrosis

IPPB Intermittent positive-pressure breathing

IPV Intrapulmonary percussive ventilation

IRBBB Incomplete right bundle-branch block

IRV Inspiratory reserve volume

IS Incentive spirometry

ISA Intrinsic sympathomimetic activity

IV Intravenous

IVCD Intraventricular conduction delay

IVS Interventricular septum

JBD Jugular venous distension

LA Left atrium

LABAs Long-acting β$_2$-agonists

LAD Left anterior descending (coronary artery), left axis deviation

LAE Left atrial enlargement

LAH(B) Left anterior hemiblock

LAO Left anterior oblique

LAP Left atrial pressure

LBBB Left bundle-branch block

LDH Lactate dehydrogenase

LDL Low-density lipoproteins

LIMA Left internal mammary artery (for CAB surgery)

LLL Left lower lobe

LM(CA) Left main (coronary artery)

LMWH Low-molecular weight heparin

Lp(a) Lipoprotein(a) (type of LDL particle)

LPH(B) Left posterior hemiblock

LTOT Long-term oxygen therapy

LTx Lung transplantation

LUL Left upper lobe

LV Left ventricle

LVAD Left ventricular assist device

LVEDP Left ventricular end-diastolic pressure

LVEDV Left ventricular end-diastolic volume

LVEF Left ventricular ejection fraction

LVESV Left ventricular end-systolic volume

LVET Left ventricular ejection time

LVH Left ventricular hypertrophy

LVOT Left ventricular outflow tract

LVRS Lung volume reduction surgery

LVSWI Left ventricular stroke work index

ⓜ Heart murmur

MAP Mean arterial pressure

MAS Meconium aspiration syndrome

MB Myocardial band (isoenzyme of creatine kinase)

MCL Midclavicular line

MDCT Multidetector-row computed tomography

MDI Metered-dose inhaler

MEP Maximal expiratory pressure

MET(s) Metabolic equivalent of energy expenditure

MetS Metabolic syndrome

MH Manual hyperinflation

MHR Maximal heart rate (= HR$_{max}$)

MHRR Maximal heart rate reserve

MI Myocardial infarction

MIDCAB Minimally-invasive coronary artery bypass (surgery)

MI-E Mechanical insufflator-exsufflator

MIF Maximal inspiratory flow

MIP Maximal inspiratory pressure

MMFR Maximal midexpiratory flow rate (FEF 25%–75%)

MPS(PECT) Myocardial perfusion SPECT

MR Mitral regurgitation

MRA Magnetic resonance angiography

MRI or MRS Magnetic resonance imaging/spectroscopy

MS Mitral stenosis

MSCT Multislice spiral computed tomography

MUGA Multiunit gated acquisition scan (= GBPS, RNA)

MV̇O$_2$ Myocardial oxygen consumption

MV Mitral valve

MVP Mitral valve prolapse

MVR Mitral valve replacement

MVV Maximal voluntary ventilation

NO Nitric oxide

np Nasal prongs

npo Nil/non per os (nothing by mouth)

NPPV Noninvasive positive pressure ventilation

NSAIDs Nonsteroidal anti-inflammatory drugs

NSCLC Non-small cell lung cancer

NSR Normal sinus rhythm

NSTEMI Non-ST elevation myocardial infarction

NT Nasotracheal

NTG Nitroglycerin (= TNG)

O$_2$ Oxygen

O$_2$ sat Oxygen saturation (= Sao$_2$)

OGTT Oral glucose tolerance test

OMC Open mitral commissurotomy

OPEP Oscillatory positive expiratory pressure (breathing)

OSA Obstructive sleep apnea

PA Pulmonary artery

PAC Premature atrial complex/contraction (= APC)

PACAB Port-access coronary artery bypass (surgery) (= PortCAB)

Paco$_2$, Pco$_2$ Partial pressure of (arterial) carbon dioxide

PAD Peripheral arterial disease

PAH Pulmonary arterial hypertension

PA line Pulmonary artery line

P$_{alv}$ Alveolar pressure

P$_{ao}$ Pressure at airway opening

Pao$_2$, Po$_2$ Partial pressure of (arterial) oxygen

PAP Pulmonary artery pressure

PAT Paroxysmal atrial tachycardia

P$_{aw}$ Pressure at any point along airways

PAW(P) Pulmonary artery wedge pressure (= PCW[P])

P$_{bs}$ Pressure at the body surface

PCP Pneumocystis carinii pneumonia (now called PJP)

PCW(P) Pulmonary capillary wedge (pressure) (= PAW[P])

PD Postural drainage, Parkinson's disease

PDA Patent ductus arteriosus, posterior descending artery

PDPV Postural drainage, percussion, and vibration

PE Pulmonary embolus, physical examination

PEEP Positive end-expiratory pressure

PEF(R) Peak expiratory flow (rate)

PEP Preejection period, positive expiratory pressure

P$_{es}$ Esophageal pressure used to estimate P$_{pl}$

PET Positron emission tomography

PFO Patent foramen ovale

PFT(s) Pulmonary function test(s)

PH Pulmonary hypertension (= PAH)

PJP *Pneumocystis jiroveci* pneumonia (formerly PCP)

P$_L$ Transpulmonary pressure (= P$_{alv}$ − P$_{pl}$)

PLB Pursed-lips breathing

pMDI Pressurized metered-dose inhaler

PMI Point of maximal impulse

PND Paroxysmal nocturnal dyspnea

PNS Parasympathetic nervous system

PortCAB Port-access coronary artery bypass (surgery) (= PACAB)

PPH Primary pulmonary hypertension

P$_{pl}$ Pleural pressure

PR Pulmonary regurgitation

PS Pulmonary stenosis

PT Prothrombin time, physical therapy, physical therapist

PTCA Percutaneous transluminal coronary angioplasty

PTS Post thrombotic syndrome

PTT Partial thromboplastin time

PV Pulmonary valve

PVC Premature ventricular complex/contraction (= VPC)

PVR Pulmonary or peripheral vascular resistance

P$_w$ Transthoracic pressure (= P$_{pl}$ − P$_{bs}$)

PWP Pulmonary wedge pressure

Q̇ Volume of blood flow, cardiac output

Q̇s Shunt volume

Q̇s/Q̇t Ratio of shunt volume to total cardiac output

Q̇t Total volume/cardiac output

R, or RER Respiratory exchange ratio (= V̇co$_2$/V̇o$_2$)

RA Right atrium, rheumatoid arthritis

RAAS Renin-angiotensin-aldosterone system

RAD Right axis deviation

RAE Right atrial enlargement

RAO Right anterior oblique

RAP Right atrial pressure

R$_{aw}$ Airway resistance

RBBB Right bundle-branch block

RBC Red blood cell

RCA Right coronary artery

RCM Restrictive cardiomyopathy

RDS Respiratory distress syndrome (infants)

RF Rheumatic fever

RHD Rheumatic heart disease

RHR Resting heart rate

RLD Restrictive lung dysfunction/disease

RLL Right lower lobe

RML Right middle lobe

RNA Radionuclide angiography (= GBPS, MUGA)

RNV Radionuclide ventriculography (= GBPS, RNA)

RPE Rate of perceived exertion

RPP Rate–pressure product

RR Respiratory rate (= *f*)

RRT Renal replacement therapy

RSV Respiratory syncytial virus

RUL Right upper lobe

RV Right ventricle, residual volume

RVAD Right ventricular assist device

RVEDP Right ventricular end-diastolic pressure

RVEDV Right ventricular end-diastolic volume

RVH Right ventricular hypertrophy

RVOT Right ventricular outflow tract

RV/TLC Percentage of total lung capacity taken by the residual volume

S$_1$ First heart sound

S$_2$ Second heart sound

S$_3$ Third heart sound

S$_4$ Fourth heart sound

S & S Signs and symptoms

SA Sinoatrial

SAM Systolic anterior motion (re: anterior mitral valve leaflet)

Sao$_2$ Oxygen saturation (= O$_2$ sat)

SBE Subacute bacterial endocarditis (= IE)

SBP Systolic blood pressure

SCD Sickle cell disease

SCI Spinal cord injury

SCLC Small cell lung cancer

SEM Systolic ejection murmur

SGOT Serum glutamic-oxaloacetic transaminase (= AST)

SGPT Serum glutamic-pyruvic transaminase (= ALT)

SIMV Synchronous intermittent mandatory ventilation

SLE Systemic lupus erythematosus

SLTx Single lung transplantation

SNIP Sniff nasal inspiratory pressure

SNS Sympathetic nervous system

SPECT Single photon emission computed tomography

SSc Systemic sclerosis (scleroderma)

ST ST segment of the electro-cardiogram (ECG)

STEMI ST elevation myocardial infardion

SV Stroke volume

SVR Systemic vascular resistance

SVT Supraventricular tachycardia

SWI Stroke work index

TAH Total artificial heart, total abdominal hysterectomy

TC/HDL Total-to-HDL cholesterol ratio

TDI Tissue Doppler imaging

TEE Transesophageal echocardiography, thoracic expansion exercises

TEF Tracheoesophageal fistula

TGA Transposition of the great arteries

TGs Triglycerides

TI Tricuspid insufficiency

TIA Transient ischemic attack

TLC Total lung capacity

TMT Treadmill test

TNG Trinitroglycerin (= NTG)

TOF Tetralogy of Fallot

TPA Tissue plasminogen activator (or tPA)

TPR Total peripheral resistance

TR Tricuspid regurgitation

TS Tricuspid stenosis

TTI Tension–time index

TV Tricuspid valve

TVR Tricuspid valve replacement

UFH Unfractionated heparin

UIP Usual interstitial pneumonia

URI Upper respiratory infection

$\dot{V}$ Minute ventilation

$\dot{V}_A$ Alveolar ventilation

VAD Ventricular assist device

VC Vital capacity

VCG Vectorcardiogram

$\dot{V}_{CO_2}$ Volume of carbon dioxide produced per minute

V_D Dead space volume

V_D/V_T Dead space to tidal volume ratio

$\dot{V}_E$ Minute ventilation, expiratory

VEA Ventricular ectopic activity

v-fib, VF Ventricular fibrillation

VLDL Very-low-density lipoprotein

$\dot{V}_{O_2}$ Oxygen consumption or uptake (total body) per minute

$\dot{V}_{O_{2max}}$ Maximal oxygen consumption or uptake

VPB Ventricular premature beat

VPC Ventricular premature complex/contraction (= PVC)

VPIs Vasopeptidase inhibitors

$\dot{V}/\dot{Q}$ Ventilation–perfusion ratio

VSD Ventricular septal defect

V_T Tidal volume

v-tach, VT Ventricular tachycardia

VTE Venous thromboembolism

WBC White blood cell

WC Waist circumference

WHR Waist-to-hip ratio

WOB Work of breathing

WPW Wolff-Parkinson-White syndrome

XRT Radiation therapy

Glossary

A or a wave The rise in the atrial pressure curve caused by active contraction of the atria

Accessory atrioventricular pathways Internodal tracts or bundles arising from fine terminal branches that allow electrical impulses traveling from the atria to bypass the atrioventricular node and propogate reentry tachyarrhythmias

ACE inhibitors See angiotensin converting enzyme inhibitors

Acetylcholine A chemical neurotransmitter released from the preganglionic and postganglionic endings of parasympathetic nerve fibers and from the preganglionic endings of sympathetic fibers, which causes cardiac inhibition, vasodilation, gastrointestinal peristalsis, and other parasympathetic effects

Acetylcholinesterase An enzyme that catalyzes the hydrolysis of acetylcholine and thus controls its effect

Acidemia A decrease in the pH of the blood to less than normal due to an increase in hydrogen ion concentration

Acidosis A disorder of normal acid–base balance resulting from accumulation of acid (hydrogen ion) or reduction of base (bicarbonate) in the blood or tissues

Acinus The portion of the lung distal to the terminal bronchiole comprising respiratory bronchioles, alveolar ducts, alveolar sacs, and alveoli

Adipocytes Fat cells

Adrenergic Related to epinephrine (adrenaline) or substances with similar activity; pertaining to or affecting the sympathetic nervous system

Adventitia The innermost layer of connective tissue of an artery or vein; tunica adventitia

Adventitious breath sounds Abnormal sounds heard on auscultation that are superimposed over normal breath sounds

Aerobic Relating to the use of oxygen to produce energy

Afterload The load or pressure against which the ventricle must exert its contraction force to eject blood

Airway reactivity Alteration of bronchomotor tone in response to noxious stimuli

Airway resistance (R_{aw}) The force opposing the flow of gases during ventilation; results from obstruction or turbulence in the upper and lower airways

Akinesis Lack of movement; in cardiology, lack of movement of an area of myocardium

Aldosterone A steroid hormone produced by the kidneys that affects resorption of sodium and excretion of hydrogen and potassium

Alkalemia An increase in the pH of the blood above normal, resulting from a decrease in hydrogen ion concentration

Alkalosis A disorder of normal acid–base balance resulting from excessive accumulation of base (bicarbonate) or loss of acid (hydrogen ion)

Alpha sympatholytic A drug that inhibits alpha-adrenergic receptors of the autonomic nervous system

Alveolar ventilation ($\dot{V}A$) The volume of inspired air that participates in gas exchange

Alveolitis Inflammation of the alveoli

Alveolus The terminal sac-like dilations of the alveolar ducts in the lungs where alveolar air comes into contact with the pulmonary capillary blood for gas exchange

Amyloidosis A group of diseases resulting from the abnormal deposition of amyloid proteins in organs and/or tissues, such as the heart, kidneys, nervous system, and gastrointestinal system

Anaerobic Relating to the production of energy without the use of oxygen

Anaerobic threshold (AT) The onset of blood lactate accumulation that occurs as exercise intensity increases beyond the level that can be met by predominantly aerobic metabolism; also called *ventilator threshold* because of the resultant stimulation of increased ventilation

Anemia An abnormally low number of red cells in the blood

Aneurysm An area of muscular weakness and dilation occurring in an artery or cardiac chamber

Angina, angina pectoris Pain, pressure, or heaviness, occurring usually in the chest or surrounding areas, which is caused by insufficient myocardial oxygen supply

Angiography Radiologic examination of blood vessels injected with contrast medium

Antibody A class of immunoglobulins capable of attacking invading antigens

Antidiuretic hormone (ADH) A hormone, secreted by the pituitary gland, that causes the kidneys to retain water and in high concentrations causes contraction of vascular smooth muscle; also known as vasopressin

Antigen Any substance capable of causing the production of antibodies

Antihistamine A drug that inhibits the action of histamine

Antimicrobial A substance that destroys or prevents the growth or action of microbes

Antitussive A drug that inhibits or relieves coughing

Apex of the heart The conical extremity of the heart formed by the left ventrical

Apgar score A 10-point scoring system used to assess the status of newborns (heart rate, respiratory effort, muscle tone, response to stimulation, and skin color); usually performed at 1 and 5 minutes after birth

Apnea Absence of breathing; a temporary cessation of breathing

Apoptosis Programmed cell death

Arrhythmia Absence or irregularity of cardiac rhythm

Arrhythmogenic Capable of producing arrhythmias

Arteriosclerosis Hardening of the arteries

Arteriovenous oxygen difference [$(a–v)o_2$] The difference between the oxygen content of arterial blood and mixed venous blood; represents the extent to which oxygen is removed from the blood as it circulates through the body

Ascites Abnormal accumulation of fluid in the peritoneal cavity

Asthma A lung disease characterized by recurring episodes of airway narrowing due to bronchoconstriction, mucosal inflammation, and overproduction of viscous mucus induced by various stimuli or triggers

Atelectasis   Collapse and airlessness of alveoli

Atherosclerosis   Disease process characterized by irregularly distributed, progressive narrowing of large- and medium-sized arteries

Atrial gallop   The triple cadence of heart sounds caused by the presence of a late diastolic (presystolic) fourth heart sound (S_4) in addition to the normal first and second heart sounds

Atrioventricular (AV) block   Delayed or interrupted conduction of the electrical impulse as it passes from the atria through the atrioventricular node to the ventricles; also called *heart block*

Automaticity   The ability of a cell to initiate its own depolarization

Autonomic neuropathy   Abnormal function of the autonomic nervous system

Baroreceptors   Sensory nerve endings located in the walls of the auricles of the heart, vena cavae, aortic arch, and carotid sinuses that are sensitive to stretch provoked by increased pressure

Barotrauma   Injury caused by excessively high or low pressure (e.g., of the lungs due to high inspiratory pressures during mechanical ventilation)

Beta (β)-Adrenergic blocker   A substance that selectively inhibits or blocks β-adrenergic (sympathetic nervous system) stimulation of effector cells

Bicarbonate   A major buffer substance in the blood; HCO_3^-

Bigeminal   Extrasystoles occurring every other beat, as when either atrial or ventricular complexes occur between sinus beats

Bleb   Coalescent alveolar sacs formed from the destruction of alveolar septa, as in emphysema

Borg Scale   A numeric scale for rating perceived exertion

Bradycardia   A slow heart rate, usually defined as less than 60 beats per minute

Bradykinin   A potent vasodilator found in the blood that mediates the inflammatory response to tissue injury; stimulates nitric oxide and prostacyclin production

Bradypnea   An abnormal slowing of respiration

Bronchial breath sounds   The sounds normally heard when auscultating over the large bronchi, which have an inspiratory to expiratory ratio of 1:1; an abnormal sound when heard over the peripheral lung tissue

Bronchiectasis   A lung disease characterized by dilation and distortion of the bronchial and bronchiolar walls as the result of chronic inflammation or obstruction

Bronchiolitis   Inflammation of the bronchioles

Bronchitis   Inflammation of the airways

Bronchoconstriction   A reduction in the luminal caliber of a bronchus

Bronchodilator   A medication that relieves bronchoconstriction and thereby increases the lumenal diameter of the bronchi

Bronchophony   Louder, distinct voice transmission heard over areas of consolidated lung tissue

Bulla   A thin-walled, air-filled cavity larger than 1 cm in diameter resulting from destruction of alveolar septa

Capacitance vessels   The large venules and veins that form a large, variable-volume, and low-pressure reservoir

Cardiac ablation   Destruction of very small areas of cardiac tissue that propogate tachyarrhythmias; most commonly performed using radiofrequency energy (radiofrequency ablation) or intense cold (cryoablation)

Cardiac index   Cardiac output divided by body surface area ($L/min/m^2$)

Cardiac output   The amount of blood pumped from the heart each minute

Cardiac reserve   The difference between resting cardiac output and the maximal cardiac output of an individual

Cardiac tamponade   See "Pericardial tamponade"

Cardiogenic shock   A condition in which the heart is unable to pump enough cardiac output to perfuse the body tissues

Cardiomegaly   Enlargement of the heart

Cardiomyopathy   Any primary disease of the heart muscle

Cardiovascular reserve   The difference between the normal resting cardiac output and the maximal cardiac output of an individual, which is effected by increases in heart rate and stroke volume and all of the factors that determine each

Cardioversion   Restoration of the normal rhythm of the heart by electrical countershock

Carina   Specifically in the pulmonary system, the ridge separating the openings of the right and left main bronchi at their junction with the trachea

Catecholamine   Any of the compounds secreted by the adrenal medulla that affect the sympathetic nervous system

Chemoreceptor reflex   An increase in the depth and rate of ventilation in response to a lack of oxygen; it also influences heart rate

Cholinergic   Relating to nerve fibers that secrete acetylcholine; pertaining to or affecting the parasympathetic nervous system

Chordae tendineae   Fibrous cords that attach the leaflets of the heart valves to the papillary muscles and myocardium

Chronotropic   Affecting the heart rate

Chronotropic incompetence   Failure of the normal rate regulating mechanisms of the heart such that heart rate fails to increase normally with exertion

Chylomicron   A complex composed of lipid and protein that transports the water-insoluble lipids in the blood from the intestines to storage sites

Cilia   Hairlike projections from respiratory epithelial cells that propel mucus and debris toward the pharynx

Closing volume   The lung volume at which small airway closure begins during expiration

Clubbing   A proliferative change in the soft tissues of the distal fingers and toes, especially the nailbeds, with broadening, loss of the base angle at the cuticle, and increased curvature, giving a bulbous appearance

Collateral circulation   Secondary or accessory branches of blood vessels that develop in response to progressive narrowing of primary blood vessels to increase circulation

Commissurotomy   A surgical division of the junction between adjacent cusps of a cardiac valve

Compensatory pause   The suspension or delay of cardiac electrical activity that may occur following an extrasystole

Compliance   A measure of the distensibility of a tissue (i.e., increase in volume per unit of pressure change); regarding patients, adherence to prescribed medical treatment, lifestyle modifications, and so on

Congestion   Excessive accumulation of blood in the vessels of an organ

Consolidation   Solidification of a normally aerated portion of a lung, resulting from the presence of exudative fluid and cells in the alveolar spaces

Contractility   The ability of tissue, especially muscle, to shorten and develop tension; in the heart, the innate rate and intensity of force development during contraction

Coronary artery disease   Progressive narrowing of the coronary arteries by atherosclerotic plaque which causes limitation of blood flow

Coronary heart disease   Heart disease caused by coronary artery disease

Cor pulmonale   Right-sided heart failure due to pulmonary hypertension resulting from acute or chronic pulmonary disease

Coryza   Rhinitis with nasal discharge (runny nose) due to the common cold or an allergy

Costophrenic   Pertaining to the ribs and diaphragm, as in the angle between the rib cage and diaphragm on a chest radiograph

Couplet   A pair of atrial or ventricular extrasystoles

Crackles   Adventitious breath sounds heard over areas where there is fluid accumulation in the distal airways, or over collapsed alveoli, which partially reopen during inspiration; rales

Creatine phosphate   An intracellular high-energy phosphate compound that supplies the phosphate for the formation of ATP from ADP; phosphocreatine

Creatine phosphokinase (CPK)   An enzyme that catalyzes the transfer of phosphate from phosphocreatine to ADP; creatine kinase (CK)

Croup   A condition resulting from acute inflammation of laryngeal structures, causing a characteristic barking cough

Cuirass   A type of negative-pressure mechanical ventilator that covers the anterior chest wall

Cyanosis   Bluish or purple discoloration of the skin and mucous membranes as a result of insufficient oxygenation with a high concentration of reduced hemoglobin in the capillaries

Cystic fibrosis   An inherited disease affecting fluid transfer in the exocrine glands, including the sweat, pancreatic, and pulmonary mucous glands

Decongestant   A drug that reduces congestion, particularly of the mucosa of the upper respiratory tract

Decortication   Removal of the cortex or external layer, usually applied to a surgical excision of residual clot and/or newly organized scar tissue that form after a hemothorax or empyema

Decreased breath sounds   Abnormally quiet breath sounds, caused by reduced ventilation or hyperinflation

Decubitus   Side-lying position

Defibrillation   Electrical shock of sufficient power to cause a fibrillating heart to resume normal rhythm

Dehiscence   Splitting open of a surgical wound

Depolarization   Loss of a negative charge in muscle cells as ions shift across the cell membranes to produce muscle contraction

Desaturate   To produce desaturation, an increase in the percentage of unfilled oxygen-binding sites on the hemoglobin molecule

Dialysis   A form of filtration that separates the smaller molecules in a solution from the larger ones through the use of a semipermeable membrane

Diaphoresis   Perspiration, sweat

Diastole   The period of ventricular relaxation in the cardiac cycle

Diastolic blood pressure (DBP)   The lowest arterial blood pressure reached during a given cardiac cycle; occurs during ventricular relaxation

Diffusion   The passive tendency of molecules to move from an area of higher concentration to one of lower concentration, as in the movement of oxygen into and carbon dioxide out of the blood in the pulmonary capillaries

Dilated cardiomyopathy   A disease of the myocardium characterized by ventricular dilitation and impaired contractile function

Diuretic   Any agent that increases the amount of urine production and thereby decreases blood volume

Dopaminergic   Relating to those nerves or receptor sites that employ dopamine as their neurotransmitter

Dysarthria   A disturbance in articulation; usually due to brain injury or paralysis

Dyskinesis   Difficult or abnormal movement; in cardiology, abnormal paradoxic movement of an area of myocardium

Dysphagia   Pain and/or difficulty in swallowing

Dyspnea   A subjective sense of difficulty or distress in breathing; shortness of breath

Ectopy   Abnormal or aberrant origination of myocardial depolarization

Effusion   An accumulation of fluid that has escaped from its natural vessels into a body cavity, as in pleural or pericardial effusion

Egophony   Abnormal vocal transmission over areas of pulmonary consolidation characterized by the auscultation of $\bar{a}$ when the vowel sound $\bar{e}$ is spoken

Ejection fraction (EF)   The portion of filling volume that is ejected from the ventricle during systole (i.e., stroke volume/end-diastolic volume)

Electrolyte   Any substance that ionizes in solution and thus conducts electricity and is decomposed by it

Electromechanical coupling   The coupling of electrical activity in the heart and the subsequent mechanical events of myocardial contraction to produce cardiac output

Electromechanical dissociation   The presence of electrical activity in the heart without effective mechanical function; also termed pulseless electrical activity (PEA)

Electron transport chain   A series of oxidation-reduction reactions occurring in the mitochondria through which the hydrogen ions released during glycolysis and the citric acid cycle are eventually transferred to oxygen to produce energy for the phosphorylation of ADP to form ATP

Embolism   Occlusion of a blood vessel by matter carried by the blood flow from another site

Embolus   Undissolved matter (e.g., thrombus, vegetation, mass of bacteria, tumor) lodged in a vessel

Emphysema   A chronic obstructive pulmonary disease characterized by abnormal, permanent enlargement of the air spaces distal to the terminal bronchioles and destruction of alveolar walls

Empyema   Accumulation of pus in a body cavity, commonly the pleural space

End-diastolic volume   The amount of blood in the ventricles at the end of ventricular filling

Endocarditis   Inflammation of the endocardium

Endocardium   The innermost layer of the heart

Endothelium   The thin layer of cells that line the interior surface of the blood vessels, which are involved in many aspects of vascular biology, including vasoconstriction/vasodilation, inflammation, blood clotting, and atherogenesis

End-systolic volume   The amount of blood remaining in the ventricles at the end of ventricular contraction

Epicardium   The outermost layer of the heart; the visceral part of the pericardium (visceral pericardium), which produces the pericardial fluid

Epiglottitis   Inflammation of the epiglottis, the cartilage that protects the trachea from aspirating foodstuff during the normal swallowing process

Epinephrine A catecholamine that is the major neurotransmitter of the sympathetic nervous system, which stimulates alpha- and beta-adrenergic receptors

Ergometer A device of known calibration that measures the amount of work, or exercise, performed

Exacerbation An increase in the severity of the signs and symptoms of a disease

Exercise-induced asthma Airway narrowing triggering by exercise or high levels of ventilation for 5 – 7 minutes in individuals who have asthma (also called *exercise-induced bronchoconstriction*)

Exercise tolerance The maximal level of physical exertion an individual can perform before exhaustion, which is limited by the capacity of his or her oxygen transport system to provide oxygen

Expectoration The act of coughing up and spitting out materials from the lungs

Extracorporeal membrane oxygenation (ECMO) The use of an artificial membrane outside the body to provide oxygenation of the blood

Extrasystoles A premature cardiac depolarization that arises from an impulse outside the sinoatrial node, which is usually followed by a compensatory pause

Exudate Any fluid that gradually oozes out of a body tissue because of abnormal leakage, as in inflammation

Fibrosis The reactive or reparative process in which fibrous tissue is formed

Fibrothorax A chronic pleural disease characterized by formation of thick fibrous tissue and adhesion of the two layers of pleura

Fick method (principle) A method of determining cardiac output (L/min) by dividing the oxygen consumption (ml/min) by the difference between the arterial and mixed-venous blood oxygen content (ml/L)

FIO_2 The fraction of inspired oxygen; the portion of an inhaled mixture of gases that is oxygen

Fissure A clearly discernible division in lung tissue that separates two lobes of the lungs

Foramen ovale In the fetus, the oval opening in the interatrial septum secundum; normally it closes soon after birth

Foramen secundum In the fetus, the opening in the dorsal part of the septum primum that forms before the septum fuses with the endocardial cushions

Fremitus A vibration within the thorax that is felt by palpation

Fulminant Suddenly occurring

Functional capacity Another term for exercise capacity that refers specifically to the ability or power to perform particular activities

Functional residual capacity (FRC) The sum of the expiratory reserve and residual volumes, or the amount of air remaining in the lungs after a normal tidal exhalation

Glottis The fissure between the vocal cords

Glucagon A pancreatic hormone that stimulates the release of glycogen from the liver and so acts to raise blood glucose level

Gluconeogenesis The formation of glycogen from protein or fat

Glycogenesis The process of synthesizing glycogen from glucose

Glycogenolysis The process by which glycogen is broken down to glucose-1-phosphate

Glycolysis The metabolic pathway where glucose in broken down anaerobically to produce energy (ATP) and hydrogen ions, which then enter the electron transport chain to produce additional ATP

Glycosylated hemoglobin (Hb A_{1c}) Hemoglobin bound with glucose and related monosaccharides, which reflects the average blood glucose level over the preceding 2 to 3 months, serving as an indicator of diabetes control

Granulation The formation of minute, rounded connective tissue projections that occurs on the surface of a lesion during healing

Granuloma Nodular inflammatory lesions composed of modified macrophages

Heart failure A condition in which cardiac dysfunction impairs the ability of the heart to pump sufficient cardiac output to meet the body's needs at rest

Heart rate variability Assessment of the variations in heart rate by measuring the regularity between ECG complexes that occur in response to specific activities (e.g., deep breathing or position change from supine to standing) or over a 2-to-5 minute period of time; provides an indication of cardiovascular risk

Hemidiaphragm One of the two domes of the diaphragm

Hemopneumothorax The presence of blood and air in the pleural cavity

Hemoptysis The expectoration of blood from the lungs because of pulmonary or bronchial hemorrhage

Hemothorax The presence of blood in the pleural cavity

Hepatomegaly Abnormally enlarged liver

Hibernating myocardium Contractile dysfunction of a region of myocardium, manifested as a regional wall motion abnormality, resulting from prolonged ischemia

High-density lipoprotein (HDL) The major class of lipoproteins containing approximately 50% protein and lower levels of cholesterol and triglycerides than low-density lipoproteins and very low-density lipoproteins

Hilus The point at which the nerves, vessels, and primary bronchi penetrate the parenchyma of each lung

Honeycombing On chest x-ray film, a coarse reticular density

Huffing A cough assistance technique in which forced expiration is performed with an open glottis to assist in the expectoration of secretions

Hyaline membrane An eosinophilic membrane lining the alveolar ducts of infants suffering from respiratory distress syndrome

Hypercapnia The presence of an abnormally high amount of carbon dioxide in the circulating blood; hypercarbia

Hyperkalemia An abnormally high potassium ion concentration in the circulating blood

Hypernatremia An abnormally high sodium ion concentration in the plasma

Hyperpnea Rapid, shallow breathing

Hyperreactive airways Airway narrowing resulting from increased responsiveness of bronchial smooth muscle to inhaled allergens and other irritants, seen in asthma

Hypersomnolence A condition of drowsiness approaching coma

Hypertension (HTN) Elevated blood pressure of 140/90 or greater

Hypertensive heart disease Myocardial dysfunction resulting from chronic high blood pressure

Hypertrophic cardiomyopathy A disesase of the myocardium characterized by excessive hypertrophy of portions of the heart (often the left ventricle) without any obvious cause accompanied by normal or even enhanced contractile function

Hyperventilation Increased alveolar ventilation relative to metabolic carbon dioxide production so that arterial carbon dioxide level is lower than normal

Hypoadaptive Failure to achieve normal responses of any physiologic system

Hypocapnia Abnormally reduced arterial carbon dioxide level; hypocarbia

Hypokalemia An abnormally low potassium ion concentration in the circulating blood

Hypokinesis Reduced movement; in cardiology, reduced wall motion of an area of myocardium

Hyponatremia An abnormally low sodium ion concentration in the plasma

Hypotension Abnormally low arterial blood pressure or a fall in arterial blood pressure with an increase in exertion or heart rate

Hypoventilation Inadequate alveolar ventilation relative to carbon dioxide production so that arterial carbon dioxide levels are increased

Hypoxemia Abnormally low arterial oxygen levels in the blood

Hypoxia Subnormal levels of oxygen in inspired gas, arterial blood, or tissues

Idiopathic Of unknown origin or cause

Idiopathic hypertrophic subaortic stenosis (IHSS) Obstruction of the left ventricular outflow tract due to hypertrophy of the left ventricular septum; now called hypertrophic obstructive cardiomyopathy

Idiopathic pulmonary fibrosis A progressive interstitial lung disease of unknown etiology

Immunodeficiency A state of defective immune response, either humoral or cellular

Immunoglobulin (Ig) Circulating antibodies that protect the body from foreign substances

Immunosuppression A reduction in the activation or efficiency of an immunologic response

Infarction A condition in which a localized area of tissue death (necrosis) results from interruption of its blood supply

Inflammation A complex biologic response of vascular tissues to injury or foreign substances, which acts to protect the tissue by removing the injurious stimuli and initiating the healing process

Inotrope An agent that influences the contractility of muscular tissue

Intercurrent Occurring during the course of an existing process

Intermittent claudication An attack of pain or lameness, usually in the calf, caused by muscle ischemia (most commonly because of atherosclerosis)

Interpolated Occurring or inserted between two other things

Interstitial Situated between essential parts or in the interspaces of a tissue

Intima The innermost layer of a vascular wall; tunica intima

Intubation The insertion of a hollow tube through the nose or mouth into the trachea, usually for the purpose of providing assisted ventilation

Ischemia Inadequate oxygenation of a tissue relative to its demands

Isocapnia A state in which the arterial carbon dioxide tension remains constant or unchanged, despite changes in ventilation

Isovolumic contraction The early systolic phase of the cardiac cycle in which the ventricles are contracting and generating an increase in ventricular pressure without any change in ventricular volume because all cardiac valves are closed

Isovolumic relaxation The phase of the cardiac cycle immediately following aortic valve closure and continuing until the mitral valve opens in which the ventricles are relaxing and the ventricular pressure falls below atrial pressure without a change in ventricular volume

Jugular venous distention (JVD) Stretching or overfilling of the jugular vein, usually due to elevated venous pressure

Junctional rhythm The rhythm of the heart when the atrioventricular node takes over as the predominant pacemaker; nodal rhythm

Kerley B lines Seen on chest radiography, fine horizontal lines a few centimeters above the costophrenic angle, which are caused by perivascular interstitial edema

Korotkoff sounds Sounds heard over an artery when pressure over it is reduced during the determination of blood pressure by the auscultatory method

Kussmaul breathing Deep, rapid respiration characteristic of diabetes or other causes of acidosis

Laryngospasm An involuntary muscular contraction that results in closure of the glottis

Left-to-right shunt A diversion of blood from the left side of the heart to the right or from the systemic circulation to the pulmonary circulation

Lipoprotein A complex of fat and protein which allows lipids to be transported in the blood; the higher the amount of fat in the complex, the lower the density

Lobectomy Surgical resection of a lobe of the lungs

Low-density lipoprotein (LDL) A major class of lipoproteins having a relatively high molecular weight and containing proportionally less protein and more cholesterol and triglycerides than high-density lipoproteins

Manubrium The upper portion of the sternum

Maximal oxygen consumption (VO$_{2max}$) The maximal rate at which oxygen is utilized for energy production (i.e., oxygen consumption fails to increase despite an increase in exercise intensity); a quantitative measure of an individual's maximal aerobic capacity

Meconium The first stool passed by a newborn

Media The middle layer, as in the layer of a blood vessel between the intima and the adventitia

Median sternotomy An incision through the chest wall through the midline of the sternum

Mediastinal shift A shifting of the mediastinum to one side as a result of lower pressure in one hemithorax compared with the other (e.g., displacement away from a tension pneumothorax or toward an atelectatic segment)

Mediastinum The area of the thoracic cavity containing the structures between the lungs

Mediate percussion The act of tapping on the surface of the chest, using one middle finger over the other, to evaluate the resonance of the underlying structures

Melanoptysis Expectoration of black sputum, as in coal workers' pneumoconiosis

MET The abbreviation for metabolic equivalent of energy expenditure; the amount of energy or oxygen required to perform particular tasks relative to that required at rest

Metabolic acidosis A decreased level of arterial bicarbonate and pH as the result of metabolic pathological conditions

Metabolic alkalosis An elevated level of arterial bicarbonate and pH as the result of metabolic pathological conditions

Methylxanthines A class of drugs (e.g., aminophylline) that have bronchodilator and cardiac and CNS stimulant properties

Microatelectasis Airlessness of a very small part of the lungs caused by resorption of gas from collapsed or blocked alveoli

Midsystolic click A clicking sound heard on auscultation of the heart that is associated with systolic prolapse of the mitral valve leaflets

Mitral valve prolapse An abnormality of mitral valve function characterized by bulging of one or both of the mitral valve leaflets into the left atrium beyond the mitral annular plane during ventricular systole

Mucociliary transport The process of removal of mucus and debris from the airways by way of the wavelike motion of the cilia

Mucokinetic Relating to an agent capable of enhancing the mobilization of secretions

Mucolytic Capable of dissolving, digesting, or liquefying mucus

Mucopurulent Containing both mucus and pus

M$\dot{V}O_2$ Myocardial oxygen consumption

Myocardial infarction Necrosis of an area of heart muscle caused by sudden insufficient or interrupted blood flow

Myocarditis Inflammation of the muscular walls of the heart

Myocardium The muscular middle layer of tissue in the heart; also used in general reference to the heart

Myocytes Muscle cells

Myxoma A benign tumor derived from endocardial connective tissue, usually located within the left atrium

Nares Nostrils

Natriuresis The urinary excretion of sodium; commonly designated enhanced sodium excretion, as in certain diseases or resulting from diuretic therapy

Neurotransmitter A chemical substance released by a presynaptic neuron that diffuses across the synapse to bind to receptors on the post-synaptic cell where it relays, amplifies, or modulates signals between the two cells

Nitric oxide (NO) A chemical produced by vascular endothelium, respiratory epithelium, and inflammatory cells that is important in the regulation of vascular tone, inflammation, coagulation, and oxidation

Nitroglycerin (NTG) A vasodilating agent, used most often in the treatment of angina pectoris

Norepinephrine A catecholamine hormone that possesses the excitatory actions of epinephrine but has minimal inhibitory effects

Nosocomial Pertaining to or originating in the hospital; usually refers to hospital-acquired infection

Obesity hypoventilation syndrome A syndrome characterized by hypercapnia and acidemia associated with reduced alveolar ventilation secondary to massive obesity

Obstructive (airways/lung) disease Lung disease characterized by chronic airflow limitation, or increased airway resistance, which is particularly noticeable on expiration

Opening snap A diastolic sound heard on auscultation of the heart that is associated with the opening of stenotic atrioventricular valves

Opportunistic infection Infection with microorganisms that do not ordinarily cause disease, occurring in individuals whose immune systems are compromised

Orthopnea Difficulty breathing when lying flat; relieved by a more upright position, as when propped up by additional pillows or sitting

Orthostatic hypotension A fall in blood pressure that occurs with rapid changes to more upright positions

Orthotopic In the normal or usual position, as in heart transplantation where the native heart is removed and the donor heart is positioned in its place

Osteoarthropathy Joint swelling and pain caused by numerous chronic pulmonary infections and other disorders

Overfat An increase in percentage body fat above normal

Overweight An increase in body weight above normal as defined by standard height and weight tables

Oxidative phosphorylation The synthesis of ATP by electron transport in the respiratory chain within the mitochondria

Oximeter An instrument that measures oxygen saturation of arterial blood

Oxygen consumption ($\dot{V}O_2$) The volume of oxygen consumed per minute to produce energy

Oxygen desaturation A reduction in the percentage of arterial hemoglobin bound with oxygen to less than 90% or greater than 4% with respect to resting level, typically experienced during exertion or sleep by individuals with serious lung disease

Oxygen pulse The volume of oxygen consumed or extracted per heart beat

Oxygen saturation (SaO_2) The percentage of hemoglobin that is bound with oxygen

Oxygen toxicity An inflammatory response of various tissues (e.g., eyes, lungs, central nervous system) to prolonged exposure to excessively high concentrations of inspired oxygen

Oxyhemoglobin dissociation The release of oxygen from the hemoglobin molecule in peripheral tissues

Palliative Mitigating; reducing the severity of

Pallor Paleness of the skin

Palpitation A pulsation of the heart that is perceived by an individual

Panacinar or panlobular Involving the entire acinus or lobule of the lung, as in panlobular emphysema

Pancarditis Inflammation of all the structures of the heart

Papillary muscles Projections of cardiac muscle that terminate in the chordae tendineae and anchor the valves

Paradoxical Occurring contrary to the normal rule

Parasympatholytic An agent that inhibits the cholinergic receptors of the autonomic nervous system

Parasympathomimetic An agent that stimulates the cholinergic receptors of the autonomic nervous system

Parenchyma The essential functioning cells of an organ, as opposed to the supporting or connective tissue

Parenteral A means of administering medication other than via the intestinal route (e.g., intravenous, subcutaneous, intramuscular, intraarterial, or intracardiac)

Parietal pleura The serous membrane of the pleural sac that covers the inner surface of the chest wall, the exposed part of the diaphragm, and the mediastinum

Paroxysmal Occurring with a sudden onset and cessation

Paroxysmal nocturnal dyspnea (PND) The sudden onset of shortness of breath that awakens an individual in the middle of sleep, causing the person to sit upright to get relief

Partial thromboplastin time (PTT) The time it takes for a fibrin clot to form after calcium and a phospholipid have been added to a blood sample; activated partial thromboplastin time; evaluates intrinsic, or contact, activation pathway and the common coagulation pathways

Pathophysiology The science of disordered function in disease

Pectoriloquy The transmission of whispered voice sounds to the chest wall

Pectus carinatum Excessive prominence or forward projection of the sternum; pigeon breast

Pectus excavatum Excessive depression or posterior displacement of the sternum; funnel breast

Perfusion Blood flow per unit volume of tissue; in the lungs the blood flow through the pulmonary circulation that is available for gas exchange

Peribronchial In close proximity to or surrounding a bronchus or the bronchi

Pericardial (friction) rub A creaking sound caused by the rubbing together of inflamed pericardial surfaces as the heart contracts and relaxes

Pericardial tamponade Compression of the heart with restriction of ventricular filling due to accumulation of fluid within the pericardial sac; cardiac tamponade

Pericardiectomy Surgical resection of part of the parietal pericardium, usually for relief of constrictive pericarditis

Pericardiocentesis The removal of fluid from the pericardial sac, using a needle

Pericarditis Inflammation of the pericardium

Pericardium The fibroserous membrane surrounding the heart and the origins of the great vessels

Periodic respirations Alternating periods of hyperpnea and apnea

Pertussis An acute inflammation of the larynx, trachea, and bronchi characterized by recurrent bouts of exhaustive spasmodic coughing that ends in stridor; whooping cough

Petechiae Pinpoint bright red or purplish discolorations of skin or mucous membrane caused by intradermal bleeding

Physiologic dead space Areas of the lungs that are ventilated but not perfused, so there is no gas exchange; includes anatomic dead space and alveolar dead space ventilation

Pleura The serous membrane enveloping the lungs and lining the chest wall

Pleural effusion An accumulation of fluid in the pleural space

Pleural rub Inspiratory and expiratory grating, creaking sounds heard on auscultation that result from pleural inflammation

Pleurectomy Surgical resection of the pleura, usually the parietal pleura

Pleurisy Inflammation of the pleura; pleuritis

Pleurodesis Creation of an adhesion between the parietal and visceral pleurae by surgical or medical means

Plethysmograph An airtight chamber into which an individual is placed to measure various pulmonary function values

Pneumatocele A thin-walled cavity within the lung; characteristic of staphylococcal pneumonia

Pneumoconiosis An inflammatory fibrosis of the lungs due to the inhalation of dust particles, usually from occupational exposure

Pneumomediastinum Air within the mediastinal tissues

Pneumonectomy Surgical resection of an entire lung

Pneumonia An inflammation of the lungs, particularly as a result of a pathogen

Pneumothorax Air within the pleural space

Polycythemia An abnormally high number of red cells in the blood, which usually develops as compensation for chronic hypoxemia

Postperfusion syndrome A condition of decreased cardiac output in conjunction with other cardiovascular symptoms that arise after using a perfusion pump (e.g., cardiopulmonary bypass machine) during cardiovascular surgical procedures

Postpericardiotomy syndrome The occurrence, often repeatedly, of the symptoms of pericarditis, with or without febrile episodes, weeks or months after cardiac surgery

Postural drainage The use of gravity and positioning to facilitate the removal of secretions from the airways

Postural hypotension Low blood pressure that develops on assumption of upright postures; orthostatic hypotension

Prediabetes A condition characterized by higher than normal blood glucose levels, but not high enough to be diagnostic of type 2 diabetes mellitus (i.e., fasting blood glucose of 100 to <126 mg/dl or blood glucose response to an oral glucose tolerance test of 140 to <200 mg/dl)

Preinfarction angina Severe constricting chest pain, often radiating from the precordium, that often precedes a myocardial infarction

Preload The resting tension or stretch on the myocardial cells, which correlates with the volume of blood in the ventricle just before systole; the end-diastolic volume

Preprandial Before a meal

Pressor An agent that enhances vasomotor tone and increases blood pressure

Prinzmetal's angina See "Variant angina"

Proarrhythmic Capable of precipitating a new or more frequent occurrence of pre-existing arrhythmias; typically a paradoxical reaction to an antiarrhythmic drug

Prodromal An early or premonitory symptom of a disease or disease-related event

Prophylactic A measure taken to prevent disease or an unwanted consequence

Prostaglandins One of a number of physiologically active hormone-like substances that participate in a wide range of body functions, including vasodilation and vasoconstriction, contraction and relaxation of smooth muscle (e.g., intestinal, uterine, or bronchial), control of blood pressure, and modulation of inflammation

Prothrombin time (PT) The time it takes plasma to form a fibrin clot after calcium and thromboplastin are added to the blood; evaluates extrinsic pathway of coagulation

Prothombotic Clot forming

Pulmonary (vascular) congestion The presence of an excessive volume of blood in the pulmonary vasculature

Pulmonary edema The presence of an excessive amount of fluid in the interstitial and alveolar spaces of the lungs

Pulmonary embolism A blockage of blood flow through a pulmonary artery, usually by a blood clot

Pulmonary vascular resistance (PVR) The resistance to blood flow that must be overcome to pump blood through the pulmonary vasculature

Pulse pressure The difference between systolic and diastolic blood pressure

Pulsus alternans The mechanical alteration of the pulse characterized by a regular rhythm and alternating strong and weak pulses; seen with serious myocardial disease

Pulsus paradoxus A marked variation in cardiac stroke volume with respiration characterized by a stronger pulse during expiration and a weaker pulse during inspiration; seen in pericardial effusion or constrictive pericarditis

Purulent Consisting of, containing, or discharging pus

Pyogenic   Producing or able to produce pus

R-on-T phenomenon   The occurrence of a premature ventricular complex (R wave) during the relative refractory period (during or on the T wave) of the preceding beat

Rales   Discontinuous adventitious breath sounds of a crackling nature heard throughout inspiration and the first third of expiration; crackles

Rate–pressure product   The product of heart rate times systolic blood pressure; an indirect indicator of myocardial oxygen demand

Rating of perceived exertion   A subjective numerical scale used to rate exercise intensity

Reperfusion   The reestablishment of blood flow to a tissue

Reperfusion injury   Damage to tissue caused by the reestablishment of blood flow to a tissue after a period of ischemia (e.g., inflammation and oxidative damage)

Resonance   The sound produced by percussing on a part of the body that can vibrate freely

Respiratory acidosis   Retention of carbon dioxide and the subsequent decrease in blood pH caused by inadequate pulmonary ventilation

Respiratory alkalosis   Excessive loss of carbon dioxide and the subsequent increase in blood pH caused by hyperventilation

Respiratory distress   Difficulty breathing or labored breathing; perceived inability to breathe deeply, regularly, and with ease; usually associated with respiratory rate above 35 breaths per minute, oxygen saturation below 90%, and increased use of accessory muscles of respiration

Respiratory failure   The inability of the respiratory system to adequately ventilate the alveoli so that there is inadequate gas exchange, as evidenced by hypoxemia and hypercapnia

Restrictive cardiomyopathy   A disease of the myocardium characterized by marked endocardial scarring of the ventricles with resultant impairment of diastolic filling

Restrictive lung dysfunction (RLD)   An abnormal reduction in pulmonary ventilation due to restriction of expansion by the lungs or chest wall

Retinopathy   Any form of noninflammatory damage to the retina (e.g., diabetic retinopathy with damage to the retinal blood vessels by elevated blood glucose levels)

Rhinitis   Inflammation of the mucous membranes lining the nose

Rhonchi   Continuous, "snoring" adventitious sounds heard on auscultation during both inspiration and expiration; caused by air passing through midsized and larger airways with intraluminal secretions; low-pitched wheezes

Right-to-left shunt   A diversion of blood from the right side of the heart to the left without participation in gas exchange; intrapulmonary shunt

Rubor dependency test   A procedure used to assess the arterial circulation of the lower extremity by skin color responses to positional changes

Sarcoidosis   A systemic granulomatous disease that predominantly affects the lungs with resulting fibrosis

Scintigraphy   A diagnostic procedure involving the intravenous injection of a radionuclide and radiologic imaging

Sensitivity   The probability that, given the presence of a disease, an abnormal test result indicates the presence of the disease

Shock   A state of profound physiologic depression due to severe physical injury or illness

Sick sinus syndrome   A condition characterized by alternating episodes of bradycardia with recurrent extrasystoles and supraventricular tachycardia

Silent ischemia   A condition of inadequate coronary blood flow without the typical symptoms of ischemia

Silicosis   A type of pneumoconiosis that results from occupational exposure over years to silica dust

Sinus block   Failure of an impulse to be transmitted from the sinoatrial node

Sleep apnea   Episodes of breathing cessation caused by an upper airway obstruction during sleep

Specificity   The probability that, given the absence of disease, a normal test result excludes the presence of the disease

Sphygmomanometer   The device used to measure arterial blood pressure that consists of an inflatable cuff to restrict blood flow and a mercury or mechanical manometer to measure pressure

Spirometry   Measurement of pulmonary function using a device that measures air volume and flow, such as a spirometer (a counterbalanced cylindrical bell sealed via a water trough)

Sputum   Expectorated matter or secretions

Status asthmaticus   Severe, intractable asthma

Sternotomy   A surgical incision through the sternum

Stridor   A high-pitched inspiratory and expiratory sound created by obstruction of the larynx or trachea to airflow

Stroke volume   The volume of blood (ml) ejected with each heart beat

Subcutaneous emphysema   The presence of free air in the subcutaneous tissue, the result of an air leak from the lungs

Subendocardial myocardial infarction   A myocardial infarction in which there is necrosis of only the inner layer(s) of myocardium

Sudden cardiac death   Death within 1 hour of the onset of cardiac symptoms

Summation gallop   The presence of third and fourth heart sounds, which are fused, in addition to the normal first and second heart sounds

Suppuration   The formation of pus

Surfactant   A surface-active agent lining the alveolar surfaces that reduces surface tension and retards the tendency of the alveoli to collapse

Sympatholytic   An agent that inhibits adrenergic receptors of the autonomic nervous system

Sympathomimetic   An agent that produces effects similar to those produced by stimulation of the sympathetic nervous system

Syncope   Sudden, transient loss of consciousness due to inadequate cerebral perfusion

Systemic vascular resistance (SVR)   The resistance to blood flow that must be overcome to pump blood through the peripheral arterial system; total peripheral resistance (TPR)

Systole   The period of ventricular contraction

Systolic blood pressure (SBP)   The highest arterial blood pressure reached during a given cardiac cycle; occurs during ventricular contraction and ejection of blood into the arterial system

Tachycardia   An abnormally fast heart rate, usually considered greater than 100 beats per minute

Tachypnea   An abnormally fast respiratory rate; polypnea

Tamponade   Compression of the heart as a result of fluid accumulation within the pericardial sac

Tension pneumothorax   The accumulation of air in the pleural cavity as the result of a communication between the lung and the pleural space in which a valve effect exists; air leaks into the pleural space on inspiration but is trapped during expiration

Thermodilution method A method of detrmining cardiac output whereby a bolus of cold saline is injected into the right atrium and the resultant temperature change is measured in the pulmonary artery

Thoracentesis The removal of fluid from the pleural space, using a needle; pleurocentesis

Thoracoplasty The surgical resection of ribs to allow inward retraction of the chest wall, to reduce the size of the pleural space

Thoracotomy Surgical opening of the thoracic cavity

Thrombocytopenia An abnormally low number of platelets in the blood

Thrombolysis The dissolving of a thrombus

Thrombosis The formation or presence of a blood clot within a blood vessel

Tissue plasminogen activator (TPA, tPA) A genetically engineered thrombolytic agent used in conjunction with heparin to limit the amount of damage caused by a myocardial infarction or stroke

Torsades de pointes A 5- to 20-beat salvo of paroxysmal ventricular tachycardia with an undulating QRS axis that progressively changes direction

Total peripheral resistance (TPR) The force opposing the flow of blood in the systemic circulation; derived by dividing the mean arterial pressure by the cardiac output

Tracheitis Inflammation of the mucosal lining of the trachea

Tracheoesophageal fistula An abnormal communication between the esophagus and the trachea

Tracheomalacia An erosion of the trachea, usually because of excessive pressure from a cuffed endotracheal tube

Tracheostomy An opening, or the creation of an opening, into the trachea

Transmural myocardial infarction A myocardial infarction involving necrosis of the full thickness of the myocardial wall

Transudate Any liquid that passes through a membrane as a result of an imbalance between the hydrostatic and osmotic forces on the two sides of the membrane

Trendelenburg position A position with the bed inclined at an angle of 45 degrees so that the hips are higher than the head; head-down position

Triglyceride A molecule of glycerol bound to three long-chain fatty acid molecules

Triplet Three consecutive atrial or ventricular extrasystoles

Tympany A low-pitched, resonant, drumlike sound obtained by percussing the chest wall or other hollow organ

Unstable angina (pectoris) Preinfarction chest pain characterized by discomfort occurring at rest and low levels of activity

v wave The rise in the atrial pressure curve near the end of ventricular systole caused by gradual passive filling of the atria with the atrioventricular valves closed

Validity The extent to which a device or test measures what it is intended to measure

Valsalva maneuver Contraction of the muscles of the abdomen, chest wall, and diaphragm in a forced expiratory effort against a closed glottis

Valvular insufficiency Inadequate closure of one of the cardiac valves so that blood regurgitates through the valve when it is supposed to be closed

Valvular stenosis Narrowing of a valvular orifice so that blood flow across it is restricted

Valvuloplasty The surgical reconstruction of a defective valve or valve leaflet to relieve incompetence or stenosis

Valvulotomy A surgical incision through a stenosed valve or valve leaflet to relieve an obstruction

Variant angina Atypical angina; angina that is not necessarily precipitated by increased myocardial demand, is often of longer duration and more severe, and is associated with ST-segment elevation rather than depression; Prinzmetal's angina

Vasculitis Inflammation of a blood vessel

Vasopressor A substance that produces vasoconstriction or an increase in blood pressure

Ventilation Movement of gas into and out of the alveoli

Ventilation–perfusion(V̇/Q̇) matching The ratio of the amount of ventilation to the amount of blood flow in a particular region or entirety of a lung; optimal $\dot{V}/\dot{Q}$ matching occurs in the mid zones of the upright lungs where the ratio is 0.8 to 1.0

Ventilatory failure Inability of the lungs to adequately perform gas exchange because of impairment of the ventilatory pump

Ventilatory reserve The difference between normal pulmonary ventilation and the maximal breathing capacity of an individual

Ventilatory threshold The level of exercise at which there is a nonlinear increase in ventilation in relation to oxygen consumption; considered to be the estimated upper limit of aerobic exercise

Ventricular fibrillation (VF, v-fib) An erratic quivering of the ventricular myofibrils that produces no cardiac output and clinical death if untreated

Ventricular gallop The presence of an early diastolic, third heart sound (S_3) in addition to the normal first and second heart sounds

Ventriculography The radiologic visualization of the ventricles, using injection of a radiopaque material

Venturi mask A supplemental oxygen delivery device that can be adjusted to deliver a specific fraction of inspired oxygen at relatively high flow rates

Very low-density lipoproteins (VLDL) A major class of lipoproteins containing a high concentration of triglycerides and a moderate concentration of cholesterol and phospholipids

Visceral pleura The serous membrane covering the surface of each lung

Volume overload An increase in venous return and ventricular filling volume caused by excessive intravascular fluid volume

Waist circumference A measure of the circumference of the waist just above the hip bones level with the umbilicus that is used as an indicator of abdominal obesity; measurements greater than 35 in for females and 40 in for males correspond to high risk for type 2 diabetes, hypertension, high cholesterol, and heart disease

Waist-to-hip ratio The ratio of waist to hip circumference that can be used as an indicator of fatness or obesity

Wandering pacemaker An abnormal cardiac rhythm in which the site of the controlling pacemaker shifts from beat to beat, usually between the sinus and different ectopic sites in the atria nodes

Wheezes Continuous, musical sounds of variable pitch and duration heard on auscultation of the lungs, caused by airway narrowing

Whispered pectoriloquy Distinct transmission of whispered words over an area of consolidated lung tissue

Work of breathing The total amount of effort required to expand and contract the lungs; the physiological cost of breathing (e.g., normally, 2% to 3% of total body oxygen consumption during quiet breathing, increasing to slightly more than 5% at maximal exercise); affected by the amount of work required to overcome the elastic forces of the lungs and chest wall and the flow-resistive forces of the airways

Index

Note: Page numbers followed by *b* indicate boxes, *f* indicate figures and *t* indicate tables.

CARDIOVASCULAR AND PULMONARY PHYSICAL THERAPY